TEXTBOOK OF LARYNGOLOGY

TEXTBOOK OF LARYNGOLOGY

Edited by

Albert L. Merati, MD, FACS
Steven A. Bielamowicz, MD, FACS

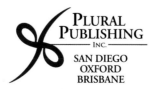

PLURAL
PUBLISHING
INC.

SAN DIEGO
OXFORD
BRISBANE

MW

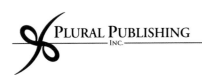

PLURAL PUBLISHING
INC.

5521 Ruffin Road
San Diego, CA 92123

e-mail: info@pluralpublishing.com
Web site: http://www.pluralpublishing.com

49 Bath Street
Abingdon, Oxfordshire OX14 1EA
United Kingdom

ISBN-13: 978-1-59756-028-3
ISBN-10: 1-59756-028-6

Library of Congress Cataloging-in-Publication Data:

Textbook of laryngology / edited by Albert L. Merati, Steven A. Bielamowicz.
        p. ; cm.
    Includes bibliographical references and index.
    ISBN-13: 978-1-59756-028-3 (hardcover)
    ISBN-10: 1-59756-028-6 (hardcover)
    1. Throat—Diseases. 2. Larynx—Diseases. I. Merati, Albert L. II. Bielamowicz,
Steven A. [DNLM: 1. Laryngeal Diseases. 2. Larynx. WV 500 T355 2006]
    RF20.T49 2006
    616.2'2—dc22

                                                                      2006015198

1/10/07

Contents

Foreword

The growing interest in the medical community for the evaluation and treatment of disorders of the larynx has evolved and matured over the last two decades. It is clear that the larynx plays a critical role in a person's quality of life through coordination of the critical functions of voice and swallowing. Deficits in either of these areas can result in dramatic functional, social and physical consequences. The following *Textbook of Laryngology* by Merati and Bielamowicz is an original and thorough treatise that brings the myriad and complex disorders of the larynx into one concise reference that can be used by the multidisciplinary group of practitioners who care for these patients.

It is apropos that a book about voice should read like a well-written play, drama, or symphony. The overture describes both the historical and contemporary aspects of the development of voice science and laryngology, and sets the stage for what is to follow. Act One describes the fundamental, basic principles of anatomy and physiology of both voice and swallowing function and provides the framework for a very comprehensive discussion of the myriad techniques and technology utilized in assessing and analyzing voice and swallowing function. These not only describe the important perceptual, radiographic, and visual assessments of voice but includes a somewhat unique chapter on swallowing evaluation techniques.

Act Two presents five excellent chapters describing the principles of therapy from prevention and hygiene to voice and behavioral therapy; from medical therapy to principles of surgical treatments including laser surgery. This is followed by an in-depth description of the many disorders that affect voice and swallowing function, including neurologic diseases and inflammatory and structural disorders. These chapters truly cover the essence of laryngology and the unique impact of the many disorders. The encore is a fascinating group of chapters that address special issues in laryngology including alaryngeal voice restoration and rhinologic disease and the larynx.

Perhaps the most remarkable aspect of this production is the performers. The Contributors List reads like a *Who's Who* in voice care, bringing decades of experience from multiple different institutions and locations to one concise but thorough reference. Merati and Bielamowicz direct these authors and orchestrate their contributions in a way that is easily readable and enjoyable. Starting with the very first chapter, you, the reader, will realize that you are in for quite a performance, from Overture to Encore. Let the show begin! Brava to the *Textbook of Laryngology*!

Michael S. Benninger, MD

Preface

"The love of learning is a pleasant and unusual bond, for it deals with what one is and not with what one has . . . "

Freya Stark, from *The Southern Gates of Arabia*, 1937

As we enter the 21st century, the re-emergence of Laryngology as a dynamic and vibrant sub-specialty has been a principal development in Otolaryngology and Speech-Language Pathology. The significance of the discipline is evident in the nature of disorders that are the subject of the *Textbook of Laryngology*; these include breathing, swallowing, and the most conspicuous laryngeal function, phonation.

With this surge of interest and discovery, it was our objective to provide a direct, cohesive, and instructional work that distills and collates the fundamentals of Laryngology in one approachable volume. Every major center of clinical and research excellence in Laryngology is represented in the *Textbook of Laryngology*.

Although there are many excellent references in Laryngology and related subjects, we believe that the *Textbook of Laryngology* is unique in its presentation of core information, key points, review material, and, in addition, the inclusion of a pretest and a post-test. For every chapter, the authors were asked to present the central themes and knowledge in their main text, while material beyond these core concepts was placed in one of the three types of "Insert Boxes" located throughout a given chapter. These include the *Thought Box*, in which an author may present an interesting idea for the reader to consider; the *Controversy Box*, in which debatable or contentious matters in the field are noted; and finally, the *Emerging Concepts* boxes, in which cutting edge information is presented. The purpose of separating these boxes from the main text was to distinguish the areas of generally accepted and common knowledge from those areas that are still controversial or in development. Of course the distinction of what belongs in an insert box and what is "established knowledge" is itself subject to debate.

The readers are encouraged to use the pre- and post-tests to assess their knowledge and to use the review questions from each chapter to evaluate their comprehension and knowledge base. We believe that the *Textbook of Laryngology* will serve well as core curriculum reading of otolaryngology training, maintenance of certification review for established otolaryngologists, or as a core textbook for graduate course work for speech-language pathologists.

The readers are welcome to contact the Editors or the authors directly for further questions. Each and every author was chosen for his or her commitment to education. We are all, first and foremost, teachers.

Al Merati
Steve Bielamowicz

Contributors

Mona M. Abaza, MD
Assistant Professor
Voice Program Director
Department of Otolaryngology
University of Colorado School of Medicine
Medical Director
National Center for Voice and Speech
Denver, Colorado
Chapter 18

Lee M. Akst, MD
Assistant Professor
Department of Otolaryngology-Head and Neck
    Surgery
Loyola University Health System
Maywood, Illinois
Chapter 1

Kenneth W. Altman, MD, PhD
Associate Professor
Department of Otolaryngology
Mt. Sinai School of Medicine
New York, New York
Chapter 31

Milan R. Amin, MD
Director, NYU Voice Center
Chief, Division of Laryngology
Department of Otolaryngology
New York University School of Medicine
New York, New York
Chapter 5

Timothy D. Anderson, MD
Department of Otolaryngology-Head and Neck
    Surgery
Lahey Clinic Voice and Swallowing Center
Burlington, Massachusetts
Chapter 24

Gerald S. Berke, MD, FACS
Professor and Chief
Division of Head and Neck Surgery
UCLA Voice Center for Medicine and the Arts
UCLA David Geffen School of Medicine
Los Angeles, California
Chapter 20

Steven A. Bielamowicz, MD, FACS
Professor and Chief
    Division of Otolaryngology
Director, Voice Treatment Center
The George Washington University
Washington, District of Columbia
Editor

Diane M. Bless, PhD
Professor, Departments of Surgery and
    Communicative Disorders
University of Wisconsin-Madison
Madison, Wisconsin
Chapters 6 and 7

Andrew Blitzer MD, DDS
Professor of Clinical Otolaryngology
Columbia University
Director, New York Center for Voice and
    Swallowing Disorders
New York, New York
Chapter 17

Joel H. Blumin, MD, FACS
Assistant Professor
Department of Otolaryngology and
    Communication Sciences
Medical College of Wisconsin
Milwaukee, Wisconsin
Chapter 20

Mary Brawley, MA, CCC-SLP
Speech-Language Pathologist
Center for Speech and Communication
    Disorders
Department of Otolaryngology and
    Communication Sciences
The Medical College of Wisconsin
Milwaukee Wisconsin
Chapter 29

Robert A. Buckmire, MD
Associate Professor of Otolaryngology-Head and
    Neck Surgery
University of North Carolina
Director, UNC Voice Center
Chapel Hill, North Carolina
Chapter 15

Bruce Campbell, MD, FACS
Professor, Department of Otolaryngology and
    Communication Sciences and the MCW
    Cancer Center
The Medical College of Wisconsin
Milwaukee, Wisconsin
Chapter 29

Nadine P. Connor, PhD
Assistant Professor
Departments of Surgery and Communicative
    Disorders
University of Wisconsin-Madison
Madison, Wisconsin
Chapter 6

Mark S. Courey, MD
Professor, Department of Otolaryngology-Head
    and Neck Surgery
Director, Division of Laryngology
The UCSF Voice and Swallowing Center
San Francisco, California
Chapter 16

Seth H. Dailey, MD
Assistant Professor
University of Wisconsin School of Medicine
University of Wisconsin Hospital and Clinics
Madison, Wisconsin
Chapter 2

Edward J. Damrose, MD
Assistant Professor, Chief of Laryngology Division
Stanford University Hospitals and Clinics
Palo Alto, California
Chapter 30

Suzy Duflo, MD
Fédération d'Otorhinolaryngology, Head and
    Neck Surgery

265 rue St Pierre, Hôspital de la Timone
Marseille France
Chapter 3

**Soh Ping Eng, MBBS, FRCSED, FRCSI, DLO,
    FAMS**
Consultant Otolaryngologist
Department of Otorhinolaryngology-Head and
    Neck Surgery
Changi General Hospital,
Singapore
Chapter 10

Reena Gupta, MD
Department of Otolaryngology
New York University School of Medicine
New York, New York
Chapter 5

Stacey L. Halum, MD
Assistant Professor of Otolarngology-Head and
    Neck Surgery
Center for Voice and Swallowing Disorders
Department of Otolaryngology, Indiana University
Chapter 11

Douglas M. Hicks, Ph.D., CCC-SP
Director, The Voice Center
Head, Speech-Language Pathology Section
Cleveland Clinic Foundation
Cleveland Ohio
Chapters 8 and 12

Jason P. Hunt, MD
Instructor
Department of Otolaryngology-Head and Neck
    Surgery
Vanderbilt University Medical Center
Nashville, Tennessee
Chapter 25

Felicia L. Johnson, MD
Director, Voice and Swallowing Clinic
Assistant Professor, Department of
    Otolaryngology-Head and Neck Surgery
University of Arkansas for Medical Sciences
Department of Otolaryngology, Head and Neck
    Surgery

Little Rock, Arkansas
Chapter 22

Joseph E. Kerschner, MD, FACS, FAAP
Associate Professor and Chief,
Division of Pediatric Otolaryngology
Academic Vice Chairman
Department of Otolaryngology and
    Communication Sciences
Medical College of Wisconsin
Medical Director, Pediatric Otolaryngology
    Children's Hospital of Wisconsin
Milwaukee, Wisconsin
Chapter 28

Marc LaCrosse, MD
Associate Head of Clinic
Department of Diagnostic Radiology
Mont-Godinne Medical Center
Université Catholique de Louvain
Yvoir, Belgium
Chapter 10

Georges Lawson, MD
Professor, Head of Clinic
Department of Otorhinolaryngology, Head and
    Neck Surgery
Mont-Godinne Medical Center
Université Catholique de Louvain
Yvoir, Belgium
Chapter 10

Elan Louis, MD, MS
Associate Professor of Neurology
Gertrude H. Sergievsky Center
Taub Institute for Research on Alzheimer's
    Disease and the Aging Brain
Department of Neurology
College of Physicians and Surgeons
Columbia University
New York, New York
Chapter 19

Christy L. Ludlow, PhD
Chief, Laryngeal and Speech Section
Clinical Neurosciences Program
National Institute of Neurological Disorders and
    Stroke

Bethesda, Maryland
Chapter 4

Nicole Maronian, MD
Assistant Professor
Department of Otolaryngology-Head and Neck
    Surgery
University of Washington Medical Center
Seattle, Washington
Chapter 9

Ted Mau, MD, PhD
Department of Otolaryngology-Head and Neck
    Surgery
University of California, San Francisco
San Francisco, California
Chapter 16

Andrew J. McWhorter, MD
Assistant Professor
Director, LSU Voice Center
Department of Otolaryngology-Head and Neck
    Surgery
Louisiana Health Sciences Center
New Orleans, Louisiana
Chapter 25

Albert L. Merati, MD FACS
Associate Professor and Chief
Division of Laryngology and Professional Voice
Department of Otolaryngology and
    Communication Sciences
Staff Surgeon
Zablocki VAMC
Medical College of Wisconsin
Milwaukee, Wisconsin
Editor, Chapter 27

Tanya Meyer, MD
Assistant Professor, Department of
    Otorhinolaryngology-Head and Neck Surgery
University of Maryland Medical Center
Baltimore, Maryland
Chapter 17

Claudio F. Milstein, PhD, CCC-SP
Speech Scientist
The Voice Center

Cleveland Clinic Foundation
Cleveland Ohio
Chapters 8 and 12

Natasha Mirza, MD, FACS
Associate Professor, Otolaryngology, Head and
    Neck Surgery
Director Penn Center for Voice and Swallowing
    at Presbyterian Hospital
Philadelphia, Pennsylvania
Chapter 21

Robert H. Ossoff, DMD, MD
Guy Maness Professor and Chairman
Vanderbilt Bill Wilkerson Department of
    Otolaryngology-Head and Neck Surgery
Nashville, Tennessee
Chapter 26

Rita Patel, MS
Research Assistant
Department of Surgery, Division of
    Otolaryngology
University of Wisconsin-Madison
Madison, Wisconsin
Chapter 7

Sachin Pawar, BBA
Medical College of Wisconsin
Milwaukee, Wisconsin
Chapter 27

Michael Pitman, MD
Director, Division of Laryngology
Director, The Voice and Swallowing Institute
    Department of Otolaryngology
New York Eye and Ear Infirmary
New York, New York
Chapter 26

Gregory N. Postma, MD
Professor, Department of Otolaryngology
Director, MCG Center for Voice and Swallowing
    Disorders
Medical College of Georgia
Augusta, Georgia
Chapter 11

James W. Ragland, MD
University of Arkansas for Medical Sciences
Department of Otolaryngology, Head and Neck
    Surgery
Little Rock, Arkansas
Chapter 22

Marc Remacle, MD, PhD
Professor, Associate Head of Department
Department of Otorhinolaryngology-Head and
    Neck Surgery
Mont-Godinne Medical Center
Université Catholique de Louvain
Yvoir, Belgium
Chapter 10

Lawrence Robinson, MD
Professor and Chair
Department of Physical Medicine and
    Rehabilitation
University of Washington Medical Center
Seattle, Washington
Chapter 9

Adam D. Rubin, MD
Director, Lakeshore Professional Voice Center
Lakeshore ENT
St. Clair Shores, Michigan
Adjunct Assistant Professor, Department of
    Otolaryngology-Head and Neck Surgery
University of Michigan Medical Center
Chapter 14

Robert T. Sataloff, MD, DMA, FACS
Professor and Chairman, Department of
    Otolaryngology-HNS
Associate Dean for Clinical Management Specialties
Drexel College of Medicine
Professor of Otolaryngology-Head and Neck
    Surgery
Jefferson Medical College
Thomas Jefferson University
Chairman, The Voice Foundation
Chairman, American Institute for Voice and Ear
    Research
Chapters 13 and 14

Sarah Marx Schneider, MS, CCC-SLP
Speech-Language Pathologist
Robert T. Sataloff, MD and Associates
Philadelphia, Pennsylvania
Chapter 13

Jennifer Spielman, MA, CCC-SLP
Speech Pathologist and Research Associate
National Center for Voice and Speech
Denver, Colorado
Chapter 18

Lucian Sulica, MD
Director, Voice Disorders/Laryngology
Department of Otorhinolaryngology
Weill Medical School of Cornell University
New York, New York
Chapter 17 and 19

Susan L. Thibeault, PhD
Research Director
Department of Surgery,
Division of Otolaryngology-Head and Neck
  Surgery
School of Medicine, The University of Utah
Salt Lake City, Utah
Chapter 3

Dana Mara Thompson, MD
Department of Pediatric Otolaryngology and the
  Aerodigestive and Sleep Center, Cincinnati
  Children's Hospital Medical Center and

The University of Cincinnati College of
  Medicine,
Cincinnati, Ohio
Chapter 28

Mai Thy Truong, MD
Stanford University Hospitals and Clinics
Palo Alto, Califonia
Chapter 30

Thierry Vanderborght, MD, PhD
Professor, Head of Division
Nuclear Medicine Division
Mont-Godinne Medical Center
Université Catholique de Louvain
Yvoir, Belgium
Chapter 10

Riitta Ylitalo, MD, PhD
Karolinska Institute,
Department of Otolaryngology
Karolinska University Hospital Huddinge
Stockholm, Sweden
Chapter 23

Steven M. Zeitels, MD, FACS
Eugene B. Casey Chair of Laryngeal Surgery:
  Harvard Medical School
Director: Center for Laryngeal Surgery and
  Voice Rehabilitation
Massachusetts General Hospital
Boston, Massachusetts
Chapter 1

Pretest for Textbook of Laryngology

1. The use of _____ therapy, emphasizing frontal tone focus, may enhance the perception of vocal loudness and allow for the voice to be more easily heard in noisy situations without excessive strain or effort.
   a. vocal function
   b. Lee Silverman
   c. botulinum toxin
   d. resonant
   e. decondition/recondition

2. Abductor spasmodic dysphonia remains a challenging disorder to treat. The most common site(s) of botulinum toxin injection for this disorder:
   a. unilateral strap muscles
   b. bilateral strap muscles
   c. posterior cricoarytenoid muscles, unilateral or bilateral
   d. interarytenoid muscle
   e. There is no role for botulinum toxin injection in abductor spasmodic dysphonia.

3. The presence of the _____ sign may help distinguish the denervated vocal fold from one that is mechanically fixed.
   a. Toohill
   b. Guttman
   c. jostle
   d. Simpson
   e. Chevalier

4. The human eye can detect up to _____ images per second.
   a. 5
   b. 10
   c. 50
   d. 100
   e. 150

5. What would you call this lesion?

   a. vocal nodule
   b. amyloidosis
   c. vocal scar
   d. intracordal cyst
   e. sulcus vocalis

6. Vocal *loudness* increases as subglottic air pressure _____ and as the duration of the closed phase of the vibratory cycle _____.
   a. increases, decreases
   b. increases, increases
   c. decreases, increases
   d. decreases, decreases
   e. increases, steadies

7. Which term is defined by periodic jerky contractions of 1 to 2 Hz that are monophasic and not suppressible with conscious effort?
   a. tremor
   b. dystonia
   c. dysdiadokinesia
   d. myoclonus
   e. asterixis

8. In its idealized form, high-speed video imaging allows for evaluation of:
   a. severely dysphonic patients
   b. patients with profound gag reflex
   c. a fractional sample of glottic cycles during the captured segment
   d. connected speech
   e. all of the above

9. The safety and utility of 585-nm pulsed dye laser energy is related to being preferentially absorbed by:
   a. skin
   b. water
   c. blood
   d. mucosa
   e. collagen

10. The cycle-to-cycle variability in *amplitude* of the voice is referred to as:
    a. perturbation
    b. jitter
    c. timbre
    d. shimmer
    e. SHR (signal-to-harmonic ratio)

11. Transnasal esophagoscopy:
    a. usually requires some sedation
    b. does not allow for therapeutic intervention
    c. is not comparable to traditional EGD for the evaluation of Barrett's metaplasia
    d. may be limited by inability to traverse the nasal vault in about 2–3% of pts
    e. is not appropriate for otolaryngologists to perform

12. _____ can be defined as using the larynx beyond its physical limits, such as may be seen with an outburst of screaming.
    a. vocal overuse
    b. vocal hyperfunction
    c. vocal misuse
    d. vocal hijinks
    e. none of the above

13. The cell bodies that supply efferent motor impulses to the cricothyroid muscle are in the:
    a. nucleus solitarius
    b. nodose ganglion
    c. superior ganglion of the vagus
    d. nucleus amibguus
    e. spinal 5th nucleus

14. These are intraoperative photos of which disorder?

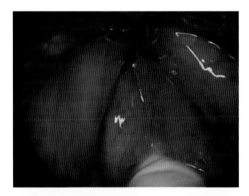

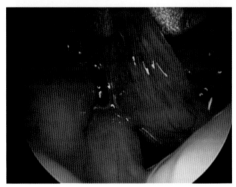

    a. laryngeal papillomatosis
    b. intracordal cyst
    c. angioedema
    d. steriod overinjection
    e. Reinke's edema

15. The photos in the above question were taken with which telescopes?
    a. 0 degree, 30 degree
    b. 0 degree, 70 degree
    c. 0 degree, 90 degree
    d. 30 degree, 70 degree
    e. 30 degree, 90 degree

16. Stimulation of the larynx may lead to coughing. The afferents are contained in the superior laryngeal nerve and have their cell bodies in the _____. Input to the brainstem from these afferent neurons terminates in the interstitial subnucleus of the _____.
    a. somatic ganglion, nucleus ambiguus
    b. nodose ganglion, nucleus ambiguus
    c. somatic ganglion, nucleus solitarius
    d. nodose ganglion, nucleus solitarius
    e. nodose ganglion, dorsal nucleus of X

17. With regard to radiographic evidence of laryngeal cartilage invasion:
    a. MRI is more sensitive and more specific than CT
    b. MRI is less sensitive but more specific than CT
    c. MRI is more sensitive but less specific than CT
    d. MRI is less sensitive and less specific than CT
    e. MRI and CT are essentially equivalent

18. LASER is an acronym for:
    a. Light Augmentation by the Simulated Emission of Radiation
    b. Light Amplification by the Stimulated Emission of Radiation
    c. Light Amplification by Stimulated Electron Radiation
    d. Light Attenuation by the Simulated Emission of Radioactivity
    e. Light Augmentation by Stimulation Energy Radiofrequency

19. Four months following a thyroidectomy, a patient has hypomobility of the left vocal fold. Laryngeal EMG reveals small polyphasic potentials in the left thyro-arytenoid. This EMG finding indicates:
    a. ongoing injury
    b. ongoing regeneration
    c. that fibrillations will be seen 2 to 3 weeks later
    d. failure of reinnervation
    e. none of the above

20. Spasticity, strain, hyperreflexia, and myoclonus are characteristic of which type of laryngeal neurological impairment?
    a. extrapyramidal
    b. upper motor neuron
    c. lower motor neuron
    d. neuromuscular junction
    e. end-organ (ie, muscle)

21. The most common error in window placement for thyroplasty surgery:
    a. too superior
    b. too posterior
    c. too anterior
    d. too small
    e. too big

22. Cricopharyngeal myotomy
    a. cannot be performed safely via the endoscopic approach
    b. has not been shown to alter UES manometry
    c. is absolutely contraindicated in the presence of reflux
    d. is dependent on division of the middle and inferior constrictors of the pharynx
    e. can be performed on either side of the neck

23. Resting vocal tremor is present in approximately what percentage of Parkinson's disease patients?
    a. 15
    b. 25
    c. 35
    d. 45
    e. 55

24. A 33-year-old male presents to your clinic with biphasic stridor. He was intubated for 16 days following a motor vehicle accident. He suffered a sternal injury from impact to the steering wheel. Your examination reveals a 3-mm airway with no detectable motion. He is in some distress. Of the following sites, which is the most likely to be the source of his obstruction?
    a. supraglottic
    b. anterior glottic
    c. posterior glottic
    d. trachea
    e. central nervous system

25. Spasmodic dysphonia and essential voice tremor have the following in common:
    a. central nervous system disorder
    b. voice breaks in connected speech
    c. clinical diagnosis only; no testing or objective findings are pathognomonic
    d. some symptomatic improvement with alcohol
    e. all of the above are true for SD and essential voice tremor

26. A laryngectomy patient undergoes a successful TE puncture. On postoperative day 14, he comes in for a prosthesis fitting. The TEP voice is halting and the patient can sustain an "ah" for only 1 or 2 seconds. He has never been radiated and is cancer-free. He has no pain. The sound is about the same whether or not the prosthesis is within the fresh puncture site. You suspect:
    a. prosthesis too long
    b. prosthesis too short
    c. pharyngoesophageal segment spasm
    d. poorly placed TE puncture
    e. flaccid neopharynx

27. Your preferred treatment for the patient in Question 26 is:
    a. prosthesis change
    b. antifungal treatment
    c. cricopharyngeal myotomy
    d. botulinum toxin injection
    e. stoma button and hands-free device

28. Menopause:
    a. occurs at a mean age of less than 50 years of age
    b. results in tremendous ovarian sensitivity to gonadotropin stimulation
    c. also results in the decline of androgen production
    d. features parallel cytological findings in the larynx and cervix
    e. May result in a drop in F_0 that is resistant to replacement therapy

29. The first successful laryngectomy was performed by which surgeon? In which year?
    a. Lynch, 1863
    b. Solis-Cohen, 1863
    c. Billroth, 1863
    d. Billroth, 1873
    e. Solis-Cohen, 1893

30. Fiberoptic endoscopic evaluation of swallowing with sensory testing (FEESST):
    a. cannot be performed in children
    b. substitutes for modified barium swallow in most cases
    c. requires cognitive participation of the subject
    d. can distinguish unilateral from bilateral sensory deficits
    e. is not useful clinically and is a research tool only

For Dr. Javad Merati and Mrs. Adele Jalali Merati, for making me an American.
For Dr. Robert H. Ossoff and Dr. Robert J. Toohill, for making me a Laryngologist.

Al Merati

For my wife Anne, my boys Matthew and Nicholas, and my parents Albin and Patricia,
with great appreciation of your support and love.

Steve Bielamowicz

PART I

Developments in Laryngology

1

Historical Developments in Laryngology

Lee M. Akst, MD
Steven M. Zeitels, MD, FACS

KEY POINTS

■ Manuel García (1855) is accepted as the father of mirror laryngoscopy although a number of physicians previously described the technique (1805–1855).

■ Johann Czermak (1857) of Budapest and Ludwig Turck (1857) in Vienna initially popularized indirect laryngoscopy and subsequently a number of others followed, including Leopold Schrötter von Kristelli and Carl Stoerk in Vienna, Morell Mackenzie in London, Louis Elsberg in New York, and Jacob Solis-Cohen in Philadelphia.

■ Local mucosal anesthesia (cocaine) was developed for the larynx by Koller and Jelinek, which facilitated substantial advancements in endolaryngeal mirror-guided surgery.

■ Topical cocaine anesthesia also facilitated Alfred Kirstein's description of direct laryngoscopy and tracheoscopy in 1895.

■ Gustav Killian and Chevalier Jackson perfected the art of rigid endoscopy of the upper aerodigestive tract; Killian also introduced suspension laryngoscopy.

■ More recent advances that have ushered in the era of modern laryngology are the developments of the surgical microscope, general endotracheal anesthesia with paralysis, and lasers along with advanced understanding of the physiologic principles of voice production.

Laryngology began in the 19th century when mirror laryngoscopy enabled visualization of the larynx. Since that time, progress in laryngology has been marked by advances in the ability to examine the larynx and manipulate laryngeal tissues. The key watershed initiatives in the history of laryngology were the development of direct and indirect laryngoscopy.[1] Improved laryngeal visualization led to enhanced understanding of laryngeal pathophysiology and new techniques of laryngeal surgery, both transoral and transcervical. Each new discovery in laryngoscopy and laryngeal surgery was followed by an expansion phase in which physicians of the era steadily advanced and applied the techniques first developed by their colleagues. More recent advances have ushered in a modern period of laryngology. This chapter describes these historical developments in laryngology thematically, rather than chronologically, to foster an understanding of the advances that have led from the birth of laryngology to the present.

INDIRECT LARYNGOSCOPY

Credit for the discovery of mirror laryngoscopy is often given to Manuel García (Figure 1–1), an opera teacher who was able to visualize his own vocal folds with the aid of two mirrors and reflected sunlight in September 1854. He described his technique to the Royal Society of London in a paper titled "Observations on the Human Voice" in 1855.[2] Although he was not the first to visualize the larynx, he was the first to utilize that imaging to provide valid concepts of human voice production.[3] These descriptions were the first to ignite widespread interest in study of the larynx and earned García recognition as "The Father of Laryngoscopy." García lived to the age of 101 and remained much celebrated throughout his career.[4] To celebrate his centennial birthday, and in honor of the fiftieth anniversary of his description of laryngoscopy, laryngologists worldwide commissioned a John Singer Sargent portrait of García.

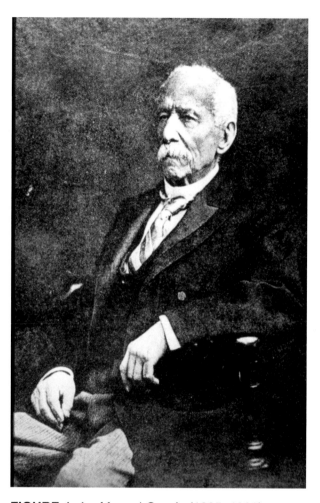

FIGURE 1–1. Manuel García (1805–1906).

Laryngoscopy Before García

Attempts to visualize the larynx were made prior to García's description, although it is thought that García himself was unaware of these previous reports. In general, these investigations may have enabled visualization of the laryngeal inlet, but the consistency and reliability of these examinations were unclear due to fogging of mirrors, marginal lighting, and inability to control the gag reflex. Regardless, these earlier investigations did not stimulate sufficient interest to initiate the field of laryngology.

One of the first reports was from Levret, a French physician who used polished metal in

1743 to visualize polyps in the "nostrils, throat, ears and other parts."[5] In 1807 Bozzini published a pamphlet concerning his invention of a double cannula with an internal mirror, which was used to visualize internal organs of the body.[6] This device included a universal handle that held a candle as a light source and a reflector; connected to this handle were a variety of different cannulae to visualize different organs/lumens of the body. Bozzini's cannula system was comprised of an extracorporeal light source for illumination contained within a universal handle to which varied examining speculae were attached. These principles of endoscopic instrument design are embodied in a majority of current instrumentation. This revolutionary instrumentation received little attention in its time and Bozzini died soon thereafter at the age of 33, prior to establishing widespread adoption of his new instrument and surgical paradigm.[7] Other physicians who reported attempts at mirror laryngoscopy in this time frame were Cagniard de la Tour in 1825 and Senn in 1827.

Following these initial descriptions of mirror laryngoscopy, Benjamin Guy Babington introduced his *glottiscope* in 1829. Babington designed an oblong mirror, which was held against the palate and used to visualize the pharynx and larynx. Although Babington likely saw the upper larynx, he never commented on vocal fold movement, physiology, or disease states so the exact degree of visualization that he attained cannot be determined with certainty.[8] He presented his results to the Hunterian Society in London and continued to use and improve his mirror for many years. However, he never published his findings so his results remained limited to his immediate circle of professional peers. Because Babington did not receive popular acclaim for his accomplishments, it is likely that García was unaware of Babington's work on laryngoscopy.

Several other descriptions of mirror laryngoscopy were reported between Babington's 1829 presentation to the Hunterian society and García's 1855 presentation to the Royal Society of London. These include Selligue in 1832, who used a speculum to see his own larynx.[9] In his

1837 surgical text Liston[10] described mirror laryngoscopy much as it is practiced today using a dental mirror warmed in hot water to see the larynx; Baumes[11] in 1838 exhibited a laryngeal mirror at the Medical Society of Lyon in France. One amusing anecdote concerns Avery, who in 1844 developed a complex device for laryngoscopy, which included a head-holder rigidly attached to a light source (candle), head mirror, and a mirrored speculum similar to Bozzini. Although he likely visualized the larynx routinely throughout the 1840s, years before García's description, Avery's[12] were not reported formally until 1862 because he first wanted to develop a system of photography to validate his claims.

Laryngoscopy After García

García's observations, which may have been the first to reliably and repeatedly describe laryngeal function, stimulated further interest in laryngoscopy and, therefore, the field of laryngology was born. Ludwig Türck[13,14] in Vienna and Johann Czermak[15,16] of Budapest remain linked as two physicians who helped popularize laryngoscopy. Turck began to explore the clinical applications of laryngoscopy in 1857 using reflected sunlight as a light source. When lack of sunlight interrupted his work, Turck loaned his laryngeal mirrors to Czermak. Czermak introduced an artificial light source and reintroduced the fenestrated mirror held by the examiner. He published the results of his clinical investigation in April 1858. Although his early publications acknowledged Turck's contributions, Czermak's later papers made no mention of Turck's role in advancing laryngology. The conflict as to which of these investigators deserved attribution for popularizing mirror laryngoscopy fueled interest in laryngology throughout the medical world.

Morell Mackenzie is one of the key physicians who studied laryngology with Czermak and then helped to develop the new field of laryngology. He visited Czermak and learned indirect laryngoscopy in 1859, when he was 21 years old. He returned to Britain and by 1863 was accomplished enough to win the Jackson Prize from the Royal College of Surgeons for his essay, "The Pathology and Treatment of Laryngeal Disease." His skills in developing new instruments and teaching laryngoscopy culminated in his 1865 textbook, *The Use of the Laryngoscope in Diseases of the Throat*.[17] By 1871 Mackenzie published his treatise on *Growths in the Larynx*[18] and his considerable skills gained him an international reputation. He opened the first hospital dedicated to diseases of the throat and is considered "The Father of British Laryngology." However, Mackenzie's legacy remains blemished by the controversy surrounding his role in the treatment of Crown Prince Frederick (see box below).

Controversy:
Mackenzie and the Crown Prince

By May 1887, Morell Mackenzie had earned an international reputation as a laryngologist based on his opening of the first hospital for diseases of the throat and his publication of treatises on topics such as *Growths in the Larynx*. Therefore, it was natural that Mackenzie was consulted when Crown Prince Frederick of Germany, who was married to the eldest daughter of Queen Victoria, suffered from chronic hoarseness. Mirror examination at that time revealed the presence of an irregular lesion, and Mackenzie counseled transoral mirror-guided biopsy. Four biopsies were performed over the next 5 weeks, and in 3, Mackenzie was able to obtain abnormal tissue. However, the esteemed pathologist Rudolf Virchow was unable to establish the diagnosis of malignancy—perhaps because Virchow believed that carcinoma arises from connective tissue rather than from epithelium, as was later demonstrated by the pathologist Waldeyer who (too late) was able to establish a diagnosis of carcinoma.[19] Regardless, despite the urgings of the Crown Prince's other surgeons, Mackenzie held firm in his refusal to recommend laryngectomy without a tissue diagnosis, Without pathologic confirmation, the clinically suspected laryngeal carcinoma was allowed to grow until it created airway obstruction. This was managed with palliative tracheotomy, but the Crown Prince died within the year, shortly after becoming emperor of Germany.

Substantial innuendo and intrigue was associated with Mackenzie's handling of the case. Mackenzie felt that the criticism arose from the Prince's private physicians. Mackenzie was so disturbed by this controversy that he published his own account of the case in a book titled *The Fatal Illness of Frederick the Noble*.[20] Although his intentions may have been honorable, Mackenzie's peers considered his actions unprofessional and unethical—he was censured by both the Royal College of Surgeons and the British Medical Society, and he resigned from the Royal College of Physicians. Ironically, Mackenzie's reluctance to allow laryngectomy may have prolonged the Prince's life—the life span of the Prince's surgeon's seven previous laryngectomy patients was only 4 months, shorter than the Prince's ultimate survival. Unfortunately, the episode of Crown Prince Frederick also led to increased speculation by opponents of transoral biopsy that Mackenzie's multiple transoral manipulations of the tissue may have induced malignant degeneration. This belief remained popular for many years, and it was not until Semon's exhaustive investigation[21] of several thousand laryngeal cancers refuted the idea that biopsies could cause cancer that Mackenzie's reputation was cleared.

As laryngology began to spread quickly throughout Europe, it did not take long for the new technique to come to America. Ernst Krackowizer, originally from Venice, was the first to perform laryngoscopy in the United States, in 1858.[22] However, it was Louis Elsberg of New York and Jacob Solis-Cohen of Philadelphia (Figure 1–2) who became the key leaders in laryngology in the United States. In 1865, Elsberg gave his prize-winning presentation on "Laryngoscopal Surgery, Illustrated in the Treatment of Morbid Growths Within the Larynx" to the American Medical Association.[23] Meanwhile, his boyhood friend Jacob Solis-Cohen became the first surgeon to become a laryngologist. Solis-Cohen (Philadelphia School of Anatomy) and Henry Kimble Oliver (Harvard Medical School) first instituted instruction in laryngoscopy in 1866. In 1869, the first academic appointment in laryngoscopy was established for Solis-Cohen at Jefferson Medical College in Philadelphia. Shortly thereafter, Frederick Irving Knight was appointed at Harvard Medical School (1870); the Massachusetts General Hospital established a clinical service for him in 1872.[24]

By 1879, through the influence of Elsberg, Solis-Cohen, and Knight, laryngologists throughout the United States united to form the American Laryngological Association (ALA).[25] Elsberg, Solis-Cohen, and Knight served as the first three presidents of the ALA. In 1880 they founded the *American Archives of Laryngology,* which ceased publication by 1884; it was followed in 1896 by *The Laryngoscope.*

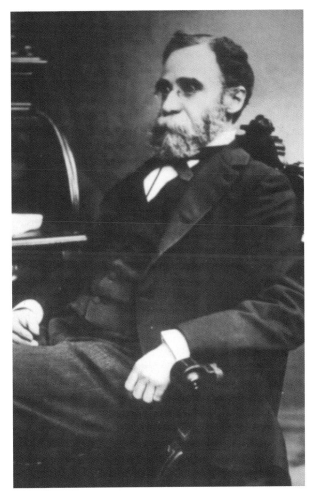

FIGURE 1–2. Jacob Solis-Cohen (1838–1927), America's first head-and-neck surgeon and second president of the American Laryngological Association. (Courtesy of the College of Physicians, Philadelphia.)

DIRECT LARYNGOSCOPY

In the 19th century, infectious diseases were a formidable problem; membranous airway obstruction was a dominant clinical issue in laryngology.[26,27] Horace Green (1802–1866) dedicated his career to this problem and spent time with Trousseau and Belloc[28] in Europe. He was the first specialist for throat and respiratory diseases in the United States. Green described transoral application of caustics to the larynx to treat infectious inflammatory disorders of the laryngeal membranes.[29,30] He was, however, maligned by his contemporaries, who did not believe that his transoral interventions were possible. Later, Green resolved this by placing a whalebone probang transorally through the glottis of a patient with a tracheotomy until the probang could be observed at the tracheotomy site.

In 1852, Green made his most seminal contribution by describing the first direct laryngoscopy and visually controlled excision of a laryngeal neoplasm. He reported the case in detail in his landmark textbook, *On the Surgical Treatment of Polypi of the Larynx.*[31] The book contained a drawing of what the artist could view of the procedure while looking over Green's shoulder. Both Bozzini and Green were courageous figures in medical history as their work was not accepted by their contemporaries, who could not replicate their techniques. They were both branded as charlatans by the general medical establishment. Although Bozzini died shortly after his manuscript was published, Green lived through the initial period of the origin of Laryngology and he was ultimately vindicated (see box below).

Following Green's description of direct laryngoscopy in 1852, the technique was largely

Controversy:
Horace Green and Direct Laryngoscopy

In 1852, Horace Green reported on the removal of a laryngeal polyp from an 11-year-old child in New York. According to his own account of the events,[31] Green used a bent tongue spatula to depress the tongue base, bringing the epiglottis into view. When the child coughed, a round white polyp appeared at the laryngeal introitus, at the lateral border of the epiglottis, just above the arytenoid. Green was able to grasp this polyp with a hook, providing enough exposure to transect the pedicle of the polyp and deliver the mass transorally. Although credit for direct laryngoscopy is sometimes given to Kirstein, this description of Green's procedure bears a remarkable similarity to Kirstein's autoscopy described several decades later; it also is a reasonable description of the exposure provided by the Macintosh blade to anesthesiologists during intubation today. Although Green did not have the advantage of a headlight as Kirstein did (instead depending on sunlight), his choice of a child (who would have had a relatively high larynx) likely allowed him to accomplish his feat. Later descriptions of direct laryngoscopy attest to the laryngeal visualization possible with a tongue blade, giving further support to the likelihood that Green did truly accomplish direct laryngoscopy.

Green was the first physician to dedicate his career to the study of the throat and respiratory diseases. Given the prevailing diseases of his era, Green spent much of his career treating inflammatory diseases of the larynx by applying caustics. He presented his technique of using a curved whale bone probang to deliver silver nitrate to the larynx to the New York Medical-Surgical Society in 1840, but in this prelaryngoscopic era his contemporaries did not believe that such application was possible.[25,32] They called for Green's resignation from the society, and attacks on Green's character grew more pronounced following Green's 1846 publication of a treatise on upper airway disease. A New York Academy of Medicine committee was appointed to study Green's claims, and they found that "the procedure was an anatomical impossibility and unwarrantable in practice." Green was not vindicated in his efforts until he had the opportunity to perform his procedure in a patient with a tracheotomy—the appearance of the probang in the subglottis, as visualized directly through the patient's tracheostoma, confirmed Green's placement. Later attempts at transoral laryngeal manipulation, enabled by the popularization of mirror laryngoscopy, which followed Green's work, further restored Green's reputation. Although he died in 1866, the founders of the American Laryngological Society later recognized Horace Green as "The Father of American Laryngology."[22]

supplanted by indirect laryngoscopy, which was redescribed by García shortly thereafter. Indirect laryngoscopy was more comfortable for the patient than direct laryngoscopy, and an adequate indirect view of the larynx did not depend on the favorable pediatric anatomy (cephalad-positioned larynx) enjoyed by Green during his index case.[7] Kirstein,[33,34] who was probably unaware of Green's work, formally reintroduced direct laryngoscopic examination. His success was based on employing electrical illumination as well as local mucosal anesthesia with cocaine.[35] Kirstein named his technique "autoscopy" to avoid academic rancor from the other laryngologists who believed that only a laryngeal mirror could be considered a laryngoscope. Kirstein performed direct examination of the larynx and trachea with the patient sitting in the classic sniffing position, using a spatula to depress the tongue base and a headlight to illuminate the lar-

ynx. Kirstein later incorporated a self-contained light source into the electrified autoscope itself, obviating the need for a separate headlight (Figure 1–3). This electrified autoscope contained all the elements of a modern laryngoscope: a universal handle, a series of detachable blades, and a self-contained light source.

Kirstein refined direct laryngoscopy and tracheoscopy by designing a variety of spatula and tubular laryngoscope speculae. Gustav Killian advanced these investigations by subsequently perfecting direct rigid bronchoscopy.[32] Killian reported that he had initially questioned Kirstein's accounts of direct laryngoscopy, but after witnessing Kirstein perform the technique Killian declared, "From that time, my entire thought became bound up in the subject."[36] Killian then developed several refinements of the laryngoscope, including an inverted-V spatula blade[37] designed to improve exposure of the anterior

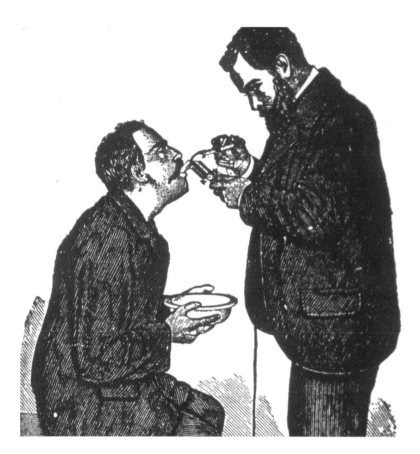

FIGURE 1–3. Alfred Kirstein (1863–1922) as he performed autoscopy (direct laryngoscopy). Note the cord hanging from the autoscope, which allowed for direct illumination. (From *Autoscopy of the Larynx* [*Direct Examination Without Mirror*][34])

commissure. Killian also developed suspension laryngoscopy as he devised a means to hold a laryngoscope stable enough to allow for anatomic illustration (Figure 1–4). In turn, he realized that this device would allow for bimanual instrumentation, which would greatly enhance precision during endolaryngeal surgery. In the United States, Lynch[38,39] further refined the Killian suspension laryngoscope. The development and popularization of chest-support-holders[7,40] was due to many surgeons' difficulty with suspension laryngoscopy with sedation and local anesthesia. True suspension laryngoscopy is enjoying revitalization because of the use of general endotracheal anesthesia along with the need to place larger laryngoscopic examining speculae for phonomicrosurgery and endolaryngeal partial laryngectomy procedures.[40,41]

Another driving force in the evolution of direct laryngoscopy was Chevalier Jackson (Figure 1–5). Jackson was greatly influenced by Killian. Jackson published the first textbook[42] of rigid endoscopy of the upper aerodigestive tract in 1907 and dedicated it to Killian. Among Jackson's many innovations was the creation of a separating laryngoscope, with a tubular design proximally and a spatula blade distally—a laryngoscope design still in routine use today. Jackson also introduced laryngoscopes with distal, rather than proximal, illumination. Jackson was instrumental in perfecting techniques for supine laryngoscopy. With the assistance of human assistants as head-holders, Jackson compared different positions and transferred the "sniffing" position of neck flexion and head extension to supine positioning. Despite these many innovations, Jackson did not use suspension laryngoscopy and instead used one hand to hold the laryngoscope while using the other to hold his instruments. In retrospect, this limited his endolaryngeal surgical accomplishments.

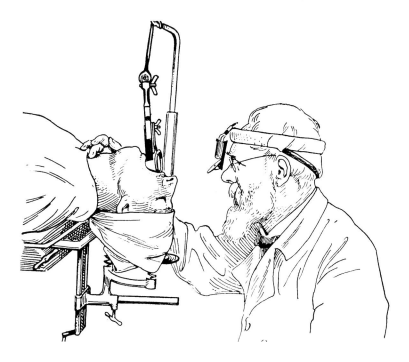

FIGURE 1–4. Gustav Killian's (1860–1921) initial suspension laryngoscopy apparatus. (From *Die Schwebelaryngoscopic und ihre praktische.*)

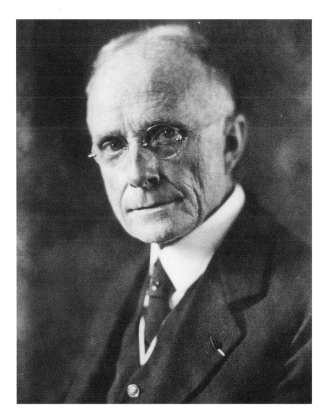

FIGURE 1–5. Chevalier Jackson (1865–1958).

ENDOLARYNGEAL SURGERY

Reports of endolaryngeal surgery predate the laryngoscopic era. As reported by Wright, for instance, Koederik used a malleable instrument to ligate a laryngeal polyp in 1770.[43] By 1852, Horace Green reported the transoral removal of a laryngeal polyp from a child in New York.[31] Shortly after the introduction of indirect laryngoscopy as a diagnostic tool, it was applied to therapeutics as well. In 1859 Stoerk[44] reported on the first laryngoscopically controlled application of silver nitrate to the larynx. By 1860, Lewin[45] reported on the mirror-guided intralaryngeal management of laryngeal tumors with application of caustics in 4 cases as well as transoral partial excision in another 3 cases. In 1865, H. B. Sands[46] reported a case of laryngoscopically directed transoral biopsy of a laryngeal tumor followed by transcervical excision; this approach of endoscopic biopsy followed by open management is still standard for many head and neck malignancies in the modern era.

From these beginnings, reports of the use of indirect laryngoscopy in the surgical diagnosis and management of laryngeal disease continued to multiply throughout the 1860s and 1870s. This growth was fueled in part by the introduction of cocaine as a mucosal anesthetic, which greatly facilitated mirror-guided laryngeal surgery.[31] By 1886, indirect laryngoscopy had allowed endolaryngeal surgery to progress to the point where the renowned German laryngologist Fraenkel became the first to report a case of transoral excision as the sole treatment for an early glottic cancer.[47] Although multiple recurrences led to repeated transoral procedures, and despite the need for subsequent neck dissection, Fraenkel's patient remained alive for at least 5 years from the time of diagnosis. The use of mirror laryngoscopy to guide biopsy and endolaryngeal surgery, however, was not without its critics, as demonstrated in the controversy surrounding Morell Mackenzie's involvement in the case of Crown Prince Frederick of Germany in 1887 (see Controversy box page 6).

Endolaryngeal surgery took another large step forward with the introduction of direct laryngoscopy. Kirstein's description of direct endolaryngeal examination was followed by Killian's introduction of suspension apparatus and Jackson's development of new instruments (despite Jackson's reliance on one-handed surgery). In 1911, Killian's disciple Brünings[48] described injection medialization laryngoplasty as a treatment for vocal paralysis, a conceptual approach that is still commonly performed today. In 1915 Lynch,[49] who used a modification of Killian suspension to increase surgical exposure, began to introduce the concept of direct removal of early vocal fold neoplasia. Unlike his predecessors, Lynch resected small unilateral lesions *en bloc* and obtained clear tumor margins; if tumors were not amenable to *en bloc* endoscopic excision, then Lynch reverted to transcervical approaches. His successes led to further reports of endolaryngeal cancer surgery, including the 1941 report of New and Dorton[50] who cured 9 of 10 patients with unilateral vocal fold carcinoma using suspension laryngoscopy and surgical diathermy. In 1910, endotracheal intubation was introduced experimentally for controlling the airway during the administration of anesthesia.[51] Eventually (1960), this was done during direct laryngoscopy, which enhanced precision of endolaryngeal surgery.[52] From these beginnings, endolaryngeal surgery continued to evolve as new equipment and techniques were developed.

Similar advances were being made in external laryngeal surgery as well.[53] Although a full accounting of the history of external laryngeal surgery is beyond the scope of this chapter, some milestones include the introduction of the anterior laryngofissure for the management of laryngeal cancer by Jacob Solis-Cohen in 1869.[54] The patient on whom Solis-Cohen performed this procedure lived for another 20 years following his surgery. Billroth performed the first successful total laryngectomy for cancer in 1873, although chronic aspiration remained a problem for his patients. Solis-Cohen explained that primary pharyngeal closure was necessary to separate the airway from the digestive tract, thereby making total laryngectomy a viable procedure. Other key advancements in transcervical laryngeal surgery were Payr's description[55] of the first medialization laryngoplasty (1915) for vocal fold paralysis, and Ballance's report[56] on neural reinnervation for the same problem.

TRANSITION TO MODERN LARYNGOLOGY

From these foundations in indirect laryngoscopy, direct laryngoscopy, and increasingly sophisticated endolaryngeal surgery, laryngology has continued to evolve. New technologies were added to the field in the late 20th century, helping laryngology to enter the modern era. From a technical standpoint, critical new advances that helped the transition into modern laryngology include use of the operating microscope and the CO_2 laser. A great paradigm shift in laryngology also occurred with the acceptance of the "body-cover" theory of voice production (see chapter 3, Anatomy of the Larynx and Physiology of Phonation). Together, the increased understanding of laryngeal physiology and the increased precision of diagnosis and surgery combined to bring laryngology from its historical roots to the present day.

The addition of the operating microscope was driven by a desire to improve surgical precision. The operating microscope was first used as part of suspension laryngoscopy by Scalco et al[57] in 1960, and by 1962, Jako[58,59] and Kleinsasser[59,60] were performing microlaryngoscopy. They recognized that use of the microscope demanded better instruments, so Jako modified otologic instruments by adding longer handles to create the first set of microlaryngeal instruments.[58] By the late 1960s, Jako,[58,61] Strong,[62,63] and Vaughan[64,65] coupled a carbon dioxide (CO_2) laser to the operating microscope, introducing laser technology both to laryngology and to surgical oncology. Since their initial results were published in 1972, the CO_2 laser has become a routine part of the armamentarium for most laryngeal surgeons. New laser technologies will continue to evolve and likely allow for a substantial volume of endolaryngeal surgery to become office-based as it was in the 19th century.[66] This is further outlined in the following chapter, Frontiers in Laryngology.

After leaving von Leden's[67-71] laboratory, Hirano pursued investigations of vocal fold histology and physiology. Connecting findings from stroboscopy, gross anatomy, and electron histology led Hirano to reintroduce the body-cover theory of voice production.[72-73] This theory had first been advanced by Bishop in 1836, who could not visualize a moving glottis and instead deduced the theory from anatomic studies: "the true vibrating surface of the glottis is the mucous membrane. The vocal cords confer on it the tension, resistance, position, and probably other conditions necessary for the vibration."[74] This was eventually proven with the use of laryngeal stroboscopy.[70,71,75,76] This prescient observation was largely forgotten until Hirano's elegant description of the layered anatomy of the vocal fold led to a renewed focus on preservation of the superficial lamina propria in laryngeal surgery.

Increased understanding of vocal fold function, coupled with the advances in surgical precision which were occurring contemporaneously, led to the development of phonomicrosurgery,[7] a term first used in 1995. In this fashion, the history of laryngology can be seen as a series of advances in technique, equipment, and knowledge extending from the early 19th century until today.

Review Questions

1. Who is generally given credit for establishing the value of indirect laryngoscopy?

2. Who were some of the other key physicians who popularized indirect laryngoscopy?

3. Who invented direct laryngoscopy?

4. Name some milestones in endolaryngeal surgery.

5. What more recent developments have helped the field of laryngology transition from its historical roots to its present state?

REFERENCES

1. Zeitels SM, Healy GB. Laryngology and Phonosurgery: past present and future. *N Engl J Med.* 2003;349:882–892.

2. García M. Observations on the human voice. *Proc Roy Soc London.* 1855;7:397–410.

3. Clerf LH. Manuel García's contribution to laryngology. *Bull N Y Acad Med.* 1956;32:603–611.

4. Mackinlay MS. *García the Centenarian and His Times: Being a Memoir of Manuel García's Life and Labours for the Advancement of Music and Science.* New York, NY: D. Appleton and Company; 1908.

5. Mackenzie M. *The Use of the Laryngoscope in Diseases of the Throat.* Philadelphia, Pa: Lindsay and Blakiston; 1865:9.

6. Bozzini P. *Der Lichtleiter oder Beschreibung einer einfachen Vorichtung, und ihrer Anwendung zur erleucht ung inherer Hohlen, und Zwischenraume des lebenden animaschen Körpers.* Weimar, Germany: Körpers; 1807.

7. Zeitels SM. Premalignant epithelium and microinvasive cancer of the vocal fold: the evolution of phonomicrosurgical management. *Laryngoscope.* 1995;105(suppl 67):1–51.

8. Babington BG. *London Med Gazette.* 1829;3:555.

9. Selligue (1832). Cited by Mackenzie M, in *The Use of the Laryngoscope in Diseases of the Throat*. London: J & A Churchill; 1865:17.

10. Liston R. *Practical Surgery*. London: J & A Churchill; 1837.

11. Baumes. *Compte rendu des travaux de la societe de medecine de Lyons*. 1836-1838;19:18.

12. Avery (1844). Cited by Mackenzie M, in *The Use of the Laryngoscope in Diseases of the Throat*. London: J & A Churchill; 1865:25.

13. Turck L. On the laryngeal mirror and its mode of employment, with engravings on wood. *Zeitschrift der Gesellschaft der Aerzte zu Wien*. 1858;26:401-409.

14. Turck L. *Chronic Inflammatory Disease of the Vocal Cord*. Wien: Wilhelm Braumuller; 1860.

15. Czermak JN. Ueber den kehlkopfspiegel. *Wiener Med Wochenschr*. 1858;8(13):196-198.

16. Czermak JN. On the laryngoscope and its employment in physiology and medicine. *New Sydenham Society*. 1861;11:1-79.

17. Mackenzie M. *The Use of the Laryngoscope in Diseases of the Throat with an Appendix on Rhinoscopy*. London: J & A Churchill; 1865.

18. Mackenzie M. *Growths in the Larynx*. London: J & A Churchill; 1871.

19. Lin JI. Virchow's pathological reports on Frederick III's cancer. *New Engl J Med*. 1984;311:1261-1264.

20. Mackenzie M. *The Fatal Illness of Frederick the Noble*. London: Sampson, Low, Marston, Searle, and Rivington Ltd; 1888.

21. Semon F. Die frage de ueberganges gutatiger kehlkopf-geschwulster in bosartige, speciell nach intralaryngealen operation. *Internationales Centralblatt fur Laryngologie, Rhinologie, Jahrgang*. 1889;4(6): 271-279.

22. Boas E. The first use of the laryngoscope in the United States. *J History Med*. 1950;5:452-454.

23. Elsberg L. *Laryngoscopal Surgery Illustrated in the Treatment of Morbid Growths Within the Larynx*. Philadelphia: Collins; 1866.

24. Snyder C. *A Tale of Four Hats or Practitioners and Professors of Laryngology and Otology*. Boston, Mass: Massachusetts Eye and Ear Infirmary; 1984.

25. Elsberg L. President's address: laryngology in America. *Trans Am Laryngological Assn*. 1879;1:30-90.

26. Green H. *A Treatise on Diseases of the Air Passages*. New York, NY: Wiley and Putnam; 1846.

27. Green H. *Observations on the Pathology of Croup*. New York, NY: John Wiley; 1849.

28. Trousseau A, Belloc H. *Phthisie Laryngie*. Paris: Chez and Bailliere; 1837.

29. Green H. On the subject of the priority in the medication of the larynx and trachea. *Am Med Monthly*. 1854;1:241-257.

30. Green, H. Report on the use and effect of applications of nitrate silver to the throat, either in local or general disease. *Trans Am Med Assn*. 1856;9: 493-530.

31. Green H. Morbid growths within the larynx. In: *On the Surgical Treatment of Polypi of the Larynx, and Oedema of the Glottis*. New York, NY: GP Putnam; 1852:46-65.

32. Donaldson F. The laryngology of Trousseau and Horace Green. *Trans Am Laryngol Assn*. 1890; 12:10-18.

33. Kirstein A. Autoskopie des larynx und der trachea (laryngoscopia directa, euthy-skopie, besichtigung ohne spiegel). *Archiv Laryngol Rhinol*. 1895;3: 156-164.

34. Kirstein A. *Autoscopy of the Larynx and Trachea (Direct Examination Without Mirror)*. Philadelphia, Pa: FA Davis Co; 1897.

35. Jelinek E. Das cocain als anastheticum und analgeticum fur den pharynx und larynx. *Wiener Med Wochenschr*. 1884;34:1334-1337, 1364-1367.

36. Killian G. Ueber direkte bronchoskopie. *Munchener Med Wochenschr*. 1898; 45:844-847.

37. Killian G. Demonstration of an endoscopic spatula. *J Laryngol Rhinol*. 1910;25:549-550.

38. Lynch RC. Suspension laryngoscopy and its accomplishments. *Ann Otol Rhinol Laryngol*. 1915;24:429-446.

39. Lynch RC. A resume of my years work with suspension laryngoscopy. *Trans Am Laryngol Assn*. 1916;38:158-175.

40. Zeitels SM, Mauri M, Burns JA, Dailey SH. Suspension laryngoscopy revisited. *Ann Otol Rhinol Laryngol*. 2004;113:16-22.

41. Zeitels SM. Instrumentation. In: *Atlas of Phonomicrosurgery and Other Endolaryngeal Procedures for Benign and Malignant Disease*. San Diego, Calif: Singular; 2001;23-36.

42. Jackson C. *Tracheobronchoscopy, Esophagoscopy, and Gastroscopy*. St. Louis, Mo: Laryngoscope Co; 1907.

43. Wright J. The first intralaryngeal operation. In: *A History of Laryngology and Rhinology*. 2nd ed. Philadelphia, Pa: Lea & Febiger; 1914;214.

44. Stoerk C. On the laryngoscope. *Zeitschrift Der Gesellschaft der Aerzte ze Wein*. 1859;46: 721-727.

45. Lewin G. Allgemeine Medicinische Central-Zeitung 1861;30:654.

46. Sands HB. Case of cancer of the larynx, successfully removed by laryngectomy; with an analysis of 50 cases of tumors of the larynx, treated by operation. *N Y Med J.* 1865:110-126.

47. Fraenkel B. First healing of a laryngeal cancer taken out through the natural passages. *Archiv Klin Chirurgie.* 1886;12:283-286.

48. Brünings W. Eine neue behandlungsmethode der rekurrenslahmungen. *Verhandl Deutsch Vereins Deutscher Laryngologen.* 1911;18:93-151.

49. Lynch RC. Intrinsic carcinoma of the larynx, with a second report of the cases operated on by suspension and dissection. *Trans Am Laryngol Assn.* 1920;40:119-126.

50. New GB, Dorton HE. Suspenion laryngoscopy in the treatment of malignant disease of the hypopharynx and larynx. *Mayo Clin Proc.* 1941;16:411-416.

51. Elsberg CA. Clinical experiences with intratracheal insufflation (Meltzer), with remarks upon the value of the method for thoracic surgery. *Ann Surg.* 1910;52:23-29.

52. Priest RE, Wesolowski S. Direct laryngoscopy under general anesthesia. *Trans Am Acad Opthalmol Otolaryngol.* 1960;64:639-648.

53. Myers EN. The evolution of head and neck surgery. *Laryngoscope.* 1996;106:929-934.

54. Solis-Cohen J. Clinical history of surgical affections of the larynx. *Med Rec.* 1869;4:244-247.

55. Payr. Plastik am schildknorpel zur behebung der folgen einseitiger stimmbandlahmung. *Deutsche Med Wochenschr.* 1915;41:1265.

56. Ballance C. Unilateral paralysis of the vocal fold: operative treatment. *Br Med J.* 1924;2:349-354.

57. Scalco AN, Shipman WF, and Tabb HG. Microscopic suspension laryngoscopy. *Ann Otol Rhinol Laryngol.* 1960;69:1134-1138.

58. Jako GJ. Correspondence documents between Geza Jako and the Stumar Instrument Company, 1962.

59. Jako GJ, Kleinsasser O. Endolaryngeal micro-diagnosis and microsurgery. Scientific Exhibition at the 115th Annual Meeting of the American Medical Association; 1966.

60. Kleinsasser O. Die laryngomicroscope (lupen-laryngoskopie) und ihre bedeutung fur die erkennung der vorerkrankungen und fruhformen des stimmlipencarcinomas. *Archiv Ohren Nasen Kehlkopfheilkunde.* 1962;724-727.

61. Jako GJ. Laser surgery of the vocal cords. *Laryngoscope.* 1972;82:2204-2215.

62. Strong MS, Jako GJ. Laser surgery of the larynx: early clinical experience with continuous CO_2 laser. *Ann Otol Rhinol Laryngol.* 1972;81:791-798.

63. Strong MS. Laser management of premalignant lesions of the larynx. *Can J Otolaryngol.* 1974;3:560-563.

64. Vaughan CW. Transoral laryngeal surgery using the CO_2 laser. Laboratory experiments and clinical experience. *Laryngoscope.* 1978;88:1399-1420.

65. Vaughan CW, Strong MS, Jako GJ. Laryngeal carcinoma: transoral treatment using the CO_2 laser. *Am J Surg.* 1978;136:490-493.

66. Zeitels SM, Franco RA, Dailey SH, Burns JA, Hillman RE, Anderson RR. Office-based treatment of glottal dysplasia and papilloma with the 585-nm pulsed dye laser and local anesthesia. *Ann Otol Rhinol Laryngol.* 2004;113:265-276.

67. von Leden H. The electronic synchron-stroboscope: Its value for the practicing laryngologist. *Ann Otol Rhinol Laryngol.* 1961;70:881-893.

68. von Leden H, Moore P. The mechanics of the cricoarytenoid joint. *Arch Otolaryngol.* 1961;73:541-550.

69. von Leden H, Moore P. Vibratory pattern of vocal cords in unilateral paralysis. *Acta Otolaryngol (Stockh).* 1961;53:493-506.

70. von Leden H, Moore P, Timcke R. Laryngeal vibrations: measurements of the glottic wave: Part III. The pathological larynx. *Arch Otolaryngol.* 1960;71:16-35.

71. von Leden H. Plastic surgery of the larynx. *Revista Panamerica de Otorrinolaringologia y Broncoesofagologia,* 1963;1:7-11.

72. Hirano M. Structure and vibratory pattern of the vocal folds. In: Sawashimi N, Cooper FS, eds. *Dynamic Aspects of Speech Production.* Tokyo: University of Tokyo Press; 1977:13-24.

73. Hirano M. Structure of the vocal fold in normal and diseased states: anatomic and physical studies. *Proceedings of the Conference on the Assessment of Vocal Pathology.* Rockville, Md: American Speech and Hearing Assn; 1981:11-27.

74. Bishop J. Experimental researches into the physiology of the human voice. *The London & Edinburgh Philosophical Magazine & Journal of Science;* 1836.

75. Oertel M. Ueber eine neues laryngostroboskopische untersuchungsmethode des kehlkopfes. *Centralblatt Medizinischen Wiss.* 1878;16:81-82.

76. Oertel M. Das laryngo-stroboskop und die laryngo-stroboskpische untersuchung. *Archiv Laryngol Rhinol.* 1895;3:1-16.

2

Frontiers in Laryngology

Seth H. Dailey, MD

KEY POINTS

■ **Benign lesions:** Prevention of vocal fold scar is of paramount importance because reparative techniques offer only partial improvement. The application of growth factors or genetic alteration of the scar may soon transform management of these challenging cases.

■ **Malignant lesions:** Office-based cytological examination and operative reconstructive techniques will allow for improved diagnostic accuracy and replacement of resected tissue.

■ **Laryngeal paralysis and reinnervation:** Neural growth factors and muscle group-specific reinnervation may ultimately produce native function of the paralyzed hemilarynx.

■ **Reflux in laryngology:** Office-based biopsy and agent-specific testing will allow for identification of specific noxious components that damage the laryngopharynx.

■ **Airway stenosis:** Tissue scaffolds and engineering of autogenous cartilage may facilitate immediate replacement of resected trachea.

The frontiers of laryngology are expanding as never before. Scientific trends such as tissue engineering, digital imaging, laser technology, and bioassays are interacting with demography to influence the way laryngology is practiced in the 21st century. Only 36 years ago flexible fiberoptic scopes were a novelty in the field, and it has been only 30 years since modern endoscopic cancer resections were described. Enhanced technologies such as distal chip cameras, office-based lasers, and vocal fold injectables have influenced the movement of procedures out of the operating room and into the office, a development that has come at a time when the population is aging and may be less likely to tolerate a general anesthetic. Within the last several years, the approaches to major challenges facing laryngology, including benign glottic lesions, laryngeal cancer, neuromuscular disorders, laryngopharyngeal reflux, and laryngeal stenosis are rapidly transforming. This makes knowledge of these technologies and techniques mandatory for ongoing education. In this chapter we examine some of the themes that will be shaping the way we practice in the years to come. Each of these areas is illustrated with a realistic contemporary scenario, a look forward to developments related to that clinical challenge, and an idealized approach that might be taken by physicians in the future.

BENIGN LESIONS OF THE VOCAL FOLDS

Today: A surgeon evaluates a patient via office mirror examination or fiberoptic laryngoscopy and finds a midmembranous vocal fold polyp. The patient is taken to the operating room for microlaryngoscopy where the pathologic vocal fold is palpated and found to have a sulcus deformity inferior to the polyp. Standard microinstruments are used to make a mini-microflap and resect the polyp. The

sulcus deformity is dissected off the vocal ligament to redrape the "cover." The epithelium and scar are torn because of a technical error and the injured segment is resected, creating a vocal fold defect. The defect heals by secondary intention over the sulcus, worsening the stiff region. Postoperatively, the patient is persistently hoarse.

Tomorrow: With these exciting advances one can envision a patient who is evaluated with high-speed color digital imaging in the office; vocal fold scarring is revealed. The depth and nature of the scar could then be immediately evaluated with in-office OCT. The surgeon, having practiced different techniques on ex-vivo surgical simulators, could then employ a robotic surgical system for precise manipulation of the vocal fold cover to reduce undesired resection. This is then followed by immediate injection of different growth factors to enhance upregulation of hyaluronic acid production and promote vocal fold pliability.

This case illustrates the shortcomings of preoperative diagnosis as well as the technical challenges of performing technically delicate surgery in a region that does not regenerate native functional capacity well. Areas of interest in the diagnosis and treatment of benign vocal fold lesions include better tools for anatomic and physiologic evaluation, improved assessment and treatment of vocal fold scarring, enhanced surgical education, and technologic advances in surgical instrumentation.

Videostroboscopy (see chapter 6, Videostroboscopy) has become the current gold standard in vocal fold evaluation and is superior to mirror examination because high resolution color images are acquired.[1] These digitally archived images can be reviewed slowly with care and offer both anatomic and viscoelastic information. Recent evidence suggests, however, that sulcus vocalis and mucosal bridges are difficult to detect even by stroboscopic office examination. In fact up to 10% of patients undergoing direct microlaryngoscopy may have additional findings noted that were not seen at videostroboscopy.[2] Differentiation of vocal fold cysts from swelling has also been identified as a common diagnostic problem.[3] This dilemma of preoperative accuracy points to the need for imaging modalities with high resolution in real time. However, the images that are derived are composite images of multiple oscillatory cycles and do not record true real-time motion. Although Bell Labs made high-speed recordings of vocal fold vibrations in 1939, the film and tape recordings were so cumbersome as to be essentially unusable. High-speed color digital imaging can now record up to 8,000 images per second and allows for cycle-to-cycle evaluation of vocal fold vibration as never before. Computer storage capacities and enhanced optics have now made this a reality, perhaps allowing for more insight into the motion of normal and pathologic vocal folds. A central advantage of high-speed imaging of the vocal folds is the evaluation of vibratory characteristics (ie, the three-dimensional plotting of vocal fold pliability). Despite these advances, the measurement of pliability is *indirect*. Studies at the University of Wisconsin, for example, are under way to determine the pliability of vocal folds—this time incorporating a tool from dermatology, the linear skin rheometer. Used ex-vivo for experimental purposes or in the operating room to enhance diagnosis and produce pliability maps of the vocal folds, this exciting technology offers insight into glottic pathology and will aid in mathematical modeling as well as surgical planning.

Anatomic definition deep to the vocal fold surface will be enhanced with the use of optical coherence tomography (OCT). Traditionally used in ophthalmology and dermatology, OCT uses tissue refraction to produce images that reliably show fluid, collagen, and other substances. It has been used in the operating room and even in the office.[4] With a high resolution and the ability of the probe to pass through the working channel of a flexible transnasal laryngoscope, OCT may provide information such as lesion size, type, composition, and three-dimensional extension within the vocal fold (Figure 2–1). This information will help pre- and intraoperative planning of both epithelial and subepithelial lesions.

Vocal fold scarring and *sulcus vocalis* remain two of the most frustrating benign pathologies. Recently, tissue engineering has been exploited to help improve vocal outcome in patients with sulcus vocalis and vocal fold scar. Animal models including rat, rabbit, pig, and dog have been used to help demonstrate the utility of injected growth factors such as TGF-beta to improve pliability of scarred vocal folds.[5] Furthermore, autologous stem cells injected into experimentally damaged canine vocal folds have demonstrated preliminary benefit in the prevention of vocal fold scar.[6] Also, the injection of hyaluronic acid variants may also inhibit vocal fold scarring after surgery. Other possible interventions include gene therapy to augment native local production of healthy components of the lamina propria.

Technical improvements may be gained through the use of enhanced surgical training and improved instrumentation. Surgical education has gained much attention recently because of a shift toward fulfilling "core competencies" in addition to a limited time (80 hours/week) for residents to learn. Laryngeal dissection stations have been designed to help answer this need and will likely couple with virtual reality stations employed already in other subspecialties for risk-free polishing of surgical skills.[7] It is natural to anticipate a time when laryngeal dissection courses will be included in the training of residents, just as modern temporal bone dissections courses have for approximately 35 years. Despite the improvements in performance that training may bring, there are inherent difficulties in performing microlaryngoscopy. The surgeon is asked to use 22-cm length instruments, a tool whose tip size is often many times the size of the lesion to be resected. With these instruments, the surgeon must preserve thin vocal fold epithelium and work through the narrow examining speculum of a laryngoscope all the while controlling any inherent technical limitations that they may have. The DaVinci surgical robotics system (Intuitive

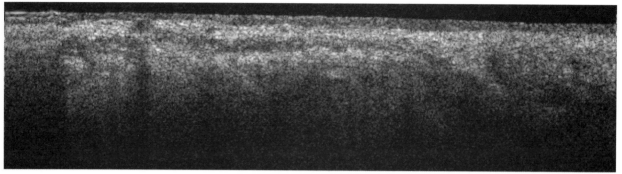

A.

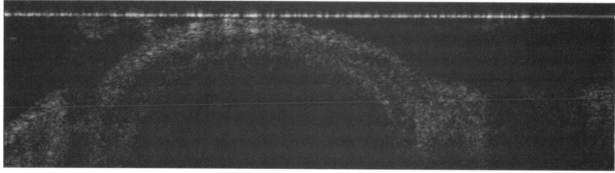

B.

FIGURE 2–1. A. Optical coherence tomography image of the membranous vocal fold. **B.** Optical coherence tomography image of intracordal cyst.

Surgical, Inc, Sunnyvale, Calif) allows the elimination of hand tremor, for example, by using robotic control of instruments inserted through a *de facto* laryngoscope.[8,9] Contemporary developments have focused on reducing the size of the instruments and developing fully rotating distal tips that assure the security of the grasped tissue.

MALIGNANT LESIONS OF THE LARYNX

Today: A former smoker is noted on mirror examination to have a white lesion of the superior surface of the vocal fold. For evaluation of the lesion, the patient under

goes microlaryngoscopy where a portion of the lesion is excised; the pathology reveals microinvasive carcinoma at one site in the epithelium. A portion of underlying superficial lamina propria is resected along with the epithelium for "margin." Postoperatively, the patient is hoarse and further resection is recommended to encompass the entire lesion for diagnostic and therapeutic purposes. The patient subsequently undergoes open cordectomy requiring tracheotomy. Although the patient is successfully decannulated, he and has breathy irregular dysphonia after healing. Pathologic examination demonstrated severe dysplasia within the rest of the surface lesion.

> *Tomorrow: A patient with a superficial white lesion of the vocal fold is imaged in the office with OCT to determine the depth of penetration. Cytobrush office biopsy reveals cancerous cells. Endoscopic combined CO_2 and Holmium laser resection performed in the operating room is immediately followed by injection of scaffolding cells though which the laminar vocal fold structure is restored.*

As in cases of benign lesions, surgeons are at a disadvantage in terms of preresection knowledge of the depth and nature of a lesion. The evaluation and treatment of laryngeal premalignancy and malignancy is dominated by several basic questions. Currently, it is still difficult to know whether a white lesion of the vocal fold has underlying epithelium that is normal, dysplastic, *carcinoma in situ,* or invasive carcinoma merely by office examination. Determination of the severity of disease requires resection of tissue to its deepest layer to determine if it is malignant and, if so, how invasive it is. Furthermore, immediately adjacent areas may have different degrees of dysplasia. In order not to miss the most severe site, surgeons have historically been aggressive in the resection of vocal fold tissue. Alternatively, radiation therapy has been preferred by many with the assumption that full knowledge of the depth of the lesion is unimportant because radiation should be effective in controlling disease, whether it is dysplasia or a T1a carcinoma. Currently, surgical biopsy is the gold standard diagnostic modality; stated simplistically, tissue is traded for knowledge. Given that the oscillatory capacity of the vocal folds is directly dependent on how much normal vocal fold cover is spared, there is a balance to be struck wherein too small a biopsy may yield insufficient diagnostic information and too large a biopsy will yield a vocal fold with a volumetric defect and reduced pliability.

Cytobrush technology, as used for white lesions of the oral cavity has been recently examined and shows promise for accurate office evaluation of the severity of dysplasia of the vocal fold with a low false-negative rate (Woo, personal communication). Office-based OCT may provide imaging sufficient to distinguish noninvasive from invasive disease prior to operative laryngoscopy. Enhanced knowledge of molecular markers and genetic characteristics is starting to transform the management of oral premalignancy and these principles will likely also affect vocal fold premalignancy.[10-12] For example, the loss of heterozygosity and of aneuploidy are negative prognostic factors for long-term outcome of oral premalignant lesions. Enhanced knowledge of these genetic markers may help to stratify patients into high and low risk groups. This stratification could be used to assign patients to aggressive or nonaggressive treatment protocols.

Management of premalignancy and early glottic carcinoma has enormous potential for development. There are limited data to support the therapeutic effects of repeated vocal fold biopsy and there is ample evidence that repeated biopsy or vocal fold stripping induces vocal fold scarring, leading to refractory dysphonia.[13-15] In an effort to avoid these repeated vocal fold "stripping" procedures, alternative treatment pathways have been sought. The use of the 585-nm pulsed dye laser has shown visual regression of keratosis with atypia without adverse voice results.[16-18] This laser can be used in the operating room and in the office with only topical anesthesia. This application offers the advantages of reducing the patient's exposure to general anesthesia, not sacrificing tissue for regression of disease, and not burning any bridges with respect to other therapies. This may eventually allow for nonsurgical treatment of premalignancy when coupled to the 585-nm pulsed dye laser.

There is increasing acceptance of endoscopic CO_2 laser techniques for treatment of early glottic carcinoma[19-21] (see chapter 25, Malignant Neoplasms of the Larynx). Generally speaking, open approaches for laryngeal malignancy have been favored in the United States; the transition to endoscopic techniques will require more centers with specialized training and experience. Hesitation to utilize endoscopic options may also be due to limited experience in reconstructive techniques.[21,22]

Furthermore, new lasers with flexible fibers will allow simultaneous cutting and coagulation with the advantage of enhanced manipulability through the laryngoscope.[23] Contact endoscopy has been used to examine diseased vocal fold epithelium and can distinguish dysplastic versus cancerous surfaces. The use of contact endoscopy is growing in popularity and reliability and may offer in-vivo real-time operative management of epithelial margins.[24,25] Tissue engineering may offer an exciting alternative to standard reconstructive techniques. Purdue et al have described reconstruction of hemilaryngectomy defects using tissue scaffolds.[26]

REINNERVATION

Today: A 35-year old woman undergoes total thyroidectomy with resultant unilateral vocal fold immobility as seen on fiberoptic laryngoscopy. A laryngeal electromyography confirms reduced motor recruitment in the distribution of the recurrent laryngeal nerve. A trial of voice therapy followed by a 9-month observation period is recommended. The patient fails to recover and is treated with a medialization laryngoplasty using a custom carved silastic implant. She has improvement in her voice at conversational levels, but is still unable to sing or to project her voice. She is unable to resume her career as a stage actor.

Tomorrow: One can envision a time when objective video capture techniques allow precise monitoring of improvement

of glottic gap. Prediction of timing and likelihood of recovery remains an ongoing challenge but could be helped by prospective studies with serial EMG recordings. Treatment of vocal fold motion impairment may be the local injection of growth factors into the area of injury and reinjection of myoblasts cultured and expanded ex-vivo back into the injured muscle groups.

Vocal fold motion impairment may be assessed by history and physical examination (including office endoscopy) as well as by laryngeal electromyography. Flexible indirect laryngoscopy in the office is superior to mirror examination given the advantages of video recording and the ability to have prolonged exams to test various gestures such as sniffing, laughing, coughing and diadochokinesis (repeated "ha, ha, ha, ha"). A paresis may be revealed by instructing the patient to perform a few minutes of whistling to tire the injured side. Recovery of motion may also be quantified using objective measurement of arytenoid motion using video capture techniques.[27] Objective acoustic and aerodynamic measures can also help to follow the severity of the glottic insufficiency. Laryngeal electromyography (EMG) can be used to counsel the patient about whether spontaneous reinnervation is likely and, therefore, if they should delay before intervention (see chapter 9, Laryngeal Electromyography). Laryngeal EMG is incapable at this time, however, of predicting *when* function will return. Fine-wire EMG offers specific information related to the individual intrinsic muscle groups and may help in surgical planning (eg, thyroplasty vs thyroplasty plus arytenoid adduction).

Teflon has served as the gold standard injectable given with benefits of long duration and predictability of effect.[28,29] It is still in use as we begin the 21st century. Migration into the neck, the inevitable development of granuloma, and stiffening of the vocal folds has led to the demise of Teflon as a mainstay for glottic augmentation. This has stimulated the introduction of collagen, micronized dermis, Gelfoam, fat, and hyaluronic acid derivatives[30] for the treatment of glottic insufficiency. Many of the latter can be injected in the office and thus obviate the need for general anesthesia. Furthermore, immediate visual feedback, audio feedback, and subjective patient feedback is possible with office injection and is safe and usually well tolerated. Open thyroplasty with various implants and arytenoid procedures have a long record of safety and efficacy but do not restore mobility or tone to the denervation vocal fold. Most are revisable but not necessarily reversible. Reinnervation techniques using the *ansa cervicalis* or nerve-muscle pedi-

cles have been pursued and are also successful in restoring tone to the denervated vocal fold but also do not restore mobility. The "Holy Grail" of unilateral vocal fold paralysis continues to be specific reinnervation of the different intrinsic laryngeal muscle groups allowing for preinjury function that is task-appropriate and symmetric to the unaffected side. Tissue engineering techniques to help support devervated muscle groups may boost laryngeal function even in the setting of neural damage.[31,32] Early work on neural growth factors may provide pathways for study.[33] Laryngeal pacing with an implantable electrodes also offers promise albeit not as elegantly as tissue engineering techniques, which employ the host's native tissues.[34]

Cross-Pollination

Ideas enter laryngology from many predictable and sometimes unpredictable sources. Historically this "cross-pollination" is not surprising given that a singing teacher (Manuel García, see chapter 1) and not a physician was the first to visualize the larynx in the awake state. Indeed, the rigid endoscope using the rod lens system was adapted from urology for use in the larynx, as another example of historical adaptation from another discipline.

This influx of ideas has added greatly to our ability to solve problems previously thought to be unsolvable. For example, molecular biology has identified exogenously produced growth factors that may allow vocal fold scar to be softened; Optical coherence tomography and the pulsed dye laser, both products of dermatology, are tools that cross over with use in the larynx; the nascent field of tissue engineering may allow us to use exogenously grown and shaped cartilage for replacement in the body. Mitomycin-C was first used as a chemotherapy agent against malignancy—it was first adapted for use in ophthalmology to reduce recurrence following ptergyium surgery and ultimately used in the larynx for simular reasons based on its preferential inhibition of fibroblast proliferation.

Students of laryngology should monitor advances in related and not-so-related fields; the possible adaptation of these innovations may prove beneficial for all patients.

REFLUX AND THE LARYNX

Today: A 40-year-old man presents with a chief complaint of hoarseness, cough, and throat clearing with excessive "phlegm." Prior treatment with 1 month of proton pump inhibitors proved ineffective in the reduction of symptoms. A Reflux Symptom Index score of 15 was recorded on presentation and flexible fiberoptic laryngoscopy revealed a Reflux Finding Score of 10. A trial for 3 months with 40 mg twice a day proton pump inhibitors did not completely reduce the symptoms; his pH probe test performed by his gastroenterologist is "negative" for reflux. The patient refuses further acid suppression treatment when he has no "heartburn." His symptoms worsen.

Tomorrow: Patients with laryngeal and pharyngeal symptoms related to reflux can have immediate visualization of the larynx in the office with tissue biopsy to confirm or disprove the diagnosis, their genetic susceptibility to injury, as well as their likelihood of responding to medical therapy. Immediately disproving the diagnosis would save thousands of patients the needless time and expense of adhering to a regimen of drug therapy. Also, patients with confirmed diagnosis would be started on a maximal pharmacotherapeutic regimen. Furthermore, tissue levels of pepsin or other noxious agents could be followed to assess the efficacy of treatment. Pepsin and bile salt binding agents could limit exposure of the laryngopharynx.

Increased awareness of the otolaryngology community to the existence of laryngopharyngeal reflux along with the development of better drugs has allowed patients to be treated more successfully.[35-44] Confusion with gastroesophageal reflux or GERD ("heartburn") symptoms often leads to diagnostic dilemmas. GERD is characterized by heartburn and epigastric symptoms, often at night. Extraesophageal reflux, on the other hand, is predominantly an upright, daytime phenomenon that produces throat clearing, globus pharyngeus, and hoarseness. Recent studies have suggested that a course of 40 mg of a proton pump inhibitor must be carried out faithfully for 4 months to establish whether someone is a nonresponder.[45] Validated instruments such as the Reflux Symptom Index and the Reflux Finding Score (see chapter 23, Reflux and Its Impact on Laryngology) have helped to correlate symptoms to double pH probe studies, currently the gold standard for diagnosis.[37,38]

Specific assays for bile salts are not currently available. In-office biopsies for tissue concentrations of the destructive enzyme pepsin within the laryngopharynx are in development as a specific and sensitive indicator for the presence of tissue damage related to reflux. Understanding the variability of tissue sensitivity to refluxate and the patient's ability to resist injury may be an important discriminator in treating extraesophageal reflux.[41,46] Other office diagnostic tests may theoretically become available for the detection of bile salts and other potentially destructive agents. Although the pharmacotherapeutic regimen of proton pump inhibitors is certainly the mainstay of therapy, Nissen fundoplication is a viable alternative when conservative measures have failed. Future strategies may include binding agents to pepsin enzyme or bile salts.

AIRWAY STENOSIS

Today: A 60-year-old man presents for evaluation with a complaint of increasing difficulty breathing. He has been intubated for congestive heart failure twice in the last 2 months for a period of 6 days each time. Chest x-ray shows narrowing of the trachea and he is taken to the operating room for examination and dilation. Surgical endoscopy at that time shows a six-ring segment of stenosis extending into the thoracic trachea. No dilation is performed. The patient is awakened for discussion of further planning options.

Tomorrow: Patients with airway stenosis undergo readily available 3-D CT reconstructions of the airway for diagnosis and surgical planning. A small amount of native cartilage is harvested in the office, grown in culture, and molded to fit the anticipated surgical defect in the case of tracheal stenosis. Complementary use of office injection of growth factors that reduce scar may obviate the need for surgery entirely. Meanwhile, in the intensive care unit, stenoses are prevented with the use of specially treated endotracheal tubes.

Airway stenosis is often the product of prior endotracheal intubation. Although the diagnosis is made largely by history of prior intubation or trauma, the specifics related to surgical planning and timing are in evolution. In addition to improvements in the quality and availability of flexible laryngoscopic imaging, airway evaluation has been greatly enhanced by the use of three-dimensional computed tomography (3-D CT) that can provide precise representations of the injured airway, effectively replacing plain radiographs.[47-49] The high-resolution images provide accurate measures of the length and degree of stenosis. Using office endoscopy and 3-D CT, the patient in the scenario above could have had better planning and a discussion of tracheal resection with anastomosis could have been undertaken. Tracheal resection and airway expansion procedures of the subglottis and trachea are limited by availability of autogenous tissue for reim-

plantation. For example, if more than half the trachea were irreversibly narrowed then resection with tension-free reanastomosis would be difficult (see chapter 26, Laryngotracheal Stenosis). Tissue engineering may allow the growth of autogenous cartilage ex-vivo; this cartilage could be shaped into new tracheal rings and reimplanted after resection of diseased trachea.[50] Similarly, instead of using ear cartilage or rib, the preformed cartilage could be used, thereby limiting morbidity. Tissue scaffolds also offer promise as they allow for the ingrowth of native cells and then are absorbed.[26] Mitomycin-C has been used topically for the prevention of scarring with some success in the airway.[51,52] Growth factors or transfection of genes that down-regulate scar may be possible with evolving technologies.

Review Questions

1. Which anomaly of the vocal folds is the most likely to be missed during office endoscopy?
   a. vocal fold polyp
   b. sulcus vocalis
   c. vocal fold cyst
   d. vocal fold hemorrhage
   e. vocal fold nodule

2. What is the current method of identifying the nature of epithelium with overlying leukoplakia?
   a. videostroboscopy
   b. office cytology
   c. surgical biopsy
   d. optical coherence tomography
   e. CT

3. Which management option(s) can restore tone to the denervated vocal fold?
   a. injection of Teflon
   b. arytenoid adduction
   c. thyroplasty
   d. observation
   e. ansa cervicalis neurorrhaphy

4. Lack of reduction of symptoms to a 3-month course of proton pump inhibitors could mean which of the following *except*:
   a. a submaximal dose was prescribed
   b. the course was not long enough
   c. the patient has sinonasal "post nasal drip" producing the symptoms
   d. H-2 blockers should have been prescribed instead
   e. the patient has nonacid reflux

5. When considering repair of tracheal stenosis the following pieces of information are essential *except*:
   a. degree of stenosis
   b. length of stenosis
   c. plain radiography of the airway
   d. CT scan of stenosis
   e. function of the glottis

REFERENCES

1. Sataloff RT, Spiegel JR, Hawkshaw MJ. Strobovideolaryngoscopy: results and clinical value. *Ann Otol Rhinol Laryngol.* 1991;100:725-727.

2. Poels PJ, de Jong FI, Schutte HK. Consistency of the preoperative and intraoperative diagnosis of benign vocal fold lesions. *J Voice.* 2003;17:425-433.

3. Rubin JS, Lee S, McGuinness J, Hore I, Hill D, Berger L. The potential role of ultrasound in differentiating solid and cystic swellings of the true vocal fold. *J Voice.* 2004;18:231-235.

4. Burns Jea. Imaging the mucosa of the human vocal fold with optical coherence tomography. *Ann Otol Rhinol Laryngol.* 2006: in review.

5. Hirano M, Bless DM, Nagai H, et al. Growth factor therapy for vocal fold scarring in a canine model. *Ann Otol Rhinol Laryngol.* 2004;113:777-785.

6. Kanemaru S, Nakamura T, Omori K, et al. Regeneration of the vocal fold using autologous mesenchymal stem cells. *Ann Otol Rhinol Laryngol.* 2003;112:915-920.

7. Dailey SH, Kobler JB, Zeitels SM. A laryngeal dissection station: educational paradigms in phonosurgery. *Laryngoscope.* 2004;114:878-882.

8. Hockstein NG, Nolan JP, O'Malley BW, Jr, Woo YJ. Robot-assisted pharyngeal and laryngeal microsurgery: results of robotic cadaver dissections. *Laryngoscope.* 2005;115:1003-1008.

9. Hockstein NG, Nolan JP, O'Malley BW, Jr, Woo YJ. Robotic microlaryngeal surgery: a technical feasibility study using the daVinci surgical robot and an airway mannequin. *Laryngoscope.* 2005;115: 780-785.

10. Sudbo J, Bryne M, Johannessen AC, Kildal W, Danielsen HE, Reith A. Comparison of histological grading and large-scale genomic status (DNA ploidy) as prognostic tools in oral dysplasia. *J Pathol.* 2001;194:303-310.

11. Sudbo J, Ried T, Bryne M, Kildal W, Danielsen H, Reith A. Abnormal DNA content predicts the occurrence of carcinomas in non-dysplastic oral white patches. *Oral Oncol.* 2001;37:558-565.

12. Scully C, Sudbo J, Speight PM. Progress in determining the malignant potential of oral lesions. *J Oral Pathol Med.* 2003;32:251-256.

13. Schweinfurth JM, Powitzky E, Ossoff RH. Regression of laryngeal dysplasia after serial microflap excision. *Ann Otol Rhinol Laryngol.* 2001;110: 811-814.

14. Leonard RJ, Kiener D, Charpied G, Kelly A. Effects of repeated stripping on vocal fold mucosa in cats. *Ann Otol Rhinol Laryngol.* 1985;94:258-262.

15. Leonard RJ, Gallia LJ, Charpied G, Kelly A. Effects of stripping and laser excision on vocal fold mucosa in cats. *Ann Otol Rhinol Laryngol.* 1988; 97:159-163.

16. Franco RA, Jr., Zeitels SM, Farinelli WA, Anderson RR. 585-nm pulsed dye laser treatment of glottal papillomatosis. *Ann Otol Rhinol Laryngol.* 2002; 111:486-492.

17. Franco RA, Jr., Zeitels SM, Farinelli WA, Faquin W, Anderson RR. 585-nm pulsed dye laser treatment of glottal dysplasia. *Ann Otol Rhinol Laryngol.* 2003;112:751-758.

18. Zeitels SM, Franco RA, Jr., Dailey SH, Burns JA, Hillman RE, Anderson RR. Office-based treatment of glottal dysplasia and papillomatosis with the 585-nm pulsed dye laser and local anesthesia. *Ann Otol Rhinol Laryngol.* 2004;113:265-276.

19. Steiner W. Results of curative laser microsurgery of laryngeal carcinomas. *Am J Otolaryngol.* 1993; 14:116-121.

20. Steiner W, Vogt P, Ambrosch P, Kron M. Transoral carbon dioxide laser microsurgery for recurrent glottic carcinoma after radiotherapy. *Head Neck.* 2004;26:477-484.

21. Zeitels SM. Optimizing voice after endoscopic partial laryngectomy. *Otolaryngol Clin North Am.* 2004;37:627-636.

22. Zeitels SM, Jarboe J, Franco RA. Phonosurgical reconstruction of early glottic cancer. *Laryngoscope.* 2001;111:1862-1865.

23. Devaiah AK, Shapshay SM, Desai U, et al. Surgical utility of a new carbon dioxide laser fiber: functional and histological study. *Laryngoscope.* 2005; 115:1463-1468.

24. Andrea M, Dias O, Santos A. Contact endoscopy during microlaryngeal surgery: a new technique for endoscopic examination of the larynx. *Ann Otol Rhinol Laryngol.* 1995;104:333-339.

25. Andrea M, Dias O, Santos A. Contact endoscopy of the vocal cord: normal and pathological patterns. *Acta Otolaryngol.* 1995;115:314-316.

26. Huber JE, Spievack A, Simmons-Byrd A, Ringel RL, Badylak S. Extracellular matrix as a scaffold for laryngeal reconstruction. *Ann Otol Rhinol Laryngol.* 2003;112:428-433.

27. Dailey SH, Kobler JB, Hillman RE, et al. Endoscopic measurement of vocal fold movement during adduction and abduction. *Laryngoscope.* 2005;115:178-183.

28. Dedo HH. Injection and removal of Teflon for unilateral vocal cord paralysis. *Ann Otol Rhinol Laryngol.* 1992;101:81-86.

29. Dedo HH, Urrea RD, Lawson L. Intracordal injection of Teflon in the treatment of 135 patients with dysphonia. *Ann Otol Rhinol Laryngol.* 1973;82:661-667.

30. Nakayama M, Ford CN, Bless DM. Teflon vocal fold augmentation: failures and management in 28 cases. *Otolaryngol Head Neck Surg.* 1993;109: 493-498.

31. Flint PW, Nakagawa H, Shiotani A, Coleman ME, O'Malley BW, Jr. Effects of insulin-like growth factor-1 gene transfer on myosin heavy chains in denervated rat laryngeal muscle. *Laryngoscope.* 2004;114:368-371.

32. Shiotani A, O'Malley BW, Jr, Coleman ME, Alila HW, Flint PW. Reinnervation of motor endplates and increased muscle fiber size after human insulin-like growth factor I gene transfer into the paralyzed larynx. *Hum Gene Ther.* 1998;9: 2039-2047.

33. Rubin A, Mobley B, Hogikyan N, et al. Delivery of an adenoviral vector to the crushed recurrent laryngeal nerve. *Laryngoscope.* 2003;113:985-989.

34. Zealear DL, Swelstad MR, Sant'Anna GD, et al. Determination of the optimal conditions for laryngeal pacing with the Itrel II implantable stimulator. *Otolaryngol Head Neck Surg.* 2001;125: 183-192.

35. Koufman JA. The otolaryngologic manifestations of gastroesophageal reflux disease (GERD): a clinical investigation of 225 patients using ambulatory 24-hour pH monitoring and an experimental investigation of the role of acid and pepsin in the development of laryngeal injury. *Laryngoscope.* 1991;101:1-78.

36. Koufman J, Sataloff RT, Toohill R. Laryngopharyngeal reflux: consensus conference report. *J Voice.* 1996;10:215-216.

37. Belafsky PC, Postma GN, Koufman JA. The validity and reliability of the reflux finding score (RFS). *Laryngoscope.* 2001;111:1313-1317.

38. Belafsky PC, Postma GN, Koufman JA. Validity and reliability of the reflux symptom index (RSI). *J Voice.* 2002;16:274-277.

39. Koufman JA, Aviv JE, Casiano RR, Shaw GY. Laryngopharyngeal reflux: position statement of the committee on speech, voice, and swallowing disorders of the American Academy of Otolaryngology-Head and Neck Surgery. *Otolaryngol Head Neck Surg.* 2002;127:32-35.

40. Westcott CJ, Hopkins MB, Bach K, Postma GN, Belafsky PC, Koufman JA. Fundoplication for laryngopharyngeal reflux disease. *J Am Coll Surg.* 2004;199:23-30.

41. Knight J, Lively MO, Johnston N, Dettmar PW, Koufman JA. Sensitive pepsin immunoassay for detection of laryngopharyngeal reflux. *Laryngoscope.* 2005;115:1473-1478.

42. Koufman JA. Laryngopharyngeal reflux is different from classic gastroesophageal reflux disease. *Ear Nose Throat J.* 2002;81:7-9.

43. Postma GN, Johnson LF, Koufman JA. Treatment of laryngopharyngeal reflux. *Ear Nose Throat J.* 2002;81:24-26.

44. Altman KW, Stephens RM, Lyttle CS, Weiss KB. Changing impact of gastroesophageal reflux in medical and otolaryngology practice. *Laryngoscope.* 2005;115:1145-1153.

45. Park W, Hicks DM, Khandwala F et al. Laryngopharyngeal reflux: prospective cohort study evaluating optimal dose of proton-pump inhibitor

therapy and pretherapy predictors of response. *Laryngoscope.* 2005;115:1230-1238.

46. Johnston N, Bulmer D, Gill GA, et al. Cell biology of laryngeal epithelial defenses in health and disease: further studies. *Ann Otol Rhinol Laryngol.* 2003;112:481-491.

47. Hoppe H, Dinkel HP, Walder B, von Allmen G, Gugger M, Vock P. Grading airway stenosis down to the segmental level using virtual bronchoscopy. *Chest.* 2004;125:704-711.

48. Toyota K, Uchida H, Ozasa H, Motooka A, Sakura S, Saito Y. Preoperative airway evaluation using multi-slice three-dimensional computed tomography for a patient with severe tracheal stenosis. *Br J Anaesth.* 2004;93:865-867.

49. Whyte RI, Quint LE, Kazerooni EA, Cascade PN, Iannettoni MD, Orringer MB. Helical computed tomography for the evaluation of tracheal stenosis. *Ann Thorac Surg.* 1995;60:27-30; discussion 30-21.

50. Kamil SH, Eavey RD, Vacanti MP, Vacanti CA, Hartnick CJ. Tissue-engineered cartilage as a graft source for laryngotracheal reconstruction: a pig model. *Arch Otolaryngol Head Neck Surg.* 2004;130:1048-1051.

51. Rahbar R, Shapshay SM, Healy GB. Mitomycin: effects on laryngeal and tracheal stenosis, benefits, and complications. *Ann Otol Rhinol Laryngol.* 2001;110:1-6.

52. Perepelitsyn I, Shapshay SM. Endoscopic treatment of laryngeal and tracheal stenosis—has mitomycin C improved the outcome? *Otolaryngol Head Neck Surg.* 2004;131:16-20.

PART II

Anatomy and Physiology

Anatomy of the Larynx and Physiology of Phonation

Suzy Duflo, MD
Susan L. Thibeault, PhD

KEY POINTS

■ Increases in length and tension of the vocal folds will result in an increase in pitch.

■ During phonation, fundamental frequency is primarily determined by activity of the intrinsic muscles and to a lesser extent by subglottal pressure.

■ The mean rate of vocal fold vibration per second represents the habitual pitch also known as fundamental frequency.

■ Phonation threshold pressure (PTP) is the minimum subglottal pressure required for initiating and sustaining vocal fold oscillation and is an indication of vocal fold function.

■ The high pitch exhibited by patients with vocal paralysis is a compensatory behavior, unconsciously developed to increase glottal contact during phonation. To achieve contact between the vocal folds, the cricothyroid muscle is activated, elongating the vocal folds and bringing them close together on adduction. This glottal position allows slightly louder and more consistent voice production in the patient with incomplete closure although it may be higher pitched.

ANATOMY OF THE LARYNX

Understanding the details of phonation requires knowledge of the anatomy of the larynx. The larynx is the principal structure for producing the vibrating airstream and the vocal folds, which are a part of the larynx, constitute the vibrating elements. The larynx is a musculocartilaginous structure located in the middle of the anterior neck region. It is suspended from the hyoid bone and sits on top of the trachea. Soft tissues and cartilage constitute the larynx. Cartilage forms a real skeleton for the larynx and the anatomy of the laryngeal muscles and ligaments can be defined in relation to this skeleton.

The Hyoid Bone

The hyoid bone is horseshoe-shaped, located immediately superior to the thyroid cartilage, and suspended in the neck by means of a sling of muscles and ligaments. It consists of a body with major and minor cornua projecting posterolaterally. Although not technically a part of the larynx, the hyoid bone plays an integral part in laryngeal motion and must be included in the laryngeal anatomy. Indeed, most of the "extrinsic" muscles of the larynx (see below) attach to the hyoid in some way.

The Laryngeal Cartilages (Figure 3–1)

Three unpaired and three paired cartilages are found in the larynx. The three unpaired are perhaps the most familiar to those outside of laryngology and speech-language pathology, the thyroid, cricoid, and epiglottic cartilages. The three smaller paired structures are the arytenoid, corniculate, and cuneiform cartilages. These cartilages articulate with each other in complex ways, including sliding and rotation in relation to one another, returning to their original positions after release of muscular forces, thus assuming different configurations to allow breathing, eating, and phonation.

The framework supports the specialized soft tissues of the larynx (ie, the vocal folds), and it is through motions of the cricothyroid and cricoarytenoid joints that the vocal folds are maneuvered into the positions for the different modes of phonation. Gross laryngeal motion can also be described in terms of degrees of freedom; it is a system with four degrees of freedom. The rotation and gliding of the cricoid and thyroid cartilages represent two degrees of freedom, and the rocking and rotation of the arytenoid cartilages represent the other two degrees of freedom.

The Thyroid Cartilage

The thyroid cartilage is made up of hyaline cartilage. This cartilage is the largest in the laryngeal skeleton, consisting of two flat plates called "laminae" that fuse together anteriorly to form an approximate 90° angle in the adult male and an approximate 120° angle in the adult female. Two pairs of horns, or cornua, extend upward (superior cornu) and downward (inferior cornu) from the posterior aspect of the thyroid cartilage. The superior horns attach to the hyoid bone via ligaments associated with the lateral aspect of the thyrohyoid membrane. On the lateral face of the laminae, there is an oblique line, which is an insert point for different laryngeal muscles. The thyroid cartilage articulates with the cricoid at the paired cricothyroid joints; this synovial joint permits the cricoid and thyroid cartilages to pitch forward around an imaginary horizontal axis drawn between the two joints.

The Cricoid Cartilage

The cricoid cartilage forms the lower part of the laryngeal framework and is located immediately above the uppermost tracheal ring. It is made of hyaline cartilage and consists of two parts: an anterior arch and a posterior quadrate lamina. It is a complete ring closed at the back where the massive lamina or plate extends vertically. Anteriorly, the cartilage becomes thinner to form the fine cricoid arch. It is connected to the thyroid cartilage by the cricothyroid membrane, the traditional site for immediate emergency surgical access to the airway. Another ligament, the *crico-tracheal* ligament, connects the cricoid cartilage to the trachea.

The Arytenoid Cartilages

The paired arytenoid (Latin for ladle or pitcher) cartilages are located on the sloping border of the cricoid cartilage. They have the shape of a pyramid with a base, an apex, and three surfaces. The anterior angle of these cartilages forms a pointed projection called the vocal process, which is the insertion point for the vocal ligament. The apices of the arytenoid are in contact with the *corniculate* cartilages. They may be fused with the arytenoid cartilages or be separated by an articulation containing synovial fluid. The corniculate cartilages are believed to be an embryonic vestige. The arytenoid cartilages are coupled to the cricoid cartilage via the cricoarytenoid joints. The movements of these cartilages on the cricoid are quite elegant; although they are thought of simplistically as opening and clos-

ing by sliding back and forth along the superior surface of the posterior cricoid, their motion is more complex. This is discussed further below.

The Epiglottis

The epiglottis is a broad fibrocartilaginous structure located just behind the hyoid bone and the base of the tongue. The space between the base of the tongue and the epiglottis forms the vallecula. The epiglottis is considered the superior edge of the larynx. Its upper edge is rounded and thin, the lower edge is narrow. It attaches to the thyroid cartilage by means of a thyroepiglottic ligament and to the arytenoid cartilages by means of the aryepiglottic folds. The aryepiglottic folds extend from the sides of the epiglottis to the arytenoids. They form a wall that separates the larynx from the lateral piriform fossae. The aryepiglottic folds extend inferiorly and medially in the larynx cavity to become the false vocal folds. The epiglottis closes over the glottal area during swallowing and prevents food from entering the larynx (Figure 3–1).

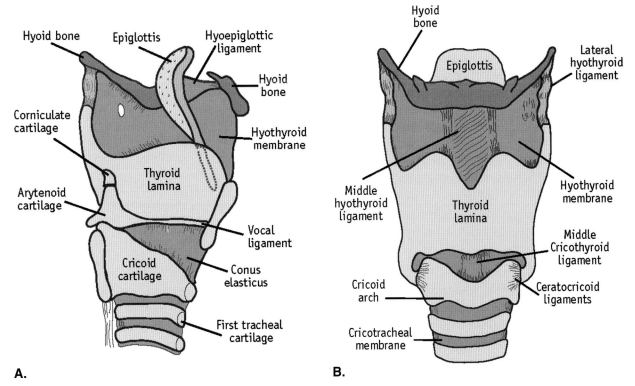

A.   **B.**

FIGURE 3–1. Laryngeal cartilages. **A.** Lateral view of the larynx (cuneiform cartilage not shown). **B.** Front view of the larynx.

Laryngeal Muscles

Two types of muscles are described in the larynx: *extrinsic* and *intrinsic* muscles. Extrinsic muscles are those that have one attachment to structures outside the larynx, intrinsic muscles have both attachments confined to the larynx. Both extrinsic and intrinsic muscles influence laryngeal function. The length and tension of the vocal folds are adjusted before and during phonation by means of rotation of the thyroid and/or cricoid cartilages as a result of the activation of laryngeal muscles.

Intrinsic Muscles (Figure 3–2)

The intrinsic muscles are attached at both ends to the cartilages of the larynx and are largely responsible for the control of sound production by moving those cartilages in relation to one another. They are abductor, adductor, tensor, and relaxer muscles and always act in pairs. Muscles on one side do not contract independently of the muscles on the opposite side. The abductor muscles, which separate the arytenoids and the vocal folds for respiratory activities, are opposed by the adductors, which approximate the arytenoid cartilages and the vocal folds for phonation and for protective purposes. The glottal tensors elongate and tighten the vocal folds. They are opposed by the relaxers, which shorten the vocal folds. They play an important role in the vibratory behavior of vocal folds. Each half of the larynx has a posterior and a lateral cricoarytenoid muscle, a cricothyroid muscle, and a thyroarytenoid muscle. There is also the interarytenoid muscle, a large, unpaired intrinsic muscle. The transverse and oblique portions extend between the two arytenoid cartilages.

Posterior Cricoarytenoid Muscle. The posterior cricoarytenoid muscle originates from a shallow depression of the posterior surface of the cricoid lamina. It is divided into two parts: a lateral vertical muscle, which inserts on the upper surface of the muscular process of the arytenoid cartilage, and a medial part that inserts via a short tendon on the posterior surface of the muscular process. It abducts the vocal folds by pulling the arytenoids cartilage through its rocking motion. It is the primary abductor muscle of the larynx and is typically active during the inspiratory phase of the respiratory cycle when the abduction of the arytenoids opens the glottis widely. It is the only muscle that *actively* opens the glottis. Two muscles act as antagonists to the posterior cricoarytenoid muscle: the lateral cricoarytenoid and interarytenoid muscles.

Lateral Cricoarytenoid Muscle. The lateral cricoarytenoid muscle originates along the upper border of the anterolateral arch of the cricoid cartilage and courses upward back to insert into the muscular process and anterior surface of the arytenoid cartilage. Some fibers blend with those of the thyroarytenoid muscle. The lateral cricoarytenoid muscle is an adductory muscle that permits rotation of the arytenoid cartilage and brings the vocal processes and vocal ligament toward midline. When the arytenoid cartilages are adducted for phonation, the lateral cricoarytenoid muscles may have the additional function of increasing the medial compression of the vocal folds.

Interarytenoid Muscle. The interarytenoid muscle is a large muscle located on the posterior surface of the arytenoid cartilages. It consists of two parts, the oblique and transverse arytenoid. The oblique arytenoid muscle is the more superficial of the two parts. It originates from the posterior surface of the muscular process and adjacent posterolateral of one arytenoid cartilage and inserts close to the apex of the opposite cartilage. A few muscle fibers continue around the apex of the arytenoid cartilage laterally, upward, and forward to insert into the lateral border of the epiglottis forming the aryepiglottic muscle. The oblique arytenoid muscles regulate medial compression of the vocal folds and permit approximation of the arytenoid cartilages. The transverse arytenoid muscle originates from the lateral margin and posterior surface of one arytenoid cartilage, courses in a horizontal direction, and inserts into the lateral margin and posterior surface of the opposite arytenoid cartilage. The deeper muscle fibers continue around the lateral margins of the arytenoid cartilages and blend with fibers of the thyroarytenoid muscle. Transverse arytenoid muscles permit approximation of the arytenoid cartilages toward the midline. The interarytenoid muscles rock the arytenoids during adduction. This action increases the medial compression of the vocal folds. Because it crosses the midline, the muscle's action on a given arytenoid is preserved even in the case of unilateral paralysis.

Cricothyroid Muscle. The cricothyroid muscle originates from the upper rim of the cricoid arch and fibers diverge to insert into the lower rim of the thyroid as two distinct groups: pars recta and pars obliqua. The pars recta forms the upper or anterior fibers and courses nearly vertically upward to insert along the inner aspect of the lower rim of the thyroid lamina. The pars oblique forms the lower or oblique fibers and courses upward and back to insert into the anterior margin of the inferior horn of the thyroid cartilage. The cricothyroid muscle lengthens the vocal folds, decreasing fold thickness and increasing pitch. It is the primary antagonist of the thyroarytenoid muscle.

Thyroarytenoid Muscle. The thyroarytenoid muscle comprises the main mass of the vocal fold. The thryomuscularis muscle (or *vocalis* muscle) inserts into the lateral and inferior aspect of the vocal process of the arytenoid cartilage and into the interior face of the thyroid angle cartilage. The contraction of the thyroarytenoid muscle permits a shortening and slackening of the vocal folds. It exerts an anterior traction on the vocal process, increasing vocal fold tension, thickness, and stiffness. Contraction of the thyroaryepiglottis muscle pulls the arytenoid cartilages forward, closing the glottis anteroposteriorly. The thyroarytenoid muscle also draws the arytenoid and thyroid cartilage toward one another, to shorten and relax the vocal folds. This action plays a role in pitch lowering. The thyroarytenoid muscle does not function as a single unit but in combination with the other laryngeal intrinsic muscles (Figure 3-2).

Extrinsic Muscles (Figure 3–3)

The extrinsic muscles are attached to structures outside the larynx. They are primarily responsible for the support of the larynx, for fixing it in position, and also for moving the larynx as a total unit, thereby changing its position in the neck. The elasticity of the trachea places a passive extrinsic force on the larynx. Three muscles are considered extrinsic: the sternothyroid, thyrohyoid muscle, and inferior pharyngeal constrictor. The suprahyoid and infrahyoid muscles play a role in deglutition and phonation.

Sternothyroid Muscle. The sternothyroid muscle inserts into the posterior surface of the sternal manubrium and first rib; it then extends itself upward and slightly laterally in the anterior neck to insert on the oblique line of the thyroid cartilage. The sternothyroid muscle is a depressor muscle and its principal action is to draw the thyroid cartilage downward.

Thyrohyoid Muscle. The thyrohyoid muscle is located in the anterior neck. This muscle originates from the oblique tendon or line of the thyroid cartilage and courses vertically upward to insert into the inferior edge of the greater horn of the hyoid bone. This muscle is an elevator as it decreases the distance between the hyoid bone and the thyroid cartilage. With the thyroid cartilage fixed, it depresses the hyoid bone and with the hyoid bone fixed, it elevates the thyroid cartilage.

Inferior Pharyngeal Constrictor. The inferior pharyngeal constrictor consists of cricopharyngeus and thyropharyngeous muscles. These muscles influence the phonation by forming a principal resonating cavity of the vocal mechanism. They are also active during deglutition.

Suprahyoid and Infrahyoid Muscles. Other extrinsic muscles, which for the most part have one attachment on the hyoid bone, may also influence the larynx. They are divided into suprahyoid and infrahyoid muscles. Functionally they are classified as laryngeal elevators and depressors.

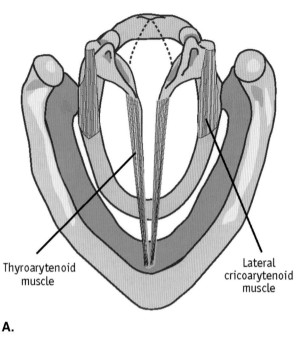

Thyroarytenoid muscle

Lateral cricoarytenoid muscle

A.

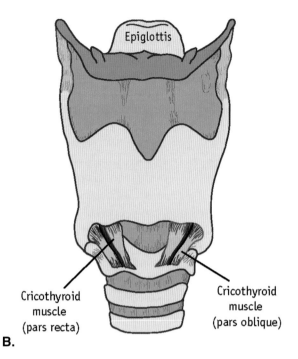

Epiglottis

Cricothyroid muscle (pars recta)

Cricothyroid muscle (pars oblique)

B.

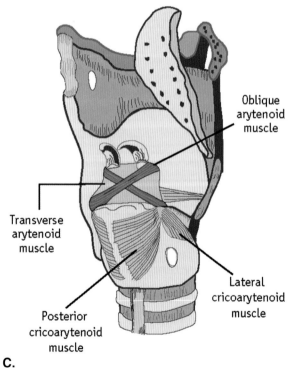

Oblique arytenoid muscle

Transverse arytenoid muscle

Posterior cricoarytenoid muscle

Lateral cricoarytenoid muscle

C.

FIGURE 3–2. Intrinsic laryngeal muscles. **A.** Thyroarytenoid muscle and lateral cricoarytenoid muscle. **B.** Cricothyroid muscle (pars recta and pars oblique). **C.** Posterior view of the larynx showing posterior cricoarytenoid muscle and lateral cricoarytenoid muscle.

The suprahyoid muscles are the laryngeal elevators (digastric, stylohyoid, mylohyoid, geniohyoid, hyoglossus, and genioglossus muscles), which play a role in deglutition. The infrahyoid muscles are laryngeal depressors (sternohyoid and omohyoid muscles). The sternohyoid muscle acts to draw the hyoid bone downward and the omohyoid muscle prevents the neck region from collapsing during deep inspiratory efforts and from compression of the vessels.

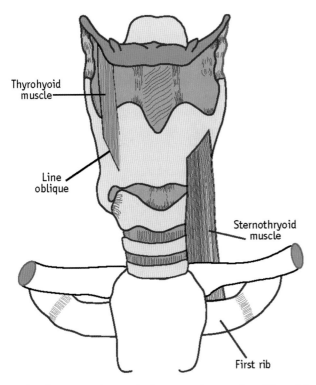

Thyrohyoid
muscle

Line
oblique

Sternothryoid
muscle

First rib

FIGURE 3–3. Extrinsic laryngeal muscles: Thyroid muscle and sternothyroid muscle (inferior pharyngeal constrictor, suprahyoid, and infrahyoid muscles not shown).

Larynx Cavity

The cavity of the larynx extends from the aditus laryngis to the inferior border of the cricoid cartilage. The aditus is a triangular opening including the epiglottis, aryepiglottic folds laterally, and apexes of the arytenoid cartilages. The vocal folds are oriented in the anterior/posterior direction and sit over the lower airway. The membranous vocal folds consist of mucosa and thyroarytenoid muscle, which is continuous with the conus elasticus. The cornus elasticus is represented by a membrane that arises in a full circle from the top of the cricoid cartilage.

The vocal folds are long, smoothly rounded bands of muscle tissue and can be lengthened, shortened, tensed, relaxed, abducted, or adducted. The medial borders of the vocal folds are free and they project like a shelf into the cavity of the larynx in a medio-lateral direction. In reference to the level of the vocal folds, the larynx can be divided into three areas: glottic, supraglottic, and subglottic areas. The space between the true vocal folds is designated the glottis or glottal area. Immediately superior to the vocal folds is a groove known as the laryngeal ventricle extending almost the entire length of the vocal folds. Superior to the ventricule is the paired ventricular or *false vocal folds*, which contain muscle fibers. The false vocal folds are not typically involved during normal phonation. The false vocal folds move with the arytenoid cartilages but they stand farther apart than the vocal folds. The space between the ventricular folds and the aditus is referred to as the vestibule of the larynx. The area superior to the true vocal folds, with the ventricle, the false vocal folds, and the vestibule, is called the supraglottis. The area immediately inferior to the true vocal folds down to the inferior aspect of the cricoid is called the subglottic region (Figure 3-4).

Laryngeal Motion[1,2]

When the glottis opens, each vocal fold changes shape by putting itself in abduction. The arytenoid cartilages rotate so that the vocal process moves outward, upward, and posteriorly. Abduction is accomplished by the posterior cricoarytenoid muscle pulling the muscular process posteriorly and inferiorly. Adduction is accomplished by the combined action of the lateral cricoarytenoid, interarytenoid, and thyroarytenoid muscles. The most powerful adductor is the lateral cricoarytenoid muscle which pulls the muscular process anteriorly and inferiorly. In addition to adduction and abduction, laryngeal muscle activity also changes vocal fold length, tension, and shape. The thyroarytenoid and cricothyroid muscles have opposing actions in this regard. Contraction of the thyroarytenoid muscle shortens and thickens the vocal fold whereas cricothyroid action stretches the vocal folds increasing length and tension and decreasing thickness. Simultaneous contraction to these two muscles can increase tension independent of length (Figure 3-5).

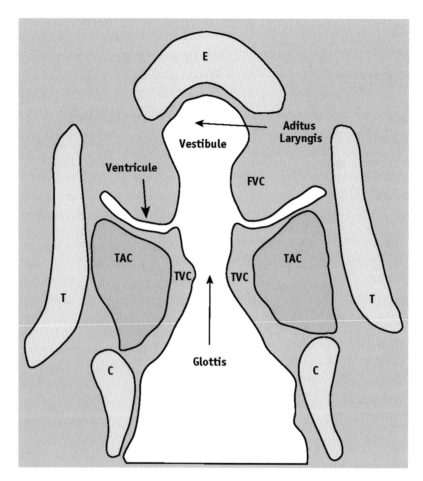

FIGURE 3–4. Larynx cavity: coronal view of the larynx. (E = epiglottis, FVC = false vocal fold, TAC = thyroarytenoid component, T = thyroid cartilage, C = cricoid cartilage, TVC = false vocal fold).

Criocoarytenoid (CA) Joint Motion

The CA joint is a diarthrodial joint that includes a synovial lining and a fluid-filled bursa. The joint capsule and the ligamentous attachments, including the CA ligament, vocal ligament, and false vocal folds, limit normal motion of the joint. The CA plays a crucial role in the adduction and abduction of the vocal folds. The rotation in which the anterior vocal process deviates medially causes adduction of the vocal folds, whereas a lateral rotation causes abduction. The vocalis ligament, CA ligament, and conus elasticus are most important in controlling abduction, whereas the posterior CA muscle and conus elasticus are crucial in limiting adduction. The vocalis ligament prevents posterior displacement of the vocal process, while the CA ligament and the posterior capsular ligament, restrict anterior vocal process migration. The anterior capsular ligament limits backward arytenoid cartilage tilting and lateral movement of the arytenoid cartilage on the cricoid cartilage facet.

VOCAL FOLD HISTOLOGY[3–5]

Most of the upper airway is lined by respiratory epithelium and contains mucous glands. The cover of the free edge of the vocal folds is adapted for vibration; subsequently the vibratory epithelium is squamous cell epithelium without mucous glands.

Hirano described five histologically distinct layers for the true vocal fold. The epithelium consists of stratified squamous cells. The superficial

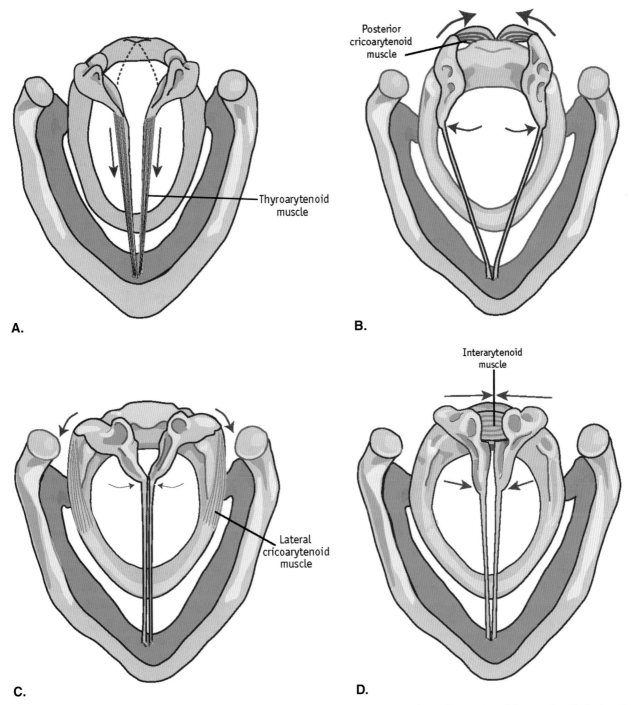

A.

B.

C.

D.

FIGURE 3–5. Laryngeal motion. **A.** Thyroarytenoid muscle. **B.** Posterior cricoarytenoid muscle. **C.** Lateral cricoarytenoid muscle. **D.** Interarytenoid muscle.

layer of the lamina propria (also known as *Reinke's space*), consists of loose fibrous components (elastin, collagen) and matrix. The intermediate layer of the lamina propria consists chiefly of elastic fibers, collagen, fibronectin, and hyaluronan. The deep layer of the lamina propria consists of collagenous fibers. The intermediate and deep layers together comprise what is clinically referred to as the *vocal ligament*. The deeper layer of the vocal fold is the vocalis muscle (Figure 3-6).

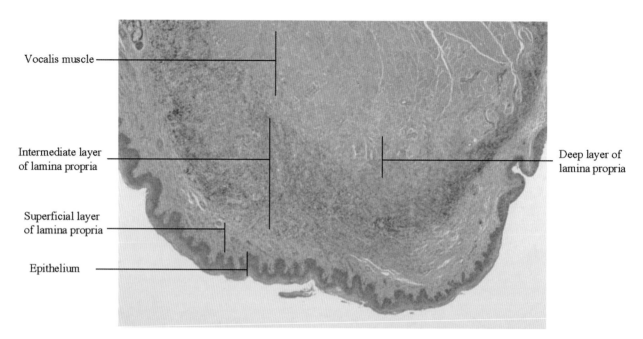

Vocalis muscle

Intermediate layer
of lamina propria

Superficial layer
of lamina propria

Epithelium

Deep layer of
lamina propria

FIGURE 3–6. Coronal histologic section through membranous portion of vocal folds.

LARYNGEAL VASCULAR SUPPLY AND LARYNGEAL INNERVATIONS[6]

Vascular Supply

The arterial vascularization of the larynx is provided by the inferior laryngeal artery, a small branch of the inferior thyroid artery and by the superior laryngeal artery, which comes from the superior thyroid artery. The superior laryngeal vein empties into the jugular vein and the inferior laryngeal vein joins the inferior thyroid vein. The lymphatic system of the larynx drains along the vessels both upward and downward into the deep cervical nodes.

Innervation

The vagus nerve (CN X) innerves the intrinsic laryngeal muscles and the trigeminal (CN V), facial (CN VII), and hypoglossal (CN XII) nerves are responsible for the innervation of the extrinsic muscles.

The vagus nerve comes from the *nucleus ambiguus* in the medulla and carries the motor and sensory supply of the larynx via two branches: the superior and recurrent laryngeal nerves. The superior laryngeal nerve exits the vagus just below the nodose ganglion and then branches into two divisions: the internal branch, which carries sensory fibers from the supraglottis and vocal folds, and the external branch, which carries motor fibers to the cricothyroid muscle. The recurrent laryngeal nerve follows a circuitous route, arising from the vagus nerve in the upper mediastinum and then ascending to the larynx in the tracheoesophageal groove. On the right side the nerve courses around the subclavian artery. On the left side the nerve curves around the aortic arch. The recurrent nerve carries motor fibers to the intrinsic muscle except for the cricothyroid muscle. The differences in intrinsic muscle innervation of the recurrent and superior laryngeal nerves are secondary to their embryonic etiology; branchial arches IV and VI form the superior laryngeal and the recurrent nerves, respectively.

Superior Laryngeal Nerve

The internal branch (ISLN) and external branch (ESLN) of the superior laryngeal nerve are supplied by their accompanying arteries in the upper pole of the thyroid gland. A topographic relationship between the ESLN, the superior thyroid artery, and the upper pole of the thyroid gland exposes the ESLN to high surgical risks during thyroidectomy[7-9] and anterior approach to the cervical spine.[10] The clinical evaluation of SLN lesions allows the diagnosis of vocal fold's hypomobility, with incomplete glottic closure and can result in detrimental voice changes, loss of airway protection, and effortful swallowing with aspiration in some cases. Injury of the ESLN produces no problem of respiration and deglutition but may result in changes in the quality of voice or even voicelessness. The consequences are important for patients like professional singers and speakers who depend on control of pitch and a clear and forceful voice. Several precautions when dissecting the superior pole of the thyroid gland seem to be necessary and sufficient to respect the ESLN. Moreover, neuromonitoring proved to be a reliable method to identify the nerve, prevent its injury,[11] and subsequently maintain optimal function of the larynx. During swallowing, the airway is protected from the aspiration of ingested material by brief closure of the larynx and cessation of breathing.

Mechanoreceptors innervated by the ISLN are activated by swallowing and connect to central neurons that generate swallowing, laryngeal closure, and respiratory rhythm. The injured ISLN causes effortful swallowing and an illusory globus sensation in the throat, sometimes with penetration of fluid into the larynx during swallowing. In contrast to the insufficient closure during swallowing after ISLN injury, laryngeal closure can be robust during voluntary challenges with the Valsalva, Muller, and cough maneuvers.[12] An afferent signal from the ILSN receptor field is necessary for normal deglutition by providing feedback that facilitates laryngeal closure during swallowing, but is not necessary for initiating and sequencing the swallow cycle, for coordinating swallowing with breathing, or for closing the larynx during voluntary maneuvers. A recent publication has also suggested that the ESLN supplies innervation to the cricopharyngeus muscle, which would further support SLN injury as a source of dysfunction in patients with dysphagia.[13]

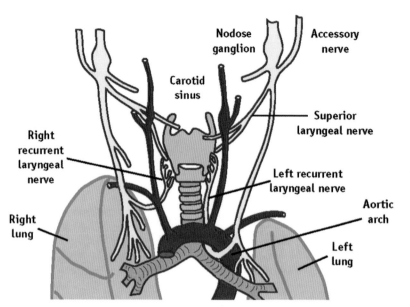

FIGURE 3–7. Nerve and blood supply of the larynx.

The trigeminal nerve supplies motor innervation to the mylohyoid muscle and the belly of the digastric. The facial nerve supplies motor innervation to the digastric and stylohyoid muscles. The hypoglossal nerve supplies motor innervation to geniohyoid, sternohyoid, omohyoid, thyrohyoid, and sternothyroid (Figure 3-7).

PHYSIOLOGY OF PHONATION

With the laryngeal anatomy detailed above, this chapter now reviews the physiology of phonation. The chapters that follow present aspects of laryngeal physiology related to airway regulation (chapter 4) and swallowing (chapter 5).

Although phonation is not the most critical domain of the larynx, it continues to draw interest due to its elegance and close association with human communication. The phenomenon of phonation is defined by a rapid opening and closing of the vocal folds that periodically interrupt the airstream to produce a vocal or glottal tone within the pharyngeal, oral and nasal cavities.[14]

Galen (AD 130–200) was among the first to recognize the glottis as the source of vocal production. He suggested that vocal intensity was dependent upon the adjustment of the soft palate and uvula.[15] In 1543, the larynx was illustrated by Andreas Vesalius in *De Humani Corporis Fabrica*. Since then, others have contributed to our understanding of the physiology of phonation. Ferrein (1776) was the first to prove that vocal fold vibration was responsible for sound.[16]

Laryngeal Function

The larynx is used for speech but also to control and ensure the flow of air into and out of the lungs. Respiration is the primary function of the larynx. (This is reviewed in detail in the following chapter.) Effortful closure, also called the *Valsalva* maneuver, is another vital function of the larynx. This seals the larynx preventing air escaping from the lungs during physical effort such as coughing, throat clearing, vomiting, urination, and defecation. There is great contrast between the position of the vocal folds during phonation and effortful closing. During phonation, only the true vocal folds adduct, but during effortful closing, there is a massive undifferentiated adduction of the laryngeal walls, including both true and false vocal folds by means of the adductory muscles and the arytenoid cartilages. During effortful closing, the thyroid cartilage is elevated, approximating the hyoid bone, as subglottic pressure increases. Another function of the larynx is to prevent and avoid ingestion of solids and liquids in the trachea and consequently in the lungs, during swallow.

Physiology of Phonation[1,2,17,18]

Phonation must be coordinated with respiration. Phonation is a dynamic process. To drive vocal folds into vibration, a minimal subglottal pressure is required. This minimal subglottal pressure is referred to as phonation threshold pressure (PTP). The configuration of the glottal aperture and viscoelasticity of the vocal folds are both important factors that can alter PTP. Because vocal folds are shelflike elastic protuberances of muscles and mucosa, their tension and elasticity can be varied. They can be thinner, thicker, and shorter or longer, open wide, close together, or come together into an intermediate position. Additionally they can be elevated and depressed in their vertical relationship to the cavities above.

During normal breathing the vocal folds are spaced widely apart. During quiet inhalation, the vocal folds abduct moving away from the midline and widen the glottis. These movements are small and inconspicuous during quiet inhalation and they are extensive during forced inhalation. During exhalation they adduct slightly toward the midline. The entire larynx also moves during respiration. It moves downward during inhalation increasing the airway capacity allowing a larger volume of air to be inhaled. This movement is coupled with downward movement of the entire bronchial tree. During exhalation the larynx elevates readying for phonation.

During prephonation, the vocal folds are adducted slightly or completely but loosely, to restrict the flow of air from the lungs but always maintaining an open glottal airway. At the same time, the forces of exhalation produce an increasing amount of air pressure beneath the folds and when the pressure becomes sufficient, the vocal folds are literally blown apart, thus releasing a puff of air into the vocal tract. This release of air results in an immediate decrease of pressure beneath the vocal folds. The elasticity of the tissues and the reduction of air pressure simply allow the folds to snap back into their adducted position ready to be blown apart once again. At this moment, the air pressure has again built up, completing one cycle of vocal fold vibration. The vocal folds can then repeat the cycle. Lieberman (1975)[19] described this behavior as the *myoelastic-aerodynamic theory*. The muscle activity needed to adduct and tense the vocal folds simply readies them for vibration but *does not* cause the vibration itself. According to Lieberman, the two aerodynamic forces which produce vibration of the vocal folds are the positive subglottal air pressure applied to the lower part of the folds, forcing them open and the negative pressure which occurs as air passes between the folds increasing the velocity of airflow (Bernouilli effect). These positive and negative pressures set the vocal folds into vibration due to the elasticity of the folds.

To understand the negative air pressure, we need to refer to Bernouilli who formulated the following aerodynamic law:

$$d \times \tfrac{1}{2}(v^2 p) = c$$

$$(d = \text{density}; p = \text{pressure}, v = \text{velocity}, \\ c = \text{a constant})$$

This means that if volume fluid flow is constant, velocity of flow must increase at an area of constriction, but with a corresponding decrease of pressure at the constriction. The Bernouilli effect applied to phonation assumes that the vocal folds are nearly approximated at the instant the airstream is released by the forces of exhalation. The airstream will have a constant velocity until it reaches the glottal constriction. Velocity will increase, as air passes through the glottis. The result of the Bernouilli force is a negative pressure between the medial edges of the vocal folds, producing a suction phenomenon. This suction and the static forces counterbalance the subglottic pressure from the lungs bringing the folds in a movement inward. The narrow channel causes an increase in suction snapping the vocal folds shut. Because the folds vibrate quickly, one puff of air follows another in an equally rapid succession. This repetition of air sets up a pressure wave at the glottis, which is audible. A necessary condition for voicing is that the air pressure below the folds must exceed the pressure above the folds. The vocal folds' elasticity permits them to be blown open for each cycle but the elastic recoil force works along with the Bernouilli principle to close the folds for each cycle of vibration (Figures 3–8 and 3–9).

Vertical Phase Difference in Vibration

Vocal folds begin to open posteriorly, and then anteriorly. Closure follows with the posterior, followed by anterior. Horizontally, typically the vocal folds close along the entire medial edge, with the posterior portion closing last. It is normal to have a gap in the posterior glottis that does not close. The posterior glottal gap (PGG) is more obvious and prominent in the female than the male. Young women demonstrate PGG and incomplete closure significantly more frequently than elderly women. This PGG is prominent in high phonation compared to normal phonation.

Voice Production, Frequencies and Harmonics, Loudness and Pitch, Voice Register, Quality of Voice

Frequencies and Harmonics

Phonation varies in intensity, frequency, and quality. As above, production of voice is the result of a steady flow of air from the lungs segmented at the laryngeal level into a series of air puffs at a fundamental frequency that generates harmonics in the cavities of the upper airway. The fundamental frequency is defined by the number of times the vocal folds open and close per second. The cavity resonation allows acoustic energy concentrations called "formant frequencies." Lieberman (1975)[19] has shown that a relationship between the fundamental frequency and the configuration of the supraglottic cavities does not exist. Increasing the subglottal pressure increases the intensity of the sound produced.

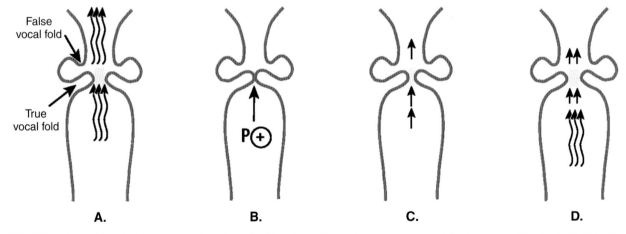

FIGURE 3–8. Vocal fold cycle vibration. **A.** Prephonation phase, the vocal folds are adducted slightly to restrict the flow of air from the lungs. An open glottal airway is maintained. **B.** The vocal folds are closed and the forces of exhalation produce an increasing amount of air pressure beneath the folds. **C.** The pressure is sufficient. Vocal folds are blown apart thus releasing a puff of air into the vocal tract. The velocity airflow is increasing and the pressure is decreasing (Bernouilli effect). **D.** The vocal folds are adducted again ready for another vocal fold cycle. The air pressure is again building up.

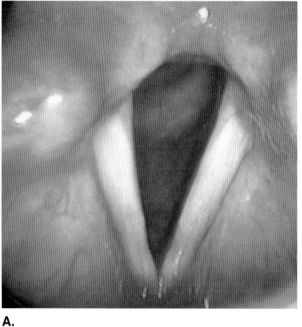

A.

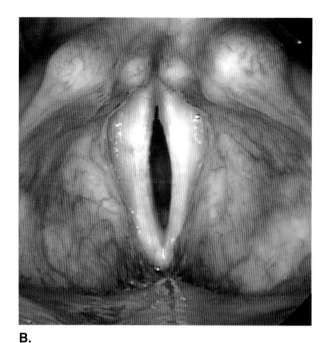

B.

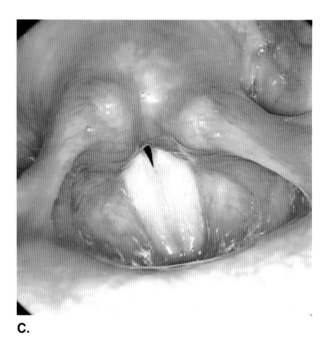

C.

FIGURE 3–9. Photographic sequence of the open and closed phases of one vibratory cycle. **A.** Vocal folds are abducted in rest position during normal breathing. **B.** Vocal folds adducted, open phase of vibration. **C.** Vocal folds adducted, closed phase of vibration.

In addition to subglottal pressure, the other major source of voice control is the larynx itself. Changes in the physical dimensions and characteristics of the vocal folds influence the sound that is produced. The fundamental frequency will change whenever the vocal folds are changed in some way that will allow them to move faster or slower. Increasing the subglottal pressure raises the fundamental frequency. According to the aerodynamic-myoelastic theory of voice production the tension of the vocal folds is considered to be one of the important forces of restoring the glottal closure. Longitudinal tension is a force that acts along the length of the vocal folds.

Physiology of Vocal Paralysis

Adequate diagnosis and treatment of unilateral paralysis of the vocal fold requires determining the cause of the immobility. The most common causes of unilateral vocal fold paralysis are surgical resection or injury of the recurrent laryngeal nerve (RLN). Examination of the larynx will show the affected vocal fold positioned in the paramedian position on the side of the paralysis. It is quite common for the aryepiglottic (AE) fold on the paralyzed side to collapse over into the glottis. Rarely, this causes symptoms of airway obstruction due to adequate abduction of the opposite vocal fold. However, in extreme cases, the AE fold on the paralyzed side may be pulled into the airway with vigorous respiratory exchange. The malposition of the arytenoid cartilage on the paralyzed side is caused by the lack of tension on the adductor muscles innervated by the RLN, which results in a rotation of the cartilage out of its normal physiologic position. The mobile vocal fold adjusts its length to match that of the paralyzed vocal fold on adduction. This is possible by reducing its length and descending inferiorly toward the midline such that the vocal processes are opposite one another during the glottal closure. However, this adaptation is insufficient to allow a normal phonation. The absence of muscle motion on one side involves a modification of pitch range and poor voice. Moreover, the larynx cannot prevent and avoid aspiration of solids and liquids because of insufficient glottal closure. Subsequently, there is a risk of increased morbidity (pneumonia) and mortality.

Many approaches have been proposed for the treatment of unilateral paralysis: speech therapy, expectant observation, intracordal injections, medialization laryngoplasty, arytenoid adduction, arytenopexy, and reinnervation of paralyzed muscle groups. None of the available methods are capable of restoring physiologic adduction and abduction to the paralyzed vocal fold. Medialization allows insertion of an implant deep to the thyroid cartilage displacing the vocal fold toward the midline. As the medialization has gained popularity, many different variations have been described.[20-22] Even in very experienced hands, some patients will obtain less than desired results or the initial good result may weaken over the follow-up period for many different reasons. Laryngeal reinnervation has been done using different nerves and methods with good results.[23,24] Studies have shown that reinnervation and medialization are both effective in the treatment of vocal fold unilateral paralysis, but the reinnervation also allows recovery of the thickness, elasticity, and tension of the vocal fold better than medialization.[25] Voice deterioration (6 months to 2 years postsurgery) is more common after medialization than reinnervation.[26] To avoid and prevent long-term deterioration of voice, combined surgical medialization and nerve-muscle pedicle reinnervation have been reported.[27] The results were significant, showing an improvement and a better quality of voice both short- and long-term. This is reviewed in detail in chapter 17.

The stretching of the vocal ligament will increase its longitudinal tension, which will accelerate the vocal fold movement and increase the rate of vocal fold vibration to raise the fundamental frequency.

Determinants of Loudness and Pitch

Vocal *loudness* increases as subglottic air pressure increases and as the duration of the closed phase of the vibratory cycle increases. Additionally, lateral excursion will increase with intensity. Glottal resistance is the resistance that the glottis places on airflow. When the vocal folds are closed longer, glottal resistance increases. Subsequently, increases in glottal resistance (with increased intensity) will be compensated with increased subglottal resistance.

For constant loudness during speech, subglottic pressure must be held constant. Frequency increases as (1) subglottic pressure increases; (2) the larynx rises in the neck, shortening the pharyngeal dimensions; and (3) vocal fold length and tension increase. In a study of excised human larynges, Kitajima et al (1979)[28] found that vocal pitch increased almost linearly with approximation of the cricoid and thyroid cartilages.

Photographic and x-ray studies have proved that fundamental frequency of phonation increases systematically with increased vocal fold length, which causes a decrease in cross-sectional area of the vocal fold. The decrease in mass causes an increase in frequency. The increase in length also creates an increase in tension that contributes to the increase in frequency. Vocal fold length

increases and thickness decreases with rising frequency in the modal registers. Pitch lowering is the result of a decrease in tension, and/or increase in mass per unit length (or the vocal folds shorten).

Vocal Registers. Although conceding that there are possibly more than three vocal registers, Hollien (1974)[29] recognizes the following:

1. *Pulse* register, the lowest range of phonation along the frequency continuum.
2. *Modal* register, the range of fundamental frequencies normally used in speaking and singing.
3. *Loft* register, the higher range of fundamental frequencies, including the *falsetto*.

In the untrained singer, transitions between registers are heard as changes in quality and even as a "break" in the voice.

Quality of Voice and Elastic and Viscoelastic Properties. The vocal tissues have two properties: elastic and viscoelastic. *Elastic* properties of vocal folds tissues are a key factor in the control of fundamental frequency in phonation,[30] but also a major determinant of the quality of voice. In 1974, Hirano[3] recognized that the morphological structure of the vocal folds is important for the control of tension in vibration; he called this the *cover-body* theory. The *cover* (epithelium and superficial layer of the lamina propria) is pliable, elastic, and noncontractile, whereas the body (muscle) is relatively stiff and has active contractile properties. The vocal ligament, composed of the intermediate and deep layers of the lamina propria, serves as a transitional layer between the two. The importance of the undulatory function of the mucosal covering of the vocal folds for normal phonation has been demonstrated in patients who have scarred vocal folds, where the mucosa has lost its mobility, resulting in breathiness and elevated pitch. Quality of voice depends on the quality of the cover and is also influenced by changes in the subglottal pressure. Normal vocal fold oscillations are an important precondition for a healthy voice.

Understanding normal laryngeal anatomy and physiology is imperative in the diagnosis and management of voice, airway, and swallowing disorders. This first chapter of the Anatomy and Physiology section (chapters 3-5) presented the basic anatomy and physiology information for the two chapters that follow.

Review Questions

1. The phenomenon of phonation:
   a. consists of a rapid opening and closing of the vocal folds which periodically interrupt the airsteam
   b. is independent and is not coordinated with respiration
   c. does not require air pressure to drive the vocal folds into vibration
   d. does not involve the Bernoulli effect
   e. requires the vocal folds to be in the abducted position

2. The range of fundamental frequencies normally used in speaking and singing is called:
   a. pulse register
   b. loft register
   c. vocal pitch
   d. modal register
   e. formant frequencies

3. The fundamental frequency of voice:
   a. depends on the configuration of the supraglottic cavities
   b. is always the same whatever the increase of the subglottal pressure
   c. will rise whenever the vocal folds move more slowly
   d. is the highest frequency which can be generate by the larynx
   e. is determined by the elasticity, tension, and mass of the vocal folds

4. The recurrent laryngeal nerve innervates:
   a. the thyrohyoid muscle
   b. the posterior belly of the digastric muscle
   c. the cricothyroid muscle
   d. the stylopharyngeus muscle
   e. the posterior cricoarytenoid muscle

5. The false vocal folds:
   a. allow the phenomenon of phonation
   b. move with the arytenoid cartilages
   c. are located in the subglottal area
   d. contain no muscle fibers
   e. move faster when the subglottal pressure increases

6. All the following occur during phonation except:
   a. the arytenoid cartilages rotate and the vocal process move outward, upward, and posteriorly
   b. adduction is accomplished by the posterior cricoarytenoid muscle
   c. the subglottal pressure increases and blows apart the vocal folds
   d. the release of air into the vocal tract entails a decrease of pressure beneath the vocal folds
   e. the Bernoulli effect results in an increase in airflow velocity

REFERENCES

1. Bless D, Abbs J. *Vocal Fold Physiology*. San Diego, Calif: College-Hill Press; 1983.
2. Titze I. *Vocal Fold Physiology*. San Diego, Calif: Singular Publishing Group; 1993.
3. Hirano M. Morphological structure of the vocal cord as a vibrator and its variations. *Folia Phoniatr.* 1974;26:89-94.
4. Hirano M. Structure of the vocal fold in normal and disease states: anatomical and physical studies. *ASHA Reports.* 1981;11:11-30.
5. Hirano M, Sato, K. *Histological Color Atlas of the Human Larynx*. San Diego, Calif: Singular Publishing Group; 1993.
6. Zemlin W. *Speech and Hearing Science Anatomy and Physiology*. Boston, Mass: Allyn and Bacon; 1998.
7. Furlan JC, Cordeiro AC, Brandao LG. Study of some "intrinsic risk factors" that can enhance an iatrogenic injury of the external branch of the superior laryngeal nerve. *Otolaryngol Head Neck Surg.* 2003;128(3):396-400.
8. Page C, Laude M, Legars D, Foulon P, Strunski Y. The external laryngeal nerve: surgical and anatomic considerations. Report of 50 total thyroidectomies. *Surg Radiol Anat.* 2004;26(3):182-185.
9. Friedman M, LoSavio P, Ibrahim H. Superior laryngeal nerve identification and preservation in thyroidectomy. *Arch Otolaryngol Head Neck Surg.* 2002;128(3):296-303.
10. Netterville JL, Koriwchak MJ, Winkle M, Courey MS, Ossoff RH. Vocal fold paralysis following the anterior approach to the cervical spine. *Ann Otol Rhinol Laryngol.* 1996;105(2):85-91.
11. Timmermann W, Hamelmann WH, Meyer T, et al. Identification and surgical anatomy of the external branch of the superior laryngeal nerve [in German]. *Zentralbl Chir.* 2002;127(5):425-428.
12. Jafari S, Prince RA, Kim DY, Paydarfar D. Sensory regulation of swallowing and airway protection: a role for the internal superior laryngeal nerve in humans. *J Physiol.* 2003;550(pt 1):287-304.
13. Halum S, Shemirani N, Merati AL, Jaradeh S, Toohill RJ. Electromyography findings of the cricopharyngeus in association with ipsilateral pharyngeal and laryngeal muscles. *Ann Otol Rhinol Laryngol.* In press.
14. Mimifie F, Hixon T, Williams F. *Normal Aspects of Speech, Hearing, and Language*. Englewood, NJ: Prentice-Hall; 1973.
15. Stroppiana L. Galen's treatise on section of the organs which produce sounds (translation and comment) [in Italian]. *Riv Stor Med.* 1970;14(2):131-148.
16. Joutsivuo T. Veraliu and De humani corporis fabrica: Galen's errors and the change of anatomy in the sixteenth century [in Finnish]. *Hippokrates.* 1997:98-112.
17. Borden G, Harris, K. *Speech Science Primer: Physuiology, Acoustics and Perception of Speech*. Baltimore, Md: Williams and Wilkins; 1980.
18. Van den Berg JW. Myoelastic-aerodynamic theory of voice production. *J Speech Lang Hear Res.* 1958;1:227-244.
19. Lieberman P. *On the Origin of Language*. New York, NY: Macmillan; 1975.
20. Odland RM, Wigley T, Rice R. Management of unilateral vocal fold paralysis. *Am Surg.* 1995;61(5):438-443.
21. Schneider B, Denk DM, Bigenzahn W. Functional results after external vocal fold medialization thyroplasty with the titanium vocal fold medialization implant. *Laryngoscope.* 2003;113(4):628-634.
22. Zheng H, Zhou S, Chen S, et al. Laryngeal reinnervation for unilateral recurrent laryngeal nerve injuries caused by thyroid surgery [in Chinese]. *Zhonghua Yi Xue Za Zhi.* 2002;82(15):1042-1045.
23. Zheng H, Li Z, Zhou S, Cuan Y, Wen W. Update: laryngeal reinnervation for unilateral vocal cord paralysis with the ansa cervicalis. *Laryngoscope.* 1996;106(12 pt 1):1522-1527.
24. Sercarz JA, Nguyen L, Nasri S, Graves MC, Wenokur R, Berke KS. Physiologic motion after laryngeal nerve reinnervation: a new method. *Otolaryngol Head Neck Surg,* 1997;116(4):466-474.
25. Wen W, Zhou S, Li Z Treatment of the unilateral paralysis of vocal fold—comparison between laryngeal framework surgery and reinnervation [in Chinese]. *Zhonghua Er Bi Yan Hou Ke Za Zhi.* 1998;33(4):237-239.
26. Tucker HM. Long-term preservation of voice improvement following surgical medialization and reinnervation for unilateral vocal fold paralysis. *J Voice.* 1999; 13(2):251-256.
27. Tucker HM. Combined surgical medialization and nerve-muscle pedicle reinnervation for unilateral vocal fold paralysis: improved functional results and prevention of long-term deterioration of voice. *J Voice.* 1997;11(4):474-478.
28. Kitajima K, Tanabe M, Isshiki N. Cricothyroid distance and vocal pitch: experimental surgical

study to elevate the vocal pitch. *Ann Otol Rhinol Laryngol.* 1979;88(1 pt 1):52-55.

29. Hollien H. On vocal registers. *J Phonet.* 1974;. 2:125-143.

30. Titze IR, Talkin DT. A theoretical study of the effects of various laryngeal configurations on the acoustics of phonation. *J Acoust Soc Am.* 1979; 66(1):60-74.

Physiology of Airway Regulation

Christy L. Ludlow, PhD

KEY POINTS

- Each of these systems is controlled by overlapping neuronal circuits in the brainstem.

- These functions interact in awake humans. Dependent upon a certain state, one system may be dominant and modulate the function of other systems through suppression and/or excitation. Alterations in one system can alter the regulation of other upper airway systems.

- Sensory feedback from the larynx to the brainstem can trigger and/or enhance activity in several systems simultaneously.

- Abnormalities in sensory feedback from the larynx may cause both short- and long-term changes in each of the upper airway systems. Chronic abnormalities in laryngeal sensation due to inflammation, irritation, or injury may produce neuroplastic changes in brainstem function. Synaptic changes in brainstem circuits can produce long-term facilitation of some brainstem functions altering airway regulation.

- A better understanding of upper airway regulation both in normal human function and in disorders should lead to better diagnosis and treatment in patients with upper airway regulation abnormalities.

The upper airway is composed of the larynx, hypopharynx, oropharynx, nasopharynx, and nasal and oral cavities. These regions are involved in respiration, swallowing, cough, voice, and speech. Each of these activities modulates the muscles of the upper airway to change the shape and function of this region. These functions are controlled by brainstem regulatory systems in addition to cortical volitional control. This chapter reviews each of the functions involved in upper airway regulation.

Respiration

During the two phases of respiration, inspiration and expiration, the airway is under control to enhance air exchange in the lungs. During inspiration, a traveling wave of muscle contractions develops to open the tract and reduce airflow resistance, starting at the nares, through the oral cavity, the hypopharynx, and finally the glottis. In this chain of muscle contractions from the alae nasi and genioglossus, to the posterior cricoarytenoid in the larynx all serve to maintain and enhance the opening of the upper airway on each inspiration. Inspiratory widening of the upper airway is often enhanced during sleep and exercise. If the levels of carbon dioxide in the blood are increased during hypercapnia, the drive to each of these airway-dilating muscles will increase.[1,2] On the other hand, if muscle tone decreases in the genioglossus, as occurs during some phases of sleep, tongue relaxation into the hypopharynx can interfere with airway opening producing an obstruction, which can be one cause of obstructive sleep apnea.[3]

During expiration, the vocal folds partially adduct[4] due to increased activity in the thyroarytenoid muscles.[5,6] The respiratory control system in the brainstem includes a dorsal sensory input region involving the nucleus tractus solitarius and the ventral respiratory control centers. These include the pre-Bötzinger region, which provides rhythm generation, and the Bötzinger complex and rostral ventral respiratory groups, which contain premotor neurons with inputs to each of the motor neuron pools involved (Figure 4–1A).[7]

Swallowing

Swallowing also modifies the upper airway to prevent the entry of food or liquid through the vocal folds into the trachea during ingestion. After entry of food or liquid bolus into the oral cavity and mastication, the bolus is formed and moved to the posterior oral cavity where its presence triggers the initiation of the pharyngeal phase of swallowing. The pharyngeal phase involves elevation of the velum (preventing entry of the bolus into the nasal cavity), and anterior and superior movement of the hyoid bone and larynx to close the vestibule along with vocal fold closure. Cocontraction of the posterior tongue and the wall of the oropharynx push the bolus downward while reflexive and mechanical opening of the upper esophageal sphincter allows entry of the bolus into the esophagus and clearance from the hypopharynx. This coordinated pattern of multiple movements is rapid, smooth, and tightly coordinated, taking less than 1 second in healthy adults, and is under the control of central pattern generators in the brainstem. The medulla contains both a dorsal swallowing group, which receives sensory inputs and cortical control, and a ventral swallowing group, which provides input to the motor neurons for each of the upper airway muscles involved (see Figure 4–1B).[8]

Cough

Aspiration of a bolus through the glottis will produce tracheobronchial cough when contact is made with receptors in the trachea. Cough involves a chain of muscle actions to clear the bolus or a foreign body from the upper airway: first a quick inspiration to intake air, a rapid vocal fold closure to build up pressure in the subglottal region, and then a rapid expiratory expulsion of air involving the abdominal muscles with a

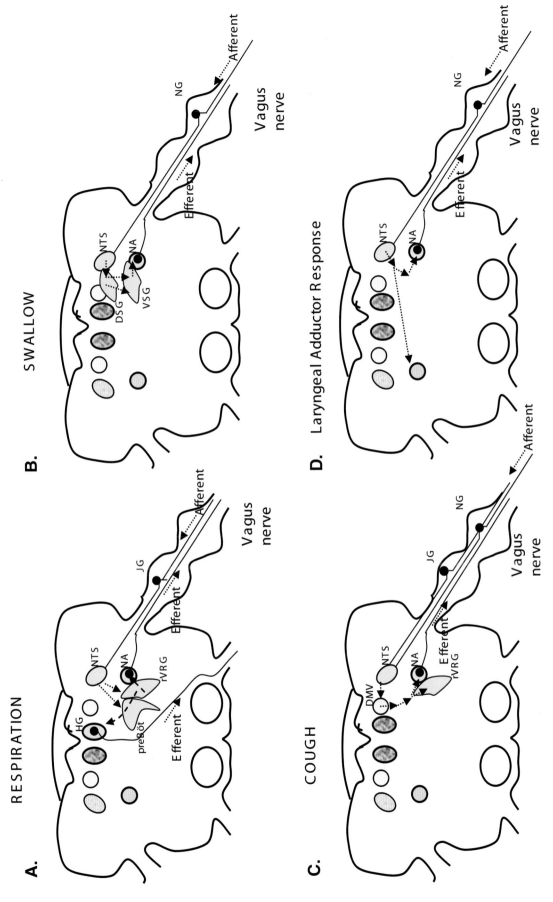

FIGURE 4–1. A schematic representation of the neural pathways involved in respiration (**A.**), cough (**B.**), swallow (**C.**), and the laryngeal adductor response (**D.**). In each diagram the control pathway is only represented on the right side of the medulla oblongata at the level of entry of the vagus. (Abbreviations: DMV = dorsal motor nucleus of the vagus; DSG = dorsal swallowing group; HG = hypoglossal nucleus; JG = jugular ganglion; NA = nucleus ambiguus; NG = nodose ganglion; NTS = nucleus tractus solitarius; preBöt = pre-Bötzinger complex; rVRG = rostral ventral respiratory group; and VSG = ventral swallowing group.)

rapid abduction of the vocal folds. Laryngeal cough is elicited by stimulation of receptors in the mucosa overlying the arytenoid cartilages in the posterior glottis. There may be differences in the chemical and sensory regulation of tracheobronchial and laryngeal cough.[9] For laryngeal cough, the afferents are contained in the superior laryngeal nerve and have their cell bodies in the nodose ganglion.[10] Input to the brainstem from these afferent neurons terminates in the interstitial subnucleus of the nucleus tractus solitarius (see Figure 4–1C).[11,12] There is some interaction between the tracheobronchial and laryngeal cough systems; persistent stimulation of the trachea can increase the sensitivity of the larynx to stimulation lowering the threshold for laryngeal cough elicitation.[13] Chronic application of several stimuli such as smoke, sulfur dioxide and allergens will produce hypersensitivity of the trachea to stimulation, resulting in enhanced cough.[14] Although not as well studied, it is likely that chronic irritation in the larynx could similarly produce hypersensitivity and enhanced cough.

Laryngeal Adductor Response

The laryngeal adductor response is a spasmodic burst of thyroarytenoid muscle activity producing a rapid vocal fold closure of a short duration (less than 100 ms) following a single short stimulation of afferents in the superior laryngeal nerve.[15-17] In awake humans responses to a single electrical stimulation of the superior laryngeal nerve includes an ipsilateral early response around 17 ms referred to as an R1 and bilateral R2 responses around 60 ms (Figure 4–2), which produce bilateral vocal fold closure.[18] An air puff presented to the mucosa overlying an arytenoid cartilage will produce a short duration bilateral glottic closure due to bilateral thyroarytenoid muscle bursts similar to an R2 response in healthy adults.[19] In the event of strong or prolonged stimulation to the posterior glottis, this reflex can become prolonged producing a laryngospasm, which can be life threatening due to prolonged airway obstruction. Hypercapnia may reduce laryngospasm,[20] as well as depress thyroarytenoid

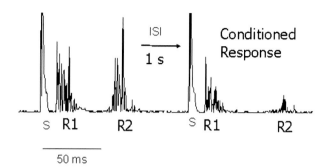

FIGURE 4–2. An example of a laryngeal adductor response to an initial electrical stimulus (*S*) to the superior laryngeal nerve and a response to a second pulse presented at an interstimulus interval (*ISI*) 1 second later.

muscle activity,[21] and was the basis for administering a carbon dioxide air mixture prior to extubation to prevent laryngospasm in pediatric anesthesia.[22] The laryngeal adductor response pathway in the brainstem involves inputs to the interstitial subnucleus in the nucleus tractus solitarius in the brainstem, the same sensory input region that is involved in cough and swallowing elicitation (see Figure 4–1D).[23]

Phonation

Vocalization can be elicited in mammals by electrical or chemical stimulation of neuronal pools in the central nervous system including the anterior cingulate and/or the periaqueductal gray, which projects to the brainstem, referred to as the indirect vocalization pathway (Figure 4–3).[24] Others have demonstrated that muscle patterning for vocalization may also be present in the nucleus retroambiguus[25] that projects to the nucleus ambiguus containing the motor neurons for the laryngeal muscles. The extent to which the indirect pathway that produces vocalization in animals (anterior cingulate, periaqueductal gray, nucleus retroambiguus) also controls voice production in humans during speech is not yet known and a matter of some controversy.[26] Jurgens proposed that voice during speech involves a direct corticobulbar pathway that may bypass the indirect system; whereas the indirect control

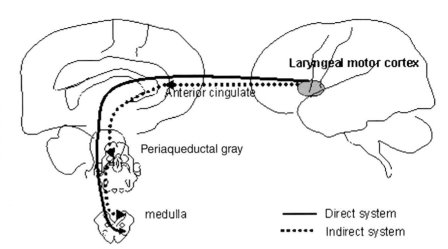

FIGURE 4–3. A schematic representation of the direct and indirect central pathways possibly involved in vocalization in humans.

system may be involved in emotional vocal expression in both humans and other mammals.[24] This may explain why patients with spasmodic dysphonia have symptoms during voice for speech while laughter and cry are symptom free. The disorder may affect the direct pathway but not the indirect pathway for voice production. Likely, both the direct and indirect systems are involved in speech while only the indirect system may be used during laughter and crying.

INTEGRATION OF UPPER AIRWAY SYSTEMS

Each of the upper airway systems involve several regions in the central nervous system from the cortex to the brainstem, where central pattern generators can produce these behaviors in an automatic fashion.[27–29] Studies in anesthetized or decerebrated animals have identified the location of neuronal pools in the brainstem, which can produce these behaviors in isolation. However, in awake humans, each of these systems must be regulated so that they do not interfere with each other. For example, every time a speaker is producing a word, he or she must maintain a controlled smooth flow of air on expiration and not swallow, cough, or inspire. In recent years, animal studies have begun to address how changes in neuronal firing within the same regions in the medulla are affected as

control is shifted between the different upper airway systems of cough, swallowing, respiration, and phonation.

Swallowing has a powerful influence on the other upper airway systems. The suppression of respiration occurs in the middle of expiration during the pharyngeal phase of swallowing. After the pharyngeal phase is complete, expiration resumes. Swallowing also has a suppressive influence on the laryngeal adductor response in humans. When electrical stimuli were presented to the superior laryngeal nerve prior to, during, and up to 5 seconds after a water swallow in healthy adults, the laryngeal adductor response was suppressed by swallowing. Both the frequency and amplitude of R1 and R2 responses were reduced when the subjects were swallowing and up to 3 seconds after they completed a swallow.[30] This demonstrates a suppression of neuronal activity in the laryngeal adductor response neural pathway during swallowing. The laryngeal adductor response is a subcomponent of the cough reflex pathway[23] (see Figure 4-1). The suppression of this pathway during swallowing may explain why coughing is reduced by taking a sip of water.

Cough also modifies respiratory control by producing a quick inspiration followed by forceful expiration. This demonstrates a modification of the neuronal firing in the ventral respiratory control system as the cough system modulates respiratory control within the medulla (see Figure 4-1B).[31]

The usual modulation of one airway system by another may be altered in certain states. If respiratory drive is increased by hypercapnia, for example, then swallowing can only occur at certain intervals within the respiratory cycles.[29] Such interactions between upper airway systems may play a role in patients with chronic obstructive pulmonary disease where patients' respiratory-swallowing coupling is altered so that more swallows occur during inspiration placing them at greater risk of aspiration.[32-35]

Effects of Sensory Inputs in Regulating Upper Airway Physiology

Each of the upper airway systems is triggered or modified by sensory feedback to the central nervous system. Stimulation of the laryngeal afferents plays a role in each of these systems. As mentioned earlier, mechanical stimulation of the mucosa overlying the arytenoid cartilages will elicit the laryngeal adductor response in the thyroarytenoid muscles.[19,36] Mechanoreceptors are contained in the superior laryngeal nerve, as are chemosensory and C fibers. Water applied to the larynx will produce both a laryngeal adductor response and a central apnea[37]; both being the result of stimulation of afferents contained in the superior laryngeal nerve.[38] Capsaicin has a powerful effect on the larynx causing vocal fold adduction and central apnea both when it is applied topically to the larynx or to the pulmonary C fibers by intravenous injection.[39-42] This may be one of the factors involved in heightened laryngeal reactivity when patients eat spicy foods.

Swallowing is highly dependent on the central effects of laryngeal sensation for the normal triggering of the pharyngeal phase. This was demonstrated in healthy adults following a bilateral block of the superior laryngeal nerve, which not only increased laryngeal penetration and aspiration[43] but also causes normal persons to feel incapable of initiating a swallow.

Although all the upper airway systems are affected by afferent input from the superior laryngeal nerve, the degree and effects of such stimulation on each system depend on the intensity and duration of stimulation. This has been carefully studied in animals where the rate of electrical stimulation to the superior laryngeal nerve may determine whether a swallow or a cough is produced.[44] A rapid rate of 30 stimuli per second can evoke repeated swallowing,[29] whereas slower rates of the same stimuli will produce coughing.[11,27,45] A central apnea due to a suppression of respiration rhythm generation will occur with high rates of electrical stimulation, between 10 and 50 stimuli per second, being presented to the superior laryngeal nerve.[46-49] Similarly the intensity of nerve stimulation will alter the effects on the central control of swallowing, cough, and respiration.[50] Inhibition of respiration occurs at a lower intensity of superior laryngeal nerve stimulation than elicitation of swallowing, indicating that some part of the same brainstem neural pathways may be involved in each.[29]

Laryngospasm, a prolonged laryngeal adductor response, is usually only elicited when a strong stimulus is applied to the larynx. This response is normally suppressed, most likely because of inhibitory mechanisms within the brainstem pathways. Conditioning studies are used to quantify inhibition of a response in central pathways. An initial stimulus excites a brainstem pathway producing a response while also activating inhibitory interneurons in the same pathway. If a second stimulus is then presented at a short interstimulus interval of 1 second or less, the responses to the second stimulus are reduced because of the active inhibition in the brainstem (see Figure 4-2). This was demonstrated in healthy adults by presenting paired air puff stimuli to the laryngeal mucosa. Each time, the response to the second puff was reduced in both occurrence (by about 50%) and amplitude.[51]

Besides brainstem inhibition of these responses, the responses are also modulated at higher levels in the central nervous system. With anesthesia, laryngospasm is less likely to occur, indicating that these responses are facilitated by brain mechanisms above the brainstem. Sasaki and his colleagues demonstrated that the bilateral laryngeal adductor response (the R2) producing a vocal fold closure is reduced with anesthesia both in an animal model as well as in humans.[52-54]

During phonation for speech, a speaker must use proprioceptive feedback in addition to audition for fine control of the laryngeal musculature. Activation levels must be controlled in all the laryngeal muscles simultaneously to control vocal fold length and tension and for accurate timing of vocal fold closing and opening to allow onset and offset of vowel production. The powerful role of hearing in the laryngeal muscle control was demonstrated by shifting the pitch of a speaker's own voice as it is fed back to him or her. This produces a rapid change in the speaker's pitch within about 100 ms.[55,56]

It has been postulated that speakers also use muscle and joint receptors to control muscles when initiating a target pitch for voice onset before they receive auditory feedback. A servomotor was used to push the thyroid cartilage and stretch the cricothyroid muscle and then release it to stretch the thyroarytenoid muscle, which altered voice pitch by muscle stretch in healthy adults. However, this did not produce any reflex responses in the laryngeal muscles, indicating that muscle stretch receptors (spindles) do not contribute to phonatory control in humans.[57] The role of other sensory feedback mechanisms, such as mechanoreceptors in the vocal fold mucosa and subglottal tracheal pressure receptors, need to be evaluated for their contribution to phonatory control in humans.

Effects of Abnormalities in Sensory Modulation on Upper Airway Regulation

Given the powerful effects of sensory and chemical stimuli to the larynx on each of the upper airway systems, it is not surprising that abnormalities affecting laryngeal sensation may produce disorders in respiration, cough, swallow, and voice.

A loss of laryngeal sensation produces swallowing deficits in healthy controls,[43] and patients with laryngeal sensory deficits often have swallowing disorders. Aviv and colleagues have shown that, when a stroke interferes with the central perception of laryngeal sensation, patients are at a greater risk of having aspiration pneumonia.[58] This is not because of any injury to the superior laryngeal nerve or the vagus, but rather due to a brain lesion disrupting sensory input to the central pathways involved in swallowing generation at the brainstem and/or cortex.[59]

Laryngopharyngeal reflux will produce low pH stimulation of the posterior larynx that can increase thyroarytenoid muscle tone producing laryngospasm.[60] Laryngopharyngeal reflux may be responsible for paradoxical laryngospasm in some patients[61] and should be considered when patients present with a history of intermittent laryngospasm. Long-term exposure to irritants may cause a hyperreactivity in the brainstem pathways involved in the laryngeal adductor response and has been postulated to be the basis for the "irritable larynx" syndrome.[62]

There may be two different effects of chronic laryngopharyngeal reflux on laryngeal function. First, acute application of low pH to the laryngeal mucosa can produce a central potentiation of the brainstem pathways involved in the laryngeal adductor response.[60] In addition, there may be long-term chronic effects due to inflammation or injury. In respiration, as a result of heightened sensory stimulation of the brainstem respiratory system with heightened serotonin release, long-term facilitation of respiratory control has been demonstrated in animal models.[63] Similarly, animals models of prolonged exposure to smoke, sulfur dioxide, and allergens in the trachea produced increased neural reactivity in the brainstem pathways involved in cough.[14] Similar mechanisms may be involved in neuropathic pain when central abnormalities continue long after the initial injury has resolved.[64] Such effects may occur in the laryngeal brainstem pathways with chronic inflammation.

Aviv and his colleagues have shown that the chronic effects of low pH to the laryngeal mucosa due to laryngopharyngeal reflux result in reduced sensory function on air-puff testing. Presumably the mucosal inflammation and edema

> ### Peripheral or Central?
>
> Patients with chronic laryngophargeal reflux may also develop a central abnormality because of the prolonged mucosal injury due to either low pH and/or peptic injury. Patients with pharyngeal sensory complaints may have both a peripheral loss of sensory function and a centrally based hypersensivity in the brainstem pathways.

interferes with air pressure changes affecting the mechanoreceptors in the mucosa.[65]

Paradoxic breathing disorder, when the vocal folds approximate in the midline during inspiration rather than opening, is often associated with chronic cough. When such disorders are refractory to proton pump inhibitors, hyperreactivity may have resulted from chronic irritation.[14,66] Such patients may need behavioral training involving upper airway regulation to restore normal function, as was demonstrated in a small case series in which patients benefitted from respiratory patterning through retraining.[67] The central mechanisms for the hyperactivity of the laryngeal adductor muscles during inspiration are not yet known. One animal study demonstrated that chemically blocking glycine receptors, normally involved in inhibition in the brainstem, increased laryngeal thyroarytenoid activity during inspiration.[68]

CURRENT AND FUTURE DIRECTIONS

Most of our understanding of central nervous system control for the upper airway systems comes from research using anesthetized or decerebrate animals. We have limited knowledge about how these systems are regulated in awake humans. Many patients have complaints of sensory abnormalities in the larynx for which we need additional diagnostic testing methods and additional treatments. With the development of air-puff testing,[58] we can now determine whether patients can sense pressure changes to the laryngeal mucosa. However, as is known from animal models of chronic cough,[14] significant disturbances in airway physiology can also come from central changes producing increased drive to the neuronal pathways in the brainstem. At present, we have few resources for diagnosing exaggerated responses to sensory stimulation and treating central increases in sensitivity, except for withdrawal of the irritating stimulus. Patients who fail a trial of proton pump inhibitors may have also developed central abnormalities affecting their responses to sensory stimulation.

Little is known about the neural mechanisms involved in the regulation of upper airway functions above the brainstem. Recent noninvasive brain imaging methods such as functional magnetic resonance imaging and other methods of study of central neurophysiology such as magnetoencephalography can be used to probe the role of central cortical control mechanisms in upper airway abnormalities. Such knowledge is needed for improved treatment approaches to disorders affecting the upper airway.

Acknowledgments. Support for preparation of this manuscript was from the Intramural Program, National Institutes of Health, National Institute of Neurological Disorders and Stroke. Both Keith Saxon, MD, and Sandra Martin, MS, provided helpful comments on earlier versions of this manuscript.

Review Questions

1. Name two effects of prolonged stimulation of the sensory fibers in the laryngeal mucosa.

2. Which two upper airway functions activate the posterior cricoarytenoid muscle?

3. Name two disorders that are often associated with reduced responses to sensory stimulation at the larynx.

4. Name two functions that are suppressed during swallowing.

5. Names two types of cough.

REFERENCES

1. Haxhiu MA, van Lunteren E, Mitra J, Cherniack NS. Comparison of the response of diaphragm and upper airway dilating muscle activity in sleeping cats. *Respir Physiol.* 1987;70(2):183-193.

2. Strohl KP, Hensley MJ, Hallett M, Saunders NA, Ingram RH Jr. Activation of upper airway muscles before onset of inspiration in normal humans. *J Appl Physiol.* 1980;49:638-642.

3. Strohl KP, Saunders NA, Feldman NT, Hallett M. Obstructive sleep apnea in family members. *N Engl J Med.* 1978;299(18):969-973.

4. Bartlett DJ, Remmers JE, Gautier H. Laryngeal regulation of respiratory airflow. *Respir Physiol.* 1973;18:194-204.

5. Kuna ST, Insalaco G, Woodson GE. Thyroarytenoid muscle activity during wakefulness and sleep in normal adults. *J Appl Physiol.* 1988;65:1332-1339.

6. Insalaco G, Kuna ST, Cibella F, Villeponteaux RD. Thyroarytenoid muscle activity during hypoxia, hypercapnia, and voluntary hyperventilation in humans. *J Appl Physiol.* 1990;69:268-273.

7. Rubin A, Mobley B, Hogikyan N, et al. Delivery of an adenoviral vector to the crushed recurrent laryngeal nerve. *Laryngoscope.* 2003;113(6):985-989.

8. Jean A. Brainstem control of swallowing: neuronal network and cellular mechanisms. *Physiol Rev.* 2001;81(2):929-969.

9. Bolser DC, Davenport PW. Functional organization of the central cough generation mechanism. *Pulm Pharmacol Ther.* 2002;15(3):221-225.

10. Yoshida Y, Tanaka Y, Hirano M, Nakashima T. Sensory innervation of the pharynx and larynx. *Am J Med.* 2000;108(Suppl 4a):51S-61S.

11. Gestreau C, Bianchi AL, Grelot L. Differential brainstem fos-like immunoreactivity after laryngeal-induced coughing and its reduction by codeine. *J Neurosci.* 1997;17:9340-9352.

12. Ohi Y, Yamazaki H, Takeda R, Haji A. Functional and morphological organization of the nucleus tractus solitarius in the fictive cough reflex of guinea pigs. *Neurosci Res.* 2005;53(2):201-209.

13. Hanacek J, Porubanova M, Korec L, Beseda O. Cough reflex changes in local tracheitis. *Physiol Bohemoslov.* 1979;28(4):375-380.

14. Bolser DC. Experimental models and mechanisms of enhanced coughing. *Pulm Pharmacol Ther.* 2004;17(6):383-388.

15. Suzuki M, Sasaki CT. Laryngeal spasm: a neurophysiologic redefinition. *Ann Otol Rhinol Laryngol.* 1977;86:150-158.

16. Ikari T, Sasaki CT. Glottic closure reflex: control mechanisms. *Ann Otol.* 1980;89:220-224.

17. Sasaki CT, Suzuki M. Laryngeal reflexes in cat, dog and man. *Arch Otolaryngol.* 1976;102:400-402.

18. Ludlow CL, VanPelt F, Koda J. Characteristics of late responses to superior laryngeal nerve stimulation in humans. *Ann Otol Rhinol Laryngol.* 1992;101:127-134.

19. Bhabu P, Poletto C, Mann E, Bielamowicz S, Ludlow CL. Thyroarytenoid muscle responses to air pressure stimulation of the laryngeal mucosa in humans. *Ann Otol Rhinol Laryngol.* 2003;112(10):834-840.

20. Nishino T, Yonezawa T, Honda Y. Modification of laryngospasm in response to changes in $PaCO_2$ and PaO_2 in the cat. *Anesthesiology.* 1981;55(3):286-291.

21. Kuna ST, Vanoye CR, Griffin JR, Updegrove JD. Effect of hypercapnia on laryngeal airway resistance in normal adult humans. *J Appl Physiol.* 1994;77(6):2797-2803.

22. Ahmad I, Sellers WF. Prevention and management of laryngospasm. *Anaesthesia.* 2004;59(9):920.

23. Ambalavanar R, Tanaka Y, Selbie WS, Ludlow CL. Neuronal activation in the medulla oblongata during selective elicitation of the laryngeal adductor response. *J Neurophysiol.* 2004;92(5):2920-2932.

24. Jurgens U. Neural pathways underlying vocal control. *Neurosci Biobehav Rev.* 2002;26(2):235-258.

25. Zhang SP, Bandler R, Davis PJ. Brainstem integration of vocalization: role of the nucleus retroambigualis. *J Neurophysiol.* 1995;74(6):2500-2512.

26. Holstege G, Ehling T. Two motor systems involved in the production of speech. In: Davis PJ, Fletcher NH, eds. *Vocal Fold Physiology: Controlling Complexity and Chaos.* San Diego, Calif: Singular Publishing Group; 1996:153-169.

27. Bolser DC. Fictive cough in the cat. *J Appl Physiol.* 1991;71:2325-2331.

28. Nakazawa K, Umezaki T, Zheng Y, Miller AD. Behaviors of bulbar respiratory interneurons during fictive swallowing and vomiting. *Otolaryngol Head Neck Surg.* 1999;120:412-418.

29. Dick TE, Oku Y, Romaniuk JR, Cherniack NS. Interaction between central pattern generators for breathing and swallowing in the cat. *J Physiol.* 1993;465:715-730.

30. Barkmeier JM, Bielamowicz S, Takeda N, Ludlow CL. Modulation of laryngeal responses to superior laryngeal nerve stimulation by volitional swallowing in awake humans. *J Neurophysiol.* 2000; 83(3):1264-1272.

31. Shannon R, Baekey DM, Morris KF, Lindsey BG. Ventrolateral medullary respiratory network and a model of cough motor pattern generation. *J Appl Physiol.* 1998;84(6):2020-2035.

32. Martin-Harris B, Logemann JA, McMahon S, Schleicher M, Sandidge J. Clinical utility of the modified barium swallow. *Dysphagia.* 2000;15(3): 136-141.

33. Langmore SE. *Endoscopic Evaluation and Treatment of Swallowing Disorders.* New York, NY: Thieme; 2001.

34. Good-Fratturelli MD, Curlee RF, Holle JL. Prevalence and nature of dysphagia in VA patients with COPD referred for videofluoroscopic swallow examination. *J Commun Disord.* 2000;33(2): 93-110.

35. Shaker R, Li Q, Ren J, et al. Coordination of deglutition and phases of respiration: effect of aging, tachypnea, bolus volume, and chronic obstructive pulmonary disease. *Am J Physiol.* 1992;263(5 pt 1): G750-755.

36. Aviv JE, Spitzer J, Cohen M, Ma G, Belafsky P, Close LG. Laryngeal adductor reflex and pharyngeal squeeze as predictors of laryngeal penetration and aspiration. *Laryngoscope.* 2002;112(2):338-341.

37. Goding GS, Richardson MA, Trachy RE. Laryngeal chemoreflex: anatomic and physiologic study by use of the superior laryngeal nerve in the piglet. *Otolaryngol Head Neck Surg.* 1987;97:28-38.

38. Van Vliet BN, Uenishi M. Antagonistic interaction of laryngeal and central chemoreceptor respiratory reflexes. *J Appl Physiol.* 1992;72(2): 643-649.

39. Kaczynska K, Szereda-Przestaszewska M. Superior laryngeal nerve section abolishes capsaicin evoked chemoreflex in anaesthetized rats. *Acta Neurobiol Exp (Wars).* 2002;62(1):19-24.

40. Szereda-Przestaszewska M, Wypych B. Laryngeal constriction produced by capsaicin in the cat. *J Physiol Pharmacol.* 1996;47(2):351-360.

41. Diaz V, Dorion D, Renolleau S, Letourneau P, Kianicka I, Praud JP. Effects of capsaicin pretreatment on expiratory laryngeal closure during pulmonary edema in lambs. *J Appl Physiol.* 1999;86(5): 1570-1577.

42. Palecek F, Sant'Ambrogio G, Sant'Ambrogio FB, Mathew OP. Reflex responses to capsaicin: intravenous, aerosol, and intratracheal administration. *J Appl Physiol.* 1989;67(4):1428-1437.

43. Jafari S, Prince RA, Kim DY, Paydarfar D. Sensory regulation of swallowing and airway protection: a role for the internal superior laryngeal nerve in humans. *J Physiol.* 2003;550(pt 1):287-304.

44. Harada H, Sakamoto T, Kita S. *Role of GABAergic control of swallowing and coughing movements induced by the superior laryngeal stimulation in cats.* Paper presented at: Society for Neuroscience; 2002; Orlando, Fla.

45. Satoh I, Shiba K, Kobayashi N, Nakajima Y, Konno A. Upper airway motor outputs during sneezing and coughing in decerebrate cats. *Neurosci Res.* 1998;32(2):131-135.

46. Lawson EE. Prolonged central respiratory inhibition following reflex-induced apnea. *J Appl Physiol.* 1981;50(4):874-879.

47. Sutton D, Taylor EM, Lindeman RC. Prolonged apnea in infant monkeys resulting from stimulation of superior laryngeal nerve. *Pediatrics.* 1978; 61(4):519-527.

48. Bongianni F, Corda M, Fontana G, Pantaleo T. Influences of superior laryngeal afferent stimulation on expiratory activity in cats. *J Appl Physiol.* 1988;65(1):385-392.

49. Bongianni F, Mutolo D, Carfi M, Fontana GA, Pantaleo T. Respiratory neuronal activity during apnea and poststimulatory effects of laryngeal origin in the cat. *J Appl Physiol.* 2000;89(3): 917-925.

50. Miller AJ, Loizzi RF. Anatomical and functional differentiation of superior laryngeal nerve fibers affecting swallowing and respiration. *Exp Neurol.* 1974;42(2):369-387.

51. Kearney PR, Poletto CJ, Mann EA, Ludlow CL. Suppression of thyroarytenoid muscle responses during repeated air pressure stimulation of the laryngeal mucosa in awake humans. *Ann Otol Rhinol Laryngol.* 2005;114(4):264-270.

52. Kim YH, Sasaki CT. Glottic closing force in an anesthetized, awake pig model: biomechanical effects on the laryngeal closure reflex resulting from altered central facilitation. *Acta Otolaryngol.* 2001;121(2):310-314.

53. Sasaki CT, Ho S, Kim YH. Critical role of central facilitation in the glottic closure reflex. *Ann Otol Rhinol Laryngol.* 2001;110(5 pt 1):401-405.

54. Sasaki CT, Jassin B, Kim YH, Hundal J, Rosenblatt W, Ross DA. Central facilitation of the glottic closure reflex in humans. *Ann Otol Rhinol Laryngol.* 2003;112(4):293-297.

55. Larson CR, Burnett TA, Kiran S, Hain TC. Effects of pitch-shift velocity on voice Fo responses. *J Acoust Soc Am.* 2000;107(1):559-564.

56. Burnett TA, Freedland MB, Larson CR, Hain TC. Voice F_0 responses to manipulations in pitch feedback. *J Acoust Soc Am.* 1998;103(6):3153-3161.

57. Loucks TM, Poletto CJ, Saxon KG, Ludlow CL. Laryngeal muscle responses to mechanical displacement of the thyroid cartilage in humans. *J Appl Physiol.* 2005;99(3):922-930.

58. Aviv JE, Sacco RL, Mohr JP, et al. Laryngopharyngeal sensory testing with modified barium swallow as predictors of aspiration pneumonia after stroke. *Laryngoscope.* 1997;107:1254-1260.

59. Aydogdu I, Ertekin C, Tarlaci S, Turman B, Kiylioglu N, Secil Y. Dysphagia in lateral medullary infarction (Wallenberg's syndrome): an acute disconnection syndrome in premotor neurons related to swallowing activity? *Stroke.* 2001;32(9): 2081-2087.

60. Loughlin CJ, Koufman JA, Averill DB, et al. Acid-induced laryngospasm in a canine model. *Laryngoscope.* 1996;106:1506-1509.

61. Loughlin CJ, Koufman JA. Paroxysmal laryngospasm secondary to gastroesophageal reflux. *Laryngoscope.* 1996;106:1501-1505.

62. Morrison M, Rammage L, Emami AJ. The irritable larynx syndrome. *J Voice.* 1999;13(3):447-455.

63. Feldman JL, Mitchell GS, Nattie EE. Breathing: rhythmicity, plasticity, chemosensitivity. *Ann Rev Neurosci.* 2003;26:239-266.

64. Coderre TJ, Katz J, Vaccarino AL, Melzack R. Contribution of central neuroplasticity to pathological pain: review of clinical and experimental evidence. *Pain.* 1993;52:259-285.

65. Aviv JE, Liu H, Parides M, Kaplan ST, Close LG. Laryngopharyngeal sensory deficits in patients with laryngopharyngeal reflux and dysphagia. *Ann Otol Rhinol Laryngol.* 2000;109(11):1000-1006.

66. Altman KW, Simpson CB, Amin MR, Abaza M, Balkissoon R, Casiano RR. Cough and paradoxical vocal fold motion. *Otolaryngol Head Neck Surg.* 2002;127(6):501-511.

67. Murry T, Tabaee A, Aviv JE. Respiratory retraining of refractory cough and laryngopharyngeal reflux in patients with paradoxical vocal fold movement disorder. *Laryngoscope.* 2004;114(8):1341-1345.

68. Dutschmann M, Paton JF. Inhibitory synaptic mechanisms regulating upper airway patency. *Respir Physiol Neurobiol.* 2002;131(1-2):57-63.

5

Physiology of Swallowing

Milan R. Amin, MD
Reena Gupta, MD

KEY POINTS

■ Swallow function involves the coordinated function of oral, pharyngeal, and laryngeal structures to allow passage of a food bolus.

■ Simultaneous motion of the related structures prevents aspiration and facilitates deglutition.

■ Swallow is divided into three phases: oral, pharyngeal, and esophageal.

■ While the oral phase is voluntary, the pharyngeal and esophageal phases are involuntary. The latter phases are triggered by sensory impulses from the food bolus.

■ Dysphagia can result from dysfunction of any component along this complex pathway.

The ingestion of nutritive substances is one of the most basic requirements of any life form. In lower animal species, the digestive tract is relatively simple, often consisting of a long tube. In higher animal species, the digestive tract takes on increasing complexity, often combining with the breathing apparatus to form a "shared" aerodigestive tract. This arrangement, however, requires complex coordination to prevent improper entry of ingested substances into the breathing apparatus. This level of coordination is certainly evident in the anatomy and physiology of the human upper aerodigestive tract.

ANATOMY

To understand the pathologic processes associated with swallow dysfunction, the anatomy of the involved structures must be understood. Of particular concern to the otolaryngologist are the oral cavity, the larynx, and the pharynx. Laryngeal anatomy, particularly as it relates to phonation, has been described in chapter 3.

Oral Cavity

The first structures involved in the completion of coordinated swallow are the lips, which are composed of skin externally and mucous membrane (stratified squamous epithelium) internally. Between these are the orbicularis oris muscle, labial vessels, nerves, fatty tissue, and numerous labial glands. Adequate closure of the lips, provided by sphincteric tightening of the orbicularis oris, prevents anterior escape of the bolus from the mouth.[1]

The 32 permanent teeth are responsible for mastication: 4 incisors, 2 canines, 4 premolars, and 6 molars each in the mandible and maxilla. Masticatory forces are applied by the masseter, temporalis, and the medial and lateral pterygoid muscles.[1] Their origins and insertions describe the applied forces and, therefore, the direction of movement of the jaw (Table 5–1). All of the muscles of mastication are innervated by branches of the trigeminal nerve.

Medial and lateral movement of the mandible is accomplished by unilateral contraction of the lateral pterygoid muscle, which deviates

TABLE 5–1. Function of Muscles of Mastication

Muscle	Origin	Insertion	Jaw Movement
Masseter			Translation of condyle; lateral fibers elevate and protrude mandible; medial fibers elevate and retrude; assists in medial/lateral movement
1. superficial	1. Zygomatic process of maxilla, anterior two-thirds of zygomatic arch	1. Angle and lower half of ramus of mandible	
2. deep	2. Posterior third and medial surface of zygomatic arch	2. Upper ramus and coronoid process	
Temporalis	Frontal, temporal, parietal, and sphenoid bones (along the superior temporal line); deep surface of temporalis fascia	Medial and lateral coronoid process, anterior border of ramus	Elevate mandible; retrude condyle; medial/lateral movement
Medial pterygoid	Lateral pterygoid plate (medial surface)	Medial surface of ramus and angle of mandible	Assists in mandibular protrusion
Lateral pterygoid	Lateral pterygoid plate (lateral surface)	Neck of condyle of mandible	Mandibular protrusion; medial/lateral movement

the mandible to the contralateral side. In contrast, unilateral contraction of the temporalis muscle results in ipsilateral mandible deviation. This directional movement is important for grinding the food bolus by the teeth.[2]

Although not a muscle of mastication, it is important to recognize the function of the *buccinator* muscle in retaining a food bolus between and medial to the teeth. Functional loss of this muscle causes food trapping in the oral vestibule, as seen in facial nerve paralysis.

The tongue, more than being simply the principle organ for sensation of taste, serves an important role in mastication and deglutition. The base of the tongue is attached to the hyoid bone by the hyoglossus, to the mandible by the genioglossus, to the epiglottis by glossoepiglottic folds, to the soft palate by glossopalatine arches, and to the pharynx by the pharyngeal constrictors. A median fibrous septum divides the tongue into lateral halves through its length, and attaches to the hyoid bone inferiorly. Each half contains intrinsic muscles, which are confined within the tongue, and extrinsic muscles, which have origins outside the tongue.[1] All are innervated by cranial nerve XII (hypoglossal) (Figure 5-1).

The extrinsic muscles are:

Genioglossus
Hyoglossus
Styloglossus
Glossopalatinus

The intrinsic muscles are:

Longitudinalis superior
Transversus
Longitudinalis inferior
Verticalis

The extensive musculature of the tongue allows it to position food for mastication between the teeth, clear the oral vestibule of food remnants, and propel the food bolus posteriorly to the hypopharynx.

Finally, the hard and soft palates serve as the roof of the oral cavity. The soft palate contains muscle fibers, fat, and soft tissue. The soft palate musculature includes the levator veli palatini, tensor veli palatini, the glossopalatine muscle, and the pharygopalatinus. This series of muscle attachments provides for velopharyngeal closure during the swallow, thereby preventing nasal regurgitation.

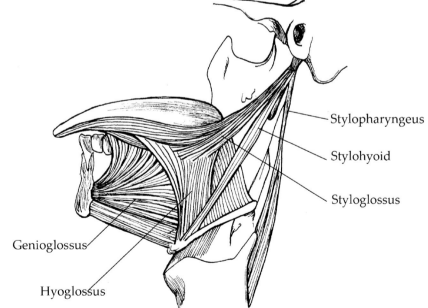

FIGURE 5–1. Extrinsic muscles of the tongue.

Stylopharyngeus

Stylohyoid

Styloglossus

Genioglossus

Hyoglossus

Larynx

For a complete description of laryngeal anatomy, refer to chapter 3. Several points are particularly important in understanding swallowing physiology. Laryngeal musculature is often divided into intrinsic and extrinsic musculature depending on whether or not both ends of the muscle are contained within the laryngeal framework. Although most commonly regarded for their phonatory function, the brisk laryngeal adductor closure reflex[3] executed by the intrinsic laryngeal muscles is a critical element to safe swallowing. Although these physiologic reflexes have been carefully described, clarifications continue to be made. Ludlow et al, for example, have shown recently that the laryngeal closure reflex, which occurs following stimulation by puffing air onto the laryngeal mucosa, results in a different muscular reaction than the traditional reflex initiated by stimulation of the superior laryngeal nerve.[4]

One group of extrinsic muscles, the "strap" muscles, must be considered in the discussion of swallowing muscles (Table 5–2). The suprahyoid group act as elevators of the hyolaryngeal complex. These muscles act to passively open the pharyngoesophageal segment (PES). These muscles are the focus of attention in the Shaker exercises, directed at strengthening these muscles for swallowing rehabilitation.[5,6] Shaker exercises are performed by having the patient lay in a supine position and perform either sustained or repeated head raising maneuvers. Another reminder of the strap muscles' role in swallowing can be seen in the dysphagia that may be experienced by patients who undergo botulinum toxin injection to these muscles for the treatment of laryngeal tremor (see chapter 19).

TABLE 5–2. Extrinsic Muscles of the Hyolaryngeal Complex

- Suprahyoid: anterior and posterior digastric, geniohyoid, mylohyoid, stylohyoid

- Infrahyoid: omohyoid, thyrohyoid, sternothyroid, sternohyoid

---

The Pharynx

The pharynx is a fibromuscular tube that extends from the base of skull to the inferior border of the cricoid cartilage, where the transition to the esophagus begins. It consists of an outer circular muscular layer and inner longitudinal muscular layer. The outer layer is arranged, superiorly to inferiorly, such that the superior muscle fibers nestle inside the superior edge of the next muscle. These muscles, called the *constrictors*, are named based on their location (*superior*, *middle*, and *inferior*). The superior constrictor originates on the pterygoid plate and hamulus; it inserts, as do the other constrictors, in the median raphe posteriorly. The middle constrictor originates from the hyoid bone and the inferior constrictor from the cricoid and thyroid cartilages. The inner longitudinal layer of the pharynx consists of the stylopharyngeus, palatopharyngeus, and salpingopharyngeus.[1] The motor innervation to the pharyngeal constrictors is derived from the pharyngeal plexus branches of the vagus nerve. This is detailed further below. The internal lining of the pharynx transitions from respiratory epithelium at the posterior nasal choanae superiorly to stratified squamous epithelium with submucosal mucous glands inferiorly.

The Esophagus

The cricopharyngeus muscle (upper esophageal sphincter) is a true sphincter of striated muscle. It originates from the lateral borders of the cricoid cartilage and forms a sling around the superior aspect of the cervical esophagus. It is located immediately distal to the inferior constrictor. Functionally, however, it is difficult to distinguish the lower parts of the inferior constrictor from the cricopharyngeus muscle. In contrast, the lower esophageal sphincter, between the distal end of the esophagus and the stomach, consists of tonically contracted smooth (involuntary) muscle, which relaxes to allow passage of a food bolus. The innervation of the cricopharyngeus muscle has been the source of some controversy for years; recent functional studies, including the use of electromyography, have implicated the superior laryngeal nerve as a likely source of innervation.[7]

The esophagus is a 23- to 25-cm long muscular tube that connects the pharynx to the stomach. It originates opposite the sixth cervical vertebra and descends along the front of the vertebral column to end at approximately the level of the eleventh thoracic vertebra. The wall of the esophagus has four layers:

■ External (fibrous) layer
■ Muscular layer: external longitudinal and internal circular fibers
■ Submucosal (areolar) layer: blood vessels, nerves, mucous glands
■ Internal (mucous) layer: longitudinal folds, stratified squamous epithelium; immediately deep to this epithelium, particularly inferiorly, is another muscular layer (muscularis mucosa).[8]

Neural Anatomy

Vagus Nerve (Cranial Nerve X)

The vagus nerve exits the skull base at the jugular foramen and enters the carotid sheath, in which it descends through the neck. The pharyngeal branch of the vagus nerve joins branches of the glossopharyngeal nerve as well as sympathetic fibers to form the pharyngeal plexus on the pharyngeal constrictors. Branches from this plexus innervate pharyngeal and soft palate musculature (except the tensor veli palatini, which is innervated by the 5th cranial nerve).

The next major branch is the superior laryngeal nerve, which descends behind the carotid artery and divides into an internal and external branch. The external branch, the smaller of the two, supplies the cricothyroid. The internal branch pierces the thyrohyoid membrane alongside the superior laryngeal artery and provides sensory innervation to the mucous membranes of the larynx.

The path of the vagus at this point differs on the two sides of the body. On the right side, the nerve sends a branch around the subclavian artery, which ascends as the recurrent laryngeal nerve. The right recurrent laryngeal nerve travels obliquely in its path back to the larynx. The left recurrent laryngeal nerve passes around the arch of the aorta and ascends in the tracheoesophageal groove. Both nerves pass under the inferior constrictor and enter the larynx at the cricothyroid joint, where they innervate all intrinsic muscles of the larynx except the cricothyroid. It also provides sensation to the lower larynx. Additionally, the recurrent nerves send branches to the esophageal musculature and mucosa. As the vagus continues inferiorly, both sides contribute to form an esophageal plexus, which provides neural control of peristalsis.[9]

Glossopharyngeal Nerve (Cranial Nerve IX)

The glossopharyngeal nerve also exits the skull through the jugular foramen and contains sensory and motor fibers. It provides sensation to the pharynx and taste to the posterior tongue. It descends anterior to the internal carotid artery, curving forward at the inferior border of the stylopharyngeus to lie upon that muscle and the middle constrictor. It passes deep to the hyoglossus to supply the pharynx. As previously mentioned, the glossopharyngeal nerve contributes to the pharyngeal plexus. Branches of the glossopharyngeal also innervate the stylopharyngeus muscle.[9]

Other Cranial Nerves

Other cranial nerves relevant to swallow function include the hypoglossal and trigeminal nerves. The hypoglossal nerve innervates the intrinsic muscles of the tongue, as described above. The trigeminal nerve has motor and sensory components. Of particular interest as it relates to the swallow is the motor function. Branches of the anterior portion of the mandibular division of CN V innervate the muscles of mastication. Its branches include the masseteric, deep temporal, and external pterygoid nerves. The inferior alveolar nerve is the largest branch of the mandibular nerve and innervates the mylohoid and the anterior belly of the digastric. The trigeminal also supplies the tensor veli palatini.[10]

NORMAL SWALLOWING FUNCTION

The swallow mechanism is traditionally divided into three phases. The *oral* phase involves mastication and formation of the bolus and propulsion of the bolus to the pharynx (Figure 5-2). The *pharyngeal* phase involves transfer of the bolus past the larynx and into the esophagus (Figure 5-3). The *esophageal* phase involves transport of the bolus through the esophagus and into the stomach (Figure 5-4).

During the oral phase, the lips, teeth, tongue, and muscle of mastication mix the ingested food with saliva to morselize the bolus into the proper consistency for ingestion. These muscles are necessary to redirect portions of the bolus back toward the teeth for mastication. The trigeminal nerve, through its second division, provides sensory innervation to the soft and hard palates, mucosa of the lips, gingivobuccal sulcus, buccal mucosa, and tongue. The trigeminal nerve, through its third division, provides motor innervation to the muscles of mastication. Once the bolus is formed in the oral cavity, it is propelled into the oropharynx by the tongue; this completes the oral phase of swallowing.

The presence of the bolus at the level of the anterior tonsillar pillars triggers the pharyngeal phase of the swallowing reflex. This phase of the swallow mechanism is completely involuntary. The sensory arm of this reflex is initiated when mucosal sensors within the oropharynx are activated by the presence of the bolus. Sensory information is then carried via the vagus and glossopharyngeal nerves to the swallowing center within the brainstem. These nerves have cell bodies in the *nucleus tractus solitarius*. There are connections to the *nucleus ambiguus*, where cell bodies of the motor neurons of the vagus nerve reside. Suprathreshold stimulation of the sensory neurons will lead to a complex set of events

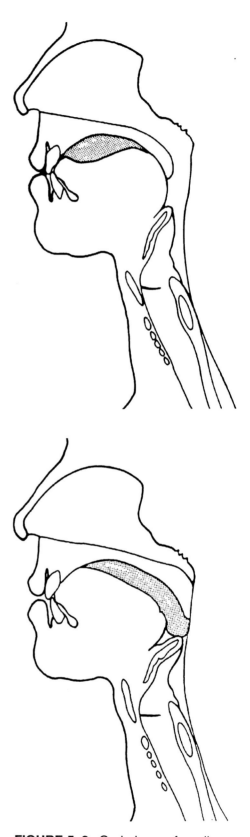

FIGURE 5–2. Oral phase of swallow.

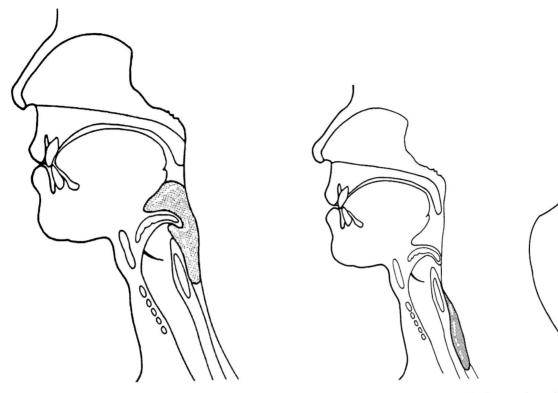

FIGURE 5–3. Pharyngeal phase of swallow.   **FIGURE 5–4.** Esophageal phase of swallow.

Infant Versus Adult Anatomy and Physiology

Although similar in many ways, the anatomy and physiology of the infant swallow differ from that described in the adult (see chapter 28, Pediatric Laryngology). In the infant, the larynx occupies a more cephalad position, such that the tip of the epiglottis makes contact with the soft palate. The consequence of this is that there is an additional "valve" present in the upper aerodigestive tract that is not present in the adult. This serves to close off a portion of the oropharynx during swallowing.

During bottle and breast feeding, the infant uses the oral cavity and facial musculature to suck milk from the nipple in a pistonlike action. The bolus is transported to the oropharynx, where is it is held in the valleculae by the "valve" described earlier. After several sucks, enough bolus accumulates to trigger a pharyngeal swallow. During accumulation of the bolus in the valleculae, the infant continues to breathe. The advantage of this for the infant is that fewer swallows are required, decreasing the obligatory apneic periods that are associated with the pharyngeal phase of the swallow.

comprising the pharyngeal phase of the swallow reflex. In this phase of the swallow, several events are occurring in rapid succession:

1. The soft palate closes against the posterior pharyngeal wall (velopharyngeal closure).
2. The false and true vocal folds close.
3. The pharyngeal constrictor muscles contract.
4. The larynx elevates and moves anteriorly toward the tongue base. During this, the epiglottis tilts posteriorly, covering the glottic inlet.
5. The cricopharyngeus muscle relaxes transiently.

Velopharyngeal closure occurs as a result of contraction of the levator veli palatini muscles. Action of this muscle causes posterosuperior displacement of the soft palate. The soft palate comes in contact with the posterior pharyngeal wall, effectively closing off the nasopharynx to prevent nasopharyngeal reflux. This closure also provides for a surface against which the bolus can be propelled downward, as it makes its turn into the lower pharynx. Dysfunction of the velum will result in characteristic hypernasal voice quality but may also contribute to dysphagia as the pharynx is impaired in its ability to generate bolus pressure in the face of leakage into the nasopharynx.

Velopharyngeal closure is followed very shortly by closure of the laryngeal inlet. During this step, the true and false vocal folds adduct in preparation for the passing bolus. At this point, there is a period of apnea, which may last 0.30 to 2.5 seconds.[11] The movement of the bolus is initiated with contraction of the tongue base, which pushes the bolus toward the posterior pharyngeal wall. From here, the pharyngeal constrictors direct the bolus inferiorly. In sequence, the superior, middle, and inferior constrictors contract to propel the bolus toward the esophageal inlet. The action of the constrictors is involuntary, but neural control and coordination occur via the pharyngeal plexus, as described above.

Simultaneous with the action of the constrictors, the larynx is brought anteriorly and superiorly by the strap muscles, which are innervated mostly by the ansa cervicalis. This motion, in turn, causes the epiglottis to retrovert, further covering the laryngeal inlet, and directing the bolus around the larynx. At this moment, the cricopharyngeus muscle relaxes from its tonically contracted state to allow the food bolus entry into the esophagus. The entire pharyngeal phase of the swallow lasts approximately 1 second.

The final phase of the swallow is the esophageal phase. Once the food bolus enters the esophagus, it is transported via peristaltic waves to the stomach. The peristaltic waves are created by a combination of muscle activity from both the circular and the longitudinal muscle fibers in the esophageal wall. The esophagus is innervated by a plexus formed by branches of the vagus nerve. Swallowing is complete when the bolus passes the lower esophageal sphincter and into the stomach. The lower esophageal sphincter relaxes reflexively as the peristaltic wave approaches. The timing and coordination of the lower esophageal sphincter is important not only in allowing proper transport of the food bolus into the stomach but also in preventing reflux.[12]

In addition to the neural innervation of the swallow mentioned above, there are some additional connections to supratentorial centers of the brain. Cortical and subcortical regions of the brain play a role in the voluntary initiation of swallowing and in the control of the oral phase of swallowing. As mentioned previously, the pharyngeal and esophageal phases of the swallow are involuntary and control lies within the brainstem.

Problems during any of the phases of the swallow reflex can cause dysphagia and aspiration, as will be outlined in the chapters ahead. In the oral phase, poor bolus formation can lead to a segmented bolus, which may affect the handling of the food during the pharyngeal phase and possible spillage into the laryngeal inlet. As alluded to above, the pharyngeal phase is particularly complex. Slowed reflex latency can lead to poor initiation of the pharyngeal phase; this occurs fairly commonly in the elderly population. Poor pharyngeal and laryngeal sensation can lead to premature spillage of the food bolus into the laryngeal inlet. The laryngeal adductor reflex[13] is affected by age[14] and the presence of laryngeal inflammation.[15] Similarly, incoordination or weakness of the pharyngeal musculature can cause poor pharyngeal stripping, which can also lead to penetration or aspiration. Poor velopharyngeal closure can cause nasopharyngeal reflux and a loss of pressure necessary for bolus transport through the pharynx. Problems such as poor epiglottic eversion or weak laryngeal elevation can lead to penetration (the presence of ingested materials beyond the vocal folds into the subglottis or trachea) or aspiration (the presence of ingested materials into the vestibule of the larynx) as well. Poor cricopharyngeal opening can lead to an increase in pooling within the piriform sinuses and subsequent spillage into the laryngeal inlet. Although the esophageal phase is often ignored in the evaluation, problems during this phase can lead to many dysphagia complaints including a feeling of food sticking within the chest or regurgitation. Problems frequently encountered during this phase include Zenker's diverticulum, and cricopharyngeal achalasia. These are reviewed in chapter 27.

Swallowing physiology is highly complex and requires intricate coordination between many specialized structures within the head and neck. Because of the dynamic nature and rapidity of the reflex, it is difficult to analyze. This presents hardships in terms of clinically evaluating and treating patients with dysphagia. Frontiers in understanding dysphagia will involve better understanding of the interrelatedness of foregut structures and the neuromuscular control that these reflexes exert over normal and disordered swallowing.[16]

Review Questions

1. List the muscles of mastication and describe their function and innevation.

2. What are the muscular attachments of the hyoid bone?

3. How does the vagus nerve contribute to swallow function?

4. How does the trigeminal nerve contribute to swallow function?

5. What are the three phases of swallow?

REFERENCES

1. Gray H. *Anatomy of the Human Body.* Philadelphia, Pa: Lea & Febiger; 1918.

2. Koolstra JH. Dynamics of the human masticatory system. *Crit Rev Oral Biol Med. 2002*;13(4): 366-376.

3. Aviv JE, Martin JH, Kim T, Sacco RL, Thomson JE, Diamond B, Close LG. Laryngopharyngeal sensory discrimination testing and the laryngeal adductor reflex. *Ann Otol Rhinol Laryngol.* 1999;108(8): 725-730.

4. Bhabu P, Poletto C, Mann E, Bielamowicz S, Ludlow CL. Thyroarytenoid muscle responses to air pressure stimulation of the laryngeal mucosa in humans. *Ann Otol Rhinol Laryngol.* 2003; 112(10):834-840.

5. Shaker R, Kern M, Bardan E, et al. Augmentation of deglutitive upper esophageal sphincter opening in the elderly by exercise. *Am J Physiol.* 1997; 272(6 pt 1):G1518-G1522.

6. Easterling C, Grande B, Kern M, Sears K, Shaker R. Attaining and maintaining isometric and isokinetic goals of the Shaker exercise. *Dysphagia.* 2005;20(2):133-138.

7. Halum S, Shemirani N, Merati AL, Jaradeh S, Toohill RJ. Electromyography findings of the cricopharyngeus in association with ipsilateral pharyngeal and laryngeal muscles. *Ann Oto Rhino Laryngol.* In press.

8. Bailey B, ed. *Head and Neck Surgery—Otolaryngology.* Philadelphia, Pa: Lippincott Williams & Wilkins; 1993.

9. Mu L, Sanders I. Sensory nerve supply of the human oro- and laryngopharynx: a preliminary study. *Anat Rec.* 2000;258(4):406-420.

10. Shankland WE 2nd. The trigeminal nerve. Part IV: the mandibular division. *Cranio.* 2001;19(3): 153-161.

11. Martin-Harris B, Brodsky MB, Price CC, Michel Y, Walters B. Temporal coordination of pharyngeal and laryngeal dynamics with breathing during swallowing: single liquid swallows. *J Appl Physiol.* 2003 94(5):1735-1743.

12. Logemann JA. Swallowing physiology and pathophysiology. *Otolaryngol Clin North Am* 1988; 21(4):613-623.

13. Aviv JE, Kim T, Thomson JE, Sunshine S, Kaplan S, Close LG. Fiberoptic endoscopic evaluation of swallowing with sensory testing (FEESST) in healthy controls. *Dysphagia.*1998;13(2):87-92.

14. Aviv JE, Martin JH, Jones ME, et al. Age-related changes in pharyngeal and supraglottic sensation. *Ann Otol Rhinol Laryngol.* 1994;103(10): 749-752.

15. Aviv JE, Liu H, Parides M, Kaplan ST, Close LG. Laryngopharyngeal sensory deficits in patients with laryngopharyngeal reflux and dysphagia. *Ann Otol Rhinol Laryngol.* 2000;109(11):1000-1006.

16. Shaker R, Hogan WJ. Normal physiology of the aerodigestive tract and its effect on the upper gut. *Am J Med.* 2003;115(suppl 3A):2S-9S.

PART III

Diagnostic Procedures in Laryngology

6

Videostroboscopy

Nadine P. Connor, PhD
Diane M. Bless, PhD

KEY POINTS

■ Video imaging of the larynx is a standard and critical part of a complete functional laryngeal and voice examination; Videostroboscopy is a video imaging method that is effective in most clinical situations.

■ Videostroboscopy provides information on both laryngeal structure and function, and also provides a permanent record that can be stored and referred to in the future to track changes in structure or function over time.

■ Videostroboscopy allows imaging and recording of apparent vocal fold motion, rather than actual cycle-to-cycle motion of the vocal folds.

■ Specialized, high-quality equipment is needed for videostroboscopy and is commercially available; training is necessary for performing and interpreting videostroboscopic examinations of the larynx.

■ Videostroboscopy scoring instruments are available in the literature and are recommended for ensuring that a complete examination protocol is followed, and that observations are recorded in a systematic manner. However, reliability of ratings is always a concern with any instrument.

Videostroboscopy is a technique that allows the clinician to image the larynx and the vocal folds, and also view the apparent motion of the vocal folds during a variety of phonatory tasks. In this manner, videostroboscopy offers a means of determining the etiology of the dysphonia.[1,2] For most clinical assessments of voice, videostroboscopic examination of the larynx is a critical and necessary part of obtaining an understanding of laryngeal structure and function. It is considered to be part of a basic, or minimal set, of procedures performed as part of a complete laryngeal and voice evaluation.[2]

A complete voice evaluation must include imaging of the vocal folds during phonation and videostroboscopy is an effective method for most clinical situations.[1] In a recent survey of speech-language pathologists specializing in voice disorders, 81% indicated they were likely to use videostroboscopy in voice assessments.[3] In addition, 94% of speech-language pathologists found videostroboscopy important in defining voice therapy goals, and 81% reported that videostroboscopy was an important tool to use in educating patients.[3] These are remarkable levels of utility, particularly in contrast to other voice

---

Does Videostroboscopic Examination Really Matter in Terms of Outcomes?

Videostroboscopic examination of the larynx assists the otolaryngologist and speech-language pathologist in forming a diagnosis and in planning treatment for individual patients. The presence of laryngeal pathology and the effect of that pathology upon vibratory function of the vocal folds can be directly discerned. In this vein, establishment of an accurate diagnosis is vital in formulating appropriate treatment decisions, and hence encouraging a positive treatment outcome. Studies completed by Woo et al[4] and Sataloff et al[13] demonstrated that videostroboscopy made a difference in diagnosis in approximately 30 to 47% of cases with voice disorders. Uncertain diagnoses were often confirmed with this procedure. To the extent that diagnosis is important in making correct management decisions and positive patient outcomes, the use of videostroboscopy appears critical.

Extensive use of videostroboscopy for determining voice therapy goals by the speech-language pathologist and for patient education has also been reported.[3] Specifically, Behrman reported that 94 and 81% of speech-language pathologists used videolaryngostroboscopy for these purposes, respectively. To the extent that definition of appropriate therapy goals and patient education are important to patient outcomes, the use of videostroboscopy appears to be a widely used and important assessment and educational method.

To summarize, it is the opinion of these authors that videostroboscopic imaging of the vocal folds is an essential part of a complete voice assessment and greatly influences patient outcomes due to its role in diagnosis, management, and patient education.

assessment modalities, such as aerodynamic assessments and electroglottography, where only 17% and 6% of speech-language pathologists, respectively, reported that these types of assessment methods were valuable.[3] As such, videostroboscopy is in common use, and has been found to be a valuable tool in diagnosing and treating patients with voice disorders. Videostroboscopic examination is completed by both speech pathologists and otolaryngologists, but only otolaryngologists use the images to make medical diagnoses.

By definition, a stroboscope is a device for studying the motion of a body in rapid vibration or revolution. In laryngeal examinations, the stroboscope causes vocal fold motion to appear to slow down or stop by periodically illuminating the larynx with pulses of light.[1] It is important to recognize that "apparent motion" is imaged with videostroboscopy, not actual cycle-to-cycle vibratory motion. Because humans cannot perceive more that 5 images per second, even 6 cycles per second is too rapid to observe. Thus, the vocal folds vibrating at a rate of 100 to 300/sec is clearly too rapid to allow vocal fold vibration to

be observed on a cycle-by-cycle basis. Furthermore, most available video recording equipment does not allow greater than 33 frames per second to be recorded, which is well below the habitual fundamental frequency of the human voice (see chapter 7, Laryngeal High-Speed Digital Imaging and Kymography). Videostroboscopy capitalizes on the limitations of human observation and recording frames. Depending on the mode selected, videostroboscopy allows the examiner to observe a composite vibratory cycle that appears to be the same point in time within a cycle to evaluate a particular phase of vibration or to examine vibration at different points of time within a cycle for appreciation of many points within the vibratory cycle.[1] In the former situation, a light is pulsed at a rate identical to the fundamental frequency of the voice. In the latter case, the light is pulsed at a frequency slightly faster than the actual fundamental frequency of vibration. This asynchronous light pulse allows the vocal folds to be observed at a different point in time within the vibratory cycle across many cycles of vibration. A schematic of this effect is shown in Figure 6–1. The net result is that the vocal fold vibration

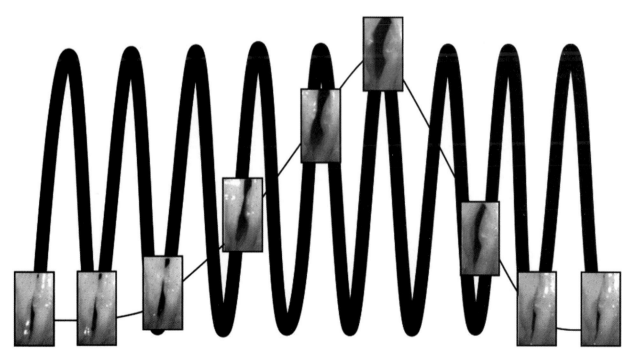

FIGURE 6–1. Apparent vocal fold motion.

appears to slow down. The eye is tricked into perceiving a continuous, slow-motion sequence of vocal fold vibration.[1,5]

EQUIPMENT

Specialized equipment is needed for videostroboscopy, as shown in Figure 6–2. This equipment includes a monitor, digital or video recording system, camera with microphone for recording an audio signal, a lens adaptor connected to either a flexible or rigid endoscope, a stroboscope that encompasses a pitch extractor and a light source, and a microphone or electroglottography (EGG) for pitch extraction. A speaker and printer are also necessary for complete functionality.[5]

The success of the technique is highly dependent on the quality of the equipment.[4] The light has to be bright enough, and pitch extraction must be accurate, have adequate range and speed, and must lock onto the patient's fundamental frequency quickly because many dyspho-

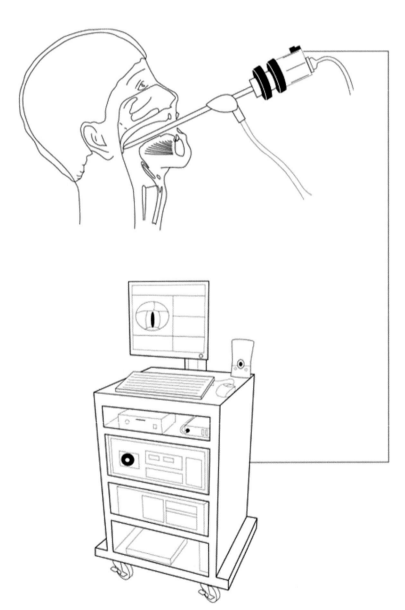

FIGURE 6–2. Diagram of equipment needed for videostroboscopy.

nic patients cannot sustain voice for long periods of time. In addition, the recording and camera equipment must be compatible and of high resolution. The resultant image will only be as good as the weakest link of the system.

Either flexible or rigid endoscopes can be used in videostroboscopy, with the goal of providing a bright image free of distortion. A flexible endoscope is passed through the nose, past the velum, and into the pharynx and has the advantage of imaging vocal fold vibration during connected speech, which is not possible with a rigid endoscope. The flexible endoscope is often better for individuals who tend to gag with something in their posterior oral cavity, those with a high tongue posture, or with young children (see

further discussion below concerning children). A flexible endoscope can be used to examine a variety of exposure angles and also to examine velopharyngeal function.[6] However, its disadvantages include the need for anesthetic spray in the nose, lower magnification, and less light delivered to the vocal folds. As such, the resolution of the vocal fold images can be compromised. In rigid videostroboscopy, a 70-degree rigid endoscope is commonly used and generally obtains images of higher resolution than a flexible endoscope, and is less invasive. The high resolution chip-tip flexible endoscope with a built-in miniature chip video camera embedded in the end of the endoscope is an exception to resolution concerns expressed above for flexible endoscopy. The

Do Patients Need to Undergo Both Flexible and Rigid Endoscopic Examination with Videostroboscopy?

Ideally, most patients would benefit from receiving both rigid and flexible endoscopic exams with videolaryngostroboscopy due to the higher resolution images generally obtained via rigid endoscopy, and the greater variety of phonatory tasks that can be accommodated by flexible endoscopy. In this manner, rigid endoscopy could be used to document the presence of pathology and the vibratory correlates of the pathology on tissue mechanics during simple phonatory tasks, such as extended vowel production, whereas voicing during connected speech could be assessed via flexible endoscopy. However, time often prohibits this practice and the endoscopist must choose either a flexible or rigid endoscope for the videolaryngostroboscopic examination. For patients presenting with signs of spasmodic dysphonia and other neurologic disease without pathology, flexible endoscopy is indicated due to the need to evaluate vocal fold behavior during connected speech. While tip-chip endoscopes make it possible to obtain well-illuminated, high-resolution images of laryngeal tissue dynamics via flexible examination, not all clinics have access to this expensive equipment.

In summary, it is the authors' opinion that use of both flexible and rigid endoscopic examination with videostroboscopy is an ideal situation that is often not clinically realistic and likely not necessary for accurate observation of vocal fold behavior by the experienced clinician.

tip-chip endoscope provides good illumination and high resolution, but is significantly more expensive than a standard rigid or flexible endoscope.

Electroglottography (EGG) is often recorded in conjunction with videostroboscopy. There are two purposes for this simultaneous recording: (1) it can be used to trigger the strobe and (2) it provides a record of every cycle of vibration helping clinicians to interpret the apparent motion from the stroboscopic images. The EGG is strapped onto the neck and functions by recording the impedance to passage of a very low current across the glottis. The EGG activates the strobe, and triggers the device to turn on the light pulse, either at the fundamental frequency of the voice or slightly faster. As mentioned, when synchronous with the fundamental frequency, the resultant glottal image appears to stand still and the recorded image is very similar to that recorded with direct, rather than pulsed, light. In other words, when vibration is regular no motion is observed. However, if vibration is irregular the pulsed light appearing at slightly different places on the vibratory cycle will result in a slight shimmering of the image rather than the static image observed during regular vibration. When asynchronous, the light is pulsed at one or two cycles faster than the fundamental frequency, thus illuminating slightly different points along the vibratory cycle (albeit from different cycles of vibration). When these illuminated images are then presented in sequence at a rate of 33 frames per second, apparent vocal fold motion is created. The addition of the EGG signal to the recorded and displayed image provides a real time cycle-to-cycle signal of vocal fold vibration.[5]

EXAMINATION PROTOCOL AND TECHNIQUES

Direct imaging of the larynx during phonation, in a variety of tasks, is needed to ascertain the effect of a lesion, a particular laryngeal structure, or mode of vibration on phonatory function. Videostroboscopy is a very practical and widely used clinical technique for this purpose.[3] Although

quantitative measures of acoustic and aerodynamic parameters of voice production provide valuable information about laryngeal function, clinicians can only infer, not directly observe, vocal fold vibratory information from these other quantitative measures.[5]

To perform videostroboscopy with rigid endoscopy, the patient should be seated and asked to lean forward with the chin extended at a 45-degree angle.[5] The EGG should be strapped gently on the neck. Patients should then be instructed to protrude the tongue and hold it out of the mouth with gauze. Then, the endoscope is inserted and a bright laryngeal image is obtained. A basic protocol can be followed during a videostroboscopic examination, with sufficient leeway for examining particular facets of a patient's case that are specific to the individual. At a minimum, a basic protocol should include the following tasks: inspiration, a gentle cough, a sustained vowel (usually the vowel /i/ is used), a sustained vowel with pitch and then loudness variations, a sniff immediately followed by a vowel, laryngeal diadochokinesis, and inspiratory phonation. For singers, it is useful to observe the singing of scales.[5] Flexible endoscopy does not necessitate an open mouth and permits adding connected speech tasks and whistling to the protocol. Connected speech tasks should be structured to include sentences loaded with vowels in contrast to sentences loaded with consonants.

The examiner should rate several parameters concurrently during the videostroboscopic examination. Recording the ratings and observations on a videostroboscopic protocol form can assist in data management, recall of the examination details at a later time, and also serve as a set of prompts to ensure that all examination tasks have been recorded. Several rating scales and forms have been proposed for use in videostroboscopic examination.[1,7-9] Use of these types of forms can allow observations of diagnostic importance to emerge during the examination. Intrajudge and interjudge reliability is always a concern in any type of perceptual rating instrument and has been shown to be variable for videostroboscopy evaluation forms, particularly when visual judgments need to be expressed as numerical entities or categories.[7,10] As mentioned throughout the literature on videostroboscopy, the training level of the rater is of primary importance to the validity and reliability of the use of an evaluation instrument. In developing the SERF, or Stroboscopy Evaluation Rating Form, Poburka[7] incorporated visual rating methods directly onto a drawing of a superior laryngeal view to remove the need to translate visual observations into numerical judgments.

Complete instructions and description of the examination to patients prior to starting is very important, so that patients know what to expect. Patients should be told at the onset that they can inform you if they experience discomfort. Instructions and a complete description will also assist in alleviating anxiety in patients and are particularly important when working with children.

VIDEOSTROBOSCOPIC EXAMINATIONS OF CHILDREN

Videostroboscopic examinations of children are generally undertaken via use of a flexible fiberoptic endoscope. Although cooperation can be limited, a rapid examination is generally sufficient to yield necessary information regarding vocal fold structure and function. Although higher resolution vocal fold images are generally obtained with a rigid endoscope, successful use of videostroboscopy can be negatively affected by gag reflexes in children, short phonation time, a highly oriented/posteriorly inclined epiglottis, increased pitch perturbation, and soft voice.[6] However, in a recent report, 74% of 42 children within the age range of 6 to 16 years old were successfully imaged via rigid videostroboscopy. Most of the failures in completing the rigid videostroboscopic examination were in children younger than 10 years old.[6] As such, flexible videostroboscopy is recommended for use in young children, whereas children over the age of 10 may benefit from a rigid videostroboscopic examination. These issues are discussed in further detail in chapter 28, Pediatric Laryngology.

INTERPRETATION OF EXAMINATION RESULTS

Direct imaging of the larynx is critically important in obtaining a description of mass lesions or other pathophysiologic manifestations underlying the presence of a dysphonia. In most cases, videostroboscopy is a valuable addition to imaging with a straight light because it also provides information about laryngeal function.

Videostroboscopy must be performed, and resultant images interpreted, by an individual trained in the technique. The importance of training and experience cannot be overstated for obtaining excellent images and for correct interpretation of findings.[11]

Interpretation of videostroboscopic data involves a visual-perceptual task on the part of the examiner.[10] For this reason, experience in performing these types of interpretations is necessary. Knowledge of normal vocal fold anatomy and vibratory characteristics, and how anatomy and vibratory characteristics are altered by phonatory tasks or pathology is also critical for accurate interpretation.[10] Clinicians should recognize that a patient's history may introduce bias.[10] However, use of the patient's history to guide the examination is often necessary and certainly appropriate. Images should be recorded and saved for review after the examination has been completed.

When viewing the stroboscopic image, the examiner should evaluate all aspects of the appearance of the vocal folds, including the color (although this might be difficult to appreciate depending on the effectiveness of the light source, position of the velum, and characteristics of reflecting tissue), appearance of blood vessels, lesion location and size, mucus (amount, consistency), vocal fold free-edge characteristics, appearance of a microweb at the anterior commissure, symmetry of vocal fold motion during opening and closing phases, periodicity of vocal fold vibration, degree of vocal excursion for inspiration, glottic closure pattern such as presence of a glottal gap or other incomplete closure, closing phase, phase of motion, and vertical level differences between the left and right vocal folds.

Who Should Perform and Interpret Videostroboscopy?

Videolaryngostroboscopy should be performed by clinicians, whether otolaryngologists or speech-language pathologists, who have been trained to perform the examination and interpret the results. In clinical reality, local traditions and staff availability often dictate whether a speech-language pathologist or otolaryngologist performs and interprets the examinations. Performance of videolaryngostroboscopic examinations is within the scope of practice of speech-language pathologists, provided that they have appropriate training and experience.[12] A speech-language pathologist experienced in the role of performing video-stroboscopic examination can increase efficiency in the clinic, allowing the physician's time to be dedicated to aspects of diagnosis and treatment not within the scope of practice of the speech-language pathologist. Interpretation of findings and treatment planning should involve a team approach.

To summarize, it is the opinion of these authors that speech-language pathologists, who are focused on acquiring an understanding of the physiologic mechanisms of vocal fold vibration, should perform recordings of laryngeal vibratory mechanics and also engage in the interpretation of findings, along with the otolaryngologist. The otolaryngologist, then, will have more time and better information to share with the patient when reviewing the medical diagnosis and surgical implications of the full voice assessment.

Most importantly, the presence and consistency of the mucosal wave and the stiffness of the vocal folds should be noted.[1,13]

During vocal fold vibration, symmetry is rated by observing the degree to which the vocal folds vibrate as mirror images of each other and reflects timing and extent of lateral excursions. Periodicity is observed during sustained phonation. Aperiodicity appears as vocal fold movement when the stroboscope is set to the patient's fundamental frequency. At this setting, the vocal folds appear to stand still when phonation is periodic, and aperiodicity is manifested as a noticeable quiver in the vocal folds. However, some caution should be used with this interpre-

tation, as the apparent aperiodicity may also reflect difficulty with pitch tracking of the stroboscope. Vocal fold closure patterns refer to glottal shape when maximally closed for phonation and include entities such as glottal gaps and whether the closed phase is abnormally long or short indicating the pressence or absence of glottal hyper- or hypofunction. Vertical level differences between the right and left vocal fold are often best observed, or inferred, from out-of-phase motion. Mucosal wave is rated as absent if the normal traveling wave present on the superior surface of the vocal folds is not observed. Any particular areas of absent mucosal wave on the vocal folds should be noted as adynamic segments of the vocal fold. These adynamic segments likely have diagnostic significance and contribute to an overall rating of vocal fold stiffness. Similarly, limits in amplitude of vibration, or how much the vocal folds move laterally from the adducted position, also may reflect vocal fold stiffness. Limited amplitude of vibration may also result from high pitch, low effort, or poor respiratory support.

Particular attributes observed via videostroboscopy for various laryngeal pathologies are summarized in multiple volumes and cannot be discussed in proper detail here. The reader is directed to the interactive video textbook by Cornut and Bouchayer [13] and the interactive training CD by Bless and Poburka [5] for video samples of laryngeal pathologies recorded during videostroboscopic examination and the descriptions of laryngeal pathologies observed via videostroboscopy in the volume by Hirano and Bless. [1]

Because vocal fold vibration must be periodic or quasiperiodic for the stroboscope to track the fundamental frequency of vibration, videostroboscopy may not work well with severe voice disorders or aphonia. High-speed video imaging of the vocal folds is recommended in these cases, as discussed in detail in the following chapter.

In conclusion, it is critical to view the laryngeal structures, and record an image of the vocal folds in motion as part of a complete voice evaluation. Information gained during this type of procedure greatly enhances diagnosis, treatment, and patient education. Videostroboscopy is an imaging technique that is effective for this purpose for most patients with dysphonia. However, videostroboscopy requires that either a synchronized microphone or electroglottograph signal effectively tracks the fundamental frequency of the voice to trigger the light pulses in either a synchronous or asynchronous fashion. If fundamental frequency tracking cannot be done, for instance, in cases of very severe dysphonia or aphonia, then videostroboscopic examination is not the video imaging method of choice. Other methods, such as high-speed video imaging, should be used with severely aperiodic voices. In most clinical situations, however, videostroboscopy provides important information on both laryngeal structure and function, and also provides a permanent record that can be stored and referred to in the future to track changes in structure and/or function over time.

Review Questions
True or False?

1. Videostroboscopy does not track aphonic or highly dysphonic voices.

2. Videostroboscopy is a research, not a clinical, tool.

3. Videostroboscopic images are based on optical illusions.

4. Videostroboscopy does little more than straight light endoscopy recording.

5. Videostroboscopy takes too long to use in routine clinical practice.

6. Videostroboscopy need not be performed when an obvious lesion is present.

7. Videostroboscopy need not be performed over the entire range of voice.

8. Videostroboscopic interpretations do not take special training.

9. Videostroboscopy can be performed with pediatric patients.

Questions for Further Review

1. Describe the manner in which vocal fold motion is tracked by the stroboscope, and the way in which an optical illusion is generated that appears to result in slow motion.

2. What equipment and training is necessary for performing a videostroboscopic examination of the larynx?

3. What is included in a videostroboscopic examination protocol?

4. Describe aspects of laryngeal structure and function that should be observed, rated, and recorded during a videostroboscopic examination.

5. From further reading and observation, such as from the book by Hirano and Bless,[1] the training CD by Bless and Poburka,[4] and the video textbook by Cornut and Bouchayer,[11] appreciate and describe the aspects of laryngeal structure and function most commonly observed with different dysphonias and laryngeal pathologies.

REFERENCES

1. Hirano M, Bless DM. *Videostroboscopic Examination of the Larynx.* San Diego, Calif. Singular Publishing Group Inc; 1993.

2. Dejonckere PH, Bradley P, Clemente P, et al. A basic protocol for functional assessment of voice pathology, especially for investigating the efficacy of (phonological) treatments and evaluating new assessment techniques: guideline elaborated by the Committee on Phoniatrics of the European Laryngological Society (ELS). *Eur Arch Otorhinolaryngol.* 2001;258:77–82.

3. Behrman A. Common practices of voice therapists in the evaluation of patients. *J Voice.* 2005; 19:454–469.

4. Woo P, Casper J, Colton R, Brewer D. Diagnostic value of stroboscopic examination in hoarse patients. *J Voice.* 1991;5:231–238.

5. Bless DM, Poburka B. *Video Laryngeal Stroboscopy* [book on CD-ROM]. Clifton Park, NY: Thomson Delmar Learning; 2002.

6. Wolf W, Primov-Fever A, Amir O, Jedwab D. The feasibility of rigid stroboscopy in children. *Int J Pediatr Otorhinolaryngol.* 2005;69:1077–1079.

7. Poburka B. A new stroboscopy rating form. *J Voice.* 1999;13, 403–413.

8. Poburka BJ, Bless DM. A multi-media, computer-based method for stroboscopy rating training. *J Voice.* 1998;12:513–526.

9. Rosen CA. Stroboscopy as a research instrument: development of a perceptual evaluation tool. *Laryngoscope.* 2005;115(3):423–428.

10. Teitler N. Examiner bias: influence of patient history on perceptual ratings of videostroboscopy. *J Voice.* 1995;9:95–105.

11. American Speech-Language Hearing Association. Vocal tract visualization and imaging: technical report. *ASHA Suppl.* 2004;24:140–145.

12. American Speech-Language-Hearing Association. Vocal tract visualization and imaging: position statement. *ASHA Suppl.* 2004;24:140–145.

13. Cornut G, Bouchayer M. *Assessing Dysphonia. The Role of Videostroboscopy* [An Interactive Video Textbook]. Lincoln Park, NJ: KayPENTAX; 2004.

14. Sataloff RT, Spiegel JR, Hawkshaw MJ. Strobovideolaryngoscopy: results and clinical value. *Ann Otol Rhinol Laryngol.* 1991;100:725–727.

7

Laryngeal High-Speed Digital Imaging and Kymography

Rita Patel, MS
Diane M. Bless, PhD

KEY POINTS

■ Video imaging of laryngeal motion is critical to understanding the structure and function of the larynx.

■ High-speed digital imaging and kymography provide a permanent record of the actual cycle-to-cycle motion of the vocal folds.

■ High-speed digital imaging and kymography can be used with all voice disorders regardless of the degree of dysphonia; the images can be used for both qualitative and quantitative descriptions of laryngeal behavior.

■ Training is necessary for both recording and analyzing the images.

■ Measures of vocal function can be obtained with high-speed digital and kymographic recordings that cannot be obtained with stroboscopy or acoustical analysis.

Fundamental to appropriate diagnoses and treatment of vocal fold pathology is direct visualization of vocal fold vibratory patterns. In the last several years, new concepts in the area of voice, voice diagnostics, image analysis, and modeling have been developed to shed light on mechanisms of irregular vocal fold vibrations.

Videostroboscopy, as detailed in the preceeding chapter, is routinely used in clinic for examination of vocal fold dynamics, but it is designed to examine periodic vocal fold vibrations, making it less valid for aperiodic voices. Moreover, videostroboscopy provides an *appar-*ent motion* making it impossible to assess cycle-to-cycle vocal fold motions that are especially critical for comprehensive clinical appraisal of subjects with hoarseness. *High-speed digital imaging* (HSDI) and *kymography* appear to overcome these limitations because they are not limited to periodic voices, and initiate recording immediately regardless of vocal frequency or loudness,[1] or degree of dysphonia, a feat that cannot be said for stroboscopy. A comparison of advantages and disadvantages of videostroboscopy and clinical high-speed imaging are listed in Table 7–1.

TABLE 7–1. A Comparison of Advantages and Disadvantages of Stroboscopy and Clinical High-Speed Imaging Systems

No.	Stroboscopy	Clinical High Speed Imaging
1.	Sampling rate: 25 to 30 frames per second.	Sampling rate: 2000 to 4000 frames per second. Research systems with temporal resolution of up to 8000 fps available.
2.	Dependent on stable phonation. Fails in voiceless cases or very hoarse voice qualities.	Not dependent on stable phonation. Can analyze extremely aperiodic voice qualities.
3.	Requires phonation duration times of at least 2–3 seconds. Phonation of >1 second needed to observe one vibratory cycle as the frequency of strobe motion is about 1 to 2 Hz.[2]	No minimum requirements of phonation duration. Analysis of phonations >1 second possible. This permits observation of momentary breaks in phonation, vocal onset, and vocal offset.
4.	Maximum resolution of about 750 × 500 pixels.	Maximum resolution of about 256 × 256 pixels.
5.	Recording duration limited only by size of recording media (tape, computer memory, or disk).	Recording duration ranges limited from 2 to 8 seconds depending on selected resolution.
6.	Routinely used in clinic, but poor research tool for gaining insights into cycle-to-cycle variations of vocal fold motion.	Excellent for use in both clinic and research.
7.	Observing transient phenomena like voice breaks, extremely small aphonic segments, vocal tremor,[3] and onset of phonation impossible.	Detailed analysis of phenomena like voice breaks, extremely small aphonic segments, vocal tremor,[3] voice onset and voice offset possible.
8.	Yields an apparent vibratory motion.	Yields real time cycle-to-cycle vibratory motion.
9.	Quantification of "actual" glottal gap size, amplitude of vibrations, and size of vocal pathology[4] is difficult due to the resultant apparent vibratory motion.	Quantification for "actual" glottal gap size, amplitude of vibrations, and size of pathology possible.
10.	Availability of reliable and valid semi-automated software programs for easy extractions of glottal parameters limited.	Semi-automated software programs for easy extractions of glottal parameters readily available.
11.	Rigid and flexible endoscopy possible.	Color HSDI limited to 90° endoscope. Use of 70° endoscope possible for black and white HSDI. Flexible endoscopy not possible at this time.
12.	Simultaneous sampling of acoustic and electroglottographic signals possible.	Simultaneous sampling of acoustic and electroglottographic signals possible.

HISTORICAL REVIEW

High-speed imaging was first developed in 1942 by Bell Telephone Laboratories.[5] The early high-speed systems were bulky, difficult to use, recorded films required subsequent development that often revealed no usable data and usable recordings, and required laborious frame-by-frame analysis. Also the camera noise, limited recording duration, and problems with synchronizing additional signals for voice measurements prevented widespread clinical acceptance of high-speed imaging. Moore, von Leden, and Timcke in the late 1960s first used the above prototype high-speed system to study the vocal fold dynamics of normal and pathologic (unilateral vocal fold paralysis, edema, unilateral polyp, bilateral polyps, benign neoplasm, hematoma, vocal fold web) voices under various phonatory conditions (pitch and loudness variations).[6-9] Using high-speed recordings, these authors were also able to describe transient but complex vocal fold behavior for phenomena like cough, inspiratory phonation, laughter, and vocal fry. Nevertheless, the combination of difficulties encountered with equipment, recordings and analysis resulted in analysis of only a few seconds of phonation obtained from a few subjects. In fact, most of our current knowledge of normal dynamic vocal fold vibration is derived from a small number of subjects ranging from one subject[6,8] to a maximum of four subjects.[7] Even as late as the 1970s, attempts at quantification of vocal parameters and data reduction of high-speed images were technologically improved but still cumbersome and clinically impractical.[10-12]

Contemporary development of digital technology has led to much needed improvements in the camera, sensor systems, recording capabilities, and memory of the recording systems that were originally designed for nonmedical purposes, such as car crash tests,[9] thereby extending its application to clinical assessment of voice. As a result of technologic advancements, since the middle to late 1990s, there has been a surge of laboratory-based studies[13-17] investigating the research and clinical applications of high-speed digital imaging especially in the European literature. Efforts to develop semi-automated motion tracking and motion analysis software like the high-speed toolbox[18] and multidimensional voice analysis system (MVAS)[19] were initiated. More recently, Yan et al[20] proposed the glottal area waveform (GAW) method to analyze normal and abnormal vocal fold vibrations. These systems are fast, generally taking no more than a couple of minutes, and yield quantitative measurements of vocal fold vibratory patterns. One example of a commercially available program for extraction of quantitative glottal parameters is depicted in Figure 7-1.

Currently available high-speed systems reach a maximum speed of 8,000 frames per second but vary with duration and resolution. Commonly commercially available clinical systems record 2000 to 4000 frames per second with recording durations ranging from 2 to 8 seconds. Spatial resolution ranges from 160×140 pixels to 256×256 pixels for clinical high-speed systems. Simultaneous recording of both acoustic and electroglottographic signals are also possible. Measures identical to those obtained with stroboscopy are possible but represent *every cycle of vibration*. Interpretation of vocal fold amplitudes, glottal width, left-right asynchrony, temporal change of vibrations, mucosal waves, vertical plane difference between the vocal folds, and closure patterns can be judged using high-speed recordings. Characterizing the three-dimensional movement of the vocal fold vibrations in the lateral plane (adduction vs abduction), vertical phase shift (mucosal wave), and the inferior and superior margins, is also possible using high-speed imaging.

APPLICATIONS OF HSDI FOR LARYNGEAL IMAGING

Applications of HSDI for clinical imaging of the larynx are broad. However, because of recording limitations in its current form, it augments rather than replaces stroboscopy. Nevertheless, it is a valuable clinical tool that can be successfully used to evaluate various types of vocal fold vibrations, even extremely aperiodic voice qualities and phonations of less than 1 second.

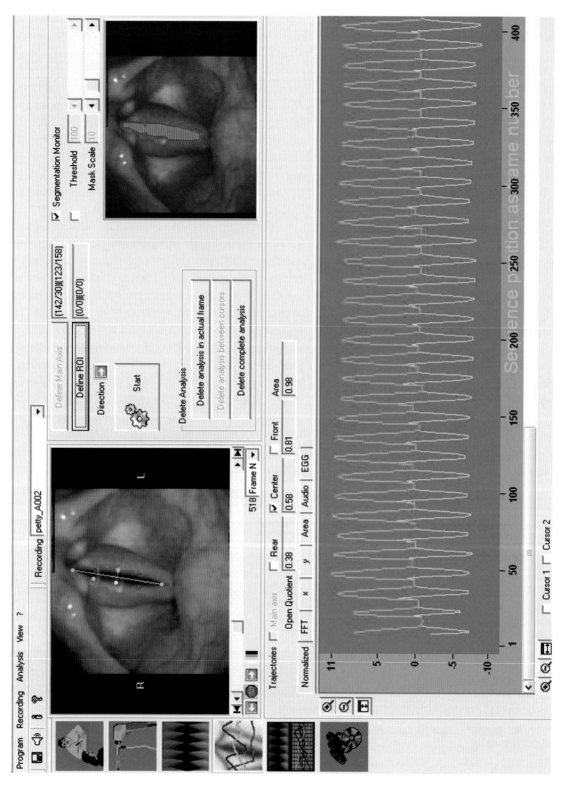

FIGURE 7-1. One example of commercially available automatic glottal feature extraction program. Vocal fold image on the left shows six points along the length of the vocal fold that tracts vocal fold amplitude across the anterior section, mid-membranous section, and posterior section of the right and left vocal fold. The graph below shows the extracted vocal fold amplitude of the mid-membranous section of the right (*green*) and left (*yellow*) vocal fold. (Courtesy of Richard Wolf Medical Instruments Corporation.)

Clinically, it is particularly useful in the setting of hoarseness that may not be explained or well characterized by stroboscopy; these abnormalities may include nonlinear dynamics such as subharmonics and bifurcations.

HSDI excels at the examination of phonatory onset and offset.[14] Traditional stroboscopy is not capable of delineating these subtleties. Furthermore, HSDI can simultaneously analyze vibratory motion with acoustic, electroglottographic, and inverse filtered signals.[21] The refined information from these imaging modalities may be able to detect even the minute return of function in cases of paresis and paralysis, as well as providing independent assessment of right and left vocal fold motions, glottal symmetry, and glottal area estimates. Specific transient vibratory phenomena, such as glissando, are better seen with these modalities as opposed to stroboscopy.[22]

In the area of basic research, high-speed imaging has been used for obtaining insights into glottal properties with use of the excised larynx setup,[23,24] as well as for the precise, noninvasive measurement of vocal fold length through the projection of two parallel laser beams onto the vocal fold.[25] In addition to the general vibratory dynamics and voice assessment applications, HSDI has been documented to be of particular

---

Do Clinical Impressions of Disorders Differ as a Function of Imaging Technique?

It is intriguing to contemplate how images of various voice disorders would differ between stroboscopy, high-speed imaging, and kymography. Would a malingering patient be more easily identified by one and not the other? The relatively long sample recorded from stroboscopy might make it more difficult for a speaker to maintain a false voice. On the other hand, the ability of kymography and HSDI to record initiation, whispering, and sudden but brief duration shifts in sustained vibratory modes (characteristics that may be present in malingerers) allows for subtle characterization not possible with stroboscopy. Even though HSDI is in its technological infancy, recordings of spastic dysphonic patients have already shown that laryngeal profiling of subgroups such as adductor, abductor, and mixed spastic dysphonia are possible with as little as 2 seconds of high-speed recording. The highly irregular patterns of severely dysphonic paralysis patients cannot be tracked longitudinally with stroboscopy because of high perturbation levels. Because this is not a limitation with HSDI or kymography, these findings may be used to predict return of function and aid in management decisions. Kymography makes interpretation of some of the images more objective consequently reducing observer bias. With kymography, it is straightforward to determine when there is no amplitude or a reduced mucosal wave, out-of-phase movement, or other aperiodicities of vibratory cycles. Software programs can be applied to both strobe and high-speed images to provide similar measures but one must question validity of measurements when the signal is highly irregular.

benefit to specific clinical cases. In some cases, it characterizes the disorder; in others it differentiates it from pathology with similar vocal characteristics; and in still others, it provides a means to document changes resulting from treatment.

The specific clinical indications reported for HSDI are numerous, and include the presence of diplophonia[26] and tremor,[4] as well as the detailed examination of benign vocal lesions and scar and stiffness of the vocal fold. HSDI is used for the assessment of moderate to severe voice disturbances[27] that cannot be reliably recorded with stroboscopy. Some authors have advocated its utility in distinguishing muscle tension dysphonia from spastic dysphonia.

At the extremes of vocal performance, HSDI has been investigated in determining the vibratory source of neoglottis and the pharyngoesophageal segment in laryngectomees.[28,29] Singers may be evaluated by these modalites, particularly for singing styles whose ranges may fall outside standard stroboscopy, such as rock singing[30] and Mongolian throat singing.[31] Finally, HSDI is useful in the investigation of low frequency or slow vibrations such as present in ventricular fold vibrations[32] and glottal fry. HSDI is relatively new; it is likely that future study will reveal additional clinical applications.

Although contemporary laryngology clinics would not function without stroboscopy, few have embraced high-speed imaging. This may be due, at least in part, to the cost of available high-speed systems and clinicians wishing to be responsible in helping control the rising costs of medical care. It also may be related to some of the current limitations of high-speed imaging. High-speed imaging requires greater skill from the examiner than does stroboscopy because: the recorded samples are shorter, flexible endoscopes cannot be used, some systems do not have color, it is difficult to use with pediatric cases, playback does not include simultaneous audio, and interpretations requires additional training. However, because technology is changing rapidly, some of the above limitations of high-speed imaging will likely be overcome in the near future.

KYMOGRAPHY

Recognition of the clinical importance of imaging every cycle of vibration in combination with the often prohibitive cost of these technologies motivated the development of video kymography, referred to as the "poor clinician's" HSDI because it has some of the advantages of high-speed imaging over stroboscopy but does so at one-fourth the cost. A kymogram or kymograph is a spatiotemporal image that shows a fixed horizontal line in the vocal fold image over time (see Figure 7–2). As the successive line images are presented in

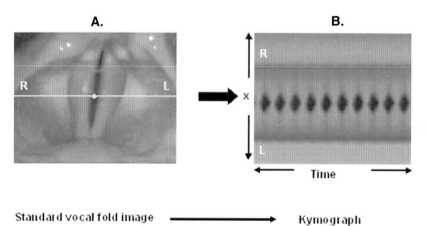

A. **B.** Standard vocal fold image ⟶ Kymograph

FIGURE 7–2. Generation of kymograph from high-speed digital imaging. **A.** A horizontal line along the mid-membranous portion of the vocal fold image obtained using high-speed digital imaging is used to generate a kymograph. **B.** When a kymograph is generated from high-speed imaging it is also called a digital kymograph.

real time, the system makes it possible to observe left-right asymmetries, open quotient, propagation of mucosal waves, and anterioposterior modes of vocal fold vibration.[33] Gall et al in 1970 first used a technique called "photokymography" to record vocal fold oscillations. Subsequent modifications of the above techniques in the 1970s were called larynx-photokymography, strip-kymography, and microphotokymography.[34] Modern kymographic techniques can be divided into two types: videokymography[35] and digital kymography.[34]

Videokymography

In 1994 videokymography (VKG) was developed by Švec and Schutte as a low-cost and better time resolution (8,000 frames per second) alternative to high-speed imaging.[35] VKG is obtained using a specialized CCD video camera that operates in two modes: standard and high-speed. In the standard mode, it records black and white images at 25 to 60 frames per second. In the high-speed mode, the system records black and white kymographic images at 8000 frames per second of an

Where We Have Come From: High-Speed Film

Paul Moore once said that there have been miles of high-speed film taken but only seconds of voice analyzed. This is not surprising when one takes a historical perspective. The development of HSDI is not unlike that of computer development. The early recordings required that a whole room be devoted to the large bulky recording apparatus. The systems needed to be table- or wall-mounted as they were far too heavy to be hand-held. They required a large water bath to cool the hot light so as not to burn the laryngeal tissue, camera housing to reduce the loud noise, and a rigid imaging apparatus that reflected light on a mirror used to illuminate the larynx. Subjects were positioned over the mirror with both neck and tongue extended. Once the larynx was visualized, they were asked to phonate /i/; when the camera was activated, a loud bang occurred followed by the buzz of the camera. The noise was sufficiently loud that it startled many patients so that they physically jumped and, in so doing, modified image placement. After the recording session was completed, the film was sent out to be developed and returned by the developers a week or so later. Often the recording started too early or late to record the phenomenon of interest. Sound synchronization was often not possible. The useful footage would be placed over a tracing, and later, a digitizing, plate, and laboriously traced frame-by-frame. *One second* (several thousand frames of film) would take hours and hours of measurement. New technology has made the current HSDI systems appear to be distant cousins. The ability to visualize the image while recording from a handheld instrument and subsequently use semiautomated software to analyze the waveform would have seemed impossible in the not too remote past.

examiner-selected single horizontal line section along the length of the vocal fold (Figure 7–3). It is critical to position this horizontal line perpendicular to the glottal axis for accurate interpretation of kymographs obtained from VKG. (Gross movements of the larynx could make the recording position inaccurate.) In VKG, positioning this horizontal line is achieved more readily with the use of a 90° rigid endoscope. To view oscillations across multiple horizontal sections along the length of the vocal fold separate endoscopic recordings are required for each horizontal section. The spatial resolution of the resultant kymographs is 768 pixels per line. Recording duration is virtually unlimited because fewer data have to be stored and processed when compared to HSDI. However, VKG lacks a full video image of the vocal folds.

Digital Kymography

Kymographs obtained from high-speed video recordings using software analysis methods of

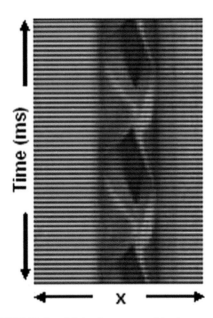

FIGURE 7–3. Videokymographic image obtained using a specialized CCD camera. Particularly note the black and white image and time along the ordinate compared to digital kymography where time is often depicted along the abscissa.

image processing are called digital kymographs (DK) or functional images.[34] In 1999, Wittenberg et al first reported extractions of multiplane kymographs from high-speed digital videos.[36] As the DK kymographs are obtained from high-speed digital video recordings the resultant DK are limited to the color, spatial, and temporal resolution of the original high-speed recordings. Presently the maximum possible spatial, and temporal resolution for clinical digital kymographs is 4,000 frames per second and 256 pixels per line, respectively. Both black and white and color DK can be obtained. Although more expensive than VKG, the DK are attractive because of the ease of examining vocal fold oscillations simultaneously from multiple horizontal sections along the vocal fold length from a single phonatory sample (Figure 7–4). This allows the examiner to easily study the tissue across a lesion and to compare anterior and posterior and lateral vibratory modes without making multiple recordings. Moreover, although general applications of VKG and DK are similar to those of HSDI, they can better define the extent of mucosal wave propagation, visibility of upper and lower margins of the vocal folds, glottal axis movement during closure, assess changes in opening and closing phases, and detect ventricular fold movements during phonation.[37]

In summary, HSDI and kymography allow for physiologically based interpretations of irregular vocal fold vibrations that can be based on the classic body cover theory[38] of vocal fold vibration. Interpretation involves the use of labels similar to those used in stroboscopy ratings (eg, mucosal wave, phase symmetry). Examiner retraining is required to make the finer qualitative vibratory pattern judgments made not from stroboscopic optical illusions of apparent motion obtained from frames of several segments of different cycles, but of thousands of frames reflecting individual vibratory cycles. Two sequential recordings, stroboscopy/endoscopy for structural examinations and simultaneous high-speed/kemographic, audio, and electroglottographic recordings may aid in complete analysis of vocal fold vibrations.

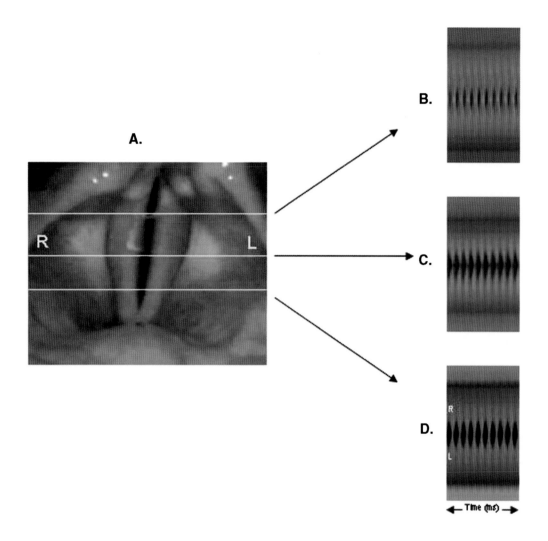

Standard vocal fold image ⟶ Multi-plane Kymography

FIGURE 7–4. Multiplane kymography from high-speed digital recording. **A.** Horizontal lines along the length of the vocal fold across to generate simultaneous multiplane kymography to compare vibratory characteristics across the anterior commissure, mid-membranous section, and posterior section of the vocal fold. **B.** Kymograph of the posterior section of the vocal fold **C.** Kymograph of the mid-membranous region. **D.** Kymograph of the anterior section of the vocal fold.

Review Questions

True or False:

1. High-speed imaging is not better than stroboscopy.

2. High-speed imaging is a research, not a clinical tool.

3. High-speed imaging and kymography give you the same information.

4. High-speed imaging depends on each and every cycle of vibration.

5. Kymographic imaging can be done with image processing software on high-speed images.

6. Kymographic imaging is unique in its ability to visualize the upper and lower lip of vibration.

REFERENCES

1. Eysholdt U, Mergell P, Tigges M, Wittenberg T, Proschel U. Direct evaluation of high-speed recordings of vocal fold vibrations. *Folia Phoniatr Logoped.* 1996;48:163–170.

2. Hertegård S. What have we learned about laryngeal physiology from high-speed digital videoendoscopy? *Curr Opin Otolaryngol Head Neck Surg.* 2005;13:152–156.

3. Colton R, Casper J. Understanding voice problems. 2nd ed. Baltimore, Md: Williams & Wilkins; 1996.

4. Hertegård S, Larsson H, Wittenberg T. High-speed imaging: applications and development. *Logoped Phoniatr Vocol.* 2003;28:133–139.

5. Fransworth DW. High-speed motion pictures of human vocal folds. *Bell Tel Rec.* 1940;18:203–208.

6. Moore P, von Leden H. Dynamic vibrations of the vibratory pattern in the normal larynx. *Folia Phonatr.* 1958;10:205–238.

7. Timcke R, von Leden H, Moore P. Laryngeal vibrations: measurements of the glottic wave. Part I.

The normal vibratory cycle. *Arch Otolaryngol.* 1958;68:1–19.

8. Timcke R, von Leden H, Moore P. Laryngeal vibrations: measurements of the glottic wave. Part II Physiologic variations. *Arch Otolaryngol.* 1969; 69:438–444.

9. von Leden H, Moore P, Timcke R. Laryngeal vibrations: measurements of the glottic wave. Part III The pathologic larynx. *Arch Otolaryngol.* 1960; 71:16–35.

10. Booth JR, Childers DG. Automated analysis of ultra high-speed laryngeal films. *IEEE Transactions Biomed Eng.* 1979;26(4):185–192.

11. Tanabe M, Kitajima K, Gould W, Lambiase A. Analysis of high-speed motion pictures of the vocal folds. *Folia Phonatr.* 1975;27:77–87.

12. Koike Y, Hirano M. Glottal area time functiona and subglottal-pressure variations. *J Acoust Soc Am.* 1973;54(6):1618–1627.

13. Wittenberg T, Mergell P, Tigges M, Eysholdt U. Quantitative characterization of functional voice disorders using motion analysis of high-speed video and modeling. *IEEE Trans.* 1997;10:1663–1666.

14. Wittenberg T, Moser M, Tigges M, Eysholdt U. Recording, processing and analysis of digital highspeed sequences in glottography. *Mach Vis Applic.* 1995;20:100–112.

15. Tigges M, Wittenberg T, Mergell P, Eysholdt U. Imaging of vocal fold vibration by digital multiplane kymography. *Comp Med Imag Graphics.* 1999;23:323–330.

16. Eysholdt U, Mergell P, Tigges M, Wittenberg T, Proschel U. Direct evaluation of high-speed recordings of vocal fold vibrations. *Folia Phoniatr Logoped.* 1996;48:163–170.

17. Kiritani S, Hirose H, Imagawa H. High-speed digital image analysis of vocal cord vibration in diplophonia. *Speech Comm.* 1993;13:23–32.

18. Larsson H, Hertegård S, Lindestad P-A, Hammarberg B. Vocal fold vibrations: high-speed imaging, kymography, and acoustic analysis; a preliminary report. *Laryngoscope.* 2000;110:2117–2122.

19. Köster O, Marx B, Gemmar, Hess M, Künzel H. Qualitative and quantitative analysis of voice onset by means of a Multidimensional Voice Analysis System (MVAS) using high-speed imaging. *J Voice.* 1998;13(3):355–374.

20. Yan Y, Ahmad K, Kunduk M, Bless D. Analysis of vocal-fold vibrations from high-speed laryngeal images using a hilbert transform-based methodology. *J Voice.* 2005;19(2):161–175.

21. Granqvist S, Hertegård S, Larsson H, Sundberg J. Simultaneous analysis of vocal fold vibration and transglottal airflow; exploring a new experimental set-up. *Speech Music Hear.* 2003;45:33–46.

22. Hoppe U, Rosanowski F, Dollinger M, Lohscheller J, Schuster M, Eysholdt U. Glissando: laryngeal motorics and acoustics. *J Voice.* 2003;17(3):370–376.

23. Jiang JJ, Yumoto E, Lin SJ, Kadota Y, Kurokawa H, Hanson DG. Quantitative measurement of mucosal wave by high-speed photography in excised larynges. *Ann Oto Rhinol Laryngol.* 1998;107: 98–103.

24. Berry DA, Montequin DW, Tayama N. High-speed digital imaging of the medial surface of the vocal folds. *J Acoust Soc Am.* 2001;110(5 pt. 1): 2539–2547.

25. Schuberth S, Hoppe U, Döllinger M, Lohscheller J, Eysholdt U. High-precision measurement of the vocal fold length and vibratory amplitudes, *Laryngoscope.* 2002;112(6):1043–1049.

26. Kiritani S, Hirose H, Imagawa H. High-speed digital image analysis of vocal cord vibration in diplophonia. *Speech Comm.* 1993;13:23–32.

27. Titze I. R. (1995). *Workshop on Acoustic Voice Analysis, Summary Statement.* Iowa City: NCVS, Wendell Johnson Speech and Hearing Center, The University of Iowa; 1995.

28. Van As CJ, Op De Coul BM, Eysholdt U, Hilgers FJ. Value of digital high-speed endoscopy in addition to videofluroscopic imaging of the neoglottis in tracheoesophageal speech. *Acta Otolaryngol.* 2004;124:82–89.

29. Lundstrom E, Hammarberg B. High-speed imaging of the voicing source in laryngectomees during production of voiced-voiceless distinctions for stop consonants. *Logoped Phoniatr Vocol.* 2004; 29(1):31–40.

30. Borch DZ, Sundberg J, Lindestad PA, Thalen M. Vocal fold vibration and voice source aperiodicity in 'dist' tones: a study of a timbral ornament in rock singing. *Logoped Phoniatr Vocol.* 2004; 29(4):147–153.

31. Lindestad PA, Sodersten M, Merker B, Granqvist S. Voice source characteristics in Mongolian "throat singing" studied with high-speed imaging technique, acoustic spectra, and inverse filtering. *J Voice.* 2001;15(1):78–85.

32. Lindestad PA, Blixt V, Olsson JP, Hammarberg B. Ventricular fold vibration in voice production: a high-speed imaging study with kymographic, acoustic and perceptual analyses of a voice patient and a vocally healthy subject. *Logoped Phoniatr Vocol.* 2004;29(4):162–170.

33. Tigges M, Wittenberg T, Mergell P, Eysholdt U. Imaging of vocal fold vibration by digital multi-plane kymography. *Comp Med Imag Graphics.* 1999;23:323–330.

34. Wittenberg T, Tigges M, Mergell P, Eysholdt U. Functional imaging of vocal fold vibration: digital multislice high-speed kymography. *J Voice.* 1997; 14(3):422–442.

35. Švec JG, Shutte HK. Videokymography: high-speed line scanning of vocal fold vibration. *J Voice.* 1996;10:201–205.

36. Tigges M, Wittenberg T, Mergell P, Eysholdt U. Imaging of vocal fold vibration by digital multi-plane kymography. *Comp Med Imag Graphics.* 1999;23:323–330.

37. Švec JG, Sram F. Kymographic imaging of the vocal fold oscillations. In: Hansen JHL, Pellom B, eds. *ICSLP-Conference proceedings.* Vol 2. 7th International Conference on Spoken Language Processing. September 16-19, 2002; Denver, Colo; Boulder, Colo: Center for Spoken Language.

38. Hirano M. *Clinical examination of voice.* 5th ed. Berlin: Springer-Verlag, 1981.

Clinical and Instrumental Evaluation of the Voice Patient

Claudio F. Milstein, PhD
Douglas M. Hicks, PhD

KEY POINTS

■ An optimal voice evaluation is accomplished by teamwork between an otolaryngologist and an SLP with expertise in voice disorders.

■ A mirror exam alone is not adequate for comprehensive evaluation of a voice patient. Videostroboscopy is the most useful instrumental tool for evaluation of voice disorders.

■ The core voice evaluation is comprised of a thorough case history, perceptual assessment, and videoendoscopic examination, complemented by other objective diagnostic techniques.

Regardless of discipline or training, all practitioners routinely employ fundamental evaluation and management methods that are not unique to the laryngology patient, such as taking a case history, generating a clinical diagnosis, and offering treatment recommendations. The focus of this chapter, however, is to address more fully components unique to the voice disordered population to maximize patient outcome and clinical efficiency.

The chapter follows the format of the management tree outlined in the next section. Some of the points are self-explanatory and require no additional comment; whereas others will be the focus of more detailed discussion.

The gold standard of clinical care for laryngology patients involves a team approach between an otolaryngologist and a speech-language pathologist (SLP) with expertise in voice care. The assumption is that the combination of both disciplines renders better treatment than can be obtained by either discipline in isolation. This philosophy is implied in a joint statement between the American Academy of Otoloaryngology and the American Speech-Language-Hearing Association.[1]

OUTLINE OF EVALUATION— MANAGEMENT TREE

1. Training requirements
2. Review of information from referral sources and previous medical records
3. Case history
   a. Questionnaire
      i. Past and present symptoms
      ii. Onset and duration
      iii. Clinical course and variability
      iv. Previous treatments
      v. Vocal symptoms
      vi. Other related symptomatology
      vii. Medical history
      viii. Medications
      ix. Tobacco, alcohol, caffeine intake
      x. Family history
      xi. Voice use
      xii. Environmental issues
      xiii. Stress/anxiety
4. Patient's perception of the problem
   a. Voice quality of life measures (eg, V-RQOL, Voice Handicap Index, VHI-10)
5. Perceptual evaluation
   a. Listen to voice quality
      i. Physical appearance, age, weight, height, facial expression
      ii. Patient interaction with clinician and others
      iii. Posture
      iv. Breathing patterns
      v. Signs of musculoskeletal tension
   b. Administer standard perceptual evaluation scales (eg, GRBAS, CAPE-V)
6. Working hypothesis
7. Head and neck evaluation
8. Laryngeal and hypopharyngeal evaluation
   a. Endoscopic
   b. Videostroboscopic
9. Diagnostic probe therapy. Concept of stimulability.
10. Objective measures
    a. Acoustic
    b. Aerodynamic
    c. EMG, Sensory testing
11. Additional testing (eg, diagnostic imaging (CT, MRI, PET, blood tests, etc)
12. Diagnosis and recommendations

Training Requirements

Routine clinical interaction with voice-disordered patients confirms that their treatment requires special training and knowledge for both otolaryngologists and SLPs. It is not sufficient to simply have a grasp of normal and pathologic anatomy of the larynx and pharynx. Beyond sound fundamentals, the practitioner must keep abreast of new developments. As previewed in chapter 2, new research related to vocal fold histology, scar formation physiology, use of new biomaterials, nerve reinnervation, and implantable devices for nerve stimulation are continually advancing the field of laryngology/vocology.

Case History

The importance of a taking a complete and thorough case history cannot be stressed enough. Even in highly motivated and insightful voice patients, their inherent naiveté about laryngeal function may influence the revelation of critical information for proper diagnosis and treatment. Therefore, the burden of uncovering this information falls to the skilled clinician with a thorough case history.

Questionnaire

An invaluable tool for case history intake is a well-organized voice-related questionnaire, which serves several purposes: (a) it allows the patient to more accurately reflect on the nature and history of his or her problem before meeting with the clinician; (b) it helps the patient recall pertinent information, some of which may not seem intuitively relevant to their voice problem (eg, thyroid function, specific asthma medicines, late night eating habits); (c) it improves efficiency for the clinician by highlighting contributing factors unique to that patient. Several excellent examples of questionnaires can be found in published textbooks.[2,3]

Problem-specific questionnaires, such as the Reflux Symptom Index[4] (see chapter 23, Reflux and Its Impact on Laryngology) can be helpful. This tool conveniently addresses a number of symptoms or complaints that might suggest the presence of laryngopharyngeal reflux, which is now perceived as important to assess and treat in voice patients.

It may be helpful to have an additional questionnaire specifically designed for singers and professional voice users. Information related to the patient's level of vocal training, performance experience, as well as his or her current and upcoming professional schedule, can affect treatment, just as in the field of sports medicine with athletes.

Patient's Perception of Problem

The current trend in health care toward treatment efficacy and outcomes parallels the value in obtaining patient perception of their vocal problem. This can be accomplished effectively with several validated quality of life instruments, such as the Voice Handicap Index (VHI) and the Voice-Related Quality of Life Questionnaire (V-RQOL).[5,6]

An obvious benefit is to help patients clarify how the current vocal problem impacts their personal and professional life. This speaks to the "functional adequacy" of their voice, which directly relates to the clinician's insight for treatment recommendations. For example, a patient whose sole motivation is reassurance that they do not have a life-threatening condition may not be interested in pursuing treatment options to improve voice quality. In contrast, there are patients whose vocal demands and expectations are sufficient so even minor hoarseness cannot be tolerated, making them almost desperate for sophisticated treatment. Ultimately, with the aid of these tools, we can clarify individual patients' specific expectation for seeking help, as well as help them define their vocal problems. In this way, the clinician can provide prescriptive care, the essence of excellent clinical practice.

An extra value of these instruments is their ability to track progress as a function of treatment, as defined by patient's perception. As an example, changes in patient's ratings over time can be highly reassuring and motivate the patient for continued compliance with treatment strategies.

Perceptual Evaluation

Listening to the patient goes beyond the obvious hearing of their voice performance. It is essential that the clinician learns to attend to the message of concern, which is always expressed by the patient in some fashion. While taking the case history, the clinician informally begins a perceptual evaluation. This requires not only carefully listening to voice quality, but monitoring physical appearance, vocal behaviors, posture, breathing patterns, signs of musculoskeletal tension, and the patient's interaction with the clinician and others.

The formal perceptual evaluation represents a protocol of eliciting representative voice performance through the use of instructions, prompts, and demonstrations. This process is facilitated by categorizing the voice into various performance parameters (pitch, loudness, laryngeal quality, and resonance). Tasks specifically designed to elicit performance in these areas are standard among clinicians, although the exact protocol varies greatly from clinician to clincian. It should be strongly stated that this important step of clinical evaluation is not an objective evaluation of the voice, but rather a formal organization of one's subjective assessment of the voice.

Characterization of voice quality in terms of severity of dysphonia and specific voice parameters (such as hoarseness, breathiness, strain) can be addressed through several published classification systems such as GRBAS scale and CAPE-V (Figure 8–1).[7,8] These have evolved in an effort to establish standardization, thereby improving reproducibility of results within and across clinicians.

Working Hypothesis

The clinician should not lose sight of the fact that all information gathered to this point is a building process leading to a working hypothesis on the nature of the problem. This requires the clinician to actively evaluate this clinical information rather than simply collect it.

By the end of the case history intake and the perceptual evaluation, the clinician should be able to establish an initial working hypothesis on the nature of the problem. The remaining instrumental/objective evaluation phase allows either the confirmation or rejection of that hypothesis. Such an approach reduces the inefficiency of examining the patient out of context—avoiding diving into an exam with a blank slate.

Laryngeal and Hypopharyngeal Evaluation

A mirror examination alone is not sufficient for evaluating the complexities of phonatory function. Thankfully, the availability of sophisticated imaging tools allows any serious practitioner with voice patients to be well equipped. In particular, videostroboscopy is routinely perceived as the most valuable tool under objective voice assessment (see chapter 6, Videostroboscopy).

An important topic that transcends any endoscopic technique is garnering optimal patient cooperation. Patient participation is fostered by careful "prescoping" instructions so the patient is fully informed of the procedure (eg, briefly review the entire protocol including nose/mouth preparation, scope insertion, duration of procedure, and anticipated physical sensations). The benefits of taking a few extra moments to accomplish this cannot be underestimated. In essence, whatever the clinician can do to make the patient relax will benefit the accuracy and completeness of differential diagnosis based on the exam. Inherent in this philosophy is the additional requirement of obtaining a representative sample of voice and phonatory function, which is only possible by enlisting patient cooperation.

Is Confidence in Perceptual Evaluation Justified?

The time-honored tradition of our clinical practice is to make informed and expert judgments of a patient's voice and larynx. This requires reliance on the auditory and visual systems of the examiner. Even with intact systems and highly trained expertise, the evaluation process is still ultimately subjective. Furthermore, it is complicated by myriad factors related to anatomy, neurology, and psychology, in addition to variability introduced by technology. The practical reality of our clinical dilemma is highlighted with a

Consensus Auditory-Perceptual Evaluation of Voice (CAPE-V)

Name: _____   Date:_____

The following parameters of voice quality will be rated upon completion of the following tasks:
1. Sustained vowels, /a/ and /i/ for 3-5 seconds duration each.
2. Sentence production:

    a. The blue spot is on the key again.   d. We eat eggs every Easter.
    b. How hard did he hit him?   e. My mama makes lemon muffins.
    c. We were away a year ago.   f. Peter will keep at the peak.

3. Spontaneous speech in response to: "Tell me about your voice problem." or "Tell me how your voice is functioning."

> **Legend:** C = Consistent   I = Intermittent
> MI = Mildly Deviant
> MO = Moderately Deviant
> SE = Severely Deviant

SCORE

Overall Severity   _____   C I   ___/100
        MI   MO   SE

Roughness   _____   C I   ___/100
        MI   MO   SE

Breathiness   _____   C I   ___/100
        MI   MO   SE

Strain   _____   C I   ___/100
        MI   MO   SE

Pitch   (Indicate the nature of the abnormality): _____
  _____   C I   ___/100
        MI   MO   SE

Loudness   (Indicate the nature of the abnormality): _____
  _____   C I   ___/100
        MI   MO   SE

_____   _____   C I   ___/100
        MI   MO   SE

_____   _____   C I   ___/100
        MI   MO   SE

COMMENTS ABOUT RESONANCE: NORMAL   OTHER (Provide description):_____
_____

ADDITIONAL FEATURES (for example, diplophonia, fry, falsetto, asthenia, aphonia, pitch instability, tremor, wet/gurgly, or other relevant terms):

Clinician:_____

FIGURE 8–1. Consensus Auditory-Perceptual Evaluation of Voice (CAPE-V).

cursory review of research studies discussing intra- and interreliability outcomes, revealing low agreement. In other words, are observations reality or illusion?

Auditory perceptual evaluation of the voice is focused on characterizing both vocal quality and degree of dysphonia. This immediately relates to the field of psychoacoustics, which confirms that subjective human perception of sounds (from simple pure tones to very complex sounds such as human speech) is very complicated. While the air pressure waves of sound can be measured very accurately with sophisticated equipment, understanding how these waves are received and mapped in the brain is not easy. This process is further complicated by the filtering role of the examiner's psyche.

The problems are compounded for the field of visual perception, which is not as advanced as psychoacoustics, secondary to less research. Processing visual input not only requires the sophisticated imprinting of illumination patterns on the retina, but involves the influence of other sensory modalities, and past experiences as well. In the field of voice, routine clinical experience suggests that visual evaluation of the severity of laryngeal disease is influenced by the associated degree of perceived dysphonia—the rating is worse when we hear a poor voice. To complicate matters, one must take into account the high variability introduced by instrumentation. Factors that can potentially affect how one rates the status of laryngeal sites and signs (eg, edema, erythema, surface irregularity) include:

- Camera adjustments
- Color versus black and white
- Monitor camera adjustments
- Image focus
- Endoscope position (angle of vision and distance of the tip of the scope to structures of interest)
- Type of endoscope (flexible versus rigid).

All these factors (visual-perceptual and technologic) may account for the generally poor intra- and interreliability scores reported in studies related to visual-perceptual observation.

This points out that technology does not ultimately solve this inherently human subjective phenomenon called perception. Improved confidence in our assessment will only come with better understanding of the processes involved through careful study. Until that time, clinicians need to exercise caution by understanding their equipment, its optimal use, paired with developing rigorous evaluation protocols.

Videolaryngoscopy/Videostroboscopy

In addition to the detailed summary presented in the chapters on stroboscopy and laryngeal imaging, it should be noted that videotaped examinations can also be used as an effective biofeedback tool. A notable example of this would be in patients with vocal cord dysfunction, where they can observe laryngeal behavior and the effects of postural changes on airway management.

Therapeutic Probes

Even within the evaluation phase of clinical management, obtaining information about therapy potential is important. This can be accomplished through a variety of stimulability tasks known as therapeutic probes. These may be similar to exercises that are part of bona fide voice therapy, but are utilized here for their prognostic value. Examples of these include humming, throat clearing, digital laryngeal manipulation, pitch and loudness shifts, lips trills, laughing, and coughing. These tasks provide a quick and effective way to predict whether a patient may be stimulable for better voice production and, therefore, a candidate for voice therapy. They also may assist in determining whether there is a functional or malingering component to the problem.

Objective Measures of Vocal Function

The role of objective measures is important but complementary to the more crucial value of the evaluation components just discussed (see Table 8-1). Objective measures never provide a conclusive diagnosis but may confirm that which is suspected based on a thorough history, evaluation, and comprehensive endoscopic evaluation. This statement is not based on personal preference but rather the reality of the current instrumentation limitations: (1) both acoustic and aerodynamic measures represent indirect information about phonatory function as they capture the product at the mouth, thus requiring inference back to the voice source; (2) current technologies are restricted to sustained phonation samples of limited dura-

TABLE 8–1. Advantages and Limitations of Objective Voice Measures

Benefits of objective measures
Provide quantitative documentation of vocal function
Help understand underlying vocal mechanism
Useful in documenting treatment efficacy and outcomes
Assist with medicolegal issues
Efficacy issues regarding health insurance/managed care issues

Words of caution
The practitioner must know the equipment and its limitations
Understand the meaning of the measures, as well as normative data
Only use appropriate tasks and protocols for each technique
Limit interpretations to the scope of the information
Use the measures to complement, not dictate, clinical judgment

tion, which do not capture either representative or complex speech samples; (3) there is lack of consensus on the mathematical algorithms (eg, jitter) that generate the numerical values recorded; and (4) there is unevenness in the normative information against which a patient's profile can be compared—this is particularly true for aerodynamic measures. Although these current observations justify caution in the confidence of objective measures for everyday clinical practice, continued research may foster legitimate utility in the future. Nonetheless, it is important to be familiar with the terminology and the theoretical basis of each measure's utility in laryngology.

The following is a representative list of measures used in clinical practice and purported to be beneficial. Specific endorsement is difficult as particular selections are a function of patient population, clinician expertise, equipment availability, room acoustics, and personal preference.

Acoustic Measures (Christine M. Sapienza, personal communications, 2006)

- **Fundamental frequency (F_0)**—directly reflects the vibration rate of the vocal folds. It is the acoustic correlate of pitch.
  - unit of measure is hertz (Hz) or cycles per second
  - normative data = 100–150 Hz males; 180–250 Hz females
  - may be measured from sustained vowels, reading, or conversation
  - useful to estimate the appropriateness of F_0 for sex and age and for demonstrating pre- and post-treatment change

- **Frequency variability**—pitch sigma is the standard deviation of the fundamental frequency.
  - assesses and documents variation of F_0 during speech production

- **Phonation range**—range of frequencies from the highest to the lowest that a patient can produce.
  - may be expressed in Hz or semitones
  - normal young adults have about a 3-octave range; may vary with practice

- **Frequency perturbation**—the change of frequency from one successive period to the next.
  - unit of measurement is *jitter*; several algorithms are used to extract jitter; normative data for jitter percent is less than 1.00%
  - measures must be made from sustained vowels
  - may represent variation of vocal fold mass, tension, muscle activity, or neural activity, all of which may affect the periodicity of vocal fold vibration

- **Amplitude perturbation**—small cycle-to-cycle changes of the amplitude of the vocal fold signal.
  - unit of measurement is *shimmer*; several algorithms are used to extract shimmer; normative data for shimmer dB is less than 0.35 dB
  - measures must be made from sustained vowels
  - may represent variation of vocal fold mass, tension, muscle activity, or neural activity, all of which may affect the amplitude of vocal fold vibration

- **Intensity (I_0)**—directly reflects the sound pressure level (SPL) of voice. The direct correlate of loudness.
  - unit of measure is the logarithmic decibel (dB) scale
  - may be measured from sustained vowels, reading, or conversation
  - useful as pre- and post-treatment measure

- **Overall sound pressure level (SPL)**—average SPL in dB.
  - indication of the strength of vocal fold vibration (Norms: 75–80 dB conversation)

- **Amplitude variability**—standard deviation of the SPL during connected speech.
  - reflects loudness variability
  - Dynamic range—range of vocal intensities that a person can produce (Norms: 50–115 dB SPL).

- **Harmonics-to-noise ratio (H/N)**—a ratio measure of the energy in the voice signal over the noise energy; may be derived from different algorithms and expressed in various units.
  - greater signal or harmonic energy in the voice reflects better voice quality
  - large noise energy represents more abnormal function

- **Voice range profile (phonetogram)**—plots maximum and minimum intensities for entire frequency range.
  - resulting plot is ellipsoid-shaped frequency/intensity profile and the dimensions are expressed in semitones
  - most useful in pre- and post-treatment of professional voice users

- **Spectral analysis**—a sound spectrogram displays the glottal sound source and filtering characteristics across time.

- both formant frequency energy (vocal tract resonance) and noise components (aperiodicity) are presented in a three-dimensional scale
- horizontal axis = time
- vertical axis = frequency (lowest band = F_0; formants are above)
- gray scale (darkness) represents intensity change

Aerodynamic measures

- **Volume (vital capacity)**—available volume of air in the lungs.
  - measured in liters, will vary with age, sex, size, health
  - measured with a spirometer

- **Airflow rate**—rate at which air passes through the glottis during phonation.
  - measured in liters/sec, with normal rate = 50–200 ml/sec
  - Flow transducer

- **Maximum phonation time (MPT)**—maximum time that a vowel may be sustained while using maximum airflow volume.
  - will vary with lung capacity, age, sex, size, health

- **Subglottal air pressure (Psub)**—measure of air pressure beneath the vocal folds necessary to overcome the resistance of the approximated folds to initiate and maintain phonation.
  - measured in cm/H_2O with norm for conversational voice being 3–7 cm/H_2O
  - intraoral pressure measures reflective of Psub
  - vocal fold stiffness, hypo/ hyperfunction, incomplete glottic closure will influence Psub

- **Laryngeal (glottal) resistance**—this is a calculated measure that utilizes measures of pressure and flow in a ratio. Laryngeal resistance is the quotient of peak intraoral air pressure (from unvoiced plosive) divided by the peak flow rate (measured from a vowel) as measured from a repeated consonant + vowel syllable such as /pi/pi/pi/.
  - estimates the overall resistance of the glottis and therefore the valving characteristics (ie, too tight, too loose, normal)

- **Phonation threshold pressure (PTP)**—a measure of the effort needed to initiate phonation.
  - measure is estimated indirectly using intraoral air pressure measured at the exact moment of voice onset for barely audible phonation
  - speakers with vocal pathologies often require greater effort to initiate phonation

- **Aerodynamic recording considerations:**
  - requires airtight seals around the lips or mask to face.
  - as natural speech as possible must be encouraged in this environment.
  - multiple trials are necessary to ensure a stable baseline.
  - instrument calibration is required prior to each examination session.

Diagnosis and Recommendations

The essential final component of a comprehensive voice evaluation involves counseling with the patient, providing conclusions, recommendations, and prognosis. Whether stated or not, the patient is assumed to be looking for answers to his or her problems in terms of "what's wrong, why is it wrong, and how do we fix it?" This places a burden of completeness on the clinician to satisfy this request through careful explanation using language appropriate for the patient's level. It is understood that success with this step requires an atmosphere of time and availability for patient comfort. In general, all voice disorders are treated through a combination of the four following options: behavioral (voice therapy, lifestyle changes, vocal hygiene, dietary modifications, as well as other complementary therapies like relaxation, biofeedback, or psychotherapy), medical therapy, and surgical intervention, or a combination of the three. This paradigm is repeated throughout this book for each of the specific laryngeal disorders presented. Finally, and frequently overlooked, is a definitive statement of prognosis. It is important to inform the patient as to the expected outcome both with and without treatment.

Review Questions

1. Can one get a representative sample of voice with sustained phonation tasks?

2. Is there value in utilizing therapeutic probes during the first evaluation contact with a voice disordered patient?

3. Can a diagnosis be reached based only on acoustic and aerodynamic measures?

4. Can a professional's original training suffice for adequate care of voice patients for an entire career?

REFERENCES

1. American Speech-Language-Hearing Association. (1998). Roles of otolaryngologists and speech-language pathologists in the performance and interpretation of strobovideolaryngoscopy. *ASHA.* 1998;40(suppl 18):32.

2. Loeh Koschkee D, Rammage L. *Voice Care in the Medical Setting.* San Diego, Calif: Singular Publishing Group; 1997.

3. Sataloff RT. *Vocal Health and Pedagogy.* San Diego, Calif: Singular Publishing Group; 1998.

4. Belafsky PC, Postma GN, Koufmann JA. Laryngopharyngeal reflux symptoms improve before changes in physical findings. *Laryngoscope.* 2001;111:979–981.

5. Hogikyan ND, Sethuraman G. Validation of an instrument to measure voice-related quality of life (V-RQOL). *J Voice.* 1999;13(4):557–567.

6. Jacobson BH, Johnson A, Grywalski C, et al. The Voice Handicap Index (VHI): development and validation. *Am J Speech Lang Pathol.* 1997;6:66–70.

7. Hirano M. *Clinical Examination of Voice.* New York, NY: Springer Verlag; 1981:83–84.

8. American Speech-Language-Hearing Association (ASHA). Consensus Auditory-Perceptual Evaluation of Voice (CAPE-V). 2003 document text available from: http://www.asha.org.

Laryngeal Electromyography

Nicole Maronian, MD
Lawrence Robinson, MD

KEY POINTS

■ Laryngeal EMG can diagnose old versus new injuries to the laryngeal musculature and provide information about recovery.

■ Prognosis for recovery of recurrent laryngeal lesions remains an area of intense research effort. Key factors in eventual recovery are likely the early presence of insertional activity and motor unit action potentials under voluntary control.

■ Laryngeal dystonia is a disorder involving multiple laryngeal muscles. Fine-wire EMG provides a "roadmap" to document the most involved muscles and assist with treatment planning.

■ Laryngeal dysmotility and immobility can be related to multiple factors. LEMG is the only method to definitively diagnose a neurologic cause for impaired vocal fold movement.

■ The percentage of recruitment of the laryngeal muscles in a recovering injury is helpful in understanding the degree of nerve injury. The ability to reliably quantify recruitment by multiple practitioners may be challenging and should be actively evaluated.

This chapter focuses on the diagnostic capabilities of laryngeal electromyography (LEMG) as part of the workup and treatment of laryngeal disorders. Utilization of LEMG as well as techniques are discussed.

Electromyography provides the capability to detect electrical activity in muscles. In the case of the larynx, use of LEMG allows the practitioner to deduce information about the status of the efferent motor nerve or the recurrent laryngeal nerve (RLN), as well as the superior laryngeal nerve (SLN) and the laryngeal muscles they supply. Essentially, it can detect loss of neurons innervating a muscle. Utilizing muscle testing, information about prior injury, recovery from injury, or stability of RLN injury can be surmised. The testing provides reproducible patterns of muscle activity that can be combined with clinical information to provide a more robust understanding of the etiology of hoarseness or swallowing dysfunction.

Performing LEMG requires specialized equipment and ideally a combined effort between laryngologist and electromyographer. A standard EMG machine that can record muscle recordings either in digital or paper form is optimal. The team approach combines the expertise of the laryngologist in needle placement with the expertise of the electromyographer in interpretation of complex muscle activity patterns. Certification in electromyography requires 6 months full-time training and subspecialty boards. Thus, the team approach provides maximal information, interpretation, and reliability of the LEMG exam. Furthermore, physician expertise greatly increases with experience and time spent working as a team. Due to the complexity of interpretation, and because patient responses cannot be anticipated, the laryngologist needs to be present throughout the examination.

Laryngeal EMG was initially described in 1944 by Weddell in four patients in whom he attempted to characterize the cause of their laryngeal injury.[1] Just one year later, the first EMG machine made specifically for clinical use was introduced.[2,3] Electromyography of the limb muscles advanced steadily with eventual acceptance as the gold standard for muscle testing following injury, providing both vital diagnostic and prognostic information.

Laryngeal EMG was advanced in the 1950s by Faaborg-Andersen when he published a study detailing testing of multiple laryngeal muscles.[4] He documented muscle activity during voiced and unvoiced tasks, such as swallowing.[4] Hirano, in 1969, described the techniques currently utilized for localization of the laryngeal muscles during routine testing.[5] Concomitant with improved understanding of the electrodiagnostic findings in muscle injury, LEMG was utilized by investigators in research capacities to better understand speech production, effects of immobility, and swallow function.[6,7] In the late 1980s, LEMG became a clinical tool utilized for assessment of voice disorders and for localization of the laryngeal muscles for botulinum toxin injection in adductor laryngeal dystonia.[8,9]

EMG BASICS FOR LARYNGOLOGISTS

EMG Findings

The primary EMG responses evaluated for diagnostic and prognostic purpose include insertional activity, recruitment, denervation, reinnervation, and central response. Signs of peripheral injury are outlined with reference to central injury signs at the end of this section.

Insertional activity is the muscle activity initially identified upon advancement into a relaxed muscle. By advancing the EMG needle into the muscle, the individual muscle fibers are mechanically stimulated resulting in brief bursts of electrical activity exhibited as motor unit action potentials (MUAPs) (Figure 9–1). This pattern of response is present in normal and partially denervated muscle. In severely denervated muscle it is lacking and indicates a complete paralysis of the muscle, possibly with overlying fibrosis.

Testing then revolves around the appropriate voluntary **recruitment task** for the muscle. In the case of the adductor muscles, the thyroarytenoid, lateral cricoarytenoid, and interarytenoid, recruitment is tested by asking the patient to repeat /i/, /i/, /i/. The EMG recording shows brisk recruitment of multiple muscle fibers in response to each of the speech bursts (Figure 9-2).

Evidence of loss of neuron supply to a denervated muscle can be ascertained by specific muscle responses. **Denervation** results in spontaneous muscle fiber action potentials that occur without voluntary control while the muscle is at rest called fibrillations (Figure 9-3). They typically appear about 2 to 3 weeks following injury. Positive sharp waves are similar types of action

potentials and typically precede fibrillations by several days (Figure 9-4). This pattern will remain until regeneration begins to occur or persist in the event of severe, irreparable injury. If a muscle becomes fibrotic, loss of these activity patterns, along with loss of insertional activity, may occur. In a densely denervated muscle, no electrical activity may be seen with attempts at voluntary activation with both voice and nonvoice tasks (eg, swallow, Valsalva) (Figure 9-5). If this response is elicited greater than 1 to 2 years from injury, a permanent paralysis is diagnosed without likely ongoing recovery.

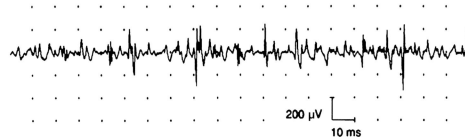

FIGURE 9–1. Normal motor unit action potentials (MUAP).

200 µV

10 ms

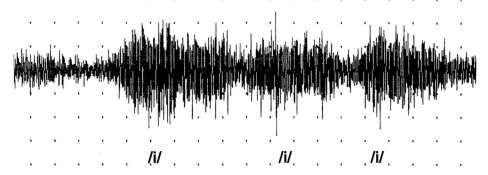

FIGURE 9–2. Normal recruitment with repeated /i/ phonation.

/i/   /i/   /i/

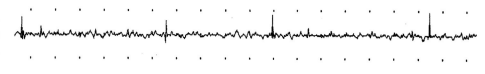

FIGURE 9–3. Denervation with fibrillations.

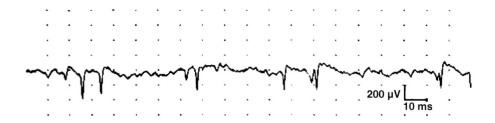

FIGURE 9–4.
Denervation pattern with positive sharp waves.

Note: By convention, the lower half of the EMG tracing is "positive," while the upper half is "negative."

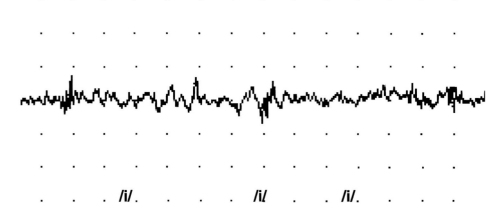

FIGURE 9–5.
Complete denervation without regeneration.

Reinnervation can occur by two different mechanisms, depending on severity of the lesion. In partial lesions, the remaining intact axons can sprout distally to reinnervate newly denervated muscle fibers, thus enlarging the existing motor unit territory. In complete lesions, axons may regrow from the point of injury to reinnervate the denervated muscle fibers. EMG evidence of reinnervation in partial lesions presents with muscle findings of polyphasic motor unit action potentials (MUAPs). These new sprouting fibers are not yet fully myelinated and thus conduct more slowly than mature nerve fibers. As the axons do not conduct at uniform speed, the motor unit becomes desynchronized and has multiple phases, characteristically more than five baseline crossings and a wider duration than a normal MUAP (Figure 9-6). Polyphasic MUAPs are signs of ongoing regeneration. They may recruit with voluntary contraction if an

adequate amount of regeneration has occurred. In complete denervation, no motor units will initially recruit. Later, as axons reach the muscle, small polyphasic MUAPs, representing just a few muscle fibers, will be recruited. Over time, these will become larger and polyphasic.

Chronically, as the new nerve sprouts mature and myelinate, they begin to conduct at faster rates. The peaks, as well as the width of the MUAP, diminish as the muscle fibers begin to discharge more synchronously. The amplitude of the response (height) increases, however, as each motor unit now contains a larger number of active muscle fibers. This unit is now called a large-amplitude MUAP. These potentials indicate a stable, chronic injury that recruits with voluntary contraction tasks. The greater the number of motor units present, the greater the degree of reinnervation that has occurred. Even though fewer units may be present, they typically fire at appropriate or faster speeds in attempts to compensate for the peripheral injury. The term, "few firing fast" implies a stable peripheral process. Large MUAPs remain indefinitely as a sign of muscle injury (Figure 9-7).

Central injuries with intact peripheral recurrent laryngeal nerves can present with essentially normal MUAPs. The central nervous system, however, acts to coordinate the peripheral response.

Thus, rate and coordination of response at the laryngeal level can be affected. Typically, with poor central nervous system control, fewer MUAPs are able to be recruited and they fire at a slow rate (Figure 9-8). In normal recruitment the individual motor units cannot be identified due to their large number and varied appearance (see Figure 9-2) With a central pattern, the motor units are sparse and slow in response because of

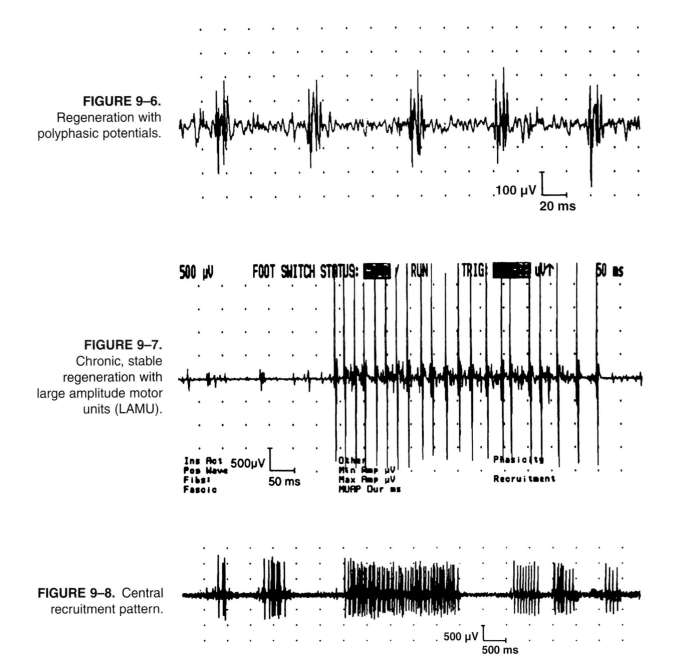

FIGURE 9–6. Regeneration with polyphasic potentials.

100 μV

20 ms

FIGURE 9–7. Chronic, stable regeneration with large amplitude motor units (LAMU).

500 μV   FOOT SWITCH STATUS: ███ / RUN | TRIG ███ μV | 50 ms

Ins Act   500μV
Pos Wave
Fibs!   50 ms
Fascic

Other
Min Amp μV
Max Amp μV
MUAP Dur ms

Phasicity

Recruitment

FIGURE 9–8. Central recruitment pattern.

500 μV

500 ms

the reduction in upper motor neuron drive. Identifying the exact upper motor neuron process based on EMG response alone is challenging. Incorporation of clinical data and further neurologic testing is typically diagnostic.

Types of EMG

Two types of EMG, needle and fine-wire (FW-EMG), are currently utilized clinically to assist in diagnosis and treatment. Needle laryngeal EMG (LEMG) is performed primarily for evaluation of MUAPs in the setting of a vocal fold dysmotility or immobility. It allows for assessment of muscle recruitment and individual MUAP characteristics. LEMG recordings can be obtained from monopolar or concentric needle electrodes. The monopolar electrodes derive signals from all surrounding motor units providing information from approximately 10 motor units at one time. This is the most common method utilized to understand what is happening in the larger context of the laryngeal muscle being tested. Bipolar or single-fiber EMG recording details firing information from one to two motor fibers, thus giving more in-depth information about individual MUAPs. Controversy remains regarding the best method of testing using either monopolar or bipolar electrodes. Many laryngologists are familiar with using a monopolar botulinum toxin injection needle and thus utilize this same needle for their EMG procedures. Upcoming vector EMG techniques combine the ability to obtain both individual muscle fiber and composite information across the muscle simultaneously. Although currently it remains primarily a research tool, it holds promise as a more well-rounded method of characterizing injury to the intrinsic laryngeal musculature.[10]

FW-EMG utilizes fine 30-gauge hooked wire electrodes. This allows for placement within the muscle in a fixed position which combats the effects of needle dislodgement with swallowing, voicing, or coughing. The FW-EMG is optimally utilized when testing speech versus simple phonatory tasks. The FW-EMG can test multiple muscles simultaneously. It is typically utilized to define muscle involvement in spasmodic dysphonia and can be utilized when testing for laryngeal synkinesis to determine timing of muscle activation and overactive, inappropriate muscle involvement.[5,7]

TECHNIQUE

Needle LEMG is typically performed with the patient in the supine position with the neck in gentle extension. The laryngologist either sits at the side of the patient's neck or above the patient's head in the same position utilized for direct laryngoscopy in the operating room. A monopolar testing needle is typically a 27-gauge hollow bore Teflon-coated injection needle attached to a tuberculin (1-cc) slip-tip syringe. This needle is familiar to most laryngologists given that it is utilized with botulinum toxin injection. The addition of the syringe allows for increased length of the needle and improved angulation to access the laryngeal muscles under the thyroid cartilage.

The testing can stimulate coughing if the needle is introduced immediately below the subglottic mucosa. Coughing can be avoided by either placing the needle lateral to the mucosa or by performing a transtracheal block with 1 cc of 2% plain Xylocaine.

Muscle testing can then proceed based on techniques previously described by Hirano.[5] The thyroarytenoid (TA) muscle is approached via the cricothyroid (CT) space. It is important to stay strictly in the midline. The needle is advanced with steady light pressure through the CT membrane with EMG guidance. One feels a loss of resistance as the CT membrane is penetrated. Once the needle tip is past the CT membrane, inserting the needle at a 15- to 30-degree angle laterally and superiorly will result in strong TA muscle activity. In the female larynx, the vocal fold is typically lower and more lateral than in the male due to their small and broader laryngeal framework. Once the needle encounters muscle, the EMG signal will dampen and transmit muscle signal. The needle should be advanced until sharp recruitment is identified. Voluntary testing of this muscle is achieved by repetitive /i/ phonation, which should reveal sharp bursts of activity on the EMG monitor.

The interarytenoid (IA) muscle is approached by placing the needle through the CT membrane and then into airspace (with an open channel electrical finding). Staying in the midline, the needle is advanced posteriorly until it reaches the posterior cricoid. The EMG signal will again dampen as tissue is reached. The examiner then advances the needle slowly upward ("walking up the posterior cricoid") until the needle falls over the superior cricoid edge into the IA muscle. A burst of muscle activity will be identified. The patient will also note more sensitivity in this area perhaps due to the greater sensory innervation at the posterior glottis. Testing again occurs with repetitive /i/ phonation to activate the adductor muscle with repeated bursts visualized on the EMG. The IA is typically felt to have bilateral innervation; however, distinct differences may be apparent even in unilateral lesions.[11]

The posterior cricoarytenoid (PCA) muscle can be reached either via the CT membrane or from a lateral approach. It can be tested along with the TA and IA using the same needle insertion. Once the needle is in the airspace, the needle is directed laterally, maintaining the same level as the CT membrane. The EMG signal is dampened as the posterior cricoid is encountered. The needle can often be advanced through the cartilage into the PCA muscle with signs of MUAPs on the EMG. In some patients, the cricoid cannot be reached due to the limits of the EMG needle or advanced through the cricoid due to calcification. In that setting, the PCA is approached laterally. The larynx is grasped and rotated to one side. The lateral edge of the thyroid lamina is palpated. The EMG needle is inserted at the lower lateral border of the larynx and advanced inferiorly and medially toward the posterior cricoid until insertional activity is identified. Appropriate testing involves asking the patient to sniff three times and observing three bursts of activity on the EMG monitor.

The cricothyroid (CT) and lateral cricoarytenoid (LCA) muscles can be approached with one needle insertion. The CT membrane is identified and the needle advanced approximately one centimeter off midline. With insertion through the skin, the CT muscle is encountered. Testing for this muscle requires the patient to phonate with a low-pitched /i/, followed by a high-pitched /i/. The motor unit recruitment will increase significantly during high-pitched phonation. If no increase in recruitment is identified, then the needle may be in the strap muscle and the patient should be asked to elevate the head. If activity increases with this maneuver, then further redirection of the needle toward the CT membrane should occur.

The LCA muscle is localized after CT testing is complete. The needle is then advanced through the CT membrane, laterally and slightly upward. The muscle is encountered and demonstrates active recruitment with repetitive /i/ phonation only at the initiation of the phonation.

UTILIZATION OF EMG IN CLINICAL PRACTICE

LEMG plays a vital role in the laryngologist's diagnostic armamentarium. LEMG is a direct extension of the laryngologist's physical exam of laryngeal motion seen on an endoscopic examination. LEMG is the only modality that can discern between complete paralysis and denervation of the RLN, versus cricoarytenoid joint fixation/scar as the etiologies of an immobile vocal fold.[12,13] It can also diagnose synkinesis within the larynx. Synkinesis occurs after a peripheral nerve injury when a nerve carries muscle activity to multiple muscles. In the larynx, the RLN carries adducting fibers to the TA and LCA muscles and abducting fibers to the PCA. With synkinesis of the larynx, these fibers become crossed in a reinnervation state resulting in a hemilarynx with immobility and good muscle tone.[14]

EMG can be utilized to determine the timing of a permanent rehabilitative procedure to the vocal folds. In the acute setting of vocal fold immobility, limited information can be gleaned about eventual recovery based on the overall lack of muscle response during very early injury. After 4 to 6 weeks, some practitioners begin utilizing EMG for prognostication of eventual recovery with 44% specificity.[15] Overall, most investigators have reported variability in correct prediction of recovery utilizing early EMG.[11,16] However, the predictive nature of laryngeal EMG in patients 3 months out from injury has not been thoroughly studied.

Unfortunately, EMG can provide only one time point in the determination of neuromuscu-lar regeneration. Thus, in injuries at a significant distance from the larynx, the regenerating axons may simply not have reached the intrinsic muscles which would result in a change in the type of motor units seen on EMG. Thus, findings on EMG may continue to show dense denervation, thereby overestimating the extent of injury if EMG is performed early. Multiple EMGs spaced out several weeks to months or an EMG at 4 to

---

Controversy: Laryngeal Reinnervation

The role of laryngeal reinnervation remains controversial in patients with vocal fold paralysis and is intimately associated with the debate over laryngeal synkinesis. As the RLN carries adductor and abductor fibers into the laryngeal muscles and branches immediately prior to the entrance into the larynx, significant injury to the RLN results in damage to both types of motor fibers. If the neural tubules remain intact, as occurs in a mild injury (eg, traction injury, mild thermal injury, compression), the proximal axons will find the appropriate target muscle and full recovery of muscle tone and appropriate function will occur. However, in patients with more profound RLN injury, nerve regeneration into the appropriate target muscle may be limited or absent. Those who argue for routine laryngeal reinnervation for patients with persistent immobility 9 to 12 months after an RLN injury assume that those patients have failed to develop a full neural recovery, have inadequate reinnervation, and would benefit from a reinnervation procedure. However, many believe that the majority of those patients have adequate muscle tone due to a synkinetic reinnervation pattern and would not benefit further by routine laryngeal reinnervation, therefore, a static medialization/augmentation is the procedure of choice. In a review of 75 patients with unilateral vocal folds paresis, only 19% of the patients demonstrated a severe level of denervation on preoperative LEMG.[30] In contrast, another study evaluated evoked EMG in patients prior to laryngeal reinnervation.[31] In this study, 15 patients with a clinical diagnosis of vocal cord "paralysis" (no preoperative diagnostic laryngeal electromyography), were tested intraoperatively for an evoked RLN response using either surface EMG via a custom endotracheal tube or bipolar concentric needles with direct stimulation of the RLN. In this study, only one patient demonstrated an evoked potential while a control group of eight patients undergoing thyroidectomy demonstrated a normal evoked potential. This clinical problem requires greater study.

6 months following initial injury will likely be more helpful in prognosticating recovery.[15] If early intervention is required for issues of aspiration or vocal requirements, then EMG can provide some guidance and reassurance particularly if early signs of recruitment are lacking. It does not, however, exclude that eventuality and ongoing recovery may occur over the next year. Clearly, the earlier that more favorable EMG signs are present (ie, preserved MUAPs with voluntary brisk recruitment), the more likely spontaneous recovery. However, lack of voluntary recruitment even at 6 months, does not preclude eventual recovery if the location of the lesion is near the skull base or the proximal aspect of the vagus nerve. The location of the lesion must be calculated into the therapeutic decision-making when applying EMG information to specific patients. In addition, the clinical interpretation of the EMG must be coordinated with the clinical findings and location of injury. For example, in patients with a vocal fold paresis after a left carotid endarterectomy, the length of time prior to reinnervation and return of motion will be much longer than in a patient who has sufferered a right vocal fold paresis after thyroidectomy.

Final characterization of the neurophysiologic state of the vocal fold yields one of the following:

1. Dense denervation with no voluntary activity which can now be termed vocal fold paralysis.
2. Partial reinnervation with diminished motor units. This can range from very few units, indicating a severe peripheral nerve lesion, to many units with robust recruitment, indicating a mild injury.
3. Normal recruitment with complete recovery.

Varying degrees of reinnervation in vocal fold recovery is much more common than complete denervation.[17] The degree of reinnervation required to achieve paretic versus normal function remains unclear. A limb muscle that has sustained up to 45% MUAP loss may preserve the appearance of near-normal mobility or strength on clinical examination.[18] In the setting of a limb paresis, partial to near normal reinnervation would be anticipated with a 50% neural injury.

It is helpful to judge the percentage of recruitment with voluntary activity. This has implications for eventual recovery and treatment planning. If near-normal recruitment is identified with standard testing but no movement is identified, then synkinesis should be suspected. If recruitment is zero or less than 10%, then reinnervation techniques should be considered.

Given that the RLN is a mixed nerve carrying abductor and adductor fibers, the consequences of a misdirected reinnervation can be significant.[19,20] This can result in a reinnervated but immobile vocal fold due to synkinesis. With simultaneous firing of the abductors and adductors, the vocal fold cannot move against these antagonistic muscle forces. The EMG definitions of synkinesis are divided into abductor and adductor types. Abductor synkinesis is commonly agreed upon to reflect PCA recruitment with phonation which is clearly abnormal.[14,19] Adductor synkinesis definitions are more challenging and variable in the literature due to the multiple glottic tasks that require TA activation.[14,19] The definition should reflect the normal function of the TA in comparison to its abnormal activation and remains an area of intense research interest.[14] Synkinesis does supply neuronal input to the vocal fold, thus resulting in improved bulk and tone and often more midline position with an upright arytenoid.[21]

Treatment decision-making will also change based on the presence of synkinesis and degree of reinnervation. In a planned therapeutic, laryngeal reinnervation procedure, the anticipated outcome is a synkinetic vocal fold that does not move but is improved in muscle tone and possibly improved position without need for a medialization implant. This approach utilizes a nonlaryngeal nerve to achieve new nerve supply to the intrinsic laryngeal muscles.[22-26] However, if a significant degree of reinnervation has occurred naturally, it is unlikely that new nerve ingrowth will be accepted by an already partially innervated muscle.[17] This has led some authors to propose that a vocal fold that is severely and permanently denervated would be the best reinnervation candidate. Other patients with partial denervation would best be served with a static repositioning procedure such as medialization with or without an arytenoid adduction suture.[21]

FW-EMG with fixed hooked-wire electrodes can also be utilized for patients with laryngeal dystonia to characterize muscle involvement and direct treatment with botulinum toxin.[27,28] In the setting of adductor laryngeal dystonia, routine testing of the TA, LCA, and IA muscles can provide a "roadmap" of predominant muscle involvement. This has been utilized to direct botulinum toxin therapy, particularly in patients less responsive to standard treatment protocols.[7,29]

EMG is a valuable adjunct to clinical decision-making in management of vocal fold movement disorders. Utilization, however, cannot occur in a vacuum. It requires amalgamation of clinical history, exam, patient needs, and EMG findings to determine the diagnosis and best treatment choice for each individual patient. It is limited by issues including patient tolerance, physician expertise, needle placement, and our present day understanding of neurolaryngeal reinnervation. Expertise in this area develops with repeated utilization and thus requires the investment of time by the laryngologist in combination with a skilled electromyographer. EMG used in context of other clinical information provides the crucial diagnosis, which cannot be gleaned from simple endoscopic observation of the vocal folds. As technical advances improve our understanding of neurophysiology, our ability to use EMG as a measurement of function will only improve our ability to care for patients with laryngeal disease.

Review Questions

1. The type of EMG utilized for diagnostic workup of vocal fold immobility or dysmotility is:
   a. needle EMG
   b. fine-wire EMG

2. In a stable, severe, longstanding paralysis of the recurrent laryngeal EMG, one may see the following EMG characteristics:
   a. fibrillations
   b. polyphasic potentials
   c. few, if any, motor unit action potentials
   d. poor insertional activity
   e. all of the above

3. EMG findings not consistent with vocal fold paresis include:
   a. polyphasic potentials
   b. reduced recruitment
   c. lack of insertional activity
   d. large motor unit action potentials

4. Adductor laryngeal dystonia involves which of the following muscles:
   a. TA
   b. LCA
   c. IA
   d. PCA

5. Laryngeal synkinesis of the abductor muscles is characterized by EMG as follows:
   a. PCA activation with phonation
   b. PCA activity with respiration
   c. TA and PCA activity with phonation
   d. cannot be characterized by EMG

REFERENCES

1. Weddell G, Feinstein B, Paattle R. The electrical activity of voluntary muscle in man under normal and pathological conditions. *Brain.* 1944;67:178–242.
2. Golseth JG. Diagnostic contributions of the electromyogram. *Calif Med.* 1950;73:355–357.
3. Golseth JG. Electromyographic examination in the office. *Calif Med.* 1957;87:298–300.
4. Faaborg-Andersen K. Electromyographic investigation of intrinsic laryngeal muscles in humans. *Acta Physiol Scand.* 1957;41:1–150.

5. Hirano MJ. Use of hooked-wire electrodes for electromyography of the intrinsic laryngeal muscles. *J Speech Hear Res*. 1969;12:363-373.

6. Sataloff RT, Mandel S, Mann EA, Ludlow CL. Laryngeal electromyography: an evidence-based review. *Muscle Nerve*. 2003;28:767-772.

7. Hillel AD. The study of laryngeal muscle activity in normal human subjects and in patients with laryngeal dystonia using multiple fine-wire electromyography. *Laryngoscope*. 2001;111:1-47.

8. Ludlow CL, Naunton RF, Sedory SE, Schulz GM, Hallett M. Effects of botulinum toxin injections on speech in adductor spasmodic dysphonia. *Neurology*. 1988;38:1220-1225.

9. Blitzer A, Lovelace RE, Brin MF, Fahn S, Fink ME. Electromyographic findings in focal laryngeal dystonia (spastic dysphonia). *Ann Otol Rhinol Laryngol*. 1985;94:591-594.

10. Roark RM, Li JC, Schaefer SD, Adam A, De Luca CJ. Multiple motor unit recordings of laryngeal muscles: the technique of vector laryngeal electromyography. *Laryngoscope*. 2002;112:2196-2203.

11. Min YB, Finnegan EM, Hoffman HT, Luschei ES, McCulloch TM. A preliminary study of the prognostic role of electromyography in laryngeal paralysis. *Otolaryngol Head Neck Surg*. 1994;111:770-775.

12. Koufman JA, Postma GN, Whang CS, et al. Diagnostic laryngeal electromyography: The Wake Forest experience 1995-1999. *Otolaryngol Head Neck Surg*. 2001;124:603-606.

13. Rontal E, Rontal M, Silverman B, Kileny PR. The clinical differentiation between vocal cord paralysis and vocal cord fixation using electromyography. *Laryngoscope*. 1993;103:133-137.

14. Maronian NC, Robinson L, Waugh P, Hillel AD. A new electromyographic definition of laryngeal synkinesis. *Ann Otol Rhinol Laryngol*. 2004;113:877-886.

15. Munin MC, Rosen CA, Zullo T. Utility of laryngeal electromyography in predicting recovery after vocal fold paralysis. *Arch Phys Med. Rehabil*. 2003;84:1150-1153.

16. Gupta SR, Bastian RW. Use of laryngeal electromyography in prediction of recovery after vocal cord paralysis. *Muscle Nerve*. 1993;16:977-978.

17. Woodson GE. Configuration of the glottis in laryngeal paralysis. II: Animal experiments. *Laryngoscope*. 1993;103:1235-1241.

18. Beasley WC. Quantitative muscle testing. Principles and applications to research and clinic services. *Arch Phys Med*. 1961;42:398-425.

19. Crumley RL. Laryngeal synkinesis: its significance to the laryngologist. *Ann Otol Rhinol Laryngol*. 1989;98:87-92.

20. Blitzer A, Jahn AF, Keidar A. Semon's law revisited: an electromyographic analysis of laryngeal synkinesis. *Ann Otol Rhinol Laryngol*. 1996;105:764-769.

21. Maronian N, Waugh P, Robinson L, Hillel A. Electromyographic findings in recurrent laryngeal nerve reinnervation. *Ann Otol Rhinol Laryngol*. 2003;112:314-323.

22. Chhetri DK, Berke GS. Ansa cervicalis nerve: review of the topographic anatomy and morphology. *Laryngoscope*. 1997;107:1366-1372.

23. Crumley RL. Update: ansa cervicalis to recurrent laryngeal nerve anastomosis for unilateral laryngeal paralysis. *Laryngoscope*. 1991;101:384-387; discussion 388.

24. Paniello RC. Laryngeal reinnervation with the hypoglossal nerve: II. Clinical evaluation and early patient experience. *Laryngoscope*. 2000;110:739-748.

25. Tucker HM. Long-term results of nerve-muscle pedicle reinnervation for laryngeal paralysis. *Ann Otol Rhinol Laryngol*. 1989;98:674-676.

26. Zheng H, Li Z, Zhou S, Cuan Y, Wen W. Update: laryngeal reinnervation for unilateral vocal cord paralysis with the ansa cervicalis. *Laryngoscope*. 1996;106:1522-1527.

27. Maronian NC, Waugh PF, Robinson L, Hillel AD. Tremor laryngeal dystonia: treatment of the lateral cricoarytenoid muscle. *Ann Otol Rhinol Laryngol*. 2004;113:349-355.

28. Hillel AD, Maronian NC, Waugh PF, Robinson L, Klotz DA. Treatment of the interarytenoid muscle with botulinum toxin for laryngeal dystonia. *Ann Otol Rhinol Laryngol*. 2004;113:341-348.

29. Klotz DA, Maronian NC, Waugh PF, Shahinfar A, Robinson L, Hillel AD. Findings of multiple muscle involvement in a study of 214 patients with laryngeal dystonia using fine-wire electromyography. *Ann Otol Rhinol Laryngol*. 2004;113:602-612.

30. Bielamowicz S, Stager SV. Diagnosis of unilateral recurrent laryngeal nerve paralysis: laryngeal electromyography, subjective rating scales, acoustic and aerodynamic measures. *Laryngoscope*. In press.

31. Damrose EJ, Huang RY, Blumin JH, Blackwell KE, Sercarz JA, Berke GS. Lack of evoked laryngeal electromyography response in patients with a clinical diagnosis of vocal cord paralysis. *Ann Otol Rhinol Laryngol*. 2001;111:563-565.

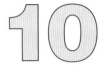

Radiology of the Larynx

Soh Ping Eng, MBBS, FRCSED, FRCSI, DLO, FAMS
Georges Lawson, MD
Thierry Vanderborght, MD, PhD
Marc LaCrosse, MD
Marc Remacle, MD, PhD

KEY POINTS

- The role of imaging is mainly complementary to clinical assessment and does not replace an accurate clinical evaluation, which includes endoscopy and biopsy.

- The aims of imaging in laryngeal oncology include radiologic diagnosis of laryngeal cancer, determining the depth and extent of tumor infiltration (especially paraglottic and pre-epiglottic space involvement, cartilage invasion, involvement of "hidden areas" such as the anterior commissure and subglottic extension), cancer staging, tumor-volumetric data for radiotherapy planning, evaluation of cervical lymph nodes, and post-treatment evaluation of treatment failures or tumor recurrence.

- The choice between CT and MRI depends on the evaluative aims of the clinician, the availability of resources, the suitability of the patient, the nature of the pathology, and the radiologist's personal experience.

- Virtual laryngoscopy has the potential for staging and presurgical assessment of laryngeal cancer but is limited due to an inability to diagnose membranous lesions or small laryngeal tumors.

- Combined FDG-PET/CT imaging systems are increasingly used as the imaging modality of choice in the management of laryngeal tumor (staging, therapy guidance, and response assessment).

Radioimaging plays an integral role in the management of laryngeal disorders today. In general, it attempts to provide the clinician with vital information concerning the nature of the lesion and the anatomic site that is involved, especially when clinical assessment is difficult such as the subglottis or anterior commissure. In so doing, imaging often assists in the diagnosis of laryngeal conditions, evaluates the extent of the disease, and even offers prognostic indicators, as in the case of laryngeal cancers.

Although the benefits of imaging are undisputed in most clinical situations, it is important to emphasize that its role is mainly complementary to clinical assessment and does not replace an accurate clinical evaluation, which includes endoscopy and biopsy.

Several reliable imaging techniques have evolved through the years and have been effectively applied in the field of laryngology. Computer tomography (CT) and magnetic resonance imaging (MRI) are among the most reliable and commonly used tools for anatomic imaging, although ultrasonography (US) and plain film radiography (x-ray) may have limited roles in specific clinical situations. In recent years, we are also witnessing an increasing role in the newer technologies of positron emission tomography (PET) and virtual laryngoscopy (VL). In the face of these myriad imaging options, the clinician should recognize the intrinsic strengths and limitations of each modality in order to choose the most effective and appropriate imaging tool for the specified purpose. Also each modality may not be mutually exclusive but may complement other studies to obtain the fullest information, such as combining PET with CT.

Anatomic imaging techniques are discussed first in this chapter, with more emphasis on CT and MRI, as they are most commonly used. A short paragraph on the latest advance with virtual laryngoscopy is included. Finally, PET is elaborated in great detail as it is an emerging technique for functional imaging.

ANATOMIC IMAGING OF THE LARYNX

Plain Film Radiography (X-Ray)

Plain film x-rays have been superceded by newer imaging modalities such as the CT and MRI for most indications. However, due to availability and cost savings, plain films are used in selected clinical situations, especially in laryngeal emergencies. For instance, epiglottitis (Figure 10–1) and retro-

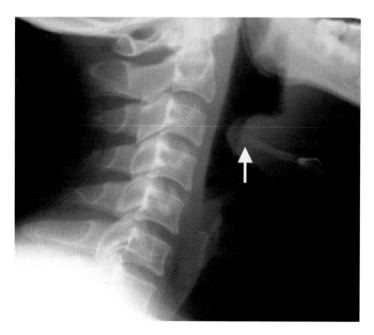

FIGURE 10–1. Acute epiglottitis: Classical "thumb" sign (*arrow*) on plain film x-ray.

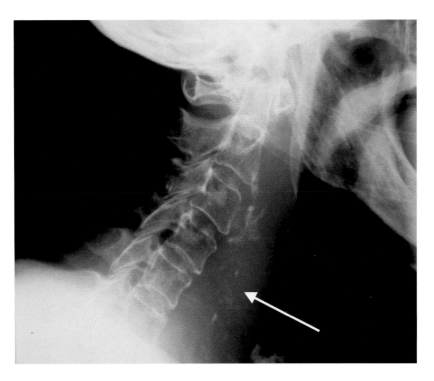

FIGURE 10–2. Plain film x-ray demonstrating a widened prevertebral space (*arrow*) secondary to a large retropharyngeal abscess.

pharyngeal abscess (Figure 10-2) can be readily diagnosed with a simple x-ray. A chest x-ray may help to identify the cause of unilateral vocal fold paresis if it is due to a mediastinal compression or an apical cancer of the lung. Some authors use x-rays to assess the accurate positioning of thyroplastic implants after surgery (Figure 10-3).

Ultrasonography (US)

In some clinical situations, clinicians may prefer ultrasound over CT or MRI because it is cheap and easy to perform in the outpatient service. The role of ultrasound is, understandably, limited and it is often reserved for selected indications only. Ultrasound could be particularly useful in pediatric cases when patient cooperation may be difficult to achieve. Ultrasound may be used to confirm the presence of cervical lymph nodes or presence of deep neck lesions or cysts. Some studies have demonstrated that ultrasound could be a more cost-effective mode of establishing pre-epiglottic space involvement in laryngeal cancer[1]; others have suggested using ultrasound for the diagnosis of epiglottic lesions such as

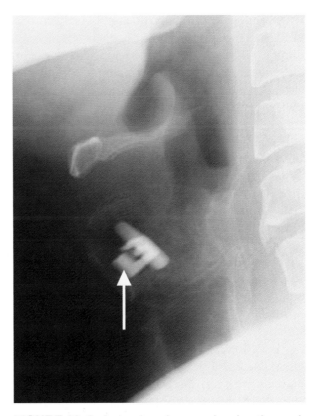

FIGURE 10–3. Lateral neck x-ray showing the position of the Montgomery prosthesis (*arrow*) after a medialization thyroplasty was performed.

cysts, epiglottitis, and for pretherapeutic staging of epiglottic cancer.[2]. In evaluating node status in laryngeal cancer, ultrasound alone (72.7%) was less accurate than CT (84.9%) or MRI (85%). However, it offers an accuracy of 89% when used in conjunction with fine-needle aspiration cytology.[3]

Computed Tomography (CT) and Magnetic Resonance Imaging (MRI)

CT and MRI have gained wide acceptance in the evaluation of the human larynx in many centers. Although one modality may be intrinsically superior to the other regarding specific anatomic detail, both are helpful in the evaluation of laryngeal anatomy.

Current CT scans have advanced over first-generation CT technology. With the advent of helical or spiral CT, more accurate details of the laryngeal and vascular anatomy are provided in a shorter examination time (less than a minute) with reduced motional artifacts.[4,5] Furthermore, utilizing three-dimensional reconstruction techniques, CT is capable of providing information on volumetric data for radiotherapy planning. It also allows better evaluation of anatomic regions that are difficult to assess clinically, such as subglottic involvement in laryngeal cancers.[6]

At the same time, developments in MRI, with multiplanar capabilities and superior soft tissue contrast resolution have made it an ideal investigative tool for tumor evaluation,[7,8] especially in assessing tumor volume, tumor infiltration, and cartilage invasion.

One may, therefore, find varying viewpoints in the literature concerning the supremacy of one modality over the other. The modality of choice should depend on the evaluative aims of the clinician, the availability of resources, the suitability of the patient, the nature of the pathology, and finally the radiologist's personal experience. For example, CT should be considered in patients with ferromagnetic implants or surgical clips because MRI is contraindicated. Conversely, MRI may be preferred if soft tissue delineation is the main interest of the investigation.

The medical literature suggests the effective applications of CT and MRI in current laryngology practice, although CT remains the main workhorse for most centers due to practical and cost-effective reasons.

Benign Laryngeal Pathologies

Both CT and MRI are used in the investigation of benign laryngeal pathologies. For example, they may provide additional information needed to assist in the differential diagnosis of tuberculosis of the larynx, which may mimic a laryngeal cancer clinically.[9,10] They also offer diagnostic hints for the clinician in managing paralaryngeal cysts like a laryngocoele[11,12] (Figure 10–4) or a thyroglossal duct cyst (Figure 10–5).

Planning and Evaluation of Laryngeal Surgery

CT has been used as an adjunct for planning and evaluating outcomes in some laryngeal surgeries. CT facilitates surgical planning by determining the limits of resection accurately in cancer surgery.[13,14]

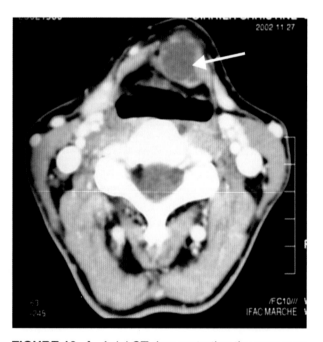

FIGURE 10–4. Axial CT demonstrating the presence of a laryngocoele (*arrow*).

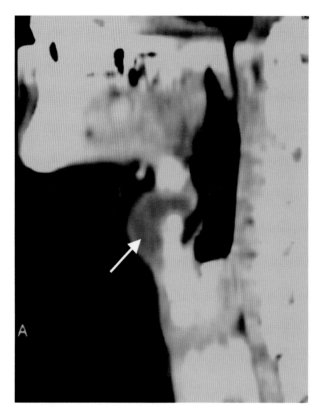

FIGURE 10–5. MRI sagittal view showing the presence of a thyroglossal cyst (*arrow*).

It is also recommended for pre- and postoperative evaluation of surgeries like thyroplasty,[15] cricothyroid approximation,[16,17] and tracheoplasty or laryngotracheal reanastomosis.[18]

Laryngeal Trauma

CT assessment is a valuable tool for the management of acute laryngeal trauma.[19,20] With well described diagnostic features,[21] it may also detect early injuries such as laryngeal perforations[22] that are not yet clinically evident. CT allows the clinician to survey the extent of injury and assist in the planning of surgical intervention.[23] Posttraumatic deformity may also be detected successfully. CT is better for visualization of ossified cartilage changes whereas MRI allows better soft tissue resolution. Fine-resolution CT may prevent explorative surgery in cases of nondisplaced laryngeal fractures.

Arytenoid Subluxation-Dislocation

As an adjunct to laryngoscopy and electromyogram, spiral-CT could aid in the diagnosis of arytenoid subluxation or dislocation (Figure 10-6). As a spiral-CT is now performed in a shortened time, the CT provides good images despite scanning a mobile structure like the larynx.[24]

Vocal Cord Paralysis

The characteristic features of a vocal cord paralysis (Figure 10-7) may include piriform sinus

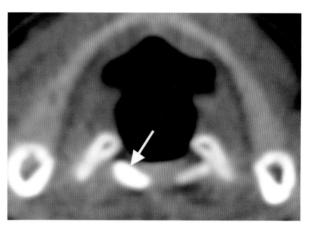

FIGURE 10–6. Subluxation of the right arytenoid (*arrow*) on CT.

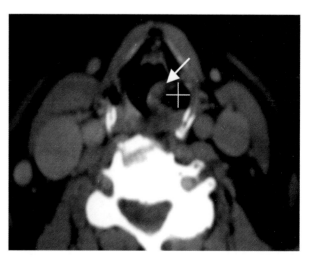

FIGURE 10–7. Left vocal cord paralysis. Features of dilatation of left piriform sinus (+) and medialization of left true cord (*arrow*) on CT.

dilatation, medial positioning and thickening of the aryepiglottic fold, laryngeal ventricle dilatation as well as atrophy of the posterior cricoarytenoid muscle.[25,26] CT or MRI is used to image the length of the laryngeal nerves from their origin in the brainstem to the larynx, including the mediastinum in the evaluation of the cause of a vocal cord paresis.[27]

Laryngeal and Tracheal Stenosis

Both CT and MRI are useful in the assessment and diagnosis of laryngeal and tracheal stenosis (Figure 10–8). They are especially useful when the narrowing is due to submucosal or extrinsic compression as endoscopic assessment may not provide this anatomic detail.[28]

Laryngeal Oncology

The aims of imaging in laryngeal oncology include radiologic diagnosis of laryngeal cancer, determining the depth and extent of tumor infiltration (especially paraglottic and pre-epiglottic space involvement, cartilage invasion, involvement of "hidden areas" such as anterior commissure and subglottic extension), cancer staging, tumor-volumetric data for radiotherapy planning, evaluation of cervical lymph nodes, and post-treatment evaluation of radiation failures or tumor recurrence.

Diagnosis of Laryngeal Cancer. In general, imaging studies have limited value in the diagnosis of early stage laryngeal cancers as the extent of these lesions is easily evaluated by clinical examination with endoscopy and biopsy. However, in atypical laryngeal cancers, CT or MRI features may help to alert the clinician to the differential diagnosis, even if the biopsy is negative.[29] For example, a rare tumor like chondrosarcoma may present with laryngeal cartilage expansion with chondroid calcifications, involving the cricoid more commonly than the thyroid or arytenoid cartilage. Although not pathognomonic, these unusual radiologic features may help to differentiate a chondrosarcoma from squamous cell carcinoma.

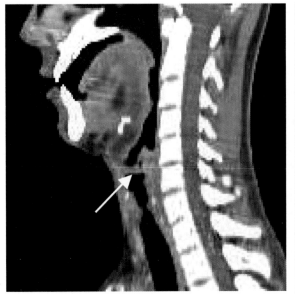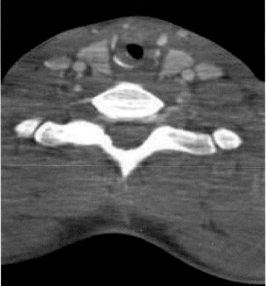

FIGURE 10–8. MRI sagittal view on the left (*arrow*) showing the extent of cricotracheal stenosis. This is correlated with axial CT on the right.

Evaluation of Tumor Infiltration. Of greater clinical importance is the role of radioimaging in the evaluation of tumor infiltration and extent of disease, as these factors indicate the prognosis as well as the surgical resectability of the tumor. These studies allow for an evaluation of laryngeal cartilage invasion, subsite extension, and evaluation of clinically hidden areas (eg, subglottic and anterior commissure, pre-epiglottic, and paraglottic spaces).

Cartilage Invasion. A crucial factor in tumor staging lies in the involvement of laryngeal cartilage, as this would imply a T4 tumor. CT and MRI are both effective, although their sensitivities and specificities may differ. CT appears to be less sensitive than MRI in detecting neoplastic cartilage invasion (up to 68% versus up to 89%, respectively) but is also more specific (up to 94% versus 84%, respectively). With CT, there is a higher risk of under estimation with resultant undertreatment, whereas MRI may detect more false positives.[30-37] These limitations should always be kept in mind when deciding on the imaging modality of choice. Further consideration should also be given to the radiologist's experience and the suitability of the patient, although CT is more commonly used because of availability, cost-savings, and claustrophobia concerns associated with MRI.

Cartilage destruction due to tumor invasion, on CT (Figure 10-9) may appear as a moderate signal interrupting the outer rim of thyroid cartilage or as a low signal focus within the cartilage. Cartilage sclerosis alone, however, should not be taken as an absolute indication of tumor invasion as degree of demineralization varies among individuals.[38,39]

Tumor Extension. Both CT and MRI are useful for detecting tumor invasion of clinically hidden areas such as the anterior commissure (Figure 10-10) and subglottis (Figure 10-11) as well as the paraglottic and pre-epiglottic spaces.[33,40] CT is able to achieve this by using multislice spiral

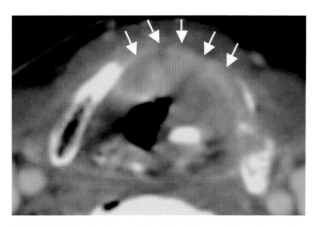

FIGURE 10-9. Extensive thyroid cartilage invasion (*multiple arrows*) from laryngeal carcinoma.

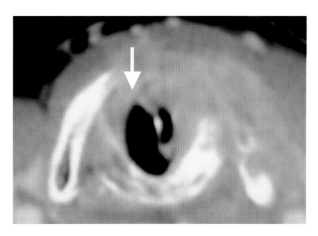

FIGURE 10-10. Laryngeal carcinoma with extension into anterior commissure (*arrow*).

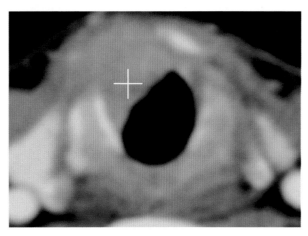

FIGURE 10-11. Subglottic infiltration (+) of laryngeal carcinoma.

CT and subse-quent multiplanar reconstruction,[41] although sagittal MRI sections have the advantage of demonstrating the anterior commissure and its relationship to the supraglottic and subglottic compartments. Generally, more than 1 millimeter thickness of the anterior commissure may suggest an abnormality.

Vocal Cord Fixation. Vocal cord fixation is considered at least a T3 tumor and cord immobility may be suggested on CT (Figure 10–12) or MRI. These features include a paramedian location of the true cord, anteromedial rotation of the arytenoid process, ipsilateral piriform sinus, and ventricle dilatation. Decreased signal in the cricoid cartilage ring could also suggest tumor invasion resulting in cord fixation.

Staging and Prognostication. Imaging studies, especially CT, are advocated for routine laryngeal staging as well as for prognostication. CT staging of laryngeal tumors has been shown to be reli-

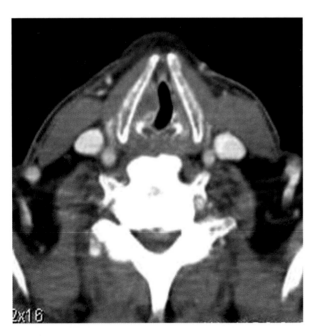

FIGURE 10–12. Squamous cell carcinoma (T3) of the right glottis, with vocal cord paralysis of the ipsilateral side. The affected cord is rotated anteriormedially and fixed in a paramedian position.

able and accurate,[42,43] although MRI may be superior for assessment of advanced T3 and T4 cancers and supraglottic tumors.[44] The accuracy is further enhanced when imaging is combined with a thorough clinical evaluation compared with relying on imaging or clinical examination alone.[45] From the radiation standpoint, image-determined factors (T stage, tumor volume, anterior commissure involvement, ventricle involvement, paraglottic and pre-epiglottic spread, subglottic extension, and thyroid cartilage invasion) may offer reliable prediction of post-irradiation local and regional recurrence.[46-52]

Evaluation of Nodal Status of the Neck. Comparisons of various modalities suggest that CT and MRI are equally accurate (CT 84.9%, MRI 85%) in the detection of nodal metastases, although ultrasound-guided fine-needle aspiration cytology and PET may provide superior diagnostic capabilities with an accuracy of 89% and 90.5%, respectively.[3]

Posttreatment Evaluation. Along with laryngoscopy, CT or MRI may be used to evaluate the larynx in posttreatment (radiotherapy and surgical resection) follow-up. CT is effective in detecting local treatment failure earlier than clinical examination.[53] Similarly, in postsurgical cases (eg, partial laryngectomy where the laryngeal anatomy is altered), CT or MRI may be chosen to evaluate tumor recurrence and treatment failures.[54,55]

FUNCTIONAL IMAGING OF THE LARYNX

Positron Emission Tomography (PET)

Treatment options for head and neck cancer include surgery, radiation therapy, and neoadjuvant or induction chemotherapy. The evaluation of tumor response to these novel treatments is

Emerging Concepts in Imaging:
Virtual Laryngoscopy

First described by Vining et al,[56] virtual laryngoscopy is an emerging radiologic tool that uses image segmentation of spiral-CT to isolate and study an anatomic area of interest. It produces visualization of luminal surfaces in three-dimensional reconstruction of air/fluid or fluid/tissue interface so that fly-through images of the ventricle, vocal fold, subglottic space, and trachea are created. According to recent studies, the accuracy and sensitivity of virtual endoscopy is comparable to fiberoptic endoscopic findings and CT-reconstructions.[57-60] These studies may suggest its potential role in the staging and presurgical assessment of laryngeal cancer, especially with subglottic assessment and with neoplastic stenosis that rendered endoscopic examination impossible.[61-63] It may also be useful for the assessment of non-neoplastic laryngotracheal stenosis or inflammation.[64] However, virtual laryngoscopy is limited in the ability to diagnose membranous lesions or small laryngeal tumors and does not provide a histologic diagnosis. Although its clinical potential seems promising, virtual endoscopy should remain adjunctive to laryngeal endoscopy for the moment.

critical. CT or MRI is used to evaluate tumors or lymph nodes by size or structural abnormalities. However, up to 15% of large lymph nodes may simply be reactive and more than 40% of metastases have been found in lymph nodes smaller than 1 cm, the cutoff generally used to differentiate benign from malignant disease.

Positron emission tomography (PET) uses 2-deoxy-2-[F-18]fluoro-D-glucose (FDG), a glucose analog, to evaluate increased glucose metabolism in tumor cells. FDG enters cells through glucose transporters, is phosphorylated into FDG-6-phosphate, and accumulated in metabolically active tumor cells because, unlike glucose-6-phosphate, it cannot undergo further metabolism. The radioactive label fluorine-18 emits positrons at the site of tumor, which, after traveling a millimetric distance, collide with electrons and emit two gamma rays at 180° to each other. With a multiring camera placed around the patient, these events are detected to reconstruct three-dimensional distribution images.

As the higher glycolytic rate of tumor cells precedes macroscopic morphologic changes, FDG-PET can establish structural abnormalities containing tumor or detect small foci of disease within otherwise normal structures. It can also assess the whole body in one study with a much lower dose of radiation than whole body CT. Physiologic uptake of FDG can make interpretation of PET data challenging despite the fact that such uptake is symmetric and in typical locations.[65,66] Intense FDG uptake is usually observed in the palatine tonsils, lingual tonsils, and soft palate, whereas uptake in the major salivary glands and vocal cords is variable but could be intense. Benign thyroid nodules or chronic thyroiditis and areas of inflammation have increased

FDG uptake and, thus, can be confused with neoplastic growth.

PET is limited by poor spatial resolution. The coregistration using fusion software for accurate designation of physiologic data obtained on PET to anatomic structures visualized on CT or MRI is particularly useful in the head and neck, especially in patients with surgically altered anatomy. Recently, dual-modality PET/CT imaging systems, combining structural and metabolic information within a single examination, may become the method of choice for assessing head and neck cancer.[67-69]

FDG-PET is increasingly used as a clinical imaging modality in the different stages of the management of head and neck cancer. At initial staging, the presence of lymph node metastases is the strongest predictor of prognosis and outcome in patients with head and neck cancer.[70,71] FDG-PET is superior to CT or MRI for detecting lymph node metastasis, with sensitivity and specificity of approximately 90% and 94%, respectively, as compared with 82% and 85% for CT, 80% and 79% for MRI, and 72% and 70% for sonography,

respectively[72] (Figure 10–13). Only micrometastasis, cystic or necrotic degeneration of metastatic lymph nodes, or lymph nodes adjacent to the primary tumor may be falsely negative on FDG-PET. However, CT is more accurate for assessing the size and local extent of the primary tumor as well as the level, number and size of nodes and the presence of extracapsular spread, factors that are important for determining the prognosis of head and neck cancer patients.

The head and neck cancer patient with a clinically N0 neck is challenging, with 30% of the patients having subclinical lymph node involvement. If a study could detect accurately patients with microscopic lymph node involvement, these patients could avoid the morbidity associated with a staging lymphadenectomy. The combination of FDG-PET and lymphoscintigraphy-guided sentinel lymph node (SLN) biopsy is currently being evaluated to address the problem.[73,74] The SLN procedure is based on the concept that a primary tumor drains via efferent lymphatic channels directly to a single lymph node, the so-called SLN, which is the first recipi-

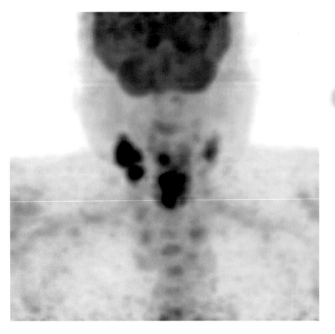
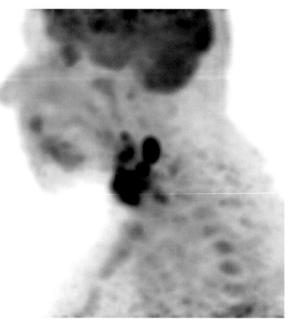

FIGURE 10–13. Maximal intensity projection of the coronal (*left panel*) and sagittal (*right panel*) FDG-PET images of a patient with a laryngeal tumor. Lymph nodes are clearly visualized bilaterally, but mainly on the right side. Note the intense brain activity and the increased uptake in bone marrow.

ent of micrometastasis. The histologic status of this lymph node should predict the nodal status of the patient. In the larynx, an endoscopic injection into the tumor of radiolabeled nanocolloid is required. The SLN localization is performed using intraoperative gamma probe radiolocalization. The thorough pathologic evaluation of the sentinel node is necessary to avoid false-negative results.[68]

Although only 1% of cancers in the head and neck present as a malignant lymph node with no known site of disease (CUP syndrome), FDG-PET has been able to reveal unknown primary tumors in approximately 30 to 60% of patients. However, false-positive findings in up to 11% of these cases have been identified.

Patients with head and neck cancers are at a 4% per year risk of another second primary cancer of the head and neck, esophagus, or lung. Also, 12 to 21% of head and neck cancer patients, especially patients with advanced stage disease, will develop distant metastases to the lungs, liver, and bones. FDG-PET significantly increases the rate of detection of simultaneous second primary tumors, usually at an early stage, and distant metastasis, which greatly affects the treatment and prognosis of patients with head and neck cancer (Figure 10–14).

Surgical treatment, radiotherapy or chemotherapy, all lead to distortion of the anatomy, which makes the distinction between post-therapy changes and recurrence or residual tumor challenging. Superior diagnostic accuracy of FDG-PET for restaging cancer and assessing response to chemotherapy and radiation therapy has been reported by many authors, with a sensitivity and specificity of approximately 88 to 100% and 75 to 100%, respectively, compared with 70 to 92% and 50 to 57% of CT and MRI,[75] Negative results obtained 4 months after completion of therapy are more reliable than imaging findings obtained earlier, as inflammation and granulation at the tumor site may induce false-positive findings.

The use of FDG-PET/CT imaging to guide head and neck intensity-modulated radiotherapy planning is currently being evaluated to selectively target and intensify treatment of head and

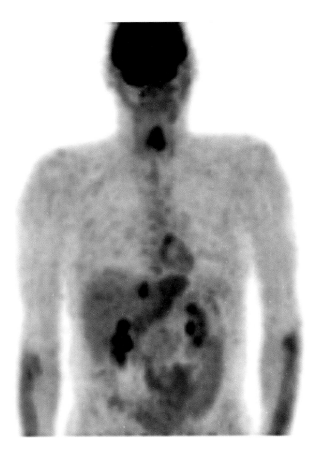

FIGURE 10–14. Maximal intensity projection of the coronal FDG-PET images shows intense uptake not only in the neck (*primary tumor*), but also in the left lobe of the liver (*metastasis*). There is normal uptake in the brain, heart, stomach, pelvis, intestine, and forearm muscles.

neck disease while reducing injury to critical normal tissue (Figure 10–15).[76,77]

The scope of laryngology has expanded exponentially in recent years. In the future, we expect further development of existing and new imaging techniques. As such, radiology will continue to be a key component to the practice of laryngology.

Acknowledgments. The authors thank Tiong Yong Tan, MBBS, FRCR, FAMS, of the Department of Radiology, Changi General Hospital, Singapore and Christian Picard, MD, of the Nuclear Medicine Division of the Université Catholique de Louvain, Belgium for their contributions of images.

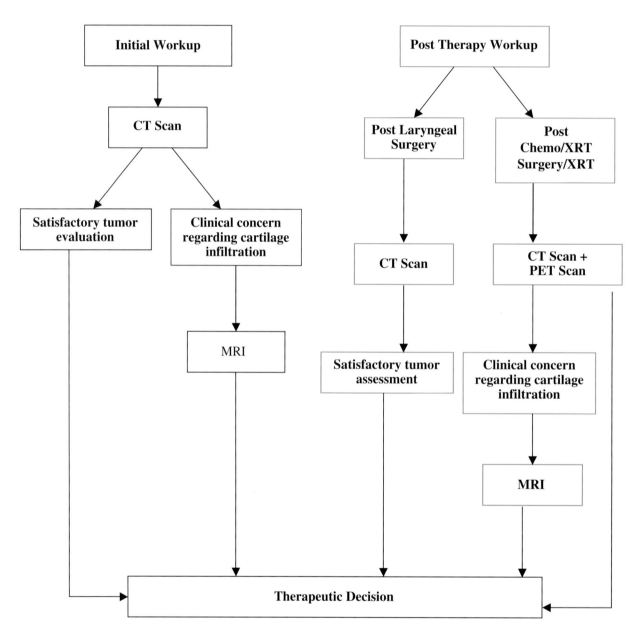

FIGURE 10–15. Algorithm for working up suspected laryngeal tumor.

Review Questions

1. The following are anatomic imaging modalities *except*:
   a. Virtual laryngoscopy
   b. CT
   c. MRI
   d. PET

2. The following are CT features of unilateral vocal cord palsy *except*:
   a. Dilatation of ipsilateral piriform sinus
   b. Thinning of ipsilateral aryepiglottic fold
   c. Dilation of the ipsilateral ventricle
   d. Thinning of ipsilateral posterior cricoarytenoid muscle

3. Concerning cartilage invasion from laryngeal cancer, the following statement is correct:
   a. Cartilage sclerosis alone is a definite indication of cartilage invasion.
   b. CT is more sensitive than MRI.
   c. MRI is less specific than CT.
   d. Invasion of thyroid cartilage will imply that the tumor is not resectable.

4. The following is true about virtual laryngoscopy (VL):
   a. VL detects membranous lesions and small cancerous lesions effectively.
   b. VL is useful for evaluation of the anterior commissure and subglottic region.
   c. VL uses helical-CT to construct its images.
   d. VL has superseded endoscopy and biopsy in the evaluation of larynx.

5. The following statement is untrue about FDG-PET:
   a. FDG-PET uses 2-deoxy-2-[F-18] fluoro-D-glucose (FDG), a glucose analog, for cancer detection.
   b. FDG-PET improves the initial staging of laryngeal tumor compared to CT or MRI.
   c. FDG-PET cannot exclude micrometastases in lymph nodes.
   d. FDG-PET has a good spatial resolution.

REFERENCES

1. Kabacinska A. Evaluation of the usefulness of ultrasonic examination of the pre-epiglottic space in patients with laryngeal carcinoma. *Ann Acad Med Stetin.* 1998;44:197–207.
2. Bohme G. Ultrasound diagnosis of the epiglottis. *HNO.* 1990;38(10):355–360.
3. Kau RJ, Alexiou C, Stimmer H, Arnold W. Diagnostic procedures for detection of lymph node metastases in cancer of the larynx. *ORL J Otorhinolaryngol Relat Spec.* 2000;62(4):199–203.
4. Korkmaz H, Cerezci NG, Akmansu H, Dursun E. A comparison of spiral and conventional computerized tomography methods in diagnosing various laryngeal lesions. *Eur Arch Otorhinolaryngol.* 1998;255(3):149–154.
5. Robert Y, Rocourt N, Chevalier D, Duhamel A, Carcasset S, Lemaitre L. Helical CT of the larynx: a comparative study with conventional CT scan. *Clin Radiol.* 1996;51(12):882–885.
6. Sakakura A, Yamamoto Y, Uesugi Y, Nakai K, Takenaka H, Narabayashi I. Three-dimensional imaging of laryngeal cancers using high-speed helical CT scanning. *ORL J Otorhinolaryngol Relat Spec.* 1998;60(2):103–107.
7. Teresi LM, Lufkin RB, Hanafee WN. Magnetic resonance imaging of the larynx. *Radiol Clin North Am.* 1989;27(2):393–406.

8. Hasso AN, Tang T. Magnetic resonance imaging of the pharynx and larynx. *Top Magn Reson Imag.* 1994l;6(4):224–240

9. Kim MD, Kim DI, Yune HY, et al. CT findings of laryngeal tuberculosis: comparison to laryngeal carcinoma. *J Comput Assist Tomogr.* 1997;21(1): 29–34.

10. Moon WK, Han MH, Chang KH, et al. CT and MR imaging of head and neck tuberculosis. *Radiographics.* 1997;17(2):391–402.

11. Morgan NJ, Emberton P. CT scanning and laryngocoeles. *J Laryngol Otol.* 1994;108(3):266–268.

12. Bootz F, Lenz M. Computerized tomography imaging of laryngocele. Its importance in the differential diagnosis of tumors of the larynx and pharynx *HNO.* 1990;38(6):220–225.

13. Saleh EM, Mancuso AA, Stringer SP. Relative roles of computed tomography and endoscopy for determining the inferior extent of pyriform sinus carcinoma: correlative histopathologic study. *Head Neck.* 1993;15(1):44–52.

14. Saleh EM, Mancuso AA, Alhussaini AA. Computed tomography of primary subglottic cancer: clinical importance. *Head Neck.* 1992;14(2):125–132.

15. Safak MA, Gocmen H, Korkmaz H, Kilic R. Computerized tomographic alignment of Silastic implant in type 1 thyroplasty. *Am J Otolaryngol.* 2000;21(3):179–183.

16. Pickuth D, Brandt S, Neumann K, Berghaus A, Spielmann RP, Heywang-Kobrunner SH. Value of spiral CT in patients with cricothyroid approximation. *Br J Radiol.* 2000;73(872):840–842.

17. Pickuth D, Brandt S, Neumann K, Berghaus A, Spielmann RP, Heywang-Kobrunner SH. Spiral computed tomography before and after cricothyroid approximation. *Clin Otolaryngol Allied Sci.* 2000;25(4):311–314.

18. Konen E, Faibel M, Hoffman C, Talmi YP, Rozenman J, Wolf M. Laryngo-tracheal anastomosis: post-operative evaluation by helical CT and computerized reformations. *Clin Radiol.* 2002;57(9): 820–825.

19. Scaglione M, Romano L, Grassi R, Pinto F, Calderazzi A, Pieri L. Diagnostic approach to acute laryngeal trauma: role of computerized tomography. *Radiol Med (Torino).* 1997;93(1–2):67–70.

20. Schaefer SD. Use of CT scanning in the management of the acutely injured larynx. *Otolaryngol Clin North Am.* 1991;24(1):31–36.

21. Lupetin AR, Hollander M, Rao VM. CT Evaluation of laryngotracheal trauma. *Semin Musculoskelet Radiol.* 1998;2(1):105–116.

22. Scaglione M, Romano L, Pinto F, Frasca P, Grassi R. Perforation of the laryngeal mucosa caused by closed trauma: comparison of laryngoscopic and CT findings. *Radiol Med (Torino).* 1997;94(6): 607–610.

23. Kuttenberger JJ, Hardt N, Schlegel C. Diagnosis and initial management of laryngotracheal injuries associated with facial fractures. *J Craniomaxillofac Surg.* 2004;32(2):80–84.

24. Alexander AE Jr, Lyons GD, Fazekas-May MA, et al. Utility of helical computed tomography in the study of arytenoid dislocation and arytenoid subluxation. *Ann Otol Rhinol Laryngol.* 1997; 106(12):1020–1013.

25. Chin SC, Edelstein S, Chen CY, Som PM. Using CT to localize the side and level of vocal cord paralysis. *Am J Roentgenol.* 2003;180(4):1165–1170.

26. Romo LV, Curtin HD. Atrophy of the posterior cricoarytenoid muscle as an indicator of recurrent laryngeal nerve palsy. *Am J Neuroradiol.* 1999;20(3):467–471.

27. Richardson BE, Bastian RW. Clinical evaluation of vocal fold paralysis. *Otolaryngol Clin North Am.* 2004;37(1):45–58.

28. Hermans R, Verschakelen JA, Baert AL. Imaging of laryngeal and tracheal stenosis. *Acta Otorhinolaryngol Belg.* 1995;49(4):323–329.

29. Becker M, Moulin G, Kurt AM, et al. Atypical squamous cell carcinoma of the larynx and hypopharynx: radiologic features and pathologic correlation. *Eur Radiol.* 1998;8(9):1541–1551.

30. Becker M. Neoplastic invasion of laryngeal cartilage: radiologic diagnosis and therapeutic implications. *Eur J Radiol.* 2000;33(3):216–229.

31. Amilibia E, Juan A, Nogues J, Manos M, Monfort JL, Dicenta M. Neoplastic invasion of laryngeal cartilage: diagnosis by computed tomography. *Acta Otorrinolaringol Esp.* 2001;52(3):207–210

32. Zbaren P, Becker M, Lang H. Pretherapeutic staging of hypopharyngeal carcinoma. Clinical findings, computed tomography, and magnetic resonance imaging compared with histopathologic evaluation. *Arch Otolaryngol Head Neck Surg.* 1997; 123(9):908–913.

33. Yousem DM, Tufano RP. Laryngeal imaging. *Mag Reson Imag Clin North Am.* 2002;10(3):451–465.

34. Castelijns JA, Becker M, Hermans R. Impact of cartilage invasion on treatment and prognosis of laryngeal cancer. *Eur Radiol.* 1996;6(2): 156–169.

35. Declercq A, Van den Hauwe L, Van Marck E, Van de Heyning PH, Spanoghe M, De Schepper AM.

Patterns of framework invasion in patients with laryngeal cancer: correlation of in vitro magnetic resonance imaging and pathological findings. *Acta Otolaryngol.* 1998;118(6):892-895.

36. Becker M, Zbaren P, Laeng H, Stoupis C, Porcellini B, Vock P. Neoplastic invasion of the laryngeal cartilage: comparison of MR imaging and CT with histopathologic correlation. *Radiology.* 1995;194(3):661-669.

37. Atula T, Markkola A, Leivo I, Makitie A. Cartilage invasion of laryngeal cancer detected by magnetic resonance imaging. *Eur Arch Otorhinolaryngol.* 2001;258(6):272-275.

38. Agada FO, Nix PA, Salvage D, Stafford ND. Computerised tomography vs. pathological staging of laryngeal cancer: a 6-year completed audit cycle. *Int J Clin Pract.* 2004;58(7):714-716.

39. Nix PA, Salvage D. Neoplastic invasion of laryngeal cartilage: the significance of cartilage sclerosis on computed tomography images. *Clin Otolaryngol Allied Sci.* 2004;29(4):372-375

40. Loevner LA, Yousem DM, Montone KT, Weber R, Chalian AA, Weinstein GS. Can radiologists accurately predict pre-epiglottic space invasion with MR imaging? *Am J Roentgenol.* 1997;169(6):1681-1687.

41. Bruning R, Sturm C, Hong C, et al. The diagnosis of stages T1 and T2 in laryngeal carcinoma with multislice spiral CT. *Radiologe.* 1999;39(11):939-942.

42. Keberle M, Kenn W, Hahn D. Current concepts in imaging of laryngeal and hypopharyngeal cancer. *Eur Radiol.* 2002;12(7):1672-1683. E-pub 2002 Feb 9.

43. Echarri RM, Rivera T, Montojo J, Bermejo C, Fraile E, Cobeta I. Correlation of clinical, radiologic, and histopathologic findings in laryngeal, hypopharyngeal, and oropharyngeal cancer. *Acta Otorrinolaringol Esp.* 2000;51(7):587-592.

44. Katsounakis J, Remy H, Vuong T, Gelinas M, Tabah R. Impact of magnetic resonance imaging and computed tomography on the staging of laryngeal cancer. *Eur Arch Otorhinolaryngol.* 1995;252(4):206-208.

45. Thabet HM, Sessions DG, Gado MH, Gnepp DA, Harvey JE, Talaat M. Comparison of clinical evaluation and computed tomographic diagnostic accuracy for tumors of the larynx and hypopharynx. *Laryngoscope.* 1996;106(5 pt 1):589-594.

46. Hamilton S, Venkatesan V, Matthews TW, Lewis C, Assis L. Computed tomographic volumetric analysis as a predictor of local control in laryngeal cancers treated with conventional radiotherapy. *J Otolaryngol.* 2004;33(5):289-294.

47. Hermans R, Van den Bogaert W, Rijnders A, Baert AL. Value of computed tomography as outcome predictor of supraglottic squamous cell carcinoma treated by definitive radiation therapy. *Int J Radiat Oncol Biol Phys.* 1999;44(4):755-765.

48. Hermans R, Van den Bogaert W, Rijnders A, Doornaert P, Baert AL. Predicting the local outcome of glottic squamous cell carcinoma after definitive radiation therapy: value of computed tomography-determined tumor parameters. *Radiother Oncol.* 1999;50(1):39-46.

49. Kraas JR, Underhill TE, D'Agostino RB Jr, Williams DW 3rd, Cox JA, Greven KM. Quantitative analysis from CT is prognostic for local control of supraglottic carcinoma. *Head Neck.* 2001;23(12):1031-1036.

50. Murakami R, Furusawa M, Baba Y, et al. Dynamic helical CT of T1 and T2 glottic carcinomas: predictive value for local control with radiation therapy. *Am J Neuroradiol.* 2000;21(7):1320-1326.

51. Ljumanovic R, Langendijk JA, Schenk B, et al. Supraglottic carcinoma treated with curative radiation therapy: identification of prognostic groups with MR imaging. *Radiology.* 2004;232(2):440-448.

52. Murakami R, Baba Y, Furusawa M, et al. Early glottic squamous cell carcinoma. Predictive value of MR imaging for the rate of 5-year local control with radiation therapy. *Acta Radiol.* 2000;41(1):38-44.

53. Hermans R, Pameijer FA, Mancuso AA, Parsons JT, Mendenhall WM. Laryngeal or hypopharyngeal squamous cell carcinoma: can follow-up CT after definitive radiation therapy be used to detect local failure earlier than clinical examination alone? *Radiology.* 2000;214(3):683-687.

54. Bely-Toueg N, Halimi P, Laccourreye O, Laskri F, Brasnu D, Frija G. Normal laryngeal CT findings after supracricoid partial laryngectomy. *Am J Neuroradiol.* 2001;22(10):1872-1880.

55. Misiti A, Macori F, Caimi M, et al. Computerized tomography in the evaluation of the larynx after surgical treatment and irradiation. *Radiol Med (Torino).* 1997;94(6):600-606.

56. Vining DJ, Liu K, Choplin RH, Haponik EF. Virtual bronchoscopy. *Chest.* 1996;109(2):549-553.

57. Magnano M, Bongioannini G, Cirillo S, et al. Virtual endoscopy of laryngeal carcinoma: is it useful? *Otolaryngol Head Neck Surg.* 2005;132(5):776-782.

58. Walshe P, Hamilton S, McShane D, McConn Walsh R, Walsh MA, Timon C. The potential of virtual laryngoscopy in the assessment of vocal cord lesions. *Clin Otolaryngol Allied Sci.* 2002;27(2):98-100.

59. Wang D, Zhang W, Xiong M, Xu J. Laryngeal and hypopharyngeal carcinoma: comparison of helical CT multiplanar reformation, three-dimensional reconstruction and virtual laryngoscopy. *Chin Med J (Engl).* 2001;114(1):54-58.

60. Gallivan RP, Nguyen TH, Armstrong WB. Head and neck computed tomography virtual endoscopy: evaluation of a new imaging technique. *Laryngoscope.* 1999;109(10):1570-1579.

61. Magnano M, Bongioannini G, Cirillo S, et al. Virtual endoscopy of laryngeal carcinoma: is it useful? *Otolaryngol Head Neck Surg.* 2005;132(5): 776-782.

62. Guazzaroni M, Turchio P, Di Rienzo L, Coen Tirelli G, Garaci F, Simonetti G. Virtual laryngoscopy of neoplastic pharyngeal and laryngeal pathology. *Radiol Med (Torino).* 2001;101(4):265-269.

63. Aschoff AJ, Seifarth H, Fleiter T, et al. High-resolution virtual laryngoscopy based on spiral CT data. *Radiologe.* 1998;38(10):810-815.

64. Rodenwaldt J, Kopka L, Roedel R, Grabbe E. Three-dimensional surface imaging of the larynx and trachea by spiral CT: virtual endoscopy. *Rofo.* 1996;165(1):80-83.

65. Burrell SC, Van den Abbeele AD. 2-Deoxy-2-[F-18] fluoro-D-glucose-positron emission tomography of the head and neck: an atlas of normal uptake and variants. *Mol Imaging Biol.* 2005;7:244-256.

66. Nakamoto Y, Tatsumi M, Hammoud D, Cohade C, Osman MM, Wahl RL. Normal FDG distribution patterns in the head and neck: PET/CT evaluation. *Radiology.* 2005;234:879-885.

67. Branstetter BF, Blodgett TM, Zimmer LA, et al. Head and neck malignancy: is PET/CT more accurate than PET or CT alone? *Radiology.* 2005;235: 580-586.

68. Muylle K, Castaigne C, Flamen P. 18F-fluoro-2-deoxy-D-glucose positron emission tomographic imaging: recent developments in head and neck cancer. *Curr Opin Oncol.* 2005;17:249-253.

69. Schwartz DL, Ford E, Rajendran J et al. FDG-PET/CT imaging for preradiotherapy staging of head-and-neck squamous cell carcinoma. *Int J Radiat Oncol Biol Phys.* 2005;61:129-136.

70. Dammann F, Horger M, Mueller-Berg M, et al. Rational diagnosis of squamous cell carcinoma of the head and neck region: comparative evaluation of CT, MRI, and 18FDG PET. *Am J Roentgenol.* 2005;184:1326-1331.

71. Hain SF. Positron emission tomography in cancer of the head and neck. *Br J Oral Maxillofac Surg.* 2005;43:1-6.

72. Kapoor V, Fukui MB, McCook BM. Role of 18F-FDG PET/CT in the treatment of head and neck cancers: principles, technique, normal distribution, and initial staging. *Am J Roentgenol.* 2005;184:579-587.

73. Ferris RL, Xi L, Raja S, et al. Molecular staging of cervical lymph nodes in squamous cell carcinoma of the head and neck. *Cancer Res.* 2005;65: 2147-2156.

74. Balkissoon J, Rasgon BM, Schweitzer L. Lymphatic mapping for staging of head and neck cancer. *Semin Oncol.* 2004;31:382-393.

75. Kapoor V, Fukui MB, McCook BM. Role of 18F-FDG PET/CT in the treatment of head and neck cancers: posttherapy evaluation and pitfalls. *Am J Roentgenol.* 2005;184:589-597.

76. Schwartz DL, Ford EC, Rajendran J et al. FDG-PET/CT-guided intensity modulated head and neck radiotherapy: a pilot investigation. *Head Neck.* 2005;27:478-487.

77. Koshy M, Paulino AC, Howell R, Schuster D, Halkar R, Davis LW. F-18 FDG PET-CT fusion in radiotherapy treatment planning for head and neck cancer. *Head Neck.* 2005;27:494-502.

11

Office-Based Instrumental Examinations in Laryngology– Including TNE, FEES, and FEESST

Stacey L. Halum, MD
Gregory N. Postma, MD

KEY POINTS

- Fiberoptic endoscopic evaluation of swallowing (FEES) and fiberoptic endoscopic evaluation of swallowing with sensory testing (FEESST) are office-based tools that may replace or be used in conjunction with videofluoroscopic swallow studies (VFSS) for evaluation of patients with dysphagia and aspiration.

- Transnasal esophagoscopy (TNE) allows a complete esophageal evaluation to be performed in the clinic without sedation.

- Indications for transnasal esophagoscopy include, but are not limited to, the evaluation of patients with dysphagia, significant extraesophageal reflux, individuals requiring chronic antireflux therapy, and head and neck cancer.

- With adequate topical anesthesia, airway evaluations such as tracheoscopy or tracheobronchoscopy can be safely performed in most adult patients in a clinic setting.

> ■ Due to its excellent safety profile, clinical utility, and time/cost savings, office-based evaluation of the aerodigestive tract will continue to emerge as the standard of care for adults.

Traditionally, endoscopic evaluation of the upper aerodigestive tract has been performed on patients under sedation or general anesthesia. Over recent years, the introduction of transnasal flexible endoscopes with high-quality optics and working channels has allowed performance of unsedated, office-based assessment and treatment of upper aerodigestive tract disorders with minimal patient discomfort. The trend toward clinic-based procedures is both safer for the patient and less expensive.[1-4] Evaluation of the awake patient also allows for superior physiologic evaluation.

The primary areas discussed include fiberoptic endoscopic evaluation of swallowing (FEES), fiberoptic endoscopic evaluation of swallowing with sensory testing (FEESST), transnasal esophagoscopy (TNE), and tracheoscopy/tracheobronchoscopy.

FEES/FEESST

Until recently, the otolaryngologist's evaluation of dysphagia was limited to standard assessment tools such as the clinical/bedside swallowing evaluation, videofluoroscopic swallow study (VFSS), and manometry. Over the past decade, FEES, the fiberoptic endoscopic examination of swallowing,[5,6] has emerged as an outstanding assessment tool for patients with dysphagia and aspiration. FEES can also be combined with sensory testing (FEESST, fiberoptic endoscopic evaluation of swallowing with sensory testing) to provide further information regarding the status of laryngeal sensation. First described by Aviv and colleagues,[7] FEESST uses a calibrated pulse of air delivered to the laryngeal mucosa. The sensation travels via the superior laryngeal nerve and, if at a supra-

threshold level, results in reflex adduction of the vocal folds via the recurrent laryngeal nerve. This laryngeal adductor reflex is an important protective mechanism that helps guard against aspiration and, thereby, provides important information regarding the protective mechanisms of the patient's swallow.

Recent studies have demonstrated that FEES is superior to bedside/clinical swallow evaluation in detecting aspiration,[8] and its findings are comparable to VFSS for dysphagia evaluation.[5,6] In a study by Langmore et al, FEES and VFSS demonstrated excellent congruence across parameters, including aspiration (90% agreement).[5] FEESST has also been found to be especially useful in developing behavioral and dietary guidelines for patients with dysphagia. Patients following behavioral and dietary guidelines based on FEESST show no difference in pneumonia incidence when compared with VFSS.[9] FEESST has also been shown to play a role in the evaluation of dysphagia in patients with laryngopharyngeal reflux (LPR), as a high rate of sensory impairment is associated with LPR-induced laryngeal edema.[10,11] With appropriate antireflux therapy, the sensory deficit resolves in the majority of patients with LPR, which can be monitored clinically with laryngeal sensory testing.[10] Finally, although FEESST and VFSS are both clinically useful assessment tools, FEESST has been shown (in a head and neck cancer population) to be a more cost-effective option when compared to VFSS.[12]

FEES/FEESST Technique

FEES or FEESST is ideally performed by two individuals, an otolaryngologist and a speech-language pathologist (SLP). The typical setup includes a flexible laryngoscope, light source, and video system. A video tower is essential for several reasons. It provides visualization for both the examiners and the patient, allows video documentation (necessary for billing purposes), and allows the physician to review the examination and to compare it to previous evaluations when available. In addition to the standard FEES equipment, two additional items are required to perform FEESST: a calibrated air pulse sensory stimulator (KayPentax, Inc, Lincoln Park, NJ) and a flexible endoscope or sheath with a side channel for the delivery of the air pulse.

These steps are included in the sensory testing portion of FEESST:

- With the patient positioned sitting upright, oxymetazoline (0.05%) without topical anesthesia is sprayed into the nasal cavity (topical anesthesia may impair laryngeal sensation).
- The lubricated endoscope is passed transnasally, evaluating nasopharyngeal closure, tongue base, hypopharynx, vocal fold motion, and possible pooling of oral secretions (the latter findings have been associated with increased aspiration risk).[9]
- The endoscope is positioned over the ipsilateral arytenoid/aryepiglottic fold junction (approximately 2 mm from the mucosa) and calibrated air pulses are administered until active laryngeal closure or LAR results, representing the stimulation threshold.
- The contralateral side is tested.
- Results are compared with normal values (less than 4 mm Hg is normal, 4 to 6 is a moderate sensory deficit, and greater than 6 mm Hg is a severe sensory deficit).[7,10]

After sensory testing, the FEES portion of the examination is performed:

- The patient is asked to perform a high pitched "ē" and pharyngeal squeeze is observed.

- The patient is asked to dry swallow while epiglottic inversion and movement of pooled secretions are assessed.
- The patient is then asked to swallow a series of color-dyed food boluses in this order: honey-thickened liquid, purees, solids, nectar-thick liquids, and thin liquids.
- Swallowing parameters are assessed including the presence of residue in the vallecula or hypopharynx, laryngeal penetration (entry of bolus into the laryngeal inlet), or aspiration (bolus below the level of the vocal folds).
- Brief tracheoscopy is performed to further confirm the presence or absence of aspiration.

After the completion of the diagnostic portion of the FEES, compensatory techniques can be tested. The endoscope remains in place, while various techniques including a supraglottic swallow, head turn, double-swallow, and head tilt are tried. This helps establish the best dietary strategy and reinforces the swallowing techniques to the patient and family.

FEES/FEESST Summary

FEES and FEESST offer many advantages over traditional methods of dysphagia assessment. FEES has comparable sensitivity with VFSS in evaluating penetration, pooled secretions, aspiration, and pharyngeal residue.[5,6,9] Furthermore, there appears to be an advantage in cost-effectiveness when comparing FEESST to VFSS.[12] Thus, FEES and FEESST provide extremely valuable assessments in dysphagia evaluation.

TRANSNASAL ESOPHAGOSCOPY (TNE)

Nearly a century ago, laryngologists such as Chevalier Jackson pioneered the technique of rigid esophagoscopy for examination, dilation, biopsy, and foreign body removal. Over recent decades, other specialties developed transoral flexible endoscopes to evaluate the upper gastrointestinal tract in sedated patients. Recently, thin, flexible TNE endoscopes that have distal-chip cameras for high-quality optics have been developed (Figure 11-1). Measuring approximately 5 mm in outer diameter, the TNE scopes can be passed safely transnasally, while providing air insufflation, irrigation, and biopsy capability. In comparison to rigid esophagoscopy and sedated flexible endoscopy, unsedated office-based TNE has been shown to be an excellent screening tool for esophageal pathology such as Barrett's esophagitis.[1,13]

TNE Indications

Although there are multiple potential TNE applications within an otolaryngologic practice, clear indications for TNE remain undefined due to the novelty of the technology. For example, it is not clear if all patients with uncomplicated laryngopharyngeal reflux should undergo esophageal screening when the prevalence of Barrett's metaplasia in persons with LPR has been reported to be as low as 7%.[14] However, Reavis et al demonstrated that symptoms of LPR were significantly more prevalent than typical gastroesophageal reflux symptoms in persons with dysplasia or adenocarcinoma of the esophagus.[15] Thus, symptoms of LPR may be the only indication of esophageal dysplasia or malignancy. Until the indications for TNE in persons with LPR can be better defined, screening such patients seems reasonable.

The following is a list of current TNE applications within an otolaryngology practice:

1. To screen patients with laryngopharyngeal reflux to evaluate for reflux esophagitis (Figure 11-2), Barrett's esophagus (Figure 11-3), or esophageal adenocarcinoma (Figure 11-4).
2. To obtain tissue specimens and perform clinical flexible panendoscopy in patients with known lesions suspicious for malignancy.
3. To assess the esophageal mucosa of patients exposed to previous sources of damage such as caustic ingestion or radiation therapy.
4. To rule out anatomic obstruction (stricture, diverticulum) and assess motility in patients with dysphagia.
5. As a therapeutic tool for procedures such as secondary tracheoesophageal puncture,[16] foreign body management, and placement of wireless pH capsules.[17]

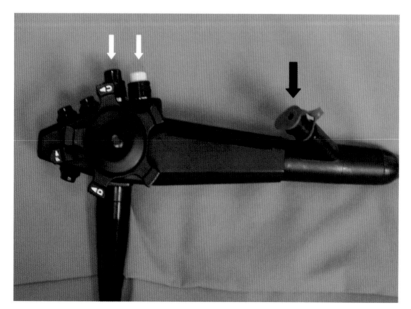

FIGURE 11–1. Transnasal esophagoscope with suction, irrigation and air insufflation (*white arrows*) as well as a working channel (*dark arrow*) to allow for passage of topical anesthesia, biopsy cups, and laser fiber.

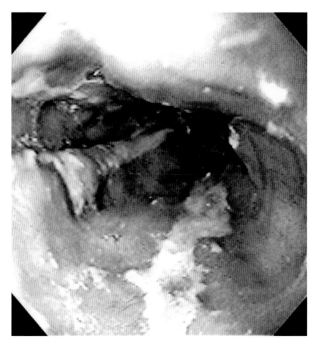

FIGURE 11–2. Severe reflux esophagitis with near-circumferential mucosal ulceration and exudate involving the distal esophagus.

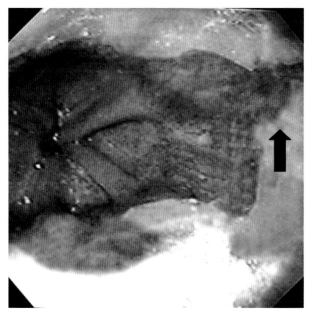

FIGURE 11–3. Long-segment (>3 cm in length) Barrett's esophagus is suspected clinically (*arrow*), but histopathologic confirmation is necessary for the diagnosis.

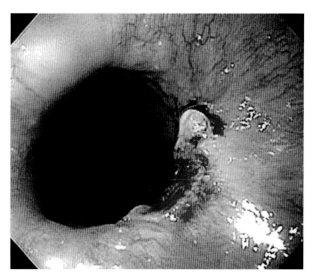

FIGURE 11–4. Early esophageal adenocarcinoma involving the distal esophagus.

TNE Technique

Transnasal esophagoscopes of adequate length to allow a retroflexed view of the gastroesophageal junction (GEJ) and gastric cardia (at least 60 cm) and a diameter small enough to allow comfortable transnasal passage are available through multiple venders (EE-1580K, Pentax Precision Instrument Corp, Orangeburg, NY; Olympus PEF-V, Olympus America Inc, Melville, NY; and Vision Sciences TNE-2000 with Endosheath, Medtronic Xomed, Jacksonville, Fla). All of the endoscopes have an air insufflation port, and working channel for biopsy and suction. Recently, endoscopes have also been created with disposable sheaths that eliminate the need for lengthy cleaning times between patients.

At the time a TNE examination is scheduled, the patient is instructed not to eat or drink for 3 hours before the TNE. This ensures that the stomach is empty. A recent meal is not an absolute contraindication to TNE, but reflux of stomach contents may interfere with visualization of the distal esophagus, GEJ, and gastric cardia.

The basic steps for successful TNE are:

■ Topical nasal anesthesia and decongestion with oxymetazoline (0.05%) and lidocaine (4%), or cocaine (2%) soaked pledget(s) for approximately 10 minutes.

- One spray of 20% benzocaine (Hurricaine, British Pharmaceuticals, Waukegan, Ill) to the oropharynx (optional).
- TNE endoscope is lubricated.
- Endoscope is advanced with visualization of nasopharyngeal closure, tongue base, hypopharynx, vocal fold motion, and possible pooling of oral secretions
- Patient is instructed to flex head forward and swallow (or belch as an alternative) as the endoscope is passed gently through the cricopharyngeus muscle.
- With gentle air insufflation and suctioning, the esophageal mucosa is visualized and the scope is advanced with the esophageal lumen always in view.
- Esophageal motility is evaluated as the patient swallows (assessment may be enhanced by feeding the patient food-colored applesauce with the TNE in place), with normal esophageal transit time less than 13 seconds.
- Lower esophageal sphincter (LES) function should be evaluated with the esophagoscope a few centimeters proximal to it, determining if the LES is closed (normal) or open at rest and whether or not it opens and then promptly closes following swallowing
- The junction of the gastric and esophageal mucosa (squamocolumnar junction or *Z-line*) (Figure 11–5) is carefully visualized to evaluate for pathology such as reflux esophagitis (see Figure 11–2), Barrett's esophagus (see Figure 11–3), or hiatal hernias.
- The endoscope is advanced into the stomach and retroflexion is performed to assist in the identification of small or medium-sized hiatal hernias (Figure 11-6).
- If mucosal lesions or irregularities are noted at any point during the TNE, biopsy forceps are passed through the working channel and multiple biopsies are obtained.

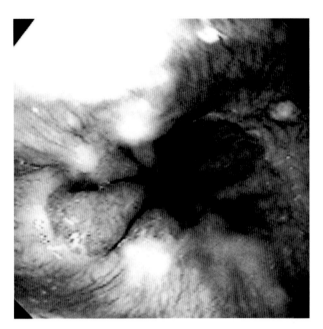

FIGURE 11–5. Normal squamocolumnar junction (*Z-line*) with regular borders and absence of mucosal irregularities.

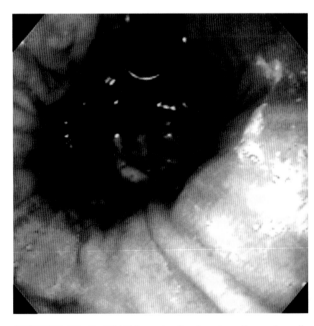

FIGURE 11–6. TNE in retroflexion to allow visualization of the scope passing through a hiatal hernia.

- The endoscope is slowly withdrawn to re-examine the mucosa of the entire esophagus.

TNE Troubleshooting

Although TNE is a relatively simple procedure, several problems can be encountered during TNE that can be warning signs to the examiner:

- **Difficulty in passing the TNE through the upper esophageal sphincter (UES)**—This should alert the examiner to the possibility of a hypertonic UES or a Zenker's diverticulum. If the endoscopist finds him- or herself in a diverticulum then suctioning, air insufflation, and gentle rotation of the scope should be used to find the lumen before continuing the examination. Perforation may occur if the tip of the esophagoscope enters a diverticulum and significant pressure is used.
- **The presence of a dilated esophagus or the retention of swallowed material**— These should alert the examiner to the potential for an esophageal motility disorder, stricture or ring, foreign body, diverticulum, mass lesion, or achalasia.
- **The patient experiences significant abdominal discomfort during the TNE**—A common error is the use of excessive air insufflation during the examination, which can result in abdominal bloating and discomfort for the patient. Air should be gently insufflated to obtain complete visualization of all mucosal surfaces and then suctioned out when possible. The majority of insufflated air is needed when evaluating the LES, and it should be suctioned out at the end of the examination.

TNE Complications

The complication rate for TNE is very low. A recent review of over 700 TNE procedures revealed only six cases of self-limited epistaxis and two vasovagal episodes.[2] Although the TNE procedure was well tolerated by most patients, failure to complete the procedure was most commonly due to the inability to pass the TNE scope through a tight nasal vault (3%). No cases of esophageal perforation have been reported with TNE performed by otolaryngologists.

TNE Conclusion

TNE is a safe and effective procedure that maintains all the advantages of previously reported flexible endoscopic techniques with regard to safety and screening, while offering the distinct advantage of performance in the clinic without sedation.

OFFICE TRACHEOBRONCHOSCOPY

Part of the popularity of flexible endoscopy, particularly in the evaluation of the tracheobronchial tree, is the ability to perform an evaluation without general anesthesia. Office tracheobronchoscopy can be used routinely and safely in most adults with topical anesthesia alone. Common indications include the evaluation of patients with known or suspected airway stenosis, hemoptysis, chronic cough, and application of flexible lasers on airway lesions such as tracheal papilloma (Figure 11-7). Its use, however, should be limited

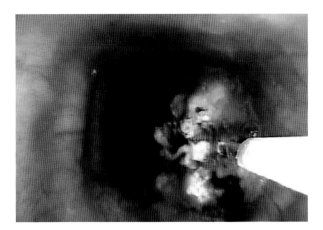

FIGURE 11–7. Tracheoscopy with the pulsed-dye fiber advanced and actively treating a large tracheal papilloma.

in patients with cardiac and reactive airway disease, as the risk of complications may be increased due to significant hemodynamic and pulmonary function changes that are associated with delivery of the topical anesthetic, passage of the endoscope through the larynx, and suctioning.[18,19] In addition, consideration should be given to the routine use of monitoring when performing lengthy procedures in the tracheobronchial tree. Many studies have recommended the routine use of pulse oximetry, but the need for cardiac monitoring is less clear.[20]

Tracheoscopy Technique

There are several basic steps to tracheoscopy in the clinic:

- The patient is first warned that he or she will experience a coughing and/or choking sensation for a few seconds.
- The examination is video-documented.
- The scope is advanced transnasally to just above the vocal folds.
- On having the patient sniff, the scope is advanced through the abducted vocal folds into the upper trachea
- The lesion or area of concern is visualized, and the scope is withdrawn within about 2 to 3 seconds as the patient coughs.
- The recorded examination can then be reviewed in slow motion or frame-by-frame to fully evaluate the findings.

Routine cursory evaluation of the upper trachea itself requires little, if any, additional anesthesia, and a standard flexible laryngoscope may be used. If a prolonged examination of the proximal trachea is necessary or a biopsy is planned, a flexible endoscope with a side channel is usually necessary. Furthermore, if a prolonged examination is required, anesthesia with the techniques described in the "Bronchoscopy" section below may be warranted.

Tracheobronchoscopy Technique

If a more detailed or distal evaluation is necessary, additional anesthesia should be used. The maximum recommended dose of lidocaine is typically 300 to 400 mg (7–10 cc of 4% lidocaine). If a prolonged examination is anticipated or extensive biopsies are planned, the lidocaine can be diluted to 2%, permitting use of a greater volume (14–20 cc) of the anesthetic.

There are several options for tracheal anesthesia:

- Topical lidocaine, usually delivered through the side channel of the endoscope or orally via an Abraham cannula, while having the patient phonate
- Nebulized lidocaine
- Cricothyroid puncture with instillation of lidocaine into the subglottic airway (this route should be avoided in patients with severe infraglottic/subglottic stenosis due to risk of edema/airway compromise).

The steps for tracheobronchoscopy are similar to those for tracheoscopy; however, a longer flexible endoscope, such as a bronchoscope or transnasal esophagoscope is necessary. A side channel is needed for delivery of topical anesthetic, biopsy, and suctioning. It is important to avoid excess suctioning, which can cause oxygen desaturation. Finally, as the endoscope is advanced into the lower airway, attention should be paid to the bronchoscopic landmarks to keep proper orientation.

Office Tracheobronchoscopy Summary

In comparison to bronchoscopy under sedation or general anesthesia, tracheobronchoscopy offers a significant cost savings by avoiding facility-based service and recovery room costs. Furthermore, office-based tracheobronchoscopy is a well-tolerated, safe, and effective technique that

Screening Endoscopy

Indications for esophageal screening with TNE are not well defined because large populations of patients with laryngopharyngeal reflux have not been screened. As multi-institutional experience with TNE increases, the prevalence and severity of esophageal disease among laryngopharyngeal reflux patients will be determined and used to create appropriate esophageal screening guidelines. The techniques for biopsy and tissue sampling have been questioned. A recent publication by the authors described the incongruence between endoscopic and histologic appearances in patients with Barrett's esophagus.[21] Finally, who should perform esophagoscopy? Many gastroenterologists have expressed concern regarding the advent of TNE and the increasing prevalence of otolaryngologists performing unsedated esophagoscopy. A recent survey of primary care providers revealed that a majority of the respondents (62%) indicated that the availability of unsedated esophagoscopy increased referral to specialists for the procedure and that 52% would be willing to perform the screening themselves in their office.[22]

has been used extensively with a very low complication rate.

This chapter has discussed the applications and techniques for office-based evaluations including FEES/FEESST, TNE, and tracheoscopy/tracheobronchoscopy. The applications for office-based aerodigestive endoscopy are rapidly evolving. Increased utilization of in-office endoscopy will help deliver improved quality of care for patients in a safer and less expensive manner. In the future, office-based evaluation of the aerodigestive tract is likely to emerge as the standard of care in adults.

Review Questions

1. Potential applications for transnasal esophagoscopy include:
   a. Esophageal screening in patients with pH probe documented laryngopharyngeal reflux
   b. Screening for the presence of a possible foreign body
   c. Evaluation of patients with dysphagia or globus sensation
   d. All of the above

2. The best method of detecting a hiatal hernia during transnasal esophagoscopy is:
   a. Have the patient swallow
   b. Retroflexing the patient in the chair
   c. Retroflexion of the TNE scope while in the stomach
   d. All of the above

3. If a patient reports abdominal discomfort during the transnasal esophagoscopy examination, the most likely etiology is:
   a. Referred pain from the upper throat

b. Esophageal perforation
c. Excessive air insufflation
d. All of the above

4. In a patient presenting to an otolaryngology clinic with dysphagia and subjective aspiration, the most appropriate evaluation that could be done in clinic is:
   a. FEES or FEESST
   b. Sensory testing alone
   c. Flexible laryngoscopy
   d. None of the above

5. Caution should be used regarding the use of office-based tracheobronchoscopy for patients with which comorbidities?
   a. Esophageal cancer
   b. Hypertension
   c. Diabetes
   d. Cardiac or reactive airway disease

REFERENCES

1. Glaws WR, Etzkorn KP, Wenig BL, Zulfigar H, Wiley TE, Watkins JL. Comparison of rigid and flexible esophagoscopy in the diagnosis of esophageal disease: diagnostic accuracy, complications, and cost. *Ann Otol Rhinol Laryngol.* 1996;105(4):262-1266.

2. Postma GN, Cohen JT, Belafsky PC, et al. Transnasal esophagoscopy: revisited (over 700 consecutive cases). *Laryngoscope.* 2005;115(2):321-323.

3. Saeian K. Unsedated transnasal endoscopy: a safe and less costly alternative. *Curr Gastroenterol Rep.* 2002;4(3):213-217.

4. Kubba H, Spinou E, Brown D. Is same-day discharge suitable following rigid esophagoscopy? Findings in a series of 655 cases. *Ear Nose Throat J.* 2003;821:33-36.

5. Langmore SE, Schatz K, Olson N. Endoscopic and videofluoroscopic evaluations of swallowing and aspiration. *Ann Otol Rhinol Laryngol.* 1991; 100(8):678-681.

6. Hiss SG, Postma GN. Fiberoptic endoscopic evaluation of swallowing. *Laryngoscope.* 2003;1138: 1386-1393.

7. Aviv JE, Kim T, Sacco RL, et al. FEESST: a new bedside endoscopic test of the motor and sensory components of swallowing. *Ann Otol Rhinol Laryngol.* 1998;1075:378-387.

8. Leder SB, Espinosa JF Aspiration risk after acute stroke: comparison of clinical examination and fiberoptic endoscopic evaluation of swallowing. *Dysphagia.* 2002;17(3):214-218.

9. Aviv JE. Prospective, randomized outcome study of endoscopy versus modified barium swallow in patients with dysphagia. *Laryngoscope.* 2000; 110(4):563-574.

10. Aviv JE, Liu H, Parides M, Kaplan ST, Close LG. Laryngopharyngeal sensory deficits in patients with laryngopharyngeal reflux and dysphagia. *Ann Otol Rhinol Laryngol.* 2000;10911:1000-1006.

11. Phua SY, McGarvey LP, Ngu MC, Ing AJ. Patients with gastro-oesophageal reflux disease and cough have impaired laryngopharyngeal mechanosensitivity. *Thorax.* 2005;60(7):488-491.

12. Aviv JE, Sataloff RT, Cohen M, Spitzer J, et al. Cost-effectiveness of two types of dysphagia care in head and neck cancer: a preliminary report. *Ear Nose Throat J.* 2001;80(8):553-556, 558.

13. Saeian K, Staff DM, Vasilopoulos S, et al. Unsedated transnasal endoscopy accurately detects Barrett's metaplasia and dysplasia. *Gastrointest Endosc.* 2002;56(4):472-478.

14. Koufman JA, Belafsky PC, Bach KK, Daniel E, Postma GN. Prevalence of esophagitis in patients with pH-documented laryngopharyngeal reflux. *Laryngoscope.* 2002;1129:1606-1609.

15. Reavis KM, Morris CD, Gopal DV, Hunter JG, Jobe BA. Laryngopharyngeal reflux symptoms better predict the presence of esophageal adenocarcinoma than typical gastroesophageal reflux symptoms. *Ann Surg.* 2004;239(7):849-856; discussion, 856-858.

16. Bach KK, Postma GN, Koufman JA. In-office tracheoesophageal puncture using transnasal esophagoscopy. *Laryngoscope.* 2003;113:173-176.

17. Belafsky PC, Allen K, Castro-Del Rosario L, Roseman D. Wireless pH testing as an adjunct to unsedated transnasal esophagoscopy: the safety and efficacy of transnasal telemetry capsule placement. *Otolaryngol Head Neck Surg.* 2004;131(1):26-28.

18. Lundgren R, Haggmark S, Reiz S. Hemodynamic effects of flexible fiberoptic bronchoscopy performed under topical anesthesia. *Chest*. 1982; 82(3):295-299.

19. Peacock AJ, Benson-Mitchell R, Godfrey R. Effect of fiberoptic bronchoscopy on pulmonary function. *Thorax*. 1990; 45(1):38-41.

20. Colt HG, Morris JF. Fiberoptic bronchoscopy without premedication. A retrospective study. *Chest*. 1990;987:1327-1330.

21. Halum SL, Postma GN, Bates DD, Koufman JA. Incongruence between histologic and endoscopic diagnoses of Barrett's esophagus using transnasal esophagoscopy. *Laryngoscope*. 2006; 116(2):303-306.

22. Boolchand V, Faulx A, Das A, Zyzanski S, Isenberg G, Cooper G, Sivak MV Jr, Chak A. Primary care physician attitudes toward endoscopic screening for GERD symptoms and unsedated esophagoscopy. *Gastrointest Endosc*. 2006;63(2):228-233.

PART IV
Principles of Therapy

12

Laryngeal Hygiene

Douglas M. Hicks, PhD, CCC-SLP
Claudio F. Milstein, PhD, CCC-SLP

KEY POINTS

■ Laryngeal hygiene does not require, and usually does not involve, direct voice manipulation through the use of traditional exercises and drills.

■ Vocal wellness encourages prevention rather than treatment.

■ The principles of vocal care and nurturing are generally common sense but not intuitive; patients will benefit from education.

■ Insufficient or incorrect information about the larynx and about the voice in particular is a major cause of vocal career problems.

Hygiene is defined as the "establishment and maintenance of health" by facilitating "conditions or practices conducive to health."[1] Vocal hygiene, in particular, is focused on promoting laryngeal health, with appropriate phonatory function and normal voice production. Achieving health involves limiting trauma to laryngeal tissues by addressing diet, lifestyle choices, and vocal demands (Figure 12-1). Hygiene does not require, and usually does not involve, direct voice manipulation through the use of traditional exercises and drills. Therapeutic intervention instructs patients to care for their vocal folds rather than teaching them voicing.[2] The impact of hygiene measures is well established in both amateur and professional voice users.[3,4] Just as importantly, the benefit of this education for teachers has been suggested,[5] although in a compelling prospective study,[6] instruction in vocal hygiene did not result in significant benefit when compared to vocal function exercises (see chapter 13, Speech-Language Intervention).

The principles of care and nurturing are often a result of common sense but not intuitive. As a result, naïveté about the larynx and vocal function becomes a major contributor to vocal

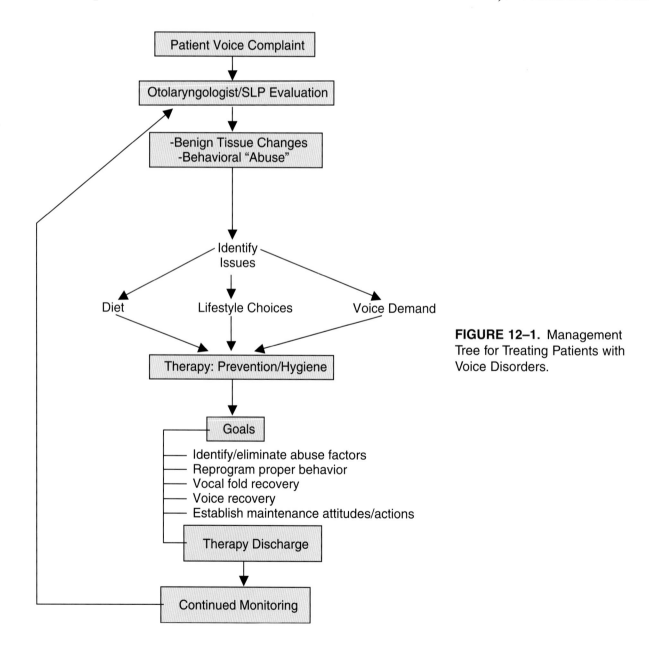

FIGURE 12–1. Management Tree for Treating Patients with Voice Disorders.

problems, sometimes chronic in nature. In all aspects of therapeutic intervention, patients are taught to be informed consumers of their problems by empowering them with knowledge that changes both their attitudes about voice and their actions. Therefore, the challenge for the patient is to increase the consistency of his or her behavior to provide a "larynx friendly" environment. This involves providing information about laryngeal function to the patient as well as reinforcing general health principles, such as the maintenance of adequate hydration.

Effective teaching of laryngeal hygiene by the speech therapist or phoniatrician, for example, is best served by initially providing several orientation concepts that explain the therapeutic process and provide a foundation for the patient's effective learning. The first concept is to clarify the nature of therapy as being cognitive—"information loading" rather than aimed at specific phonatory techniques. The "hard work" nature of therapy manifested in both consciousness and conscientiousness, is described below:

- **Consciousness:** a necessary part of any habit-changing process; requires patient to become temporarily preoccupied with a behavior previously produced unconsciously and automatically. Effective reprogramming of maladaptive behaviors demands this level of concentration.
- **Conscientiousness:** refers to an increased disciplined compliance in order to foster effective reprogramming of behavior. This process neither requires perfection nor paranoia about voice. Success should occur as long as the patient implements proper therapeutic changes "more often than not."

It is important to change as little as possible to produce the proper outcome; this reinforces the important principle that the cost of success through therapy is not for the patient to become uncomfortable with his or her new vocal profile. These principles are further discussed in chapter 13, Speech-Language Intervention. The practitioner must make it clear that ultimate success is the patient's responsibility. Patients need to take personal ownership for both creating the problem through bad choices and achieving successful recovery. That process is not easy or guaranteed as recent research implies different stages of mental readiness to behavioral changes that may complicate patient compliance.[7] The majority of laryngeal hygiene intervention does not focus directly on actual voice performance. In contrast, most activity is focused on changing enough behavior (vocal choices) to promote recovery of laryngeal structure and function, which translates into voice restoration. The essence of vocal hygiene is an indirect focus on actual voice performance rather than a direct manipulation of specific performance parameters (pitch, loudness, laryngeal quality) through traditional exercises or drills. This is in addition to dietary and general health measures that should be emphasized in all patients, such as the avoidance of irritants (tobacco, alcohol, caffeine) and the maintenance of excellent hydration. This is discussed further in upcoming sections.

Two important therapy goals in patients suffering from vocal abuse are educating them on several key hygiene concepts and identifying/eliminating specific abusive factors. This information facilitates both proper attitudes about voice and recovery action plans.

There are several general concepts to keep in mind. Many therapists find it beneficial to emphasize the association between *structure*, *function*, and *performance*. The voice outcome represents a tangible behavioral indicator of vocal fold status. It is always available to be monitored contingent on the patient going beyond simple "hearing" of voice to the next step of analysis, implied in "listening." The patient may indeed become a self-sufficient monitor of both proper and poor vocal performances. They may learn to react properly to what they hear (and feel) by implementing appropriate therapy strategies, with each day constituting a series of decision points either for or against the larynx.

Vocal abuse must be defined in the instruction of laryngeal hygiene. Misuse can be defined as using the larynx beyond its physical limits (ie, screaming). Overuse, on the other hand,

involves using the larynx within its physical limits but for too long or too often. Vocal abusers
typically have evidence of both components; it is
rare for an individual to manifest strictly one. The
"abuse threshold" is variable even within a given
individual as it may be a function of fatigue,

The Role of Complete Voice Rest in Vocal Hygiene Intervention

The traditional reliance on complete voice rest to resolve vocal
fold nodules or other benign tissue changes has been replaced
by a philosophy of conservation or caution. This is based on the
realization that abusive behaviors underlying the tissue changes are
ultimately maladaptive habit—chronically perpetuated as automatic,
unconscious, and natural behaviors. Although complete cessation of
voicing accomplishes the necessary reduction in tissue contact/
collision forces, it does nothing to reprogram the patient's bad
habits. Vocal conservation, in contrast, produces enough positive
change to promote tissue recovery that will lead to voice improvement. Furthermore, these changes are accomplished in real-life
circumstances rather than in an unrealistic world of silence.
Long-term establishment and maintenance of new, vocally healthy
habits are best formed in the very activities or settings that previously
fostered abuse. By its nature, this process takes longer than what
can be accomplished through complete voice rest. However, the
strength and permanence of behavior reprogramming through a
conservation approach is superior to the more aggressive silence
approach. Cultivating patience in the patient is a necessary step for
eventual success but acceptance is usually easy, given the benefit of
generally maintained life routines possible with conservation.

This more contemporary practice pattern does not eliminate,
however, a continued, valuable role for complete voice rest. Although
more limited, its use in certain voice and larynx circumstances can
be essential for positive outcomes with certain voice and larynx
circumstances. These typically involve more acute or significant
tissue impact as represented by acute laryngitis, laryngeal trauma,
vocal fold hemorrhaging, or postphonosurgical care. The duration
of complete rest for the first three conditions is usually dictated by
recovery, through medical management, and/or natural healing
time. Voice rest postsurgery is a far more variable time frame as a
function of several factors including the specific surgical procedure;
the extent, location, and nature of tissue insult; surgeon preference;
healing response; and the nature of expected voice demands on
recovery. In general, however, the weaning process back to normal
promotes the shortest duration of complete voice rest that the
tissue integrity and future positive vocal outcomes can allow.

In summary, complete voice rest has evolved in current practice
to a limited but well-defined role that usually is not a part of routine
vocal hygiene instructions.[11]

concurrent inflammation, and other medical and environmental issues. The important practical issue is for the patient to learn limits and operate within them.

A useful tool for managing vocal use and hygiene is the concept of "vocal finances." The patient may consider vocalization to be a tangible commodity that can be spent or saved. Although informal, the money analogy in which each use of the voice is considered a withdrawal from one's laryngeal "bank account" is highly effective with patients. It requires patient to assess the vocal expense of activities, scenarios, and life choices. The patient may ask him- or herself the following questions at each daily decision point: (1) Is there a vocal cost? (2) How much is that cost? and (3) Can I afford it?

The next major objective is to identify and eliminate specific abuse factors. The rationale is simple—focus on the major contributing factors that will increase both efficiency and effectiveness of treatment strategies. To accomplish that identification step, a simple but effective exercise can be used (Table 12–1).

The final step of hygiene intervention involves a review of numerous possible practical issues related to diet, lifestyle choices, and vocal demands. Perhaps the best studied of these factors is hydration. Several important studies have demonstrated the impact of systemic hydration on phonation threshold pressure and fatigue.[8] In a double-blinded, placebo-controlled study, Verdolini and colleagues demonstrated an inverse relation between phonatory effort and hydration level, although primarily for high-pitched phonation tasks.[9] Water should be each patient's primary beverage, with rare exception in the case of cardiac or renal disease. Even nasal obstruction and resultant oral breathing has been shown to negatively affect vocal effort.[10] In particularly harsh climates, consideration of whole house or room humidifiers is helpful.

In addition to drinking plenty of water, the patient should avoid known irritants such as caffeine, alcohol, and tobacco. See chapter 23, Reflux and Its Impact on Laryngology, for more information. Practitioners patients should be aware that decaffeinated products have their own potential liability as the chemicals used

TABLE 12–1. Exercise to Identify and Eliminate Specific Voice Abuse Factors

1. Have the patient generate a generic detailed activity schedule for a full week from wake-up to bedtime, Monday through Sunday—using 30-minute intervals. Preferably this is done as a home assignment with patient returning for the next session with a written schedule printout.

2. Together, patient and therapist review *all* activities and overlay them with voice use/demand. To generate an accurate and comprehensive voice profile, it is important to be detailed.

3. In parallel with establishing voice use, identify the activities or scenarios that represent vocal abuse—previously defined and understood as either misuse or overuse. Compile a full list of abuse factors.

4. Rank-order the worst abuse factors (limit to maximum of five—requiring the patient to address additional factors reduces their effectiveness in strategy implementation and compliance).

5. Require the patient to generate at least two strategies to address and counteract the top-ranked factors. To stimulate his or her creativity, stress that effective action plans typically involve either elimination, reduction, or change-of-form thinking. Requiring patients to generate a strategy proposal markedly increases their ownership of the plan, usually improving subsequent implementation and compliance. The therapist role is strictly as a reactant—to confirm the patient's plan and offer edits when needed (usually because patient's suggestions are overly aggressive).

6. The final strategy decision step is ideally one of negotiation rather than unilateral dictation by the therapist. Re-emphasize the prior promise of changing as little as necessary to accomplish change. The ultimate litmus test for strategies is confirming the changes are specifically matched to a particular abuse factor, are easy to implement, and will be natural for the patient's use—in other words, "doable."

for decaffeination are purported to also promote reflux. Beyond that, the general well-being related to adequate rest and physical fitness provides the ideal environment for vocal and laryngeal health. Important tips for general laryngeal health and hygiene are noted in Table 12-2.

TABLE 12–2. Vocal Wellness and Laryngeal Health

Take personal ownership of your vocal health—be accountable

1. Practice proper vocal hygiene—be guided by common sense
2. Common sense—respond to how the voice sounds/feels
3. Count the vocal "costliness" of your lifestyle choices
4. Managing your voice requires discipline plus flexibility
5. Avoid physical/emotional exhaustion (eat/sleep wisely)
6. Hydration/humidification are key
7. Reduce caffeine intake
8. No smoking—active or second-hand
9. Alcohol in moderation
10. Avoid late night eating/drinking
11. No substitute for vocal training
12. Respond promptly to upper respiratory tract infections.

It is clear from clinical experience that maintenance of laryngeal hygiene is important in preventing and treating vocal dysfunction. Hydration is a key issue but the fundamentals of patient education and daily decision-making will provide for ideal long-term maintenance of laryngeal health. Factors that predispose the patient to vocal abuse should be identified and eliminated within the framework of the patient's wishes for vocal and laryngeal health.

Review Questions

1. Can the speaking voice harm the singing voice?

2. Do caffeinated beverages provide adequate vocal fold hydration?

3. Is the temperature of beverages irrelevant for my voice?

4. Is whispering a good "voice" alternative during laryngitis?

REFERENCES

1. Hygiene Definition; *Webster's Medical Desk Dictionary*. Springfield, Mass: Merriam-Webster, Inc; 1986.
2. Verdolini, K. *Guide to Vocology*. Iowa City, Ia: National Center for Voice and Speech; 1998:27.
3. Timmermans B, Vanderwegen J, DeBodt MS. Outcome of vocal hygiene in singers. *Curr Opin Otolaryngol Head Neck Surg*. 2005;13(3):138–142.
4. Yiu EM, Chan RM. Effect of hydration and vocal rest on the vocal fatigue in amateur karaoke singers. *J Voice*. 2003;17(2):216–227.
5. Chan RW. Does the voice improve with vocal hygiene education? A study of some instrumental voice measures in a group of kindergarten teachers. *J Voice*. 1994;8(3):279–291.
6. Roy N, Gray SD, Simon M, Dove H, Corbin-Lewis K, Stemple JC. Evaluation of the effects of two treatment approaches for teachers with voice disorders: a prospective randomized clinical trial. *J Speech Lang Hear Res*. 2001;44(2):286–296.
7. Van Leer E, Hepner E. Toward a theoretical framework for patient adherence to voice therapy. *J Voice*. In press.
8. Solomon NP, DiMattia MS. Effects of a vocally fatiguing task and systemic hydration on phonation threshold pressure. *J Voice*. 2000;14(3):341–362.
9. Verdolini K, Titze IR, Fennell A. Dependence of phonatory effort on hydration level. *J Speech Hear Res*. 1994;37(5):1001–1007.
10. Sivasankar M, Fisher KV. Oral breathing increases PTH and vocal effort by superficial drying of vocal fold mucosa. *J Voice*. 2002;16(2):172–181.
11. Sataloff RT. Voice rest. In: Sataloff RT. *Professional Voice: The Science and Art of Clinical Care*. (2nd ed.) San Diego, Calif: Singular Publishing Group; 1997:453–456.

13

Speech-Language Intervention–Voice Therapy

Sarah Marx Schneider, MS, CCC-SLP
Robert T. Sataloff, MD, DMA

KEY POINTS

- ■ Diagnostic and medical treatment of voice disorders are the responsibility of physicians, ideally otolaryngologists with expertise in this area. Behavioral evaluation and treatment of dysphonia in the professional voice user are the responsibility of speech-language pathologists.

- ■ Interdisciplinary team relationships are crucial to improve patient care.

- ■ Special information should be included when gathering the history of the professional voice user compared to the nonprofessional because of differences in vocal demand and expectations.

- ■ The initial voice evaluation provides the clinician with valuable baseline information about vocal function, patient stimulability, possible therapy techniques, expectations of the voice user, and information regarding likely success and outcomes of therapy.

- ■ Voice therapy is patient specific. A common diagnosis among patients does not indicate that the same facilitators will be appropriate for each. Multiple approaches must be available.

The practice of speech-language pathology includes prevention, habilitation, and rehabilitation of communication, swallowing, or other upper aerodigestive disorders; elective modification of communication behaviors, and enhancement of communication.[1] The American Speech-Language-Hearing Association (ASHA) states that the speech-language pathologist should provide prevention, screening, consultation, assessment, treatment, intervention, management, counseling, and follow-up services for speech, voice, language, swallowing, cognition, and sensory awareness for communication, swallowing, and upper aerodigestive functions. In the area of treating voice disorders, the speech-language pathologist is concerned not with diagnosis and treatment of laryngeal diseases or other physiologic disorders, but rather with understanding, analyzing, and modifying vocal function.

If, perceptually, the voice is within normal limits for the patient and is being produced in a reasonably efficient, nonabusive manner, then intervention by a speech-language pathologist need not be conducted. It is not within the speech-language pathologist's scope of practice to provide special training that will develop range, power, control, stamina, and the esthetic quality required for artistic expression. The speech-language pathologist is concerned with the voice that presents with a current or potential problem, identifying and analyzing the problem, then helping the voice user modify vocal behaviors to use the vocal mechanism with optimal efficiency. Responsibilities in ameliorating the voice problem include: analyzing vocal behaviors perceptually and objectively; analyzing vocational, educational, and psychological factors that may interact with vocal behaviors to precipitate, maintain, or exacerbate vocal difficulty; and then designing and implementing an individual program for modifying vocal behaviors.[2]

Just as do physicians, speech-language pathologists vary in their backgrounds and experience in the treatment of voice disorders. Furthermore, the curricula that speech-language pathologists complete during education and training varies widely and typically addresses normal and disordered voice production only at a general level. Curricula rarely provide extended education or knowledge about the professional voice. Therefore, prior to making a referral to a speech-language pathologist for voice therapy, his or her background and training should be considered.

This chapter focuses on the speech-language pathologist's treatment of voice disorders with special emphasis on the treatment of professional voice users. There are many factors to consider when working with professional voice users. The following is not meant to be an inclusive list but is intended merely to provide a framework of key considerations. Evaluation and treatment of a professional voice user requires increased sensitivity from the clinician. At first, when listening to the patient's voice, it may sound "normal. However, sounding "normal" is relative. The professional voice user, typically, has increased awareness of minute changes in the voice. Therefore, a speech-language pathologist must be "supersensitive to superspeaking." The goals of the professional voice user/performer are typically different from those of a nonperformer and must be considered as such. With that in mind, it is important to learn the patient's expectations and provide a realistic perspective on the possible outcome of therapy based on the diagnosis and response to trial therapy techniques during the initial assessment.

Further consideration must be given to body and self-awareness issues in performers versus nonperformers. Body- and self-awareness, in this sense, refers to the patient's awareness of his or her own behaviors and the ability to make changes as instructed. Depending on their previous depth of training, professional voice users may have increased awareness of vocal behaviors. Body- and self-awareness are important skills to develop or maximize in the voice user. They will aid the patient in developing, recognizing, and maintaining techniques for efficient voice use.

Environmental contributions also should be noted. As a professional voice user, the patient may be in situations that may not be obvious to a treating clinician. These may include poor acoustics while performing, interference of costumes and clothing, positional factors, and so forth, which can be significant contributing factors to suboptimal voice performance. Therefore, the clinician must ask specific questions or even attend a rehearsal or performance to make a complete assessment of conditions.

Psychological factors also commonly contribute to voice problems. The voice can be described as an emotional part of each person. Studies by Fonagy, described by Sundberg, have indicated that articulatory and laryngeal structures in addition to respiratory muscle activity patterns change in relation to 10 different emotions.[3] This is indicative of the emotional/psychological connection to the voice. Psychological factors may be related to the patient's response to the voice disorder and its effect on his or her life, or the voice disorder may be the manifestation of a larger psychological issue that is causing a voice disorder, as in psychogenic voice disorders. In either case, treatment should be tailored to the needs of each patient with careful history taking and thorough examination. The speech-language pathologist may act as a patient advocate speaking with the physician and acting as a catalyst for a referral to the appropriate psychological professional as deemed by the physician.

Emotional factors also can affect the patient's overall response to the voice disorder. Is the patient able to cope with the voice disorder? How will it affect his or her current life, voice demand and expectations, and career? Are past vocal experiences, the diagnosis, or other people's responses affecting therapy sessions or outcomes?[4] These basic questions should be addressed with the patient.

Treating voice patients requires the interaction of many disciplines. Patients and clinicians alike will benefit from a team approach to the voice patient's care. In some centers, the interdisciplinary team may be in one facility, but not always. It is important to build relationships within the community to maximize patient care. Treatment by an interdisciplinary team is important when treating anyone with a voice disorder and crucial when treating the professional voice user. The members of the team may include a laryngologist, speech-language pathologist, singing voice specialist/singing teacher, acting-voice specialist, voice researcher/scientist, singing coach, and/or psychologist. Relationships with other medical specialists are also important, including neurologists, pulmonologists, gastroenterologists, endocrinologists, physiatrists, psychiatrists, and others (Table 13–1).

Additionally, in specific cases, other specialists may be included in the interdisciplinary

TABLE 13–1. Composition of a Typical Interdisciplinary Team

Member	Role
Laryngologist	Primary medical member of the team—responsible for diagnosis and medical/surgical intervention
Speech-Language Pathologist	Conducts evaluation and treatment of the voice problem by promoting efficient use of the vocal mechanism
Acting Voice Specialist	Develops singing technique and singing voice production—may be beneficial to a nonsinger in teaching more efficient breathing and coordination with voicing that can be carried over into speaking
	Focuses on honing vocal skills such as projected speech and communication skills as they relate to vocally demanding professions—typically utilized once a patient has become efficient in speaking voice production with a speech-language pathologist
The Patient	The most important member of the team—the patient must be motivated to participate in therapy, be knowledgeable about the voice disorder and techniques for treatment as instructed by the clinician, and be involved in therapy decision-making and planning

team. The *voice researcher/scientist* can provide valuable insight and perspective with regard to the care of a voice patient because of his or her specific knowledge and skill-set in acoustic measurement and voice production. Referral to a *singing voice coach* may also be useful following rehabilitation work with the speech-language pathologist and singing voice specialist. The singing voice coach will be a valuable aide in the development of artistic style and repertoire for the voice user. A *psychologist or psychiatrist* may prove valuable in a team setting, providing the patient with counseling for the management of emotional reactions to the voice disorder, as well as psychological issues that may have contributed to its occurrence. In addition, a *physiatrist* may offer contributions in the way of addressing areas of tension or other injury throughout the body.

Of note regarding the interdisciplinary team, both singing and acting-voice specialists, in addition to the singing coach, have no formal licensing or certification board. Therefore, it is important to understand that resources can vary widely from community to community, as can the backgrounds and knowledge of various voice professionals. For example, singing and acting-voice teachers/coaches are not trained to work with the injured voice and, therefore, may not have experience in this area. Singing voice specialists and acting-voice specialists are experienced teachers who have acquired such training, usually through apprenticeships.

EVALUATION

The initial voice evaluation should include a thorough review of case history, performance of objective and subjective evaluation, trial therapy,

---

Interdisciplinary Treatment of Voice Disorders

The interdisciplinary approach to the treatment of voice disorders is increasing and professional organizations are recognizing the development of these specialized relationships. The American Speech-Language-Hearing Association (ASHA) is working in conjunction with the National Association of Teachers of Singing (NATS), and the Voice and Speech Trainers Association (VASTA) to revise the joint statement, *Role of the Speech-Language Pathologists, the Teacher of Singing, and the Speaking Voice Trainer in Voice Habilitation.* This statement is intended to encourage interdisciplinary treatment of voice disorders and to encourage professionals working with voice patients to work within the scope of practice and laws regarding treatment. In addition, ASHA is working with the Speech, Voice, and Swallowing Committee of the American Academy of Otolaryngology-Head and Neck Surgery to generate a new joint statement, *The Use of Voice Therapy in the Treatment of Dysphonia,* which is currently under consideration for approval. This statement recognizes the importance of voice therapy in conjunction with medical and surgical management in treating voice disorders as supported by clinical research and expert experience.

and assembling initial impressions and recommendations. This will provide the clinician with baseline information about vocal function, patient stimulability and possible therapy techniques, expectations of the voice user, and information from which to draw conclusions regarding success of therapy and possible outcomes.

Case History

A thorough case history should be elicited from the patient beginning with the onset and development of the voice problem and the circumstances under which it ensued. The patient's previous and/or current medical diagnoses and treatments should be reviewed. The duration of the voice disorder and its constancy are also important factors. In some cases, voice problems can be intermittent over many years with the patient not having pursued treatment until the problem worsened significantly. Knowing this information can give the clinician perspective on the patient's overall voice disorder. Whether or not the patient had received voice therapy previously should be documented. If so, when the treatment took placed, its duration, techniques employed, and whether previous treatment was effective should be noted. These factors can be indicative of how receptive the patient will be to further intervention and how he or she will likely respond to different voice therapy techniques.

A complete inventory should be taken regarding vocal hygiene, abuse, and misuse including hydration, caffeine intake, yelling, shouting, loud talking, coughing, throat clearing, smoking, exposure to second-hand smoke, sleep patterns, overall rest, and other environmental factors. In addition, vocal demands should be reviewed and the patient should provide examples of voice use during a typical day. Throughout this inventory, the patient should explain the primary vocal complaints so as to provide the clinician with a possible starting point for intervention. The patient's initial concerns are addressed immediately and may increase his or her motivation to continue therapeutic intervention.

Special factors must be considered when eliciting a history from a professional voice user. Learning vocal complaints as they are related to their "performance voice" can be very helpful. The clinician should inquire about the history of professional voice use, whether it be singing, acting, public speaking, or a combination thereof. The clinician should also ask about the genre of music the patient is singing, voice classification, performance venues, and the size of his or her typical audience, if any. Knowing the extent of the professional voice user's vocal training is also valuable, particularly when and how long he or she has studied, the specific school of training and whether he or she is studying currently. This process provides information about the types of vocal techniques the patient may already employ or be aware of, or those that may need to be developed or reworked.

The clinician should request that the patient share his or her professional goals and expectations for voice. Ideally, voice therapy should be tailored to accommodate the patient's professional and career goals concurrently with satisfying the clinician's therapeutic objectives. Even though the singing voice specialist typically will perform a more thorough evaluation of the complaints of a singer, the speech-language pathologist can play an important role in singing voice rehabilitation and development. The clinician can use knowledge of a patient's background, education, and experience to assist in development of an efficient daily speaking voice and in articulating the relationship between daily speaking routines and singing or stage voice.

Objective Evaluation

Gathering and analyzing objective voice data is a crucial part of the complete voice evaluation. Completing pre- and post-therapy voice measures can supply objective data to assist in predicting therapy outcomes, for use in research, and to provide tangible voice statistics for use by insurance companies. The objective voice evaluation is discussed further in chapter 8.

Subjective Voice Evaluation

Respiration

The respiratory system is the source of power for voice production. Many voice problems can be related to uncoordinated breathing. The clinician should pay special attention to the manner in which the voice user inhales and then exhales air to produce voice during the evaluation. Observation of the patient's breathing pattern should be completed during reading and conversational speech. Breathing patterns that may be inefficient for voice production include clavicular breathing, upper thoracic breathing, or a combination of the two. So called "diaphragmatic breathing" can be the most efficient breathing pattern as it tends to provide optimal balance of inspiratory and expiratory muscle use. Speaking on residual air, shortness of breath while speaking, gasping for air during inhalation, forced exhalation, or decreased airflow during phonation are also common indicators of vocal misuse.

Phonation

Phonation is defined as the production of sound at the level of the vocal folds. A perceptual evaluation of phonation (vocal quality, loudness, and pitch) during reading and conversation should be completed. Vocal quality characteristics may include: hoarseness, breathiness, roughness, raspiness, vocal fry, diplophonia, voice breaks, pitch breaks, and others. Vocal intensity or loudness should be judged as appropriate, increased, or decreased for the particular setting. The pitch of the patient's voice should be judged as appropriate, high, or low for the age and gender. In addition, the frequency of hard glottal attacks should be assessed.

Resonance

Vocal resonance refers to the way sound is shaped acoustically as it travels through the vocal tract. Phonation begins at the level of the vocal folds and moves up through the pharynx, oral cavity, and nasal cavity. Frontal resonance or forward focus of sound is ideal for most efficient voice production. It optimizes acoustics of the vocal tract while balancing oral-nasal resonance. The use of resonant voice therapy, which places emphasis on frontal tone focus, can increase perceived vocal loudness levels which then may allow the voice to be heard better in noisy situations without excessive strain. A variety of resonance patterns may be observed while making a perceptual judgment of the voice including oral, oral pharyngeal, nasal, nasopharyngeal, and hypopharyngeal.

Articulation

A global assessment of articulation should be completed judging clarity and accuracy of articulatory movement for intelligible speech production.

Prosody

Prosody may have a subtle effect on voice production and should be assessed generally paying attention to the rhythm, fluency, rate, pauses, and intonation or inflection patterns used.

Locating Muscle Tension

Muscle tension can have an adverse affect on voice production causing vocal fatigue, pain, and/or changes in the ease and quality of voice production. Locating these areas of tension is vital in breaking patterns of tension and retraining efficient muscle patterns. Possible places of tension are outlined in Table 13–2.

Laryngeal palpation provides valuable information regarding specific areas of tension, which may include the thyroarytenoid muscle, suprahyoid area, strap muscles, and other related structures. The base of tongue should also be palpated to assess the presence and degree of tension. Digital manipulation and laryngeal massage of the extrinsic laryngeal musculature during evaluation can provide the clinician with valuable information regarding tension and may yield immediate improvement in vocal quality or an identifiable

TABLE 13–2. Possible Places of Muscle Tension

Tongue	Anterior/posterior neck
• Anterior	• Strap muscles
• Base of tongue	• Occipital area
Jaw	**Shoulders**
• Masseter	• High shoulder posture
• TMJ	• Tightness/stiffness
Laryngeal Tension	**Upper chest**
• Intrinsic laryngeal muscles	• Anterior/posterior chest muscles
	• Clavicular area

release in laryngeal tension. These changes are useful to provide the patient with an identifiable vocal change or release of tension and may be indicative of the patient's responsiveness to therapeutic intervention.

Oral Mechanism Exam

A general assessment of oral and facial structure and function should be completed to rule out abnormalities or asymmetries in strength, range of motion, and coordination that may affect functional communication. Structures include the face, mouth, dentition, tongue, and hard and soft palate. Abnormalities may be indicative of neurologic problems that warrant further evaluation.

Trial Therapy

During the initial evaluation, a period of trial therapy should be completed using facilitators to improve ease and quality of voice production. The facilitators are used to assess the patient's stimulability for improvement in voice production. Throughout the trial therapy period, the clinician attempts to provide the patient with a demonstration of possible improvement in voice production, which should in turn increase motivation and feelings of therapeutic success. While completing facilitating techniques, the clinician should gain information on the patient's self-awareness of existing habits and changes in voice production that may occur. Judgments can also

be made by the clinician on the patient's ability to learn new techniques, willingness to comply with voice therapy, and overall appropriateness for therapy. A statement of prognosis for outcomes through voice therapy should also be made.

Impressions/Recommendations

A complete voice evaluation provides the clinician with baseline data regarding voice production and the patient's view of his or her voice disorder, in addition to allowing the speech-language pathologist to develop an impression of the cause and/or contributing factors to the voice disorder. The review of vocal hygiene, vocal demand, and overall voice use provides the clinician with a place to begin educating the patient about his or her voice. Although the trial therapy portion identifies facilitators for improved ease and/or quality of voice production, it also provides an appropriate starting point for therapeutic intervention.

When a general impression has been formulated by the clinician, it should be discussed with the patient. The clinician should indicate to the patient if a course of voice therapy is recommended and identify expectations for follow-up sessions. The goals of therapy should then be discussed with the patient and consideration should be given, at that time, to the patient's personal goals. Once the goals are delineated, other referrals may be made including singing intervention, physical therapy, and so forth. Expectations for therapeutic intervention should be clear to the patient, including the approximate length of the therapy in months, weeks, or sessions, and how often the sessions should be scheduled (weekly, biweekly, monthly). The patient also should be aware that home practice is a crucial part to success in therapy. The clinician will teach the patient tools and provide support to improve vocal efficiency and carryover of efficient voice use. It is the patient's responsibility to attend sessions, complete home practice, and work to carry over efficient voice use in everyday life with the clinician's guidance so that therapy goals can be met and independence in efficient voice use can be achieved.

THERAPY

Initially, goals for therapy must be set forth. When treating the professional voice user the ultimate long-term goal is to produce an excellent speaking voice. The means to reaching this goal is to increase vocal efficiency during speaking. The therapy techniques presented in this chapter can be used to address behavioral voice problems that may or may not include organic or structural changes that have taken place in the vocal folds.

Therapy begins with educating the patient. A brief overview of the anatomy and physiology of voice production should be introduced and discussed with the patient; including coordinating breathing, phonation, and balancing oral-nasal resonance. This explanation should provide the patient with a foundation for understanding voice production and the primary focus of voice therapy. Vocal hygiene should be addressed and improved to eliminate vocal stressors and promote an optimal environment for improving vocal ease and quality. Furthermore, the voice user must be made aware of vocal habits that promote abuse and/or misuse of the vocal mechanism and should be provided with alternatives to abusive vocal behavior.

Voice conservation strategies should be taught to the patient in an attempt to manage voice use on a daily basis. Vocal exercises should then be introduced and practiced to begin retraining muscle patterns for voice production. The vocal exercises work to maximize efficiency of the vocal mechanism and promote carryover of targeted voice use into daily activities. Body- and self-awareness should be targeted from the onset of therapy to promote carryover of the efficient voice learned during therapy.

Areas of tension can have an adverse effect on efficient voice production. Areas of muscle tension that were identified during the initial evaluation should be addressed throughout therapy. The patient should be taught a daily routine for stretches and massage that may include those listed in Table 13–3. Laryngeal massage may also be taught to the patient and completed independently outside the therapy setting.

TABLE 13–3. Exercises to Reduce Muscle Tension

Sites of Tension	Sample Exercises (Partial List)
Tongue	
• Anterior	• Tongue stretches
• Base of tongue	• Base of tongue massage
Jaw	
• Masseter	• Massage
• TMJ	• Jaw stretch
	• Tension/relaxation awareness exercises
Laryngeal Tension	
• Intrinsic laryngeal muscles	• Digital manipulation of the suprahyoid area and thyrohyoid muscle
• Intrinsic laryngeal muscles	• Breathy, sighing
	• Gentle scales and glides
Anterior/Posterior Neck	
• Strap muscles	• Neck stretch
• Occipital area	
Shoulders	
• High shoulder posture	• Shoulder shrugs
• Tightness/stiffness	• Shoulder rolls

Postural alignment should also be addressed with special attention given to hip angle and shoulder and head placement. Slight misalignments in posture can cause increased muscle tension. For example, elevated chin placement will tighten laryngeal and neck muscles or an arched lower back will make relaxing the abdomen for lower abdominal breathing difficult.

Facilitators for Breath Control and Support

As respiration is the power source for phonation, the patient must be taught to balance inspiratory and expiratory muscles for efficient breathing. Exercises for breath management may start with a simple explanation of the respiratory system. This may include a description of the expansion of the lungs and diaphragm with subsequent expansion of the rib cage and abdominal area during inhalation. As exhalation takes place these areas begin to slowly deflate. Expiratory muscles may be engaged but should not be hyperfunctioning. The patient must understand that it is possible to coordinate breathing and vocalization without hyperfunctional muscle use.

Appropriate terminology should be used when teaching a new breathing pattern secondary to learned responses that many adults have to phrases such as "take a deep breath." When a patient is asked to do this, the stomach pulls in, the shoulders and chest rise, and the patient holds his or her breath. Phrases such as "expand for inhalation" versus "take a deep breath" and release/deflate for exhalation or engage the abdomen during exhalation rather than pushing/pulling in may be employed. In addition, the image of a newborn baby during quiet breathing with the belly rising on inhalation and falling on exhalation may elicit understanding of the target breathing pattern.

While establishing a more efficient breathing pattern, the patient may be placed in multiple positions to experience the targeted feeling of expansion during inhalation and active deflation during exhalation. Positions may include lying on the floor in the supine or prone position and concentrating on expansion of the lower rib cage and abdomen during inhalation and then slowly releasing air during exhalation. These two positions with the help of gravity provide tactile feedback during expansion and deflation. They also aide in decreasing shoulder and upper thoracic movement while breathing. However, these strategies alter respiratory function and should be used cautiously and with knowledge of their purposes and limitations. Another useful technique is instructing the patient to bend over at the waist with arms extended to a chair or table so that his or her back is parallel with the floor. The patient is instructed to expand the abdomen during inhalation and feel the abdomen actively deflate during exhalation. These breathing techniques/positions are not meant to be sustained but to increase body awareness of an efficient pattern of breathing that can be applied during daily activities. As the patient and clinician work through the therapeutic hierarchy and gradually introduce simple to complex exercises the patient should be instructed to use the new breathing patterns for short periods multiple times throughout the day while breathing quietly and also while talking, as appropriate.

Facilitators for Increasing Airflow During Phonation

Once an efficient breathing pattern can be replicated, breathing and voicing should be paired together, cueing the patient to produce voicing during exhalation. It is important for the patient to understand that inhalation prior to phonation is as important as releasing air during exhalation to produce phonation. To achieve appropriate airflow during phonation, muscle hyperfunction must be eliminated from the vocal tract by various exercises.

The *yawn-sigh* may be used to promote active inhalation while decreasing muscular tension in the throat in addition to creating increased oral-pharyngeal space by lifting the soft palate. The increased oral-pharyngeal space and the sensation of an open throat should be maintained during exhalation while producing a sigh. The patient may be cued to place the tongue in a relaxed position behind the bottom incisors to maintain oral space. When the targeted yawns-sigh can be replicated consistently, the yawn can then be "downsized" to an open-mouthed inhalation and voicing during exhalation may be shaped into words, phrases, and so forth.

The *stretch and flow* therapy technique, originally developed by R.E. Stone, focuses on increasing ease and quality of voice production by increasing airflow during phonation. The patient is asked to use a strip of tissue, draped over his or her finger, to provide a visual cue for airflow. The patient is instructed to blow a passive airstream onto the tissue. This should feel easy. Confirm this feeling with the patient. Once a consistent, passive airstream is achieved, the patient is instructed to add his or her voice on a /u/ vowel, while maintaining the airstream. The patient should produce a smooth, air-filled, easy voice. This voice may sound slightly more air-filled than "normal." The initial goal is to slightly overexaggerate the airflow during the exercise, so ultimately the ease of voice production is maintained and airflow can be normalized. Each trial should be modified until the targeted voice is achieved. The air-filled, easy /u/ will then be used as a facilitator into words, phrases, sentences, and so forth, through the therapeutic hierarchy. When the patient can produce the targeted voice consistently using the facilitator, its use should be gradually eliminated until the targeted voice can be produced consistently independent of the facilitator.

Lip trills, raspberries, or tongue-out trills are other facilitators to coordinate airflow and phonation. For lip trills, the patient is instructed to expand and produce a raspberry with only airflow. If this is difficult the patient may place his or her index finger on each cheek and slightly press forward to release lip tension. The patient may also be cued not to clench the back molars together. When the patient is consistent with production of the lip trill with air only, they are instructed to add voicing. Consistency should be developed on one pitch and through a range of pitches. Once this is completed the lip trill may be used as a facilitator in initial /br/ words, phrases, and so forth. Similarly with the tongue-out trill, the patient should relax the tongue over the bottom lip, expand during inhalation, and release air to produce a tongue-out trill without voicing. This facilitator requires that the tongue and jaw be relaxed and airflow coordinated to produce the targeted tongue-out trill. When consistency is achieved, voicing should be added and developed at one pitch and through a range of pitches. The tongue out-trill can then be used as a facilitator into open vowels, words, phrases, and so forth. When the targeted voicing is achieved, the use of the facilitator should be faded out.

When evaluating coordination of airflow and phonation, hard glottal attacks (abrupt abductions of the vocal folds on words with an initial vowel) should be addressed. Voicing should be initiated with airflow rather than abrupt adduction of the vocal folds. This can be addressed by targeting coordination of airflow and phonation. Easy onset exercises should be completed beginning with discrimination tasks so the patient is able to identify hard glottal attacks. Minimal pairs

should then be used (ie, hear/ear, hat/at). The patient should be made aware of the abduction of the vocal folds during an /h/ and closure of the vocal folds during the voiced cognate. Prior to each trial, cueing may be required to inhale to ensure vocal fold abduction and gentle adduction of the vocal folds to initiate voicing. The patient in then instructed to maintain the open feeling during the /h/ into the voiced cognate without producing an /h/. Complexity should be increased as appropriate. The above mentioned exercise addresses vowel-initiated words that begin a breath group. When a vowel-initiated word is found within a breath group "linking" should be employed. Linking is used to connect the last sound of the word previous to the vowel-initiated word. For singers or musicians it may be described as tying the words together, just as notes on the staff may be tied.

Facilitators for Oral Resonance

To achieve an optimal balance of oral-nasal resonance, a relaxed vocal tract must be maintained, in addition to maintaining breath support and appropriate airflow during phonation. In many hyperfunctional voice users, it is difficult to achieve forward tone focus secondary to reduced space in the oropharynx which may be caused by increased tongue and/or jaw tension. To increase oral-pharyngeal space, it may be beneficial to increase soft palatal lift, address jaw tension through stretches and massage, and decrease tongue retraction through stretches and tongue relaxation exercises.

Resonance exercises may include the use of a hum to achieve improved balance of oral/nasal resonance. The patient should be cued to maintain oral space. This may be achieved by creating space in between the back molars to release jaw tension and maintaining relaxed tongue placement behind the lower front incisors and away from the roof of the mouth. The patient is instructed to inhale and then exhale while producing a hum, or hum-sigh on a descending glide, with the lips barely touching. The patient's attention should be brought to the targeted frontal tone focus and "buzz" on the lips. This buzz can provide tactile feedback for the patient in working to maintain frontal focus while increasing complexity of trials. If the patient has difficulty achieving a hum without pressing, he or she may be cued to release air through the nose and maintain a consistent airstream. When the targeted hum is achieved consistently, it should be used as a facilitator into vowels, words, phrases, and so forth. Eventually use of the facilitator should be minimized and then eliminated.

"Honking" is used as an effective facilitator for developing awareness and maintenance of balanced oral/nasal resonance. Honking is completed by pinching the nose while phonating on any vowel. The patient is cued to allow the sound to resonate in his or her nose and release airflow through the mouth. Tactile feedback should be provided with vibration or "buzz" at the nasal bridge. When the patient is able to achieve consistent voicing and awareness of the buzzing, words and phrases may be spoken using the honking as a facilitator. The word or phrase may be spoken while occluding the nose and then repeated after releasing the nose, maintaining airflow and frontal focus of the sound production. When consistency of voice production is achieved, the use of the facilitator should be gradually eliminated.

There are multiple other resonance exercises. The last to be discussed is the use of the /f/ and /v/ or /s/ and /z/ sounds. This exercise, as with others mentioned, combines the use of abdominal breathing, use of a continuous airstream, and frontal tone focus. Initially, the /f/ or /s/ sound is used to establish a consistent stream of air coming past the lips. The patient is instructed to expand during inhalation and make an /f/ sound during exhalation with the back molars parted and the top teeth barely touching the bottom lip. Following the trial, confirm the feeling of air past the lips. The patient is then instructed to use the same airflow and breath support with voicing to produce a /v/ sound. A "buzz" should be felt on the lower lip during this trial. This should be confirmed with the patient. If the patient has difficulties achieving the buzz, recheck jaw tension and oral space. Production of a /v/ sound should become consistent and then may be used as a facilitator into /v/ words, phrases, and so forth. The /v/ may also be used as a facilitator into words and phrases that do not begin with /v/. Use of the facilitator should eventually be faded out.

There are three elements of voice production, respiration, phonation and resonance. There are multiple facilitators that target each element. Choosing an appropriate therapeutic facilitator can be challenging. Clinical judgment should be applied when choosing therapeutic techniques and modifications should be made for patients as needed. When choosing a facilitator, consider the patient's primary complaints, the perceptual and acoustic evaluation of his or her voice, and the physiology of the patient's current voice production versus the targeted efficient voice production. The clinician should be aware of the benefits and limitations of each facilitator and chose appropriately to maximize the patient's voice output and potential for improved voice production

Review Questions

1. What is not within the scope of practice for a speech-language pathologist when treating voice disorders and how does this affect the treatment of the patient?

2. Name and describe the roles of three multidisciplinary team members. Why is it necessary to cultivate professional relationships with team members?

3. Compare history taking for a professional voice user to that for a nonprofessional.

4. How do breath support during phonation and airflow during phonation differ?

5. Name three factors to consider when choosing a therapeutic facilitator.

REFERENCES

1. American Speech-Language Hearing Association. *Scope of Practice in Speech Language Pathology.* Rockville, Md: Author; 2001.
2. Sataloff RT. *Professional Voice: The Science and Art of Clinical Care.* 3rd ed., San Diego, Calif: Plural Publishing; 2005.
3. Sundberg, J. *The Science of the Singing Voice.* DeKalb, Ill: Northern Illinois University Press; 1987:146–156.
4. Smith E, Verdolini K, Gray S, et al. Effects of voice disorders on quality of life. *J Med Speech Lang Pathol.* 1997;4:223–244.

SUGGESTED READING

1. Benninger MS, Jacobson BH, Johnson AF. *Vocal Arts Medicine.* New York, NY: Thieme Medical Publishers, Inc; 1994.
2. Boone DR. *Is Your Voice Telling on You? How to Find and Use Your Natural Voice.* San Diego, Calif: Singular Publishing Group, Inc; 1994.
3. Colton R, Casper J. *Understanding Voice Problems.* Baltimore, Md: Williams & Wilkins; 1990.
4. Rosen DC, Sataloff RT. *The Psychology of Voice Disorders.* San Diego, Calif. Singular Publishing Group, Inc; 1997.
5. Rubin JS, Sataloff RT, Korovin GS. *Diagnosis and Treatment of Voice Disorders.* 3rd ed. San Diego, Calif: Plural Publishing, Inc; 2006.
6. Sataloff, Robert T., *Professional Voice: The Science and Art of Clinical Care.* 3rd ed. San Diego, Calif: Plural Publishing; 2005.
7. Sataloff RT, Castell DO, Katz PO. *Reflux Laryngitis and Other Related Conditions.* 3rd ed. San Diego, Calif: Plural Publishing; 2006.
8. Stemple, JC. *Voice Therapy Clinical Studies.* 2nd ed. San Diego, Calif: Singular Publishing Group, Inc; 2000.
9. Sundburg J. *The Science of the Singing Voice.* DeKalb, Ill: Northern Illinois Press; 1987.
10. Zemlin WR. *Speech and Hearing Science: Anatomy and Physiology.* Englewood Cliffs, NJ: Allyn & Bacon; 1998.

14

General Principles of Microlaryngeal Surgery

Adam D. Rubin, MD
Robert T. Sataloff, MD, DMA

KEY POINTS

■ The surgeon must know *when* and *when not* to operate on the vocal folds.

■ Be prepared with the appropriate instrumentation to obtain adequate exposure and perform the surgery.

■ Preserve all normal mucosa and superficial lamina propria, and do not traumatize the vocal ligament.

■ Excellent postoperative care is essential.

The goal of microlaryngeal surgery (or phonomicrosurgery) for benign vocal fold lesions is to improve voice. This is achieved through a complete understanding and respect for the multilayered structure and function of the vocal folds (see chapter 3, Anatomy of the Larynx and Physiology of Phonation) as well as meticulous surgical technique. Good clinical judgment is paramount when evaluating and planning treatment for the patient with vocal complaints and pathology.

There are four basic principles of microlaryngeal surgery; the key points listed above provide our outline for this chapter.

THE SURGEON MUST KNOW *WHEN* AND *WHEN NOT* TO OPERATE ON THE VOCAL FOLDS

The decision to proceed with surgical excision of a vocal fold mass is complex (Figure 14–1). The mere presence of a mass on the vocal fold is seldom reason enough. Of course, if malignancy is suspected, proceeding with a biopsy is appropriate. Large hemorrhagic polyps, Reinke's edema, and intracordal cysts are likely to need surgical intervention if voice improvement is desired by the patient. However, when considering a small cyst, pseudocyst, or fibrotic mass on the medial edge of the vocal fold, one must weigh the risks of anesthesia—as well as the potential for scarring and making the patient's voice worse—against the chances of voice improvement. Furthermore, there are successful singers and performers who work consistently despite the presence of a vocal fold mass (or masses). Some performers even depend on vocal fold irregularities to provide "character" to their voices. Removing masses that have been present, and perhaps stable for many years, may destroy such a patient's career.

One must be certain that a mass is not only present, but moreover, is the cause of the patient's voice difficulties. In other words, is the mass *"pathologic"*? Voice problems are often multifactorial. Vocal fold vibration and glottic closure problems may be caused by a number of underlying problems such as reflux, allergy, poor technique, and paresis. Such underlying conditions may lead to the development of vocal fold masses. However, sometimes a new insult may occur to a patient with a long-stable vocal fold mass, resulting in new voice symptoms. Recognition of all potentially contributing issues is important for devising the optimal treatment plan. Furthermore, controlling underlying pathology will improve the chances of obtaining an optimal surgical outcome, should surgery become necessary. For example, if a patient's cough from asthma or reflux is not controlled prior to surgery, it will likely lead to trauma to the surgical site and poor healing. Aggressive management of underlying medical issues that may be contributing to a patient's voice problems and impair healing is crucial.

When malignancy is suspected, biopsy should not be delayed excessively. However, recognizing what is a "benign" lesion is important, as this may prevent unnecessary biopsies and consequent scar and dysphonia. Although most often this distinction is not difficult, some pathology is less easy to distinguish. For example, longstanding ulcerative laryngitis and other inflammatory conditions may be mistaken easily for malignancy on clinical examination.[1] Repeated biopsies may reveal only inflammation; it is tempting to sample deeper tissue on subsequent trips to the operating room. A more aggressive approach may result in trauma to the vocal ligament or vocalis muscle, as well as potentially significant scarring and permanent hoarseness. Of course, if there is any doubt, it is better to biopsy than fail to detect an occult malignancy. However, making someone permanently hoarse for a self-limited inflammatory process does not do the patient justice. Rigid stroboscopy with video-documentation is useful for following masses in the office when one is determining whether biopsy is necessary.

Recognizing the patient's goals and motivations is important in the decision-making process, as well. An elderly, retired patient with a large vocal fold polyp may come to clinic with one thought—to make sure that he does not have cancer. He may be less likely to agree to medical or surgical intervention than a schoolteacher with a small cyst on the medial edge of the vocal fold and recurrent hoarseness from phonotrauma.

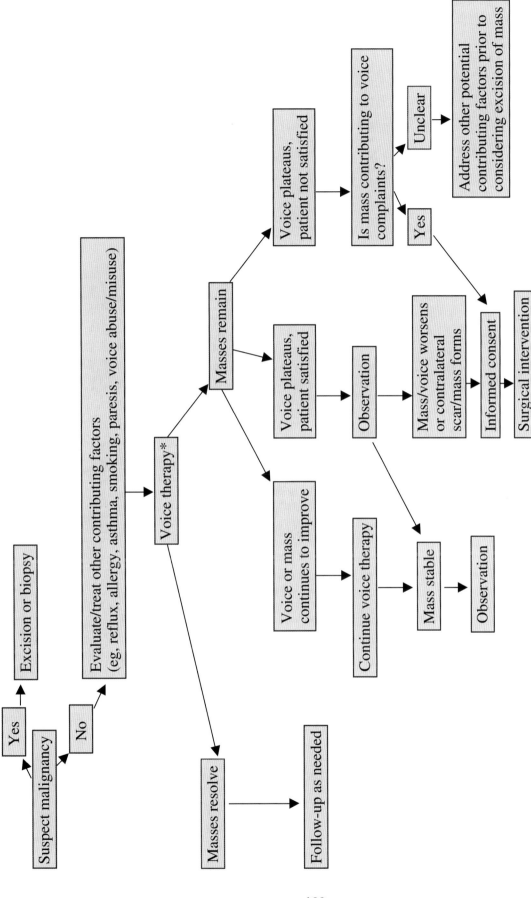

FIGURE 14–1. Voice treatment algorithm.

* Large hemorrhagic polyp, large cysts, and Reinke's edema are unlikely to have significant improvement from voice therapy, although 1 or 2 sessions preoperatively may be useful. Proceeding to surgical intervention may occur sooner than for more subtle lesions, although other underlying issues, such as reflux and smoking, should be addressed first.

Vocal Paresis and Benign Vocal Masses

Vocal fold paresis has been postulated by some to be involved in the development of benign vocal fold masses. Paresis may involve the superior laryngeal nerve, recurrent laryngeal nerve, or both. The most common etiology is a preceding upper respiratory tract infection. Subtle paresis may be missed on exam, unless it is looked for and the patient is challenged with a series of phonatory tasks. Paresis may be confirmed by laryngeal electromyography.

Supporters of this paradigm believe that a subtle paresis yields a hypofunctional larynx and voice change. Patients try to compensate for the paresis with excessive muscle tension, and become hyperfunctional. Such hyperfunction leads to chronic trauma and the subsequent development of vocal fold masses. For example, a patient with no previous voice problems complains of hoarseness that has not improved since a cold (or perhaps thyroid surgery) 6 months prior. Examination may reveal subtle asymmetry in vocal fold adduction, a small cyst or pseudocyst on the medial edge of one vocal fold, and contact fibrosis on the contralateral fold. LEMG shows reduced recruitment with evidence of chronic denervation when the electrode is inserted in the cricothyroid muscle and the patient asked to do a glissando.

Why is this patient hoarse (let us assume for our purpose that this patient has had a dual-channel pH probe which demonstrated no episodes of reflux at the upper probe)? Was this nerve injury caused by the URI or had it been present years before? The same question could be asked of the mass. If the mass developed after the onset of the URI, how long did it take to develop? Did the patient have a violent coughing fit which led to the development of the mass, or did it result from compensatory hyperfunction?

Of course, it is unlikely that we will able to answer any of the above questions with certainty in most patients. Most people do not have baseline laryngeal examinations when they are healthy with which to compare current examination results. However, it is important to think of all possible scenarios when counseling patients and planning treatment. Say this patient failed voice therapy. What would be the most appropriate surgery? The role of medialization and/or mass excision is not well studied in this clinical scenario. The subtleties and ambiguities of laryngology continue to challenge us and contribute to the "art" of our profession.[42-44]

Furthermore, patients need to be motivated to follow postoperative voice rest and care instructions. It is wise to explain to the patient that his or her treatment requires a team approach involving the patient, the voice therapist, and the surgeon. The patient must be committed to following postoperative instructions, receiving postoperative voice therapy, and complying with follow-up recommendations. Continuance of abusive vocal behavior, particularly in the early postoperative period, may increase the risk of scarring and recurrence.

The surgeon must be aware of the degree of importance of voice quality to each patient's livelihood and quality of life. The physician must weigh the potential medical-legal risks and his or her own comfort level performing this type of surgery. Although every patient's larynx should be treated with the same care and precision as a singer at the Metropolitan Opera, the surgeon with limited experience in microlaryngeal surgery or without the appropriate equipment for thorough evaluation and appropriate surgery, should consider referral to a voice specialist.

Preoperative Evaluation

Understanding a patient's disease and planning treatment begins with a thorough evaluation. A complete medical and voice history should be obtained, and the larynx should be visualized. Flexible laryngoscopy is used to assess the larynx during voice production, to observe gross movement of the vocal folds, to look for hyperfunction, and to detect any sign of paresis or neurologic dysfunction.[2] Videostroboscopy is vital to assess the fine structure of the vocal fold and the mucosal wave. Rigid telescopes currently provide the highest and clearest magnification of instruments available for videostroboscopy, and thus, they are best for evaluating subtle masses and scar. Flexible laryngoscopes using distal-chip technology are an improvement over traditional fiberoptic flexible laryngoscopes and may be used for videostroboscopy as an alternative to a rigid examination, particularly if the patient is unable to tolerate rigid endoscopy. Although the flexible distal-chip laryngoscopes provide good image quality, they still do not provide the magnification of a rigid scope.

Computerized voice analysis in the voice laboratory is useful in the treatment of voice disorders. Although the "ideal" objective voice measurements do not exist, current measures are useful for documenting severity of dysphonia, and for following and assessing treatment outcomes. Several quality of life instruments exist, including the voice related quality of life instrument (V-RQOL)[3,4] and the Voice Handicap Index (VHI).[5,6] These measures are particularly valuable because they quantify the severity of the effects of a voice problem for each individual patient, which may be the most useful measure in deciding upon treatment and assessing success (see also chapter 8, on perceptual and objective voice assessment).

Preoperative voice therapy is important for both determining whether the patient would be served best by proceeding to the operating room and improving the chances of obtaining a good, long-term surgical result. It relieves the patient of compensatory hyperfunction and helps the patient develop good vocal technique to minimize further trauma to the vocal folds. Some masses, such as nodules, may disappear with voice therapy. Others may not disappear, but the patient may learn to obtain adequate voice despite the mass, without causing further trauma to the mass or the contralateral vocal fold. *If a mass persists despite voice therapy and prevents a patient from meeting his or her vocal needs, if a mass worsens by becoming larger or more fibrotic, or if the patient begins to demonstrate evidence of trauma from the mass on the contralateral vocal fold, surgical excision is warranted in most cases.*

Once the decision to proceed with surgery is made, informed consent must be obtained. In addition to the general risks of endoscopy, such as trauma to oral structures, tongue numbness, tongue weakness, pharyngeal perforation, arytenoid cartilage dislocation/subluxation, and loss of airway, patients, particularly professional voice users, must understand that despite excellent surgical technique, scarring may occur, which can make the voice worse. Although this seldom occurs with good surgical technique, it is important to counsel the patient so that he or she understands the worst of possible circumstances and can make a well-informed decision as to whether to proceed with surgery.

BE PREPARED WITH THE APPROPRIATE INSTRUMENTATION TO OBTAIN ADEQUATE EXPOSURE AND PERFORM THE SURGERY

Performing microlaryngeal surgery well without appropriate instrumentation is difficult, if not impossible. The surgeon must be prepared to obtain adequate exposure even in the most difficult anatomic cases; in addition to these "gross" motor requirements, and to handle vocal fold mucosa in a delicate manner. Performing surgery for benign vocal fold masses with a Holinger laryngoscope and large biopsy forceps, for example, is generally inappropriate.

Adequate exposure is paramount to good surgical excision. Surgeons must be prepared to deal with the most unfavorable anatomy. Optimal positioning for laryngeal visualization is the "sniffing" position (Figure 14–2). The neck should be flexed toward the chest, and the head extended. No shoulder roll is required.[7,8] Most operating room tables have a head board that can be flexed to keep the neck flexed against the chest (Figure 14-3). Prior to each procedure, however, the surgeon should check to make sure the head board fasteners are tight, so that the board does not come out of the table while placing it in flexion. Such an event could result in a sudden posterior collapse of the patient's head and potentially result in a catastrophic cervical spine injury.

A suspension system should be used. Many varieties are available. The Lewy system is used most commonly. The arm may be lowered by an assistant; however, the primary surgeon should be holding the laryngoscope in the position he or she wishes to maintain. The system is designed to stabilize a laryngoscope that is already in proper position and should not be used as a lever. The suspension arm should be lowered only until it touches the stand. In other words, one should not use the suspension arm to "crank" the patient's head to try to improve exposure as this will risk traumatizing the patient's teeth. If one arm of the suspension device touches down

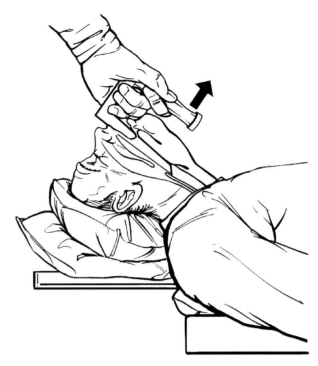

FIGURE 14–2. The "sniffing position" is ideal for visualization during laryngoscopy. Note that the neck is flexed and the head is extended. Often the neck must be flexed considerably more than illustrated. The arrow indicates correct direction of pull during laryngoscopy. (Reprinted with permission from Sataloff R. Voice surgery. In Sataloff R. *Professional Voice: The Science and Art of Professional Care.* 3rd ed. San Diego, Calif: Plural Publishing, Inc; 2005:1146.)

prior to the other, towels or gauze may be placed under the hanging footplate to provide support. Other devices, such as the Boston suspension system, are designed to actually help create the exposure. However, this system also works best when optimal exposure is obtained by the surgeon prior to application of the suspension device. Anterior pressure is often useful and can be maintained throughout the case with a broad piece of tape stretched across the neck of the patient from the operating table. It takes very little tension on the tape to effect a change in the laryngeal exposure. In addition to these maneuvers. flexing the neck further usually provides better anterior exposure for difficult cases.

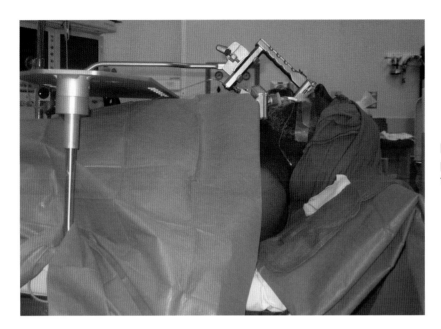

FIGURE 14–3. Patient is in sniff position with the headboard of the table flexed.

The operating table may be placed in varying degrees of Trendelenburg or reverse Trendelenburg positions to direct the opening of the laryngoscope so that the microscope and surgeon's hands may be positioned ideally. Suspending the laryngoscope from a table which attaches to, and thus moves with, the patient's operating bed will minimize the risk of dental injury and save valuable time.

Having a variety of laryngoscopes to choose from will assist the surgeon in obtaining adequate visualization. One should use the largest laryngoscope that can be inserted safely and expose the entire length of the true vocal folds (Figure 14-4). The laryngoscope should provide internal distention to push the false vocal folds out of the way and provide enough tension on the true vocal folds to ensure precise excision of the mass.

The laryngoscope must be large enough to ensure the ability to operate simultaneously with both hands (Figures 14-5 and 14-6). If exposure cannot be obtained with the largest laryngoscope available, the surgeon should try increasingly smaller scopes, until the largest insertable scope is identified We find the Ossoff-Pilling Large (Teleflex-Pilling 52-2191, Fort Washington,

Pa) laryngoscope to be the smallest scope available currently that will still permit two-handed operating. When even this scope is inadequate, exposure can be obtained in most cases with a subglottiscope (Teleflex-Pilling 52-2245, Fort Washington, Pa) or by using the Ossoff-Pilling laryngoscope and working through it with a 70-degree telescope and angled instruments.

In addition to a sufficient choice of laryngoscopes, one must have appropriate instrumentation to allow surgery on millimeter-sized masses without excessive trauma to surrounding tissue. A number of instrument sets exist with a variety of graspers, microscissors, micropics, hockeysticks, spatulas, ball-dissectors, and microalligator forceps. Disposable knife blades are available with the Medtronic-Xomed Sataloff microlaryngeal set which ensures sharp, fresh knives with each procedure. Having an array of microinstruments to choose from is useful, particularly when raising microflaps and dissecting out difficult intracordal cysts.

Microlaryngeal surgery requires magnification, typically provided by an operating microscope. Surgeons should be familiar and adept with the microscope to avoid long time delays and frustration while making adjustments.

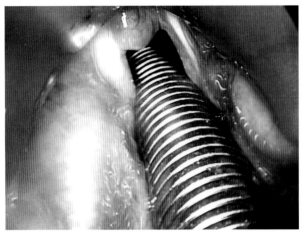

A.

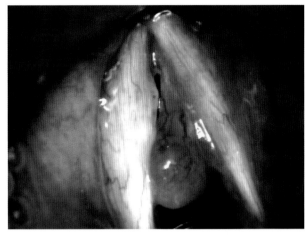

B.

FIGURE 14–4. A. Inadequate exposure of right vocal fold polyp (0-degree endoscope). **B.** Adequate exposure of right vocal fold polyp and left contact mass. The patient's neck has been flexed more and the laryngoscope adjusted, so that the entire length of the vocal folds is visualized. The extent of the right vocal fold mass cannot be appreciated in *A*. Moreover, the left vocal fold mass was not visualized at all. Of note, the endotracheal tube in *A* is a Mallincrodt. This was placed by anesthesia without discussion with the surgeon. Neither author typically uses these tubes, as they believe the ridges may be traumatic to the vocal folds. Preintubation discussion with the anesthesiologist is critical. Ideally, as small an endotracheal tube as possible for adequate ventilation should be used to leave as much room as possible for instrumentation. The authors prefer a number 5 endotracheal tube if possible. A laser-safe tube need not be used, unless the surgeon plans to operate the laser.

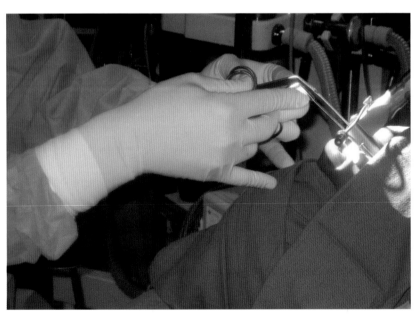

FIGURE 14–5. The fifth digits rest on the patient while performing microsurgery for stability.

Newer microscopes have autofocus and zoom controls, which facilitate procedures. However, older microscopes with knobs for stepwise magnification changes are often sufficient. For laryngologic surgery, a 400-mm lens is used most commonly. Lenses with shorter focal lengths will

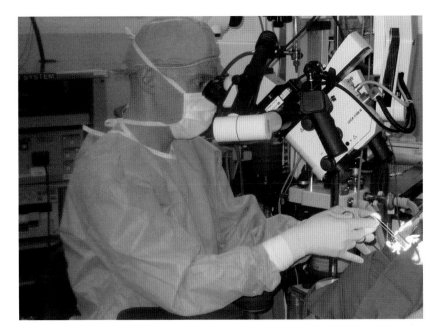

FIGURE 14–6. The surgeon's elbows and fifth digits are stabilized for multipoint stabilization.

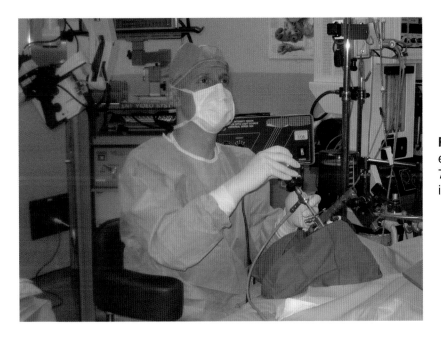

FIGURE 14–7. Surgeon examines lesions with 0- and 70-degree endoscopy. He views images on a monitor.

increase magnification. However, they require the microscope to be too close to the operating field, thereby preventing the insertion of long laryngeal instruments into the laryngoscope.

Laryngeal telescopes are useful to assess the full three-dimensional extent of mass lesions. The authors use 0-degree and 70-degree telescopes in most circumstances (Figure 14–7).[9] Some surgeons

use the telescopes during the actual excision.[10] However, someone else must hold the scope to enable the surgeon to operate with both hands. We use this technique only in cases in which good exposure cannot be obtained without a telescope.

The CO_2 laser is useful in the excision of some benign lesions of the larynx, such as amyloid. The use of CO_2 laser on medial edge lesions such as cysts and polyps remains popular, though controversial. The laser offers the advantages of hemostasis (although, hemostasis is usually achievable during cold excision with the application of cotton pledgets soaked in 1:1000 epinephrine) and ease. Many people believe that using a micromanipulator requires less dexterity in the nondominant hand. However, deft control of the "joystick" is essential; an excellent laryngeal laser surgeon generally must be trained as an excellent cold surgeon first.

The depth of tissue injury is less predictable with CO_2 laser and more tissue may be lost through thermal damage than with cold excision.[11] The use of the microspot CO_2 laser in superpulse mode reduces the zone of thermal injury from previous conventional CO_2 lasers.[12] Benninger reported no significant difference in voice outcome comparing microspot CO_2 laser to "cold-knife" excision of benign lesions limited to the medial edge of the vocal fold from a randomized, prospective study.[13]

CO_2 laser is certainly useful in some cases. The excision of malignant lesions of the vocal fold in which muscle must be excised results in bleeding and obscuring of the surgical field with cold instruments, but less trouble with a laser. Laser excision of supraglottic lesions also is appropriate in many cases. Feeding vessels to polyps may be obliterated with low-wattage laser using an unfocused beam. Ultimately, the decision to use cold instrumentation or laser is probably best determined by the individual surgeon, based on what yields his or her best results. For more information, see chapter 15, Lasers in Laryngology.

> **PRESERVE ALL NORMAL EPITHELIUM AND SUPERFICIAL LAMINA PROPRIA AND AVOID TRAUMATIZING THE VOCAL LIGAMENT**

A number of techniques have been described for the removal of benign masses. Until 1975, when Hirano described the histology of the vocal fold,[14] *vocal fold stripping* was the most common

approach. Although mucosal healing occurs and the vocal fold may appear normal under continuous light, the absence of superficial lamina propria results in loss of vocal fold vibration and voice quality in many patients.

Hirano demonstrated that the vocal fold is a multilayered structure consisting of: an epithelium; superficial, intermediate, and deep layers of the lamina propria; and the thyroarytenoid muscle (Figure 14–8).[14] The superficial lamina propria (Reinke's "space") is composed predominantly of loose fibrous tissue consisting of a network of hyaluronic acid, mucopolysaccharides, decorin, and other extracellular matrix components. It is not a "space," but a layer of the vocal fold that allows for complex vibration. It lies immediately below the epithelium, contains very few fibroblasts, and provides flexibility of the vocal fold cover. The intermediate layer of lamina propria contains mature elastin fibers arranged longitudinally and large quantities of hyaluronic acid which may act as a shock absorber. The deep layer of the lamina propria consists of collagen fibers arranged longitudinally and is rich in fibroblasts.[15] A complete review is presented in

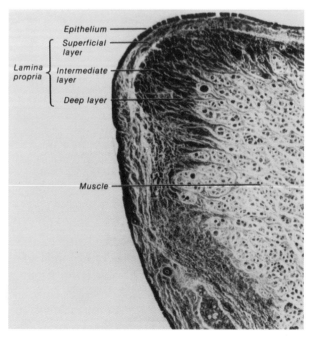

FIGURE 14–8. Structure of the vocal fold. (Reprinted with permission from Hirano M. *Clinical Examination of Voice.* New York, NY: Springer-Verlag; 1981.)

chapter 3, Anatomy of the Larynx and Physiology of Phonation.

These five histologic layers act as three mechanical layers. The epithelium and superficial lamina propria make up the "cover" of the vocal fold; the intermediate and deep layers make up the vocal ligament or the "transition"; and the thyroarytenoid muscle makes up the "body" of the vocal fold. The relationship between these three layers and the gradient of increasing stiffness provide the mechanics for the complex mucosal wave. Understanding this histology is critical when surgically excising benign vocal fold lesions. Respect for these layers is necessary for restoring and preserving the oscillatory properties of the true vocal folds. All normal mucosa and superficial lamina should be preserved, and care must be taken not to traumatize the vocal ligament. Usually it is possible to remove superficial lesions without disturbing the deeper, fibroblast-containing layers.

The classic microflap approach to the excision of vocal fold lesions involves making an incision through the epithelium on the superior surface of the vocal fold lateral to the mass about halfway to the ventricle (Figure 14-9). A plane is then created in the superficial lamina propria until the lesion is identified. The lesion is then separated from the vocal ligament and overlying cover.[16] This technique requires a long incision and is

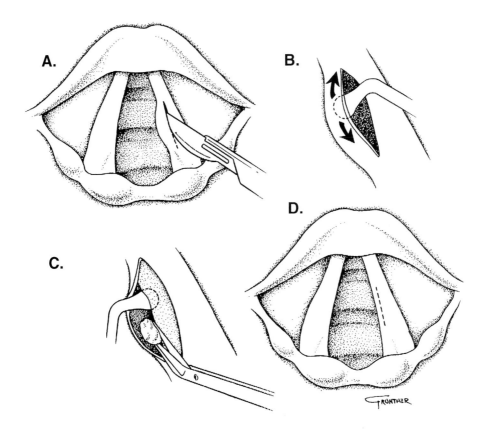

FIGURE 14–9. Microflap procedure, as illustrated by Sataloff in Cummings et al. In this technique, a superficial incision is made in the superior surface of the true vocal fold **A.** Blunt dissection is used to elevate the mucosa from the lesion **B.**, minimizing trauma to the fibroblast-containing layers of the lamina propria. Only pathologic tissue is excised under direct vision **C.** Mucosa is reapproximated **D.** without violating the leading edge. (Reprinted with permission from Sataloff RT. The professional voice. In: Cummings W, et al, eds. *Otolanyngology–Head and Neck Surgery.* Vol. 1. St. Louis, Mo: CV Mosby; 1986:2029–2053.)

difficult technically. It is now reserved for larger lesions (such as diffuse leukoplakia, papilloma, or large intracordal cysts) and for lesions in which identification of the vocal ligament is difficult.[17]

Sataloff et al reapproached the microflap procedure and fashioned the mini-microflap based on their outcomes assessment of microflap surgery and on Gray's discovery of a complex basement membrane structure between the epithelium and superficial layer of lamina propria (Figures 14-10, 14-11, and 14-12).[18] An intricate series of type VII collagen loops attach the epithelium and

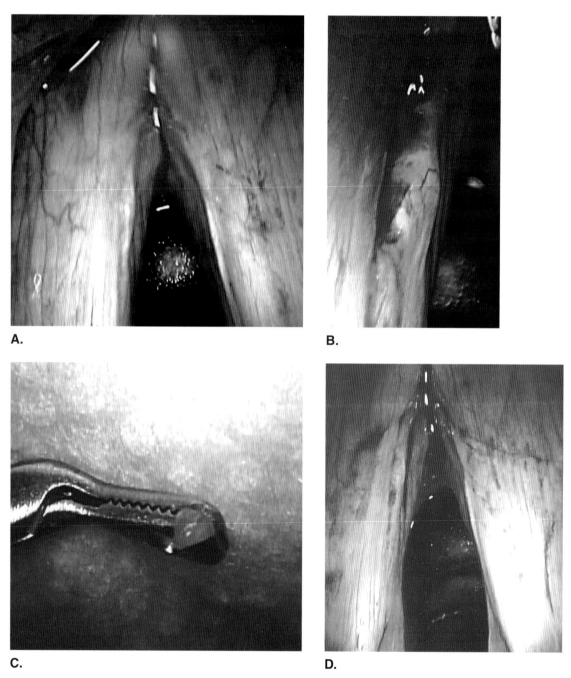

A.

B.

C.

D.

FIGURE 14–10. A. Small submucosal mass in left vocal fold. **B.** Mini-microflap incision made just lateral to the mass. **C.** Fibrovascular mass excised. **D.** Flap redraped with no secondary defect.

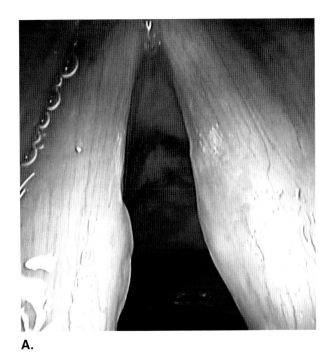

A.

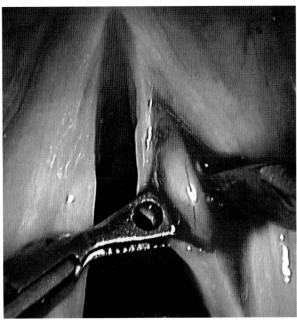

B.

FIGURE 14–11. A. Right submucosal cyst and left contact mass. **B.** Right submucosal cyst exposed after mini-microflap created. Note that the incision was made just lateral to the mass, but was made longer than the previous example to help with exposure of the cyst.

basement membrane to the superficial lamina propria.[15,19] Microflap techniques disturb this arrangement and may lead to hypodynamic segments of mucosa. In creating a mini-microflap, an incision is made at the junction of the mass and normal tissue (Figure 14–13). Small vertical anterior and posterior incisions are made if necessary and the mass is separated by blunt dissection from the superficial layer of the lamina propria. The lesion is excised preserving as much normal adjacent mucosa as possible. A small amount of mucosa directly over the lesion may be removed if necessary. Because the mass often acts as a tissue expander, an inferiorly based "mini-microflap" usually can be created to prevent a significant secondary defect.

Courey et al described the medial microflap technique as a variation of the traditional lateral microflap for submucosal lesions that involve the medial surface exclusively and are covered by atrophic and redundant mucosa. Similar to the mini-microflap, this technique emphasizes sparing all normal lamina propria and overlying mucosa, thereby avoiding any defect along the

medial edge of the vocal fold that would need to heal by secondary intention.[20]

A secondary defect is difficult to avoid in some cases. Some masses, such as broad-based polyps, have significant vertical dimension; and some masses are very difficult to separate from the overlying mucosa. Moreover, leaving redundant or deformed mucosa may result in fluid accumulation and development of a pseudocyst.

Specific Considerations for Common Vocal Fold Lesions

The following section highlights specific approaches and surgical principles for several common phonosurgical procedures. A detailed review of benign vocal fold pathology is found in chapter 24.

Reinke's Edema

Caution must be observed when operating on Reinke's edema. Overaggressive resection may lead to scarring and adherence of the epithelium to

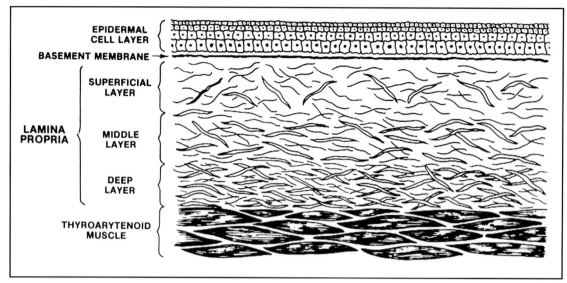

A.

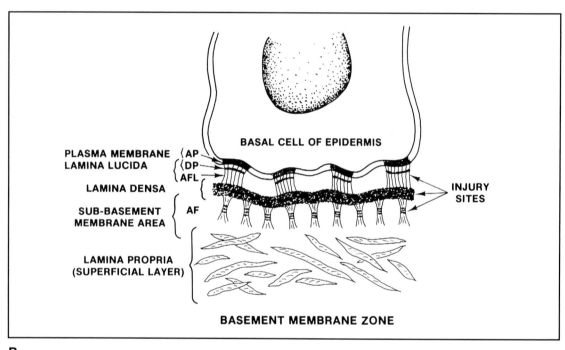

B.

FIGURE 14–12. **A.** Layers of vocal fold (not drawn to scale). The basement membrane lies between the epithelium and the superficial layer of the lamina propria. **B.** Basement membrane zone. Basal cells are connected to the lamina densa by attachment plax (*AP*) in the plasma membrane of the epidermis. Anchoring filaments (*AF*) extend from the attachment plax through the sub-basal densa plate (*DP*) and attach to the lamina densa (dark single-layer, electron-dense band just beneath the basal cell layer.) The sub-basement membrane zone consists of anchoring fibers (*AF*) that attach to the lamina densa and extend into the superficial layer of the lamina propria. Type VII collagen fibers attach to the network of the lamina propria by looping around Type III collagen fibers. (Reproduced with permission from Gray S. Basement membrane zone injury in vocal nodules. In: Gauffin, J, Hammarberg B, Eds. *Vocal Fold Physiology.* San Diego, Calif: Singular Publishing Group; 1991.)

180

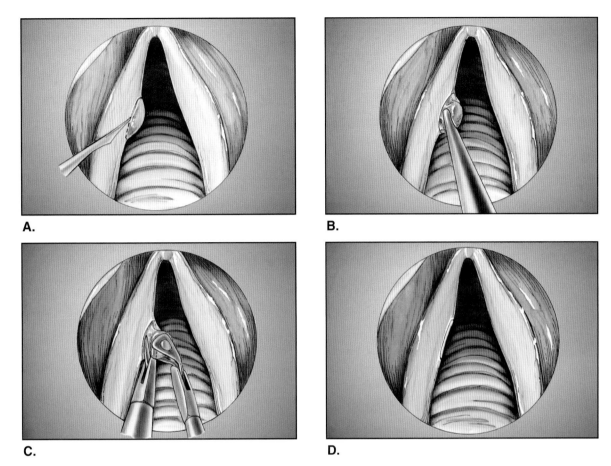

A.

B.

C.

D.

FIGURE 14–13. A. In elevating a mini-microflap, an incision is made with a straight knife at the junction of the mass and normal tissue. Small vertical anterior and posterior incisions may be added at the margins of the mass if necessary, usually using a straight scissors. **B.** The mass is separated by blunt dissection, splitting the superficial layer of the lamina propria and preserving it as much as possible. This dissection can be performed with a spatula, blunt ball dissector (*illustrated*), or scissors (*as illustrated in A*). **C.** The lesion is stabilized and a scissors (straight or curved) is used to excise the lesion, preserving as much adjacent mucosa as possible. The lesion itself acts as a tissue expander, and it is often possible to create an inferiorly based mini-microflap. **D.** The mini-microflap is replaced over the surgical defect, establishing primary closure and acting as a biological dressing. (Reprinted with permission from Sataloff R. Voice surgery. In Sataloff R. *Professional Voice: The Science and Art of Professional Care.* 3rd ed. San Diego, Calif: Plural Publishing, Inc; 2005:1165.)

the underlying vocal ligament. An incision is created along the superior surface and edematous material is removed with suction (Figure 14–14). Not infrequently, some of the fibrous stroma may need to be excised with cold instruments. Redundant mucosa is trimmed and the mucosal edges are reapproximated. This procedure was initially described by Hirano, and replaced the traditional technique of vocal fold stripping for this disease.[21]

There is some controversy as to whether both vocal folds should be operated on at one time.[22] Although bilateral surgery may be performed without an anterior web if care is taken in the anterior commissure, unilateral surgery offers other advantages. If the operated side becomes stiff postoperatively, the contralateral edematous vocal fold will usually compensate well. If a surgeon operates on both sides at once and each side suffers severe scarring, the patient

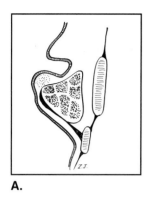 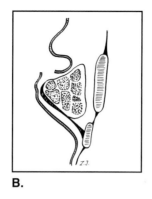 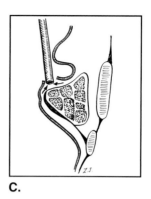 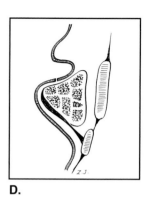

A. **B.** **C.** **D.**

FIGURE 14–14. A. Bulky vocal fold showing Reinke's edema (*small dots*) in the superficial layer of the lamina propria. **B.** Incision in the upper surface opens easily into Reinke's space. **C.** Using a fine-needle suction, the edema fluid is aspirated (*arrows*). **D.** The mucosal edges are reapproximated, trimming redundant mucosa if necessary. (Reprinted with permission from Sataloff R. Voice surgery. In Sataloff R. *Professional Voice: The Science and Art of Professional Care.* 3rd ed. San Diego, Calif: Plural Publishing, Inc; 2005:1170.)

will be left with a hoarse, breathy voice requiring high phonation pressures. This results in strained, effortful phonation, and the patient may be left unhappier than he or she was with the initial low or masculized voice. The patient can return to the operating room for the treatment of the contralateral vocal fold after healing has occurred, if symptoms warrant the additional procedure.

Ectasias and Varicosities

Although often asymptomatic, ectasias and varicosities may lead to dysphonia and/or recurrent vocal fold hemorrhages. Thus, symptomatic lesions require excision. In addition, vocal fold polyps often have a large feeding vessel that may need to be treated. Varices and ectasias may be photocoagulated with low-wattage (1–1.5 watts) CO_2 laser, defocused in interrupted single 0.1 second pulses. The beam is defocused to 300 to 400 μm. Low-power density is used to try to avoid thermal injury to the superficial lamina propria and minimize risk of injury to the vocal ligament.[23,24] Cold excision of varices and ectasias is technically more difficult, but potentially safer to the underlying lamina propria; and this procedure eliminates the risk of recanalization, which may occur after laser vaporization. An incision is created adjacent to the vessel, and the vessel is elevated with a 1-mm right-angle vascular knife

(Xomed-Medtronics) (Figure 14–15). The elevated vessel is then retracted gently to provide access to its anterior and posterior limits where it is divided sharply. Bleeding stops spontaneously, although topical 1:1000 epinephrine may be used for hemostasis.[25]

Vocal Process Granulomas

Granulomas usually result from reflux[26] and/or trauma, such as endotracheal intubation. One should resist operating on these lesions until conservative measures, such as antireflux treatment, voice therapy[27] and steroids, have been exhausted. These lesions may take months to resolve. If they do not improve with medical management, surgical excision may be performed. Laser or cold excision may be used. However, care must be taken not to traumatize the underlying perichondrium as this will likely result in recurrent granuloma formation. The authors prefer cold excision of these lesions and injection of decadron (4 mg/cc) into the surgical site. Chemical denervation with botulinum toxin may be useful, particularly in the setting of recurrent granuloma. Pre- and postoperative voice therapy and long-term antireflux therapy also help prevent recurrence. In multiply recurrent cases, mitomycin-C may have a role; and recently, one of the authors (RTS) has had success using pulsed-dye laser therapy.

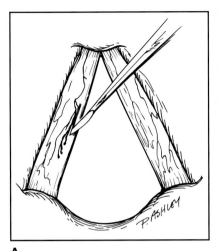 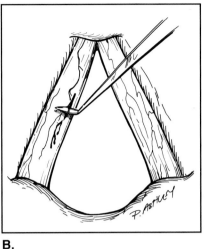 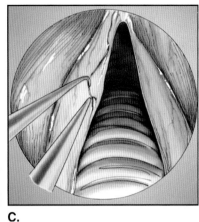

A. **B.** **C.**

FIGURE 14–15. Ectasia. **A.** This figure illustrates the technique for elevating and resecting a varicose vessel. A superficial incision is made in the epithelium adjacent to the vessel using the sharp point of the vascular knife or using a microknife (*illustrated*). **B.** The 1-mm right angle vascular knife is inserted under the vessel and used to elevate it. It may be necessary to make more than one epithelial incision in order to dissect the desired length of the vessel. **C.** Once the pathologic vessel has been elevated, it is retracted gently to provide access to its anterior and posterior limits. These can be divided sharply with a scissors or knife (bleeding stops spontaneously) or divided and cauterized with a laser, as long as there is no thermal injury to the adjacent vocal ligament. (Reprinted with permission from Sataloff R. Voice surgery. In Sataloff R. *Professional Voice: The Science and Art of Professional Care.* 3rd ed. San Diego, Calif: Plural Publishing, Inc; 2005:1169.)

Recurrent Respiratory Papillomatosis

Laryngeal papillomatosis continues to be a difficult problem for the patient and laryngologist. Much of the complexity is a result of the fact that human papilloma virus (HPV) exists in normal epithelial tissue as well as gross papillomas.[28] Recurrence is common, resulting in multiple surgical excisions and subsequent vocal fold scarring and dysphonia.

In addition to numerous medical treatments (none of which is highly effective), a variety of techniques have been described for managing laryngeal papillomatosis surgically including cold excision,[29,30] pulse-dye laser,[31] photodynamic therapy,[32] and the microdebrider or laryngeal shaver.[33,34] Injection of cidofovir is being used adjunct with or in lieu of surgical excision,[35] though concern continues to be raised with regard to the possible transforming effects of this agent.[36] Regardless of the methods used, when excising papillomas of the true vocal fold, the surgeon should remember that this is a disease of epithelium and should preserve all underlying superficial lamina propria and not traumatize the vocal ligament. In addition, the surgeon must remember that surgery is not likely to be curative. Conservative and precise excision should be performed with the hope that the patient's immune response, current adjunctive therapy (eg, cidofovir), or future treatment options (eg, vaccination) will yield complete remission of the disease. Viral subtyping is useful to determine whether there is increased risk for malignant transformation. Anal and genital papilloma data suggest that subtypes 16 and 18 are associated with a higher risk for malignant transformation and may warrant closer follow-up. However, there is evidence that subtype 11 may have a more aggressive course in the larynx than it does at other sites.[37] Otherwise, the decision to proceed to the operating room should be determined on an individualized basis, influenced by patient's desires, risk for airway obstruction, and voice disturbance.

Submucosal Infusion

Submucosal infusion technique arose from anatomic experiments which helped define the connective tissue compartments of the larynx.[38]. The benefits of submucosal infusion include elevation of the mass from the underlying superficial lamina propria and vocal ligament, increasing the tension of the epithelium, and hemostasis. In some cases, however, injection may obscure the mass or the epithelial boundary of normal and abnormal tissue.

A number of substances may be injected including a 1:10,000 dilution of epinephrine (9 cc of sterile saline with 1 cc of epinephrine 1:1000), decadron, and, in selected cases of papilloma, limited amounts of cidofovir. Steroids may be useful particularly when operating on a vocal fold with significant scar and sulcus. However, there is some evidence suggesting that steroids may not be beneficial and, in fact, may delay wound healing.[39]

EXCELLENT POSTOPERATIVE CARE IS ESSENTIAL

Postoperative care and evaluation are critical to obtaining optimal surgical results. The outcomes of voice surgery are unpredictable for any individual. Even with the best surgical technique, voice results can be compromised by postoperative inflammation and scar formation.

The use of postoperative steroids and antibiotics is not universal, but they are used by some surgeons empirically to promote healing. Certainly, underlying medical issues such as reflux and cough should be treated. Aggressive reflux control is especially important. There is little downside to using mucolytics and antitussives in the postoperative period. Patients should be discouraged from taking medications that may be irritating or otherwise harmful to the vocal folds, such as steroid inhalers, aspirin, ibuprofen, and antihistamines.

The issue of voice rest is controversial. There is no consensus as to the application of voice rest postoperatively. A recent survey suggested that, although the majority of otolaryngologists performing microlaryngeal surgery recommend voice rest postoperatively, there is lack of agreement as to duration and type of voice rest (absolute vs relative). The most common recommendation was 7 days of absolute or relative voice rest.[40] There are no adequate prospective trials comparing surgery with and without voice rest. However, it seems likely that reducing traumatic forces at the surgical site would reduce the risk of scar formation. Certainly, when we make an incision elsewhere on the body, we discourage traumatizing it while it is healing.

Phonation should probably be avoided until the epithelium has healed and can provide protection for the underlying lamina propria. The authors recommend 1 week of absolute voice rest in most cases, followed by strobovideolaryngoscopic evaluation. If resection has been very limited, reepithelization may occur within 2 or 3 days and short periods of voice rest may be acceptable in carefully selected patients. The findings of the postoperative evaluation determine how rapidly a patient may increase voice use. Useful parameters include return of mucosal wave (favorable), and the development of early postoperative complications such as hemorrhage or early scar or granuloma formation. If such complications arise, one should consider restricting voice use longer and using steroids (either systemically or by local injection). The authors typically gradually increase voice use over the following 2 to 6 weeks, under supervision of the voice team. Additional voice therapy is important in the postoperative period to prevent the development of hyperfunctional compensatory techniques, and consequent phonotrauma, and to optimize surgical outcome.

After about 6 weeks, strobovideolaryngoscopy should be repeated. If there has been good return of mucosal wave and no additional injuries, the patient should be permitted to speak freely.

Emerging Concepts

Although microsurgical techniques for removing benign vocal fold lesions have improved since the days of vocal fold stripping, there is still much room for improvement. Innovations in the treatment of papilloma, such as intralesional cidofovir injections, the careful use of the laryngeal microdebrider, and pulsed-dye laser are good examples of innovations achieved through people thinking "beyond-the-box" to improve treatment of a very difficult and often frustrating disease process. Time and well-controlled studies will determine the efficacy of these novel ideas. Current surgical treatment of other benign lesions also still leaves something to be desired. Although we can minimize scar formation in most situations by using meticulous technique, we cannot eliminate it. In addition, many patients have scar present preoperatively, that, to date, we cannot treat as well as we would like. Fat, hyaluronic acid, and collagen have all been used to try to treat scar, although the ideal injectable does not exist. Eventually, genetic screening may be able to identify people at high risk for scar formation, and genetic engineering may allow us to grow new superficial lamina propria to repair scar. We should not be satisfied until we are able to obtain maximal voice improvement in every microsurgical case.

The patient should be advised that any worsening of the voice should prompt an urgent evaluation and return to more voice restrictions. In general, singing should not be started until about 6 weeks postoperatively. Return of mucosal wave is desirable prior to return to singing. Performers should be advised that surgical results are variable, and some patients may not be able to get back to full capabilities until after 6 months to a year of rehabilitation.[41] Occasionally, full recovery does not occur at all, usually due to scar formation.

Microlaryngeal surgery for benign vocal fold lesions is a challenging and important part of care for the voice patient. The otolaryngologist must exercise good judgment before, during, and after surgery. A thorough understanding of the anatomy and physiology of the voice, as well as access to and familiarity with appropriate instrumentation, is critical to provide quality surgical care for the laryngeal surgery patient.

Review Questions

1. Optimal positioning for viewing the entire length of the vocal folds during microdirect laryngoscopy includes:
   a. Head extension, neck extension
   b. Head flexion, neck flexion
   c. Head flexion, neck extension
   d. Head extension, neck flexion
   e. None of the above

2. A young professional soprano presents to you with mild hoarseness, loss of upper range, and increased vocal fatigue since an upper respiratory tract infection 3 months ago. Her voice is becoming progressively worse. She complains of globus sensation and the

need to clear her throat frequently. Visualization of the larynx with both flexible and rigid videostroboscopy demonstrates symmetrical vocal fold adduction and abduction, posterior inflammatory changes, bilateral vocal fold edema, a small cyst on the medial edge within the left vocal fold striking zone, contralateral fibrosis, and an hourglass deformity. Which of the following would be the most appropriate initial course of action?

a. Surgical excision of the cyst and steroid injection into the contralateral vocal fold
b. Treatment of reflux followed by surgical excision of the cyst.
c. Treatment of reflux and voice therapy
d. Treatment of reflux, voice therapy, then surgical excision of the cyst.
e. Bilateral thyroplasty

3. The medial microflap and mini-microflap are similar in that they both:
a. Try to reduce scarring
b. Try to preserve as much superficial lamina propria as possible
c. Try to preserve normal overlying epithelium
d. Are useful for masses along the medial edge of the vocal fold
e. All of the above

4. Potential advantages of cold excision of benign vocal fold lesions over CO_2 laser include all of the following except:
a. Cold excision provides more control of depth of injury
b. CO^2 laser introduces a risk of airway fire
c. CO^2 laser provides better hemostasis
d. CO^2 laser requires less surgical skill
e. In the right hands, either technique can yield good results.

5. A severely dysphonic, breathy patient presents to you 6 months after having "smokers' polyps" removed. Which of the following are you most likely to see with videostroboscopy?
a. Severe scarring bilaterally
b. Bilateral hemorrhage
c. Recurrent polyposis
d. Vocal fold immobility
e. Function dysphonia

REFERENCES

1. Rakel B, Spiegel JR, Sataloff RT. Prolonged ulcerative laryngitis. *J Voice.* 2002;16(3):433–438.
2. Merati AL, Heman-Ackah Y, Abaza M, Altman KW, Bielamowicz S. Common movement disorders of the larynx: a report of the Neurolaryngology Subcommittee. *Otolaryngol Head and Neck Surg.* 2005; 133(5):654–665.
3. Hogikyan ND, Sethuraman G. Validation of an instrument to measure voice-related quality of life (V-RQOL). *J Voice.* 1999;13(4):557–569.
4. Rubin AD, Wodchis WP, Spak C, Kileny PR, Hogikyan ND. Longitudinal effects of Botox injections on voice-related quality of life (V-RQOL) for patients with adductory spasmodic dysphonia: part II. *Arch Otolaryngol Head and Neck Surg.* 2004;130(4):415–420.
5. Benninger MS, Ahuja AS, Gardner G, Grywalski C. Assessing outcomes for dysphonic patients. *J Voice.* 1998;12(4):540–550.
6. Rosen CA, Lee AS, Osborne J, Zullo T, Murry T. Development and validation of the voice handicap index–10. *Laryngoscope.* 2004; 114(9):1549–1556.
7. Zeitels SM, Vaughan CW. "External counterpressure" and "internal distension" for optimal laryngoscopic exposure of the anterior glottal commissure. *Ann Otol Rhinol Laryngol.* 1994; 103:669–676.
8. Hochman II, Zeitels SM, Heaton JT. Analysis of the forces and position required for direct laryngoscopic exposure of the anterior vocal folds. *Ann Otol Rhinol Laryngol.* 1999;108(8):715–724.
9. Anderson TD, Sataloff RT. Value of the 70 degrees telelaryngoscope in microlaryngoscopy for benign

pathology. *Ear Nose Throat J.* 2002;81(12): 821-822.

10. Yeh AR, Huang HM, Chen YL. Telescopic video microlaryngeal surgery. *Ann Otol Rhinol Laryngol.* 1999;108:165-168.

11. Zeitels SM. Laser versus cold instruments for microlaryngologic surgery. *Laryngoscope.* 1996; 106(5):545-552.

12. Garrett G, Reinisch L. New generation pulsed CO_2 laser: comparative effects on vocal fold wound healing. *Ann Otol Rhinol Laryngol.* 2002;111(6): 471-476.

13. Benninger MS. Microdissection or microspot laser for limited vocal fold benign lesions: a prospective randomized trial. *Laryngoscope.* 2000;110 (2 pt 2, suppl 92):1-17.

14. Hirano M. Phonosurgery. Basic and clinical investigations. *Otologia Fukuoka.* 1975;21:239-442.

15. Gray SD. Cellular Physiology of the vocal folds. *Otolaryngol Clin North Am.* 2000;33(4) 679-697.

16. Courey MS, Gardner GM, Stone RE, Ossoff RH. Endoscopic vocal fold microflap: a three-year experience. *Ann Otol Rhinol Laryngol.* 1995;104 (4 pt 1):267-273.

17. Ford CN. Adavances and refinements in phonosurgery. *Laryngoscope.* 1999;109(12):1891-1900.

18. Sataloff RT, Spiegel JR, Heuer RJ, et al. Laryngeal mini-microflap: a new technique and reassessment of the microflap saga. *J Voice.* 1995;9(2):198-204.

19. Gray S. Basement membrane zone injury I vocal nodules. In: Gauffin J, Hammarberg B, eds. *Vocal Fold Physiology: Acoustic, Perceptual and Physiologic Aspects of Voice Mechanics.* San Diego, Calif: Singular Publishing Group; 1991:21-27.

20. Courey MS, Garrett CG, Ossoff RH. Medial microflap for excision of benign vocal fold lesions. *Laryngoscope.* 1997;107:340-344.

21. Hirano M, Shin T, Morio M, et al. An improvement in surgical treatment for polypoid vocal cord: sucking technique. *Otologia (Fukuoka).* 1976; 22:583-589.

22. Zeitels S, Casiano R, Gardner G, Hogikyan N, Koufman J, Rosen C. Management of common voice problems: committee report. *Otolaryngol Head Neck Surg.* 2002;126(4):323-348.

23. Postma, GM, Courey, MS, Ossoff, RH. Microvascular lesions of the true vocal fold. *Ann Otol Rhinol Laryngol.* 1998;107(6):472-476.

24. Garrett G, Reinisch L. New generation pulsed CO_2 laser: comparative effects on vocal fold wound healing. *Ann Otol Rhinol Laryngol.* 2002;111(6):471-476.

25. Hochman I, Sataloff RT, Hillman R, Zeitels S. Ectasias and varices of the vocal fold: clearing the

striking zone: *Ann Otol Rhinol Laryngol.* 1999; 108(1)10-16.

26. Ylitalo R, Ramel S. Extraesophageal reflux in patients with contact granuloma: a prospective controlled study. *Ann Otol Rhinol Laryngol.* 2002;111(5 pt 1):441-446.

27. Leonard R, Kendall K. Effects of voice therapy on vocal process granuloma: a phonoscopic approach. *Am J Otolaryngol.* 2005;26(2):101-107.

28. Rihkanen H, Aaltonen LM, Syrjanen SM. Human papillomavirus in laryngeal papillomas and in adjacent normal epithelium. *Clin Otolaryngol Allied Sci.* 1993;18(6):470-474.

29. Zeitels SM, Sataloff RT. Phonomicrosurgical resection of glottal papillomatosis. *J Voice.* 1999;13(1): 123-127.

30. Courey MS, Ossoff RH. Laser applications in adult laryngeal surgery. *Otolaryngol Clin North Am.* 1996;29(6):973-986.

31. Franco RA Jr, Zeitels SM, Farinelli WA, Anderson RR. 585-nm pulsed dye laser treatment of glottal papillomatosis. *Ann Otol Rhinol Laryngol.* 2002; 111(6):486-92.

32. Shikowitz MJ, Abramson AL, Freeman K, Steinberg BM, Nouri M. Efficacy of DHE photodynamic therapy for respiratory papillomatosis: immediate and long-term results. *Laryngoscope* 1998;108:962-967.

33. Patel N, Rowe M, Tunkel D. Treatment of recurrent respiratory papillomatosis in children with the microdebrider. *Ann Otol Rhinol Laryngol.* 2003;112(1):7-10.

34. Patel RS, MacKenzie K. Powered laryngeal shavers and laryngeal papillomatosis: a preliminary report *Clin Otolaryngol Allied Sci.* 2000;25(5):358-360.

35. Bielamowicz S, Villagomez V, Stager SV, Wilson WR. Intralesional cidofovir therapy for laryngeal papilloma in an adult cohort. *Laryngoscope.* 2002;112(4):696-699.

36. Wemer RD, Lee JH, Hoffman HT, Robinson RA, Smith RJ. Case of progressive dysplasia concomitant with intralesional cidofovir administration for recurrent respiratory papillomatosis. *Ann Otol Rhinol Laryngol.* 2005;114(11):836-839.

37. Gerein V, Rastorguev E, Gerein J, Draf W, Schirren J, Incidence, age at onset, and potential reasons of malignant transformation in recurrent respiratory papillomatosis patients: 20 years experience. *Otolaryngol Head Neck Surg.* 2005;132(3):392-394.

38. Kass ES, Hillman RE, Zeitels SM. Vocal fold submucosal infusion technique in phonomicrosurgery. *Ann Otol Rhinol Laryngol.* 1996;105(5):341-347.

39. Coleman JR Jr, Smith S, Reinisch L, Billante CR, Ossoff JP, Deriso W, Garrett CG. Histomorphometric

and laryngeal videostroboscopic analysis of the effects of corticosteroids on microflap healing in the dog larynx. *Ann Otol Rhinol Laryngol.* 1999;108(2):119-127.

40. Behrman A, Sulica L. Voice rest after microlaryngoscopy: current opinion and practice. *Laryngoscope.* 2003;113:2182-2186.

41. Emerich KA, Spiegel JR, Sataloff RT. Phonomicrosurgery III: pre- and postoperative care. *Otolaryngol Clin North Am.* 2000;33(5):1071-1080.

42. Dursun G, Sataloff RT, Spiegel JR, Mandel S, Heuer RJ, Rosen DC. Superior laryngeal nerve paresis and paralysis. *J Voice.* 1996;10(2):206-211.

43. Amin MR, Koufman JA. Vagal neuropathy after upper respiratory infection: a viral etiology? *Am J Otolaryngol.* 2001;22(4):251-256.

44. Rubin AD, Praneetvatakul V, Heman-Ackah Y, Moyer C, Mandel S, Sataloff RT. Repetitive phonatory tasks for identifying vocal fold paresis. *J Voice.* 2005;19(4)702-706.

15

Lasers in Laryngology

Robert A. Buckmire, MD

KEY POINTS

■ Laser light differs fundamentally from other sources of disorganized radiant energy, such as a lightbulb, because it is of uniform wavelength (monochromatic) and unidirectional (collimated).

■ The surgical characteristics of a given laser, including depth of injury, hemostatic properties, and the available delivery systems (fiberoptic vs articulated arm), are dependent upon the inherent characteristics of the wavelength of laser light produced. These factors must be taken into account when selecting the type of laser for a laryngoscopic application.

■ The intraoperative use of a surgical laser introduces a risk to the patient and operative staff and adds complexity to the protocol for anesthetic delivery.

■ The use of "no touch" (laser) techniques is a promising development. This will allow some procedures traditionally accomplished under general anesthesia with suspension laryngoscopy to be transitioned to the outpatient office setting under local anesthesia.

■ Both laser and "cold steel" microlaryngeal surgery produce excellent safe results when employed in a thoughtful and measured manner for appropriate laryngeal indications.

Lasers have enjoyed an excellent reputation in laryngology due to their reliability and intuitive application to laryngeal disease states. The CO_2 laser has been, by far, the laser most commonly used in otolaryngology. Despite the increased complexity of the anesthetic and surgical protocols required for safe intraoperative laser use, lasers have unequivocally expanded the surgical spectrum of the laryngeal surgeon. The physics of laser light and its tissue effects are particularly well suited to a variety of ablative or destructive operative indications as well as to procedures in which hemostatic control and precision are critical. The expansion of the clinically useful types of lasers in laryngology, including CO_2, KTP, Nd:YAG, and the pulsed dye laser has opened new avenues leading to novel treatment protocols for laryngeal disease entities. These applications are discussed below. Additionally, the use of "no touch" (laser) techniques has allowed some procedures traditionally accomplished under general anesthesia with suspension laryngoscopy to be transitioned to the outpatient office setting under local anesthesia.

DEFINITION

"LASER" is an acronym for *Light Amplification* by the *Stimulated Emission* of *Radiation*. Several components are common to all lasers; each has an optical resonating chamber with two mirrors, (one fully reflective and the other allowing partial transmission). Secondly, each chamber is filled with an active medium such as CO_2. The excitement of the chosen medium by an external energy source (eg, an electrical current) causes atoms to be raised to a higher energy state, resulting in spontaneous emissions of light energy (photons) in all directions. These photons, in turn, stimulate further emissions from atoms in their excited state. The interaction yields pairs of identical photons; the pairs are in phase with one another and have equal wavelength, frequency, and energy. The reflections from the mirrors within the resonating chamber serve as a positive feedback mechanism by reflecting the stimulated emissions back and forth. The partially transmissive mirror emits some of the radiant energy as laser light. All the emitted light is of the same wavelength (monochromatic) and unidirectional (collimated). These two characteristics differentiate laser light from other sources of disorganized radiant energy such as a lightbulb (Figure 15–1).

A BRIEF HISTORY OF LASERS IN OTOLARYNGOLOGY

Albert Einstein postulated the theoretical concept of a laser in 1917. In 1960 Theodore Maiman produced a visible light laser by stimulating a synthetic ruby crystal.[1] The first experimental laser use in otolaryngology was reported in 1965. Geza Jako, credited for popularizing the use of the CO_2 laser for laryngeal surgery, first experimented on human cadaveric and canine larynges. Subsequently, in the early 1970s, he and Stuart Strong collaborated in human clinical series[2-4] (Figure 15–2). In 1968, an articulated arm necessary for the delivery of the infrared CO_2 laser was developed by Polanyi.[5]

LASER TISSUE INTERACTIONS

When laser light interacts with tissue, several potential outcomes are possible. Depending upon the characteristics of the radiation wavelength and the tissue in question, variable proportions of the light energy will be reflected, absorbed, transmitted, and scattered. The shorter the wavelength of the light, the more it tends to be scattered by the tissue. Only the absorbed energy is available to induce effects on the target tissue. The primary effect of commonly used infrared or visible laser light is tissue heating. With absorption of radiant energy and heating of tissue to approximately 100°C, vaporization of intracellular water occurs. Carbonization, disintegration

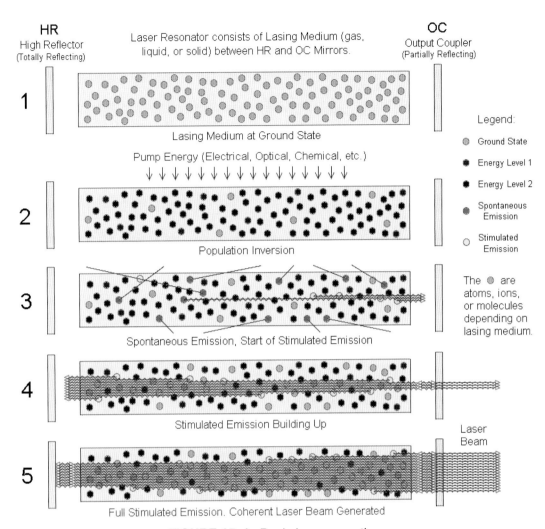

HR
High Reflector
(Totally Reflecting)

Laser Resonator consists of Lasing Medium (gas, liquid, or solid) between HR and OC Mirrors.

OC
Output Coupler
(Partially Reflecting)

1

Lasing Medium at Ground State

Pump Energy (Electrical, Optical, Chemical, etc.)

2

Population Inversion

3

Spontaneous Emission, Start of Stimulated Emission

4

Stimulated Emission Building Up

5

Full Stimulated Emission. Coherent Laser Beam Generated

Legend:

- Ground State
- Energy Level 1
- Energy Level 2
- Spontaneous Emission
- Stimulated Emission

The ⊙ are atoms, ions, or molecules depending on lasing medium.

Laser Beam

FIGURE 15–1. Basic laser operation.

smoke, and gas generation with destruction of the laser-radiated tissue occurs at several hundred degrees centigrade. In the center of the wound is an area of vaporization. Immediately adjacent to this area there is a zone of thermal necrosis and, more peripherally, an area of thermal conductivity and repair.[6]

SAFETY CONSIDERATIONS

The use of laser technology necessitates the alteration of standard anesthetic techniques for microlaryngeal surgery and adds risk, expense, and complexity to these procedures. A closed ventilatory circuit (with cuffed endotracheal tubes) reduces the possibility of ignition of surgical debris and the anesthetic gases as well. To raise the sensitivity of the detection of inadvertent injury to the closed anesthetic circuit, endotracheal tubes can be fitted with low pressure cuffs and filled with saline tinted with methylene blue. Injury to the cuff is therefore detected early as methylene blue leaks into the operative field. Further protection of the endotracheal tube cuff and distal airway structures can be accomplished by the placement of saline-soaked cottonoid pledgets between the surgical site and the endotracheal tube cuffs. This is particularly helpful

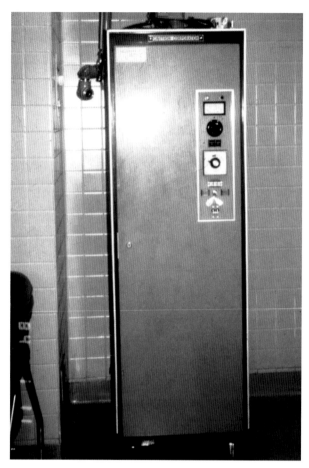

FIGURE 15–2. The original CO_2 laser. (Photo courtesy of Steven M. Zeitels, MD.)

airway fires. This constraint may potentially further complicate the delivery of a safe and effective general anesthetic in patients requiring substantial pulmonary support.

Protective measures are required for both patient (moistened eye pads, airway pledgets, and protective patient coverings) as well as for the operating room staff (goggles) to avoid inadvertent injury from stray laser emissions. The recommended protective measures are entirely dependent on the specific type and wavelength of laser and the delivery system. Eye protection is generally in the form of goggles made from glass or plastic and tinted to absorb or reflect potentially injurious misdirected light energy prior to ocular exposure. Because different laser wavelengths are absorbed by different colors of the visible spectrum, eyewear needs to be appropriate for the particular laser in use. One set of goggles is not universally protective for all lasers. In most hospitals, specialized training and personnel are required to safely operate the laser.[7]

TYPES OF LASERS

in laser laryngology procedures utilizing the CO_2 laser due to its efficient extinction in water. Low inhaled fractions of inspired oxygen (FiO_2 <.30), are recommended to minimize the risk of

The CO_2 laser is the most commonly used laser in laryngeal surgery. It produces light in the infrared range (10.6 microns). A second laser, a coaxial helium-neon laser is necessary for visible aiming of the invisible CO_2 beam. The introduction of the microspot manipulator allowed for a focused beam (as small as 0.2 mm) to be delivered at a 400-mm operative distance, ideal for

The Hot Versus Cold Controversy

There has been a longstanding debate in laryngology regarding the relative merits and drawbacks of laser use versus more traditional cold steel operative technique. One major thrust of the discussion has centered on the relative wound healing characteristics of laser and cold steel-induced injuries. This issue has been investigated by many authors with their conclusions falling on both sides of the issue. Durkin et al found that wound granulation was delayed in the laser ablated canine vocal fold epithelium in comparison to the vocal fold stripped by a cup forceps.[8] Regarding the relative rates of ongoing healing, Buell and Scheuller in 1983, found that tissue repair after CO_2 laser injury in hog skin yielded inferior tensile strength within the first 3 weeks postoperatively in comparison to scalpel wounds. After this point, however, both wounds demonstrated rapidly increasing tensile strength at similar rates.[9]

With regard to laryngeal microsurgery specifically, there has been a recent trend toward more traditional techniques (cold steel dissection) owing to the development of finer laryngeal instrumentation and obviating acceptance of the additional risk to the patient and operating room staff when the laser is employed. The potential for postoperative scar formation secondary to collateral thermal effects has been of particular concern following laser laryngeal phonosurgery. Despite these potential risks, several large series have been published demonstrating that microlaryngeal laser surgery can be performed, achieving both excellent safety and clinical outcomes.[10] Benninger compared microspot CO_2 laser surgery with cold microdissection technique in a prospective, randomized series of patients with benign vocal fold lesions and found no difference in surgical recovery time or clinical outcomes between the two groups.[4]

The effects of various parameters of the CO_2 laser have been well studied as they apply to tissue healing of the layered vocal fold tissue. The result of these data suggest that shorter pulse durations used with the CO_2 lasers (<0.10 second) produce less lateral thermal injury and wounds with greater tensile strength, resulting in earlier wound healing.[11] Additionally, a pulsed CO_2 laser delivery histologically caused less thermal injury and scar formation, and, improved vibratory characteristics in canine vocal folds when compared to a continuous wave CO_2 laser.[12]

Lasers: Pros
- hemostasis
- microspot accuracy (250 microns)
- potential for epithelial sparing in treatment of vascular lesions (PDL)
- application of "no touch" technique to laryngeal office procedures

Laser: Cons
- complicated anesthetic protocol (low FiO_2, absent use of nitrous oxide, laser safe ET tubes)
- increased complexity of surgical setup (eye protection and training for surgical staff)
- risk of peripheral thermal soft tissue damage in larynx
- risk of airway fire

suspension microlaryngoscopy.[13] The favorable characteristics of this wavelength of light include strong absorption by all tissues high in water content and negligible scatter and reflection. These factors have made the CO_2 laser a very useful tool for a variety of otolaryngologic indications. The most apparent limitation of the CO_2 laser is the inability to deliver the laser beam via a flexible fiber, necessitating the use of an articulated arm with mirrors arranged to direct the beam from the source to the target. For multiple laryngologic indications, the use of the CO_2 laser has become relatively standard. The most significant of these are detailed later in this chapter, as well as in later chapters whose focus is on the management of specific disease processes.

The KTP (potassium titanyl phosphate) laser emits light at 532 nanometers that is strongly absorbed by hemoglobin. This can be delivered through an optical fiber, facilitating its use in many flexible endoscopic procedures. Because of its strong hemoglobin absorption, this laser is useful for coagulating blood vessels or managing vascular lesions.

The Nd:YAG (neodymium: yttrium-aluminum Garnet laser) laser produces a light with a wavelength of 1.064 microns. Its light is poorly absorbed by water and hemoglobin, thus facilitating its use in fluid-filled cavities (ophthalmologic surgery). The effective extinction length in biologic tissue is usually 2 to 4 mm, making this laser ideal for indications where lateral coagulation and hemostasis are desired. On the contrary, the depth of thermal injury makes precise control and complete preservation of adjacent normal tissues practically impossible. Potential delivery via a flexible fiber and the use of a contact tip make this laser an excellent tool for vaporization of obstructing lesions with a high bleeding potential.

The 585 nanmeter pulsed dye laser (PDL) is a recent addition to the laryngeal surgical armamentarium. Light of this wavelength was designed to provide maximal hemoglobin absorption with minimal scatter of energy. It is therefore well suited for lesions with vascular characteristics different from the normal vocal fold epithelium. It, too, can be delivered through a flexible fiber, making it available for use through a flexible endoscope.

SPECIFIC LASER APPLICATIONS

With the basis of laser laryngology having been presented, the remainder of this chapter reviews its use with different categories of laryngeal surgical disorders. Several other chapters in this volume provide further detail for each category, particularly chapters 24: Benign Lesions of the Larynx; chapter 25: Malignant Lesions of the Larynx; and chapter 26: Laryngotracheal Airway Stenosis.

Lasers and Airway Stenosis

Laryngeal stenosis with respiratory embarrassment is regularly encountered by otolaryngologists. Tracheotomy provides a highly effective means of airway management providing surgical access to the airway for ventilatory support, pulmonary toileting, and a means by which a source of upper airway obstruction can be mechanically bypassed. Tracheotomy does, however, have a deleterious effect on both voice production and deglutition, and therefore is a less than desirable long-term option in patients with adequate respiratory reserve to rely on their native airway.

Many procedures short of tracheotomy including cordectomy, cordotomy, endoscopic and external arytenoidectomy, vocal fold lateralization, and laryngeal reinervation have been proposed for patients with clinically significant glottic stenosis. In these patients, several laser procedures have proven useful. In 1984, Ossoff et al reported a series of 11 patients managed with endoscopic CO_2 laser arytenoidectomy for the management of bilateral vocal fold paralysis. Ten of the 11 patients were successfully decannulated.[14] Since this report, subsequent series have confirmed the effectiveness of this operative approach in both bilateral vocal fold paralysis and other etiologies of glottic stenosis. The complete arytenoidectomy procedure, however, yields inherent phonatory deficits. Crumley in 1993 proposed a limited (medial) arytenoidectomy for the management of patients with glottic stenosis in an attempt to minimize the detrimental effects on the phonatory (membranous) portion of the glottis.[15] Based on a similar desire to

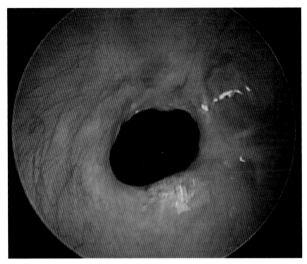

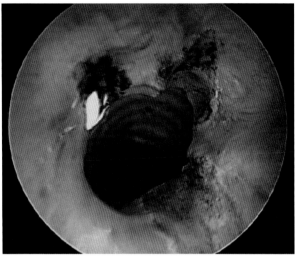

A.   **B.**

FIGURE 15–3. A. Subglottic stenosis prior to laser radial incision. **B.** Subglottic stenosis after laser radial incision, prior to dilation

limit the phonatory effects of widening the static glottic airway, Dennis and Kashima reported a small series of patients (6) successfully treated with a limited posterior CO_2 laser cordotomy with relief of their primary dyspneic symptom.[16] Reoperation with a more aggressive cordotomy was necessary in several patients and postoperative tracheotomy was required in another. More recent series of endoscopic CO_2 laser posterior transverse cordotomy suggest that a simultaneous bilateral approach is both safe and perhaps more effective in producing a long-term, patent glottic airway in a single stage procedure.[17,18] Most cases, however, are managed with unilateral procedures. Remarkably, throughout all of these series, aspiration has not presented as a significant postoperative complication.

Lasers have also been successfully applied to the treatment of weblike subglottic stenoses. A common technique utilizing the CO_2 laser is endoscopic laser radial incisions with subsequent dilation (see Figures 15-3A and 15-3B).

Lasers and Vascular Lesions

Due to the unique tissue interactions of light of different wavelengths, various lasers have become increasingly utilized in the treatment of specific laryngeal lesions. Wavelengths with a strong absorption by hemoglobin and water have been particularly useful for treatment of vascular and soft tissue laryngeal lesions.

Vascular lesions of the larynx may cause voice or airway compromise depending upon their size and location on the vocal fold mucosa. For several years, the CO_2 laser has been a mainstay of the treatment for laryngeal vascular laryngeal lesions, both small and large. Microvascular lesion of the vocal folds may present either incidentally or with symptoms of dysphonia caused by resultant mass lesion, hemorrhage or altered vibratory properties of the involved fold. In a review of the surgical management of these lesions, Postma et al found that isolated CO_2 laser treatment of the feeding vessels with a low power setting (1-2 watts) and a slightly defocused beam (300-400 microns) yielded excellent long-term results with return to full vocal activities and no findings of recurrent varices, scarring or further vocal fold hemorrhage.[19] In 2003, Hsuing et al reported on the treatment of a series of 10 patients with microvascular lesion of the vocal folds treated with a KTP laser (continuous mode, 0.4-0.6 mm beam, total energy 3-7 joules). The authors reported significant improvements in perceptual voice characteristics as well as videostroboscopic measures in the study cohort.[20]

Hemorrhagic mass lesions such as polyps have also been treated successfully by endoscopic laser modalities (Figures 15–4A and 15–4B). Despite the traditional concern for peripheral soft tissue thermal injury, no decrement in vibratory function was noted by the authors on postprocedural videostroboscopy.

In areas of the larynx where small degrees of epithelial damage are less critical to the function of the organ, many options are available to treat discrete vascular lesions. For example, in the treatment of obstructive subglottic hemangiomas, clinical series using CO_2, KTP, Argon and Nd:YAG lasers have all been reported to deliver safe and successful, functional outcomes.[21-23] The location and characteristics of the vascular lesion, surgeon preference and experience, as well as the advantages and limitations of each of these laser wavelengths, play a primary role in determining the laser type selected for treatment.

Lasers and Benign Laryngeal Lesions

Lasers have been used as a treatment modality for several other types of benign glottic lesions. Granulomata, epithelial hyperplasia, and recurrent respiratory papillomata have all been treated with laser modalities and reported in the laryngologic literature. There has been a growing trend toward the office-based laser treatment of several epithelial glottic lesions. Multiple investigators have examined the utility of the 585-nm pulsed dye laser in the treatment of benign laryngeal pathologies. The primary benefit of this laser is the ability for the energy emitted to penetrate epithelium without damage and then to be selectively absorbed by the underlying microvasculature.[24,25] In the office setting, this laser can be delivered through a small caliber fiber via a flexible transnasal endoscope with a working channel. Zeitels et al reported a 25% or greater disease regression in 77 patients treated in the office under local anesthesia for recurrent respiratory papillomatosis and glottic dysplasia. Although the procedure was on occasion aborted due to procedural difficulty, no complications were reported in the study cohort.[26] In a small series of 10 patients with laryngeal granulomas, Clyne et al reported a 50% resolution rate of lesions treated in the office with the pulsed dye laser.[24] The lack of a pathologic specimen is one important drawback of this technique, specifically with regard to treating dysplastic lesions.

Lasers and Laryngeal Carcinoma

Laser excision of small, limited laryngeal carcinomas has been a routine part of the laryngeal

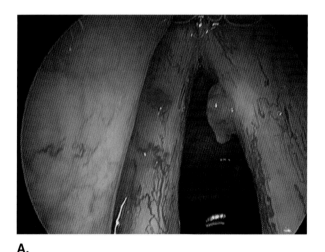
A.

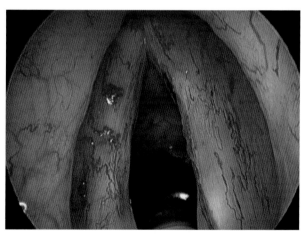
B.

FIGURE 15–4. A. Hemorrhagic polyp of the right true vocal fold in a post-radiation patient. Note the characteristic hypervascularlity of the vocal folds in this patient population. **B.** Same patient following CO_2 laser resection. The pathology was benign.

surgeon's armamentarium for many decades. However, over the last 10 years, there has been growing interest in the use of the CO_2 laser for the endoscopic treatment of locally advanced laryngeal carcinoma. Head and neck surgeons have endeavored to treat increasingly advanced laryngeal tumors with a transoral endoscopic laser approach with notable successes. The specific details of technique and outcomes are beyond the scope of this chapter but are considered separately in chapter 25.

In the 1970s Vaughn introduced the concept of the use of the CO_2 laser in the treatment of supraglottic cancer.[27] Since that time, surgeons have continued to push the boundaries of endoscopic laser excision of laryngeal carcinoma. The principles of these excisions, at times, violate several traditional surgical principles including en bloc resection of carcinoma and disease-free margins. Techniques for endoscopic supraglottic laryngectomy have been shown to be successful for the local control of early (T1 and T2) and selected locally advanced squamous cell carcinomas (SCCAs) of the larynx.[28,29]

In 2004, Steiner et al reviewed their experience with endoscopic laser treatment of selected recurrent glottic carcinoma after radiotherapy with curative intent. The authors concluded that CO_2 laser microsurgery could successfully be used as a curative organ-preservation procedure for recurrent glottic carcinomas.[30] A review of the postoperative complications seen with transoral CO_2 laser surgery for carcinoma of the larynx and hypopharynx found complications to be related to tumor extension and the surgeon experience.[31] An analysis of recurrences following CO_2 laser treatment of a large cohort of patients (n = 322) with early glottic carcinomas (T1 and T2), revealed a significant relationship between disease recurrence and lateral tumor extension with involvement of the bottom of the laryngeal ventricle.[29]

The indications for laser applications in laryngeal surgery are continually expanding. The trend toward the safe utilization of these technologies in the office setting will undoubtedly yield significant advances in both cost containment and patient convenience. One important frontier, the administration of a CO_2 laser via a small flexible fiber (waveguide), continues to be the focus of a great deal of investigation.[32,33] When achieved, this technology will open a far wider spectrum of applications of this user-friendly wavelength via flexible endoscopy in the sinonasal tract, trachea, and bronchi as well as expanded indications within the larynx. It will also facilitate realizing the potential of this laser in the outpatient office setting.

Review Questions

1. What are the common components of all lasers?

2. What safety precautions are specific to microlaryngeal laser surgery?

3. Why does the Nd:YAG laser have a limited role in the management of benign, nonobstructing epithelial laryngeal disease?

4. What is the primary limitation to the use of the CO_2 laser for office laryngeal procedures?

5. What parameters of the CO_2 laser translate into improved wound healing in experimental models?

REFERENCES

1. Maiman TH. Stimulated optical radiation in ruby. *Nature.* 1960;187:493.
2. Jako GZ. Laser surgery of the vocal cord: an experimental study with carbon dioxide lasers on dogs. *Laryngoscope.* 1972;82:2204–2216.
3. Strong MS, Jako GJ. Laser surgery in the larynx: early clinical experience with continuous CO_2 laser. *Ann Otol Laryngol Rhinol.* 1972;81:791–798.
4. Benninger, MS. Microdissection or microspot CO_2 laser for limited vocal fold benign lesions: a prospective randomized trial. *Laryngoscope.* 2000; 110(2 pt 2 suppl 92):1–17. Erratum in: *Laryngoscope.* 2000 Apr;110(4):696.

5. Polanyi TG. Laser physics. *Otolaryngol Clin North Am.* 1983;16:752-774.

6. Ossoff RH Garrett CG, Reinisch L. Laser surgery: basic principles and safety considerations. In: Cummings CW, Flint PW, Harker LA, et al, eds. *Otolaryngology-Head and Neck Surgery.* 4th ed. Philadelphia, Pa: Elsevier; 2005.

7. Courey MS, Ossoff RH. Laser applications in adult laryngeal surgery. *Otolaryngol Clin North Am.* 1996;29(6):1005-1010.

8. Durkin GE Duncavage JA, Toohill RJ, Tieu TM, Caya JG. Wound healing of the true vocal cord squamous epithelium after CO_2 laser ablation and cup forceps stripping. *Otolaryngol Head Neck Surg.*1986 95(3):273-277

9. Buell BR, Schueller DE. Comparison of tensile strength in CO_2 laser and scalpel skin incisions. *Arch Otolaryngol.* 1983;109(7):465-467.

10. Remacle M, Lawson G, Watelat J. Carbon dioxide laser microsurgery of benign vocal fold lesions: indications, techniques, and results in 251 patients. *Ann Otol Rhinol Laryngol.* 1999;108(2): 156-164.

11. Fortune DS, Huang S, Sotyo J, Pennington B, Ossoff RH, Reininsh L. Effect of pulse duration on wound healing using a CO_2 laser. *Laryngoscope.* 1998;108(6):843-848.

12. Garrett CG, Reinisch L. New-generation pulsed carbon dioxide laser: comparative effects on vocal fold wound healing. *Ann Otol Rhinol Laryngol.* 2002;111(6):471-476.

13. Shapshay SM, Wallace RA, Kveton JF Hybels RL, Bohigisn RK, Setzer SE. New microspot micromanipulator for carbon dioxide laser surgery in otolaryngology. Early clinical results. *Arch Otolaryngol Head Neck Surg.* 1988;114(9):1012-1015.

14. Ossoff RH, Sisson GA, Duncavage JA, Moselle HI, Andrews PE, McMillan WG. Endoscopic laser arytenoidectomy for the treatment of bilateral vocal cord paralysis. *Laryngoscope.* 1984;94(10): 1293-1297.

15. Crumley RL. Endoscopic laser medical arytenoidectomy for airway management in bilateral laryngeal paralysis. *Ann Otol Rhinol Laryngol.* 1993;102(2):81-84.

16. Dennis DP, Kashima H. Carbon dioxide laser posterior cordectomy for treatment of bilateral vocal cord paralysis. *Ann Otol Rhinol Laryngol.* 1989; 98(12 pt 1):930-934.

17. Laccourreye O, Escovar MI, Gerhardt J, Hans S, Biacabe B, Brasnu D. CO_2 laser endoscopic posterior partial transverse cordotomy for bilateral

18. Khalifa MC. Simultaneous bilateral posterior cordectomy in bilateral vocal fold paralysis. *Otolaryngol Head Neck Surg.* 2005;132(2):249-250.

19. Postma GN, Courey MS, Ossoff RH. Microvascular lesions of the true vocal fold. *Ann Otol Rhinol Laryngol.* 1998;107(6):472-476.

20. Hsuing MW, Kang BH, Su WF, Wang HW. Clearing microvascular lesions of the true vocal fold with the KTP/532 laser. *Ann Otol Rhinol Laryngol.* 2003;112(6):534-539.

21. Cholewa D, Waldschmidt J. Laser treatment of hemangiomas of the larynx and trachea. *Lasers Surg Med.* 1998;23(4):221-232.

22. Madgy D, Ahsan SF, Kest D, Stein I. The application of the potassium-titanyl-phosphate (KTP) laser in the management of subglottic hemangioma. *Arch Otolaryngol Head Neck Surg.* 2001;127(1): 47-50.

23. Sie KC, McGill T, Healy GB. Subglottic hemangioma: ten years' experience with the carbon dioxide laser. *Ann Otol Rhinol Laryngol.* 1994;103(3): 167-172.

24. Clyne SB, Halum SL, Koufman JA, Postma GN. Pulsed dye laser treatment of laryngeal granulomas. *Ann Otol Rhinol Laryngol.* 2005;114(3) 198-201.

25. Anderson RR, Parrish JA. Microvasculature can be selectively damaged using dye lasers: a basic theory and experimental evidence in human skin. *Lasers Surg Med.* 1981;1(3):263-276.

26. Zeitels SM, Franco RA Jr, Dailey SH, Burns JA, Hillman RE, Anderson RR. Office-based treatment of glottal dysplasia and papillomatosis with the 585-nm pulsed dye laser and local anesthesia. *Ann Otol Rhinol Laryngol.* 2004;113(4):265-276.

27. Vaughan CW. Transoral laryngeal surgery using the CO_2 laser: laboratory experiments and clinical experience. *Laryngoscope.* 1978;88(9 pt 1): 1399-1420.

28. Motta G, Esposito E, Testa D, Iovine R, Motta S. CO_2 laser treatment of supraglottic cancer. *Head Neck.* 2004;26(5):442-446.

29. Peretti G, Piazza C, Bolzoni A, et al. Analysis of recurrences in 322 Tis, T1, or T2 glottic carcinomas treated by carbon dioxide laser. *Ann Otol Rhinol Laryngol.* 2004;113(11):853-858.

30. Steiner W, Vogt P, Ambrosch P, Kron M. Transoral carbon dioxide laser microsurgery for recurrent glottic carcinoma after radiotherapy. *Head Neck.* 2004;26(6):477-484.

31. Vilaseca-Gonzalez I, Bernal-Sprekelsen M, Blanch-Alejandro JL, Moragas-Luis M. Complications in transoral CO_2 laser surgery for carcinoma of the larynx and hypopharynx. *Head Neck.* 2003;25(5): 382–388.

32. Cossman PH, Romano V, Sporri S, et al. Plastic hollow waveguide: properties and possibilities as a flexible radiation delivery system for CO_2 laser radiation. *Lasers Surg Med.1995;* 16(1):66–74.

33. Gibson DJ, Harrington JA. Gradually tapered hollow glass waveguides for the transmission of CO_2 laser radiation. *Appl Opt.* 2004;43 (11) 2231–2235.

PART V

Disorders of the Larynx

A. Neurologic Disorders

16

Voice and Speech Abnormalities in Systemic Neurodegenerative Disorders

Ted Mau, MD, PhD
Mark S. Courey, MD

KEY POINTS

■ Lesions in different parts of the nervous system produce characteristic signs. The key to neurologic diagnosis is to infer the location of the lesion or the neurosystem involved from specific findings on the physical examination.

■ The possibility of a treatable, unrelated voice disorder in a dysarthric neurodegenerative patient should not be overlooked.

■ The addition of speech tasks to a standard head and neck examination can aid in pinpointing deficits in specific muscle groups involved in articulation.

■ Patients with a breathy voice as the result of a neurodegenerative process may benefit from vocal fold augmentation if they demonstrate a glottal gap on laryngoscopic examination and have breathy dysphonia as a major contributing factor to their decreased intelligibility.

■ A significant number of patients with undiagnosed systemic neurologic disorders are seen initially by otolaryngologists for voice and speech complaints. A familiarity with neurodegenerative disorders and heightened clinical suspicion may avoid a delay in diagnosis.

Voice and speech difficulties are common in patients with neurodegenerative syndromes. More than 70% of patients with Parkinson's disease experience problems with voice and speech, and 30% of them describe these abnormalities as the most debilitating aspect of their disease.[1] Given the prevalence of these problems in this patient population, it is all the more puzzling that these disorders traditionally have received little attention in the otolaryngology literature. There are several reasons for this neglect. First, the neurodegenerative processes that underlie the voice and speech difficulties are progressive and typically not amenable to current surgical or medical intervention. Second, the patients and the medical professionals who care for them are largely unaware of the possible role of the otolaryngologists in carrying out interventions that can potentially improve, albeit temporarily, the quality of life of the patients. This chapter aims to discuss the classification of the neurodegenerative syndromes, review pertinent physical findings, and summarize the available interventions. The discussion is limited to voice and speech abnormalities as part of generalized neurologic disorders. Localized laryngeal disorders with a neurologic origin, such as spasmodic dysphonia, are mentioned for comparison here and are further detailed in the following chapters (see chapter 18, The Larynx in Parkinson's Disease; chapter 19, Essential Tremor; and chapter 20, Spasmodic Dysphonia).

VOICE AND SPEECH

We begin with a clarification of the distinction between voice and speech. Voice is the sound produced by the vibration of the vocal folds. A voice disorder has its origin in the sound-generating structures, the true vocal folds. Physical lesions of the vocal folds can produce an abnormal voice. Central or peripheral neurologic lesions that affect the innervation of laryngeal muscles can also produce a voice disorder. For example, spasmodic dysphonia, a focal dystonia of the larynx with a presumed origin in the basal ganglia, is a disorder of the voice.

Speech, on the other hand, requires four components for production: a pulmonary power supply, a vibratory source for phonation, a resonance chamber for amplification, and an articulatory system. In the source-filter model of speech production, the larynx is the source of sound production. Airflow from the pulmonary system moves past the vocal folds causing the tissue to vibrate. Vibration of the vocal folds creates local disturbances in air pressure equilibrium. These changes in air pressure equilibrium are interpreted as sound by the receiving auditory system. Sounds produced by vocal fold vibration are termed "voiced." An example of the difference between a voiced and unvoiced sound can be heard when comparing an "s" (voiceless) to a "z" (voiced). This is also true for the voiceless "f" sound and the voiced "v" sound. Vocal fold vibration creates a complex sound with a characteristic fundamental frequency of vibration related to the actual vibratory rate of vocal folds and a harmonic spectrum. As this sound is propagated through the tube created by the pharynx and oral cavity, some frequencies of the harmonic spectrum are amplified and others suppressed. The modulation of the phonated sound by the vocal tract is known as resonance and is determined by the length, shape, and openings of the vocal tract. The sound generated by the vocal folds and resonating cavity is then shaped into words by movement of the lips, tongue, palate, and pharynx through the process of articulation. It is this final product that is perceived as speech.

Motor speech disorders include both apraxia and dysarthria. *Apraxia* is the inability to execute (coordinate) a skilled motor act. Apraxia of speech is a deficit in the ability to smoothly sequence the speech-producing movements of the tongue, lips, palate, and pharynx. Apraxia of speech affects articulation, the shaping of the sounds of speech, and prosody, the patterns of stress and intonation in a language. Speech apraxia is largely due to cortical lesions. On the other hand, apraxia of voice refers to the inability to properly time the onset of voicing with vocal fold adduction. The intensity or volume of speech is often poorly coordinated with prosody, making the vocal product inappropriately loud and/or soft.

Dysarthria is the impaired production of speech due to disturbed motor control of the speech mechanism. This can originate from disturbances in the central or peripheral nervous system and manifests as a deficit in articulation. The voice in terms of intensity and pitch is usually well preserved. In generalized neurologic disorders, dysarthria can be secondary to lesions in both central and peripheral structures. Central lesions or lesions of the upper motor neuron produce slowing in speech with relatively preserved articulation, whereas lesions in the peripheral nervous system (lower motor neurons) or in the end organ muscle produce imprecise articulation with relatively well preserved rate of speech.

NEUROANATOMY OF SPEECH PRODUCTION

To understand how neurodegenerative processes produce voice and speech abnormalities, it is necessary to review the neuroanatomic pathways that lead to speech production[2] (Figure 16–1). The motor control of speech originates from the cerebral cortex and descends through the internal capsule in the corticobulbar tract. The motor outputs are modulated by the basal ganglia and the cerebellum. The basal ganglia modulates the rate of motor contractions, whereas the cerebellum is thought to coordinate the actions of the multiple muscle groups to produce speech. The "fine-tuned" motor signals arrive in the brain stem via the corticobulbar tracts, which synapse onto the motor nuclei of the respective cranial nerves. Fibers of the corticobulbar tracts are upper motor neurons (UMN), whereas the motor component of the cranial nerves is the lower motor neurons (LMN). Lesions that affect the upper motor neurons cause different physical signs than those that affect the lower motor neurons and this distinction should be noted on the physical examination. Finally, the motor signals

arrive at the neuromuscular junction. This is the site of action of botulinum toxin, a mainstay in the symptomatic treatment of the neurodegenerative patient. The anatomy and physiology of phonation, airway regulation, and swallowing are reviewed in chapters 3 through 5.

Anatomically, it is useful to think of specific locations of disease involvement: UMN, LMN, basal ganglia, cerebellum, and the neuromuscular junction. Because many neurodegenerative syndromes involve multiple structures, it is also useful to think in terms of functional groups. Although a comprehensive classification of neurologic voice disorders has been proposed,[2] for the purpose of the current discussion, three groups of diseases will be considered. The first include the extrapyramidal and cerebellar disorders, which classically are thought to be due to lesions in the basal ganglia and/or the cerebellum. The second are the motor neuron diseases with lesions in the UMN and/or the LMN. The third are diseases of the neuromuscular junction. The key to neurologic diagnosis is to infer the location of the lesion or the neurologic system involved based on characteristic signs on physical examination (Table 16–1). Before introducing specific disease entities, terms used to describe examination findings are reviewed first.

DEFINITION OF TERMS

Spasticity and flaccidity are descriptors of muscle tone. *Spasticity*, or chronically increased muscle tone, originates from lesions in the central nervous system and is specifically associated with lesions of UMN in the descending corticospinal tracts of axial nerves and/or descending corticobulbar tracts of the cranial nerves. As otolaryngologists, we are most often called to deal with symptoms affecting the bulbar musculature innervated by the cranial nerves. Examples include a strained voice as a result of a corticobulbar lesion in patients with primary lateral sclerosis and spasticity of the facial muscles contributing to labored speech in pseudobulbar palsy.

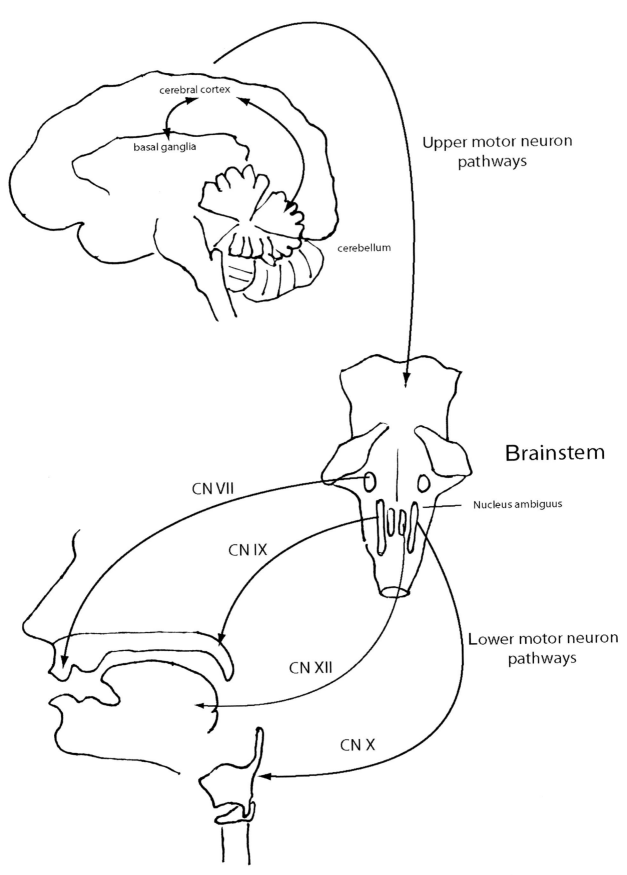

FIGURE 16–1. Neuroanatomic pathways that lead to speech production.

TABLE 16–1. Neuroanatomic Systems Involved in Voice and Speech Production

Neurologic System Involved	Examination Findings
Extrapyramidal system	Tremor
	Spasmodic contractions (eg, pitch instability)
	Excessive tension (eg, vocal strain)
	Irregular rhythm of repetition
	Hyperkinesia/hypokinesia
	Rigidity
Upper motor neuron (UMN)	Spasticity (eg, vocal strain)
	Slow but regular rhythm of repetition
	Hyperreflexia
	Myoclonus
Lower motor neuron (LMN)	Flaccidity
	Weakness
	Atrophy
	Fasciculations
	Hyporeflexia
Neuromuscular junction	Fatigue with repetitive use

Flaccidity, or chronically decreased muscle tone, is associated with lesions of the LMN. Flaccidity manifests as weakness, atrophy, and/or fasciculations. Examples include a weak voice and atrophy of the vocal folds secondary to a high vagal lesion or flaccidity of the tongue with fasciculations, known as "bag of worms," seen in patients with amyotrophic lateral sclerosis (ALS).

Tremor, dystonia, and myoclonus are terms used to describe movement disorders. *Tremors* are rhythmic oscillatory movements that occur at rest or with action. Tremors result from alternating contractions of opposing muscle groups. Pathologic resting tremor is usually in the range of 3 to 6 Hz and is exemplified by the tremor seen in Parkinson's disease. It is associated with basal ganglia lesions. *Intention tremor* occurs with action and is associated with cerebellar lesions. Intention tremor occurs at a rate between 2 and 5 Hz. The oscillations are coarse and increase in amplitude as the movement target is approached. In its most severe form, intention or kinetic tremors are present at rest and then increase in severity as the body part is activated. Multiple sclerosis is the most common cause of this cerebellar postural tremor. Other causes of this tremor include tumors and strokes, as well as neural degeneration in the cerebellum. *Essential tremor* is typically a postural tremor that occurs with sustained posture or during movement but in severe forms may also occur at rest. Essential tremor exhibits a frequency between 8 to 12 Hz and is thought to result from overactivity of the cerebellum. It most commonly affects the hands but can also affect the legs, head, tongue, or the larynx. Essential tremor of the voice is further discussed later in this chapter as well as in chapter 19.

Dystonia is broadly defined as a deviation of posture caused by involuntary sustained or spasmodic muscular contractions. It is attributed to dysfunction of the extrapyramidal system. Dystonia that occurs only during voluntary movement or is worsened by movement is called *action* dystonia. Action dystonia that occurs only with specific actions (eg, writer's cramp) is a task-specific dystonia. As a dystonic condition progresses, dystonia may occur even at rest, causing *rest* dystonia. Dystonias are also classified by the body regions affected. *Focal* dystonias affect one area of the body, *segmental* dystonias affect two or more adjacent areas, *multifocal* dystonias affect two or more nonadjacent areas, and *generalized* dystonias involve several areas on both sides of the body. Blepharospasm and oromandibular dystonia are examples of focal dystonias. The presence of both constitutes oral facial dystonia, also known as Meige's syndrome. Spasmodic dysphonia is generally thought of as a focal dystonia of the larynx. Patients with adductor spasmodic dysphonia exhibit abrupt initiation and termination of vocal production during speech caused by irregular hyperadduction of the vocal folds, whereas patients with abductor spasmodic dysphonia have aphonic, segmented speech due to irregular abduction of the vocal folds.

Myoclonus describes periodic, jerky contractions of 1 to 2 Hz that are typically multifocal. It can be associated with UMN lesions. Myoclonus is distinguished from tremor in that the former is monophasic while the latter is biphasic, involving opposing muscle groups. Myoclonus is not suppressible with conscious effort.

Tics are intermittent, nonrhythmic, patterned movements associated with an irresistible urge to perform them. Motor tics manifest as visible movements or twitches. Phonic or vocal tics can manifest as unwanted vocalizations such as throat clearing, coughing, barking, or yelling. Complex vocal tics may involve repeated words or phrases, including profanities. Unlike myoclonus, tics are suppressible with effort, and a postsuppression train of tics is characteristic. *Tourette's syndrome* is a chronic tic disorder characterized by both motor and vocal tics with onset in childhood. The disorder begins with simple tics and progresses to more complex tics. The tics have a migrating pattern, with one tic replaced by another. This distinguishes tics from dystonic movements, which do not migrate.

PHYSICAL EXAMINATION

The physical examination plays a pivotal role in the evaluation of patients with neurodegenerative disorders. Although a typical otolaryngologic office visit may not allow the type of comprehensive assessment possible during a neurology or speech pathology consultation, the diagnostic yield of a routine head and neck examination can be increased by careful, targeted observation. Even before starting a standard head and neck examination, the examiner gains valuable clues about the disease state from observing the overall appearance of the patient. Abnormal posture should be noted. Spontaneous limb or truncal movements such as tremor suggest the possibility of synchronous movements in the pharyngeal or laryngeal musculature.

The patient's speech and voice offer more insights. The rate, prosody, articulation, and resonance should be noted. Slow but fluent speech can result from a problem with rate control (eg,

basal ganglia or UMN lesion), with muscular coordination (eg, cerebellar lesion), and/or with muscular contraction (eg, UMN lesion). A flat, expressionless voice suggests the lack of fine motor control of the intrinsic laryngeal musculature needed to produce normal inflections in pitch and tone. Difficulty with articulation can result from weakness and/or incoordination. A test word such as "butterfly" can elicit deficiency in facial muscle (/b/), the tongue (/t/, /l/), or the lip (/f/). Rapid repetition of the syllables "pa-ta-ga" tests lip closure, tongue tip motion, and tongue base motion, respectively. A hypernasal quality suggests palatal weakness, and tremor in the voice cues the examiner to pay special attention to tremors of the pharyngeal and laryngeal musculature during the head and neck examination. Voice evaluation with perceptual techniques usually reveals strained sounds in UMN disease and breathy/asthenic patterns in LMN disorders. The voice is variable in extrapyramidal disorders, but typically becomes breathy and asthenic in the later stages of the disease.

The face is examined next. Involuntary facial twitches or blepharospasm should be noted. A limited range of facial expression may point to an extrapyramidal defect. Spasticity of facial movements suggests a disorder of UMNs whereas flaccidity of the facial muscles suggests an LMN disorder. The presence of either should alert the examiner to look for the same in other muscle groups controlled by the cranial nerves important in speech and swallow.

Examination of the oral cavity and oral pharynx should note symmetry and strength of tongue movement, symmetry and strength of palatal elevation, symmetry and strength of lateral pharyngeal wall motion, and any abnormal movements such as myoclonus or fasciculations. Isolated palatal myoclonus is a specific disorder associated with lesion in the Guillain-Molaret triangle in the brainstem. Tongue fasciculations imply weakness secondary to lesion in the LMN. Tongue strength can be assessed by asking the patient to push the tongue into the cheek while the examiner applies opposing digital pressure externally, by asking the patient to push the tongue out against a tongue depressor, or it can be formally measured by a pressure transducer connected to a bulb placed in the oral cavity.[3] Palatal strength should be assessed by asking the patient to say "ah" repetitively while upward and lateral motion are observed.

The evaluation continues with endoscopic examination of the nasopharynx, the posterior oropharynx, hypopharynx, and larynx. Palatal closure is assessed best with a flexible endoscope by placing the tip of the scope in the nasopharynx. Completeness of palatal closure can be visualized during production of non-voiced consonants such as sustained /ss/ or the word "popeye." A flexible scope can then be advanced into the oropharynx, or alternatively a rigid endoscope or a mirror can be used through the oral cavity. The examiner should first look for the presence of secretions or food residue in the vallecula. Retained secretions in the vallecula implies weakness of tongue base, whereas retained secretions or food in the piriform sinus suggests weakness of lateral pharyngeal wall contraction, poor laryngeal elevation, and/or the failure of the cricopharyngeal sphincter to relax completely during swallow. Tongue base strength can be assessed with words such as "ball" or "mall." In patients with normal strength of tongue base musculature, the tongue base will nearly contact the posterior pharyngeal wall during each of these tasks. Lateral pharyngeal wall strength and symmetry of motion are best evaluated during sustained high pitched /i/ or glides up in pitch. The lateral pharyngeal walls should contract symmetrically as the posterior pillars contract toward the midline. Unilateral weakness suggests LMN lesion because most pharyngeal muscles receive bilateral UMN innervation.

Finally, examination of the vocal folds and arytenoids during phonation should yield an assessment of strength and symmetry of movement. The vocal folds should abduct and adduct fairly symmetrically and briskly. Significant unilateral asymmetry usually suggests an LMN lesion such as paralysis or paresis. Bilateral slowing or motion and/or sphincteric closure patterns can be suggestive of UMN. If there are any voice complaints, then stroboscopy is required to assess the adequacy of laryngeal tissue vibratory patterns and completeness of laryngeal closure during vibration. Often atrophic vocal folds as seen

in extrapyramidal disorders, late stage UMN disease, or early LMN disease can result in asymmetric vibratory patterns and failure of complete closure of the glottis during phonation. This is often visualized during stroboscopy as a spindle-shaped glottic gap anterior to the vocal process.

EVALUATION OF SWALLOWING

Patients who present with dysphagia should undergo fluoroscopic and/or endoscopic swallowing evaluation. The modified barium swallow (MBS), or videofluorographic swallow study, is usually carried out jointly by a speech-language pathologist (SLP) and a radiologist. The patient ingests barium-coated boluses or liquid barium of varying consistencies while the oral, oropharyngeal, and hypopharyngeal phases of swallowing are observed fluoroscopically with the patient in a sitting or standing position. Abnormal tongue movement, barium pooling in the vallecula or piriform sinus, and aspiration can be easily observed. Bolus transit through the pharyngeal phases of swallow is also assessed. Opening of the cricopharyngeus muscle is best observed with barium swallow. Failure of opening is often seen as an indentation in the posterior aspect of the esophagus and cannot be well visualized by either methods of swallow evaluation. MBS provides objective evidence of swallow function and helps to identify specific functional deficits. Based on the study, recommendations for maneuvers to minimize aspiration and on food consistencies can be made.

Although the MBS provides a global view of the oral and pharyngeal structures during the swallow, endoscopic evaluation shows selected details of the swallowing process and allows simultaneous assessment of laryngeal competence. Fiberoptic endoscopic evaluation of swallowing (FEES) is performed either by an SLP or an otolaryngologist with a fiberoptic laryngoscope. Patients ingest food boluses with varying consistencies treated with food dye as the pharynx is observed before and after the pharyngeal swallow. FEES directly observes premature spillage of food into the pharynx or larynx during the oral phase, assesses airway closure during the swallow, and localizes food residue. If aspiration is present, flexible endoscopic evaluation of swallowing with sensory testing (FEESST) should be performed. FEESST delivers controlled air pulses to determine the sensory threshold in various parts of the laryngopharynx. This method of airway protection assessment is gaining popularity and has been applied to patients with neurodegenerative syndromes.[4] The technical aspects of these examinations are presented in Chapter 11, Office-Based Instrumental Examinations in Laryngology.

Whether MBS, FEES/FEESST, or both should be performed for a particular patient depends on several factors.[5] In general, FEES is preferred over MBS when access to fluoroscopy is limited, when the patient requires a bedside examination, or when the test is also used to determine therapeutic options. Most patients will tolerate the flexible endoscope for an extended period of time as different food consistencies and therapeutic maneuvers are attempted. Radiation exposure during MBS limits its usefulness for repeated swallows with different maneuvers. FEES/FEESST is also favored when there is laryngeal involvement of the disease. In addition, sensory testing is only possible with FEESST. On the other hand, MBS is indicated when the oral phase, the oral-pharyngeal transition, hyoid and laryngeal elevation, or cricopharyngeal relaxation needs to be examined. These are some of the areas not observed during FEES/FEESST. MBS is also preferred as a screening examination when the patient complaint is vague and global assessment is needed. Either the fluoroscopic or the endoscopic examination should suffice for most patients.

CATEGORIES OF NEUROGENIC DISEASES

Extrapyramidal and Cerebellar Disorders

Extrapyramidal disorders include Parkinson's disease and Parkinson-related disorders. Parkinsonism is a syndrome consisting of resting tremor,

rigidity, bradykinesia, and gait disturbance. Parkinson's disease (PD) is idiopathic parkinsonism without more widespread neurologic involvement. PD results from lesion in the substantia nigra of the basal ganglia. PD patients have characteristic hypokinetic dysarthria and vocal tremor. Speech is poorly articulated and patients may be described as mumbling. There is a typical festination pattern with delayed onset then an increased rate. The voice is usually hypophonic, but some patients have a strained voice with aphonic breaks, reflecting the rigidity component of the disease. On laryngoscopic examination, PD patients have good vocal fold mobility and usually demonstrate normal vocal process excursion.[6] However, the vocal folds have a typical atrophic appearance. The vocal process is unusually prominent. During stroboscopic assessment, the mucosal membranes do not vibrate to closure as the prephonatory gap is too wide, due to muscle atrophy that precludes the vocal folds from being placed in an adequate prephonatory position. In addition to the phonatory glottal gap, bradykinesia of the intrinsic laryngeal musculature may also contribute to Parkinson dysphonia. Delayed adduction of the "rigid" vocal folds relative to expiration allows premature air leakage, resulting in lower subglottic pressure when the vocal folds are finally brought to the phonatory position. This further aggravates the hypophonia and decreases phonation time. In terms of swallowing, patients with PD usually do not have prominent dysphagia, reflecting the brainstem mediation of most of the swallowing process. A complete review of Parkinson's disease and its effect on the larynx is presented in chapter 18.

When patients with parkinsonism do not respond to standard dopaminergic treatment and have additional signs and symptoms, other Parkinson-related disorders need to be considered. One such syndrome is *multiple system atrophy* (MSA).[7] The dominant features of MSA are parkinsonism, ataxia, and autonomic failure. MSA encompasses three previously described central nervous system degenerative syndromes that differ in the predominant neurosystem involved but have overlapping clinical manifestations.

Direct Electrical Stimulation of Denervated Laryngeal Muscles: Is It Possible?

In the future, some patients with laryngeal symptoms due to systemic neurodegenerative disorders, such as multisystem atrophy and motor neuron diseases, may benefit from a laryngeal pacemaker designed to bypass degenerated nerves and stimulate the target muscles directly. In the past, laryngeal pacing with direct electrical stimulation has been explored as a means to restore oral ventilation in patients with bilateral vocal fold paralysis who are tracheotomy-dependent. The premise of laryngeal pacing lies in the ability of the posterior cricoarytenoid (PCA) muscle to be stimulated by an external electrical signal delivered by an implanted electrode. In 1996 the first report of electrical pacing of a unilaterally paralyzed human vocal fold showed it was possible to produce stimulated abduction of the paralyzed fold of a magnitude comparable to the normal side using impulses synchronized with inspiratory effort generated by a plethysmographic transducer.[30] Subsequent studies in patients with bilateral vocal fold paralysis showed it was possible to produce sufficient increase in airflow with unilateral laryngeal electrical stimulation to achieve decannulation.[31,32] The later studies were carried out with a device that delivered programmed impulses rather than impulses synchronized with inspiration. Certain technical issues limited the clinical outcome. For example, size and spacing of the electrode channels on existing electrode devices were suboptimal for PCA stimulation, and the implanted electrode was susceptible to corrosion. Nevertheless, this innovative technology holds great promise not only for patients with paralyzed vocal folds but also for those with impaired neurologic function of the larynx.

One group of patients who may benefit from laryngeal pacing are patients with multiple system atrophy (MSA) with nocturnal stridor. These patients have inappropriate inspiratory vocal fold adduction and abductor paresis during sleep. This problem seems ideally suited for laryngeal pacing. An electrode array implanted in the PCA can be connected to an impulse generator synchronized to a chest wall sensor[30] or diaphragmatic contraction. With an external switch, the device can be turned on at night when the patients go to sleep and be turned off when the patients wake up in the morning. The additional stimulus for abduction from the pacer during inspiration can potentially reverse the unfavorable adduction-abduction balance and eliminate stridor. A more advanced design could incorporate simultaneous blocking of adductor muscles. One challenge is to implant the stimulating electrode in the PCA without jeopardizing native recurrent laryngeal nerve function.

A second group of patients who may benefit from this technology are patients with motor neuron disease (MND) who are at increased risk of aspiration due to degeneration of motor neurons that control the pharyngeal and laryngeal musculature. It may be possible to produce stimulated laryngeal closure, namely, true vocal fold abduction and false vocal fold approximation, that is triggered by swallowing. This may reduce the likelihood of aspiration. Another possibility is to synchronize glottic closure with cough. This would enable patients to generate larger subglottic pressures and produce stronger coughs to clear airway secretions or aspirated material.

Technical hurdles obviously exist, but advances in microarray technology, electronics design, and surgical implantation should make these therapeutic concepts into reality one day and produce laryngeal pacers that can benefit selected patients with generalized neurodegenerative disorders.

Patients with *striatonigral degeneration* have predominantly parkinsonism features. Patients with *olivopontocerebellar atrophy* have prominent cerebellar dysfunction. *Shy-Drager syndrome* is characterized by autonomic instability, urinary and rectal incontinence, and orthostatic hypotension. Patients with MSA may have a mixed dysarthria with variable hypokinetic, ataxic, and spastic components depending on the predominant neurosystem affected.[8] Sixteen percent of patients with MSA, particularly those with Shy-Drager, have inspiratory stridor during sleep,[9] and rarely this can be the initial manifestation of MSA.[10] The etiology of inspiratory stridor is thought to be a combination of bilateral abductor paresis and inappropriate inspiratory adduction.[11-12] Patients with Parkinsonism who are evaluated for hypophonia should be carefully questioned for the presence of stridor during sleep. If the history is positive and abductor paresis or paradoxic vocal fold movement is seen on laryngoscopy, the diagnosis of MSA should be entertained, and a polysomnograph should be obtained.[13] Such patients often demonstrate obstructive sleep apnea, presumably due to obstruction at the glottic level. Although continuous positive airway pressure (CPAP) does not usually provide relief of fixed glottal obstruction

or bilateral vocal fold paralysis due to LMN injury, some MSA patients have benefitted from CPAP for treatment of nocturnal stridor.[14] One sleep physiology study showed the application of CPAP reduced the inspiratory activity of the TA muscle.[11] The authors speculate that the inspiratory TA activation in MSA patients is an inappropriate response to negative airway pressure during sleep and that CPAP suppresses TA activation by reducing the negative airway pressure. They caution that further studies are necessary before CPAP is routinely applied to patients with MSA.

Progressive supranuclear palsy (PSP) is another Parkinson-related syndrome. In addition to bradykinesia and rigidity, patients with PSP have characteristic vertical gaze paresis, frequent falls, and blepharospasm. There may be facial weakness, dysarthria, and dysphagia. The diagnosis is usually suspected due to gait instability.

Essential tremor is a disorder characterized by tremor that occurs with sustained action and is suppressed by alcohol intake. It is thought to result from overactivity of the cerebellum. Although it is not considered a neurodegenerative disorder, it is included here for comparison. A type of essential tremor familiar to otolaryngologists is essential tremor of the voice, which involves the periodic contraction of antagonistic adductor-abductor and/or superior-inferior laryngeal muscles in an alternating or synchronous fashion resulting in a periodic tremulous voice.[15] The thyrohyoid muscle is most commonly involved, followed by the thyroarytenoid, sternothyroid, and cricothyroid.[16] Most patients with essential tremor of the voice also have tremors elsewhere in the body, most notably the upper extremity.[17] Essential tremor is detailed further in chapter 19.

Motor Neuron Diseases

Motor neuron diseases result in progressive weakness of voluntary muscles throughout the body due to degeneration and eventual loss of the cell bodies of UMNs and/or LMNs. The weakness usually starts in one muscle group then progressively involves others. Motor neuron diseases are classified according to the type of motor neurons involved. Disease in which the UMNs alone are affected is termed primary lateral sclerosis (PLS). The motor neuron deficit can primarily be limited to the LMNs, for example in progressive bulbar palsy (PBP). Finally, when both UMNs and LMNs are affected, the disease is called amyotrophic lateral sclerosis (ALS), or *Lou Gehrig's disease*.

Primary lateral sclerosis (PLS) involves predominantly the UMNs. It results from the selective loss of large pyramidal cells in the precentral gyrus and degeneration of corticobulbar projections. PLS typically presents with gradual onset lower extremity stiffness and pain due to spasticity, which may lead to imbalance. As the disease progresses, upper extremities and bulbar muscles become involved. Spasticity of the lip, tongue, pharyngeal, and laryngeal musculature results in slow, labored articulation and dysphagia. The voice is typically harsh and strained and may sound like patients with spasmodic dysphonia. Botox injection may provide some benefit. The rate of progression is usually slow, and the disease does not significantly shorten life expectancy. In most cases, the disease does progress to involve the LMNs and develop into ALS, in which flaccid weakness becomes the predominant symptom.

Patients with *pseudobulbar palsy* have prominent UMN symptoms in the bulbar muscles. Unlike PLS, pseudobulbar palsy is not a distinct disease entity. It results from bilateral corticobulbar tract lesions that can be produced by stroke, encephalitis, multiple sclerosis, or neoplasm. Spasticity of the muscles of mastication, facial expression, and speech result in characteristic difficulty with chewing, expressionless facies, hyperactive gag reflex, and inability to protrude the tongue. Patients may also demonstrate emotional lability.

Progressive bulbar palsy (PBP) involves the motor nuclei of the LMNs, predominantly the lower cranial nerves IX, X, and XII. Weakness of the pharyngeal musculature leads to nasal regurgitation, slurred, hypernasal speech, poor cough and gag reflex, and aspiration. The tongue is usually affected first and may be atrophic and show fasciculations. Facial muscles, starting with the orbicularis oris, may be affected as well. Patients with adult-onset symptoms have a variable disease course and eventually progress to ALS. PBP of childhood, or Fazio-Londe disease, is a rare entity that shows rapid progression leading to death within 1 to 3 years of diagnosis from respiratory compromise.

Amyotrophic lateral sclerosis (ALS) affects both UMN and LMN. Although patients with ALS commonly present with movement complaints involving their extremities, as many as 25% have initial speech and swallowing symptoms,[18] and a significant number of these patients are initially seen by an otolaryngologist before the neurologic diagnosis is made.[19] In ALS, idiopathic progressive degeneration of both UMN and LMN results in spasticity, weakness, atrophy, and fasciculations. Palatal weakness results in hypernasal speech and nasopharyngeal regurgitation, and tongue weakness produces dysarthria. A characteristic finding on physical examination is the "bag of worms" appearance of the tongue fasciculations. About half the patients demonstrate a glottal gap on videostroboscopic examination.[20] As the disease progresses, patients with ALS often need tracheotomy for pulmonary toilet and eventually depend on mechanical ventilation.

Swallowing difficulties in patients with motor neuron diseases manifest differently according to the site of lesion. Patients with UMN involvement may have difficulty initiating the swallow in the oral phase, a voluntary action that requires input from the corticobulbar tract. The pharyngeal and esophageal phases of swallow, which entail involuntary actions mediated by the brainstem, are relatively unaffected in early stages of the disease. The dysphagia is a consequence of predominantly incoordination rather than weakness. Therefore, in patients with PLS, swallowing is usually well preserved. On the other hand, patients with LMN disease tend to have more severe dysphagia because all phases of the swallow are affected. Swallowing difficulty can often be one of the symptoms first noted in patients with PBP or ALS and PLS presenting with initial bulbar symptoms. Some ALS patients are candidates for laryngotracheal separation, thus completely preventing aspiration at the cost of any phonation. These patients typically do not have intelligible speech due to derangement of tongue function. The procedure does not allow for efficient swallowing, but it does remove the risk of aspiration of secretions (Figure 16–2).

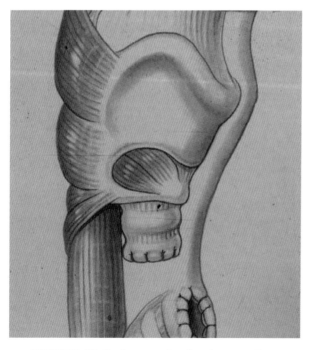

FIGURE 16–2. Laryngotracheal separation.

Diseases of the Neuromuscular Junction

The best example of a disease in this category is *myasthenia gravis.* Although it is not generally considered a neurodegenerative disorder, myasthenia gravis is included here as an example of a systemic neurologic disorder where undiagnosed patients may present with vocal complaints to an otolaryngologist. The pathophysiology underlying myasthenia gravis is the production of autoantibodies to the acetylcholine receptor, which results in easy fatigue with repetitive use. The hallmark of myasthenia gravis is the fluctuating nature of the weakness. Ocular muscles and eyelids are affected first in 40% of patients, resulting in ptosis and diplopia. Facial and oropharyngeal muscles are next commonly involved. Patients may complain of fluctuating hoarseness, and laryngeal complaints can be the presenting symptom.[21] The fatigue may be elicited by asking the patient to repeat the vocalization of "ee-ee-ee." Patients with more severe disease may demonstrate dysarthria, dysphagia, aspiration, and even stridor, although stridor as the presenting symptom is unusual and tends to be due to delayed diagnosis. Response to anticholinesterase (eg, Tensilon), establishes the diagnosis. Myasthenia gravis is most common in women between the second and fourth decades. It must be ruled out in women in this age group who present with fluctuating hoarseness.

ROLE OF THE OTOLARYNGOLOGIST

Patients with neurodegenerative disorders present significant challenges in management. Their primary disease process is irreversible, and they deteriorate over time despite the physician's best efforts. The otolaryngologist participates in their care in several ways. Patients are sent to otolaryngologists for assessment of their voice, speech, and swallowing abnormalities. Sometimes a neurologic diagnosis has already been made based on systemic symptoms. For patients who aspirate, the neurologist may seek assistance in evaluating airway protection mechanisms and the need for tracheotomy. For patients with predominantly voice and speech complaints, speech therapy may be beneficial. Not uncommonly, patients who do not carry a neurologic diagnosis are referred to a laryngologist or voice and swallowing center for management of what was perceived by the referring center as an isolated voice, speech, or swallowing abnormality. In these cases, a familiarity with the neurodegenerative disorders enables the otolaryngologist to suspect or establish the diagnosis. Timely referral for neurologic consultation is especially critical if symptoms are advanced and progressing, as sometimes seen in ALS.[22]

Although otolaryngologists traditionally have not played a major role in the management of patients with neurodegenerative disorders, interventions that already exist in the otolaryngologic armamentarium for other disorders can improve the quality of life in selected patients.

Botulinum toxin (Botox, Allergan) injection, which has an established role in the treatment of spasmodic dysphonia, has been applied to patients with essential tremor of the voice. Warrick et al reported a crossover study of unilateral versus bilateral injection of Botox for 10 patients.[15] They found that, although most patients did not have a significant improvement in objective acoustic measures, most benefitted from a subjective reduction in vocal effort, which may be attributed to reduced laryngeal airway resistance from decreased adduction. Most patients reported satisfaction with the procedure.

Botox injection may also have a role in the treatment of dysphagia in patients with neurodegenerative disorders. The cricopharyngeus (CP) muscle is tonically active at rest and relaxes during swallow. Failure of the CP muscle to relax or hypertonicity can contribute to dysphagia in patients with systemic neurodegenerative disorders. Both percutaneous[23] and endoscopic[24] injection of the CP muscle have been described, although no report specifically addresses the treatment of dysphagia in the context of neurodegenerative disorders. Of the 12 patients reported by

Parameswaran and Soliman,[24] one suffered from ALS, and another had Parkinson's disease. Both patients reported only modest improvement in their swallowing function. The limited gain from CP injection is not surprising as the dysphagia results from global pharyngeal dysfunction rather than isolated CP involvement. The use of Botox as a therapeutic and diagnostic modality in these patients, therefore, was beneficial in evaluating the potential effects of CP myotomy. If the Botox is minimally effective, then it is unlikely that myotomy will help and the patient can avoid the morbidity of the more invasive procedure. Overall, the utility of Botox injection of the CP muscle in the neurodegenerative patient requires further investigation. For patients who may be hesitant to undergo botulinum toxin injection, a "test" injection of lidocaine into the UES may provide similar diagnostic information. This is an embraceable but not well-studied approach (Figure 16–3). The test injection may be performed in the clinic or in the fluoroscopy suite. In the clinic, the patient may be asked to eat different consistencies and subjectively report any impact of the injection on his or her dysphagia. In the fluoroscopy, the patient may be imaged immediately before and after injection to more objectively determine any change on swallowing function.

Botox can also be used to treat spasticity and sialorrhea in patients with diseases of the UMN including pseudobulbar palsy and PLS. In patients with symptoms of pseudobulbar palsy, Botox injection into facial muscles may ameliorate spasticity which will lessen dysarthria and oral incompetence associated with the disorder. In one case report, Botox injection into the thyroarytenoid muscles was also found to reduce spastic vocal symptoms.[25] Clinically, Botox can be beneficial in reducing dysarthria and vocal strain in patients with PLS. In this group of patients, Botox must be used with caution. EMG of the muscles considered for injection, either facial or laryngeal, should be undertaken to document the absence of LMN findings. If there are no signs of LMN loss, then injection of Botox in small increments can result in a reduction of

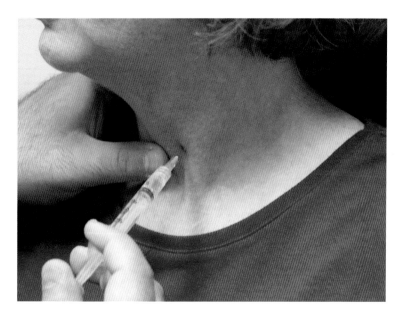

FIGURE 16–3. Percutaneous injection of lidocaine along cricoid cartilage into the UES. The left hand is on the patient's neck with the thumb on the cricoid. Lidocaine 2% without epinephrine is used.

spasticity. For reduction of laryngeal spasticity and vocal strain, Botox injections in the range of 0.3 to 0.6 mouse units into one thyroarytenoid muscle are usually effective. Vocal and often speech fluency improves and the patients report less effort required to speak. Reduction in sialorrhea in patients with ALS after salivary gland Botox injection has been reported also, but its efficacy has yet to be proven.

Parkinson's dysphonia is traditionally treated with speech therapy (see chapter 18).[26] However, when vocal training in itself is ineffective due to excessive vocal fold atrophy, augmentation of vocal fold mass with either injection laryngoplasty or bilateral type I thyroplasty may provide additional vocal improvement. Berke et al reported a series of 35 Parkinson patients with hypophonic dysphonia who underwent percutaneous injection of cross-linked collagen.[27] These patients were selected based on the finding of persistent glottic aperture on videostroboscopic examination. Parkinson patients with dysphonia but with normal glottal closure were excluded. After injection, 75% of the patients reported satisfaction with the procedure. Kim et al reported a series of 18 patients with similar findings.[28] More recently, the use of calcium hydroxylapatite as a vocal fold augmentation material for Parkinson patients has also been reported.[29] In the senior author's clinical experience, bilateral

type I thyroplasty (medialization laryngoplasty) works well in this select group of patients. The goal is to medialize the membranous portion of the vocal folds so they remain in an adducted position even during inspiration. The airway in the posterior cartilaginous portion of the glottis is preserved. Therefore, patients do not report a significant alteration in breathing and usually notice that the voice is louder with the sensation of less phonatory effort. Pre- and postoperative measures of vocal intensity can be used to objectively evaluate these changes.

Selection of Parkinson patients for any type of vocal fold augmentation must take into consideration the severity of the disease. As discussed previously, the dysphonia in patients with PD has multiple contributing factors, only one of which is addressed by vocal fold augmentation or medialization. Patients with large phonatory glottal apertures as the predominant factor for their dysphonia are more likely to benefit from augmentation than those with severe bradykinesia. Patients with advanced disease, aphonia, difficulty with speech initiation, or dysphagia are likely to have more significant bradykinesia and are less likely to benefit from augmentation.[28]

Finally, otolaryngologists are often involved in airway management in patients with motor neuron disease, although the options are largely palliative. Intractable aspiration may be managed with tracheotomy with limited efficacy. Laryngeal diversion or laryngectomy are alternatives that are rarely indicated.[22] The most common indication for tracheotomy in motor neuron disease is for mechanical ventilation as the respiratory apparatus weakens.

CONCLUSIONS

Voice and speech abnormalities are common in patients with neurodegenerative disorders. Evaluation of these patients is facilitated by an understanding of the anatomic location of the neurologic lesion and the neurologic system affected by the particular disorder. The care of the patient with neurodegenerative disorder is multidisciplinary. The neurologists are the specialists of the primary disease process and direct the medical therapies. The speech pathologists perform detailed functional assessments of voice, speech, and swallowing functions and carry out behavioral therapies. The otolaryngologists have the potential to improve the quality of life in selected patients with interventions already familiar to them. A familiarity with the neurodegenerative disorders will enable the otolaryngologist to potentially make the initial diagnosis in patients with isolated voice and speech complaints.

Review Questions

1. A 33-year-old business consultant presents with a 2-month history of intermittent hoarseness. She complains that she often "loses her voice" during meetings. On examination, her voice is mildly asthenic but otherwise normal. Videostroboscopic examination shows vocal folds without lesions and apparent normal mobility. What disease entity should you consider, and what other diagnostic maneuver would you perform?

2. Which of the following findings on laryngoscopic examination of a patient with Parkinson's disease indicates possible benefit from vocal fold augmentation?
   a. Atrophic, bowed vocal folds
   b. Vocal cord paresis
   c. Glottal gap
   d. Laryngeal tremor

3. Which of the following is not a sign of LMN lesion?
   a. Tongue fasciculations
   b. Voice strain
   c. Hypernasality
   d. Vocal cord paresis

4. A patient with parkinsonism is sent to you for the evaluation of dysphonia. Laryngoscopic examination shows limited abduction of bilateral vocal cords. What specific history should you query, and what disease entity should you consider?

5. Botox injection of vocal cords has been found to be beneficial for some patients with which of the following conditions?
   a. Parkinson's disease
   b. ALS
   c. Shy-Drager
   d. Essential tremor of the voice

REFERENCES

1. Hartelius L, Svensson P. Speech and swallowing symptoms associated with Parkinson's disease and multiple sclerosis: a survey. *Folia Phoniatr Logop.* 994;46:9–17.
2. Hanson DG. Neuromuscular disorders of the larynx. *Otolaryngol Clin North Am.* 1991;24:1035–1051.
3. Robin DA, Goel A, Somodi LB, et al. Tongue strength and endurance: relation to highly skilled movements. *J Speech Hear Res.* 1992;35:1239–1245.

4. Aviv JE, Murry T, Zschommler A, et al. Flexible endoscopic evaluation of swallowing with sensory testing: patient characteristics and analysis of safety in 1,340 consecutive examinations. *Ann Otol Rhinol Laryngol.* 2005;114:173-176.

5. Langmore SE, Aviv JE. Endoscopic procedures to evaluate oropharyngeal swallowing. In: Langmore SE, ed. *Endoscopic Evaluation and Treatment of Swallowing Disorders.* New York, NY: Thieme; 2001: chap 5.

6. Perez KS, Ramig LO, Smith ME, Dromey C. The Parkinson larynx: tremor and videostroboscopic findings. *J Voice.* 1996;10:354-361.

7. Siemers E. Multiple system atrophy. *Med Clin North Am.* 1999;83:381-392.

8. Kluin KJ, Gilman S, Lohman M, Junck L. Characteristics of the dysarthria of multiple system atrophy. *Arch Neurol.* 1996;53:545-548.

9. Wenning GK, Tison F, Shlomo YB, et al. Multiple system atrophy: a review of 203 pathologically proven cases. *Mov Disord.* 1997;12:133-147.

10. Hughes RG, Gibbin KP, Lowe J. Vocal fold abductor paralysis as a solitary and fatal manifestation of multiple system atrophy. *J Laryngol Otol.* 1998; 112:177-178.

11. Isono S, Shiba K, Yamaguchi M, et al. Pathogenesis of laryngeal narrowing in patients with multiple system atrophy. *J Physiol.* 2001;536:237-249.

12. Merlo IM, Occhini A, Pacchetti C, et al. Not paralysis, but dystonia causes stridor in multiple system atrophy. *Neurology.* 2002;58:649-652.

13. Blumin JH, Berke GS. Bilateral vocal fold paresis and multiple system atrophy. *Arch Otolaryngol Head Neck Surg.* 2002;128:1404-1407.

14. Iranzo A, Santamaria J, Tolosa E, et al. Long-term effect of CPAP in the treatment of nocturnal stridor in multiple system atrophy. *Neurology.* 2004; 63:930-932.

15. Warrick P, Dromey C, Irish JC, et al. Botulinum toxin for essential tremor of the voice with multiple anatomical sites of tremor: a crossover design study of unilateral versus bilateral injection. *Laryngoscope.* 2000;110:1366-1374.

16. Koda J, Ludlow CL. An evaluation of laryngeal muscle activation in patients with vocal tremor. *Otolaryngol Head Neck Surg.* 1992;107:684-696.

17. Brown JR, Simonson J. Organic voice tremor: a tremor of phonation. *Neurology.* 1963;13:520-525.

18. Kent RD, Kent JF, Weismer G, et al. Impairment of speech intelligibility in men with amyotrophic lateral sclerosis. *J Speech Hear Disord.* 1990;55: 721-728.

19. McGuirt WF, Blalock D. The otolaryngologist's role in the diagnosis and treatment of amyotrophic lateral sclerosis. *Laryngoscope.* 1980;90: 1496-1501.

20. Chen A, Garrett CG. Otolaryngologic presentations of amyotrophic lateralsclerosis. *Otolaryngol Head Neck Surg.* 2005;132:500-504.

21. Mao VH, Abaza M, Spiegel JR, et al. Laryngeal myasthenia gravis: report of 40 cases. *J Voice.* 2001;15:122-130.

22. Hillel A, Dray T, Miller R, et al. Presentation of ALS to the otolaryngologist/head and neck surgeon: getting to the neurologist. *Neurology.* 1999;53 (8 suppl 5):S22-S25.

23. Blitzer A, Brin M. Use of botulinum toxin for diagnosis and management of cricopharygeal achalasia. *Otolaryngol Head Neck Surg.* 1997;116: 328-329.

24. Parameswaran MS, Soliman AM. Endoscopic botulinum toxin injection for cricopharygeal dysphagia. *Ann Otol Rhinol Laryngol.* 2002;111:871-874.

25. McHenry M, Whatman J, Pou A. The effect of botulinum toxin A on the vocal symptoms of spastic dysarthria: a case study. *J Voice.* 2002;16:124-131.

26. Ramig LO, Fox C, Sapir C. Parkinson's disease: speech and voice disorders and their treatment with the Lee Silverman Voice Treatment. *Semin Speech Lang.* 2004;25:169-180.

27. Berke GS, Gerratt B, Kreiman J, et al. Treatment of Parkinson hypophonia with percutaneous collagen augmentation. *Laryngoscope.* 1999;109: 1295-1299.

28. Kim SH, Kearney JJ, Atkins JP. Percutaneous laryngeal collagen augmentation for treatment of parkinsonian hypophonia. *Otolaryngol Head Neck Surg.* 2002;126:653-656.

29. Belafsky PC, Postma GN. Vocal fold augmentation with calcium hydroxylapatite. *Otolaryngol Head Neck Surg.* 2004;131:351-354.

30. Zealear DL, Rainey CL, Netterville JL, et al. Electrical pacing of the paralyzed human larynx. *Ann Otol Rhinol Laryngol.* 1996;105:689-693.

31. Zealear DL, Billante CR, Courey MS, et al. Electrically stimulated glottal opening combined with adductor muscle Botox blockade restores both ventilation and voice in a patient with bilateral laryngeal paralysis. *Ann Otol Rhinol Laryngol.* 2002;111:500-506.

32. Zealear DL, Billante CR, Courey MS, et al. Reanimation of the paralyzed human larynx with an implantable electrical stimulation device. *Laryngoscope.* 2003;113:1149-1156.

17

Vocal Fold Paralysis

Tanya Meyer, MD
Lucian Sulica, MD
Andrew Blitzer, MD

KEY POINTS

■ Vocal fold paralysis implies immobility as a result of injury to the vagus or the recurrent laryngeal nerve. Although nerve injury is usually the cause of immobility, it is important to consider potential causes of mechanical fixation in the differential.

■ Laryngeal EMG can help differentiate neurogenic from mechanical immobility and can help prognosticate return of function.

■ The *need* for the treatment of glottic insufficiency resulting from a vocal fold paralysis is determined by symptomatology: adequacy of cough, presence of dysphagia, and defects in phonatory function. The *type* of treatment offered to the patient is determined by the patient's overall prognosis, the potential for spontaneous return of glottic function, and the glottic configuration.

■ Most patients are well served by medialization of the vocal fold; an arytenoid adduction suture is often needed for individuals with a large posterior glottic gap and flaccid arytenoid.

■ Reinnervation procedures can enhance the tone of the paralyzed vocal fold, but will not recover meaningful vocal fold motion.

As a dynamic organ, the larynx and associated structures are responsible for regulating the major functions of the upper aerodigestive tract. Proper laryngeal valving is therefore essential in voice, breathing, swallowing, coughing, as well as stabilization of the thorax (*Valsalva*) during upper limb activity. When the proper function of the larynx is disturbed, any or all of these domains may be affected.

This chapter provides a summary of the clinical evaluation and management of vocal fold paralysis, focusing on adult unilateral vocal fold paralysis. In the final sections of the chapter, key issues related to bilateral vocal fold paralysis, isolated superior laryngeal nerve dysfunction, and pediatric issues are reviewed.

TERMINOLOGY

In common parlance, "vocal fold paralysis" is used to describe the *sign* of vocal fold motion impairment, regardless of cause. More precise usage would restrict the term to compromised mobility due to loss of motor innervation. Although paralysis is by far the most common cause, "vocal fold immobility" is a more accurate term until the etiology of the motion impairment has been determined. For example, although a patient with acute voice changes and "paralysis" following a carotid enarterectomy very likely has suffered a neuropathic injury, the proper descriptor is "immobility" until nerve damage can be confirmed by laryngeal electromyography (see chapter 9) fold excursion due to the neuropathy could properly be called "vocal paralysis."

"Recurrent laryngeal nerve paralysis" is often used interchangeably with "vocal fold paralysis"; although the recurrent nerve is almost always involved, vocal fold paralysis may or may not also involve the superior laryngeal nerve. "Paresis" is used clinically to refer to a vocal fold that retains some mobility despite partial dysfunction.

CAUSES OF VOCAL PARALYSIS

Vocal fold immobility may be broadly categorized as neurogenic or mechanical in nature. Unilateral immobility is usually the result of nerve dysfunction, the causes of which fall into four broad categories: neoplastic (compression or infiltration by tumor), trauma (surgical and nonsurgical trauma), medical disease, and those that are idiopathic in nature (Table 17–1).

Neoplasms along the course of the cervical or thoracic vagus and recurrent laryngeal nerve may cause paralysis. Mediastinal tumors, often metastases from primary lung malignancies, account for the majority of paralyses from neoplastic causes. The roster of surgical procedures that place the laryngeal nerves at particular risk includes thyroidectomy and a variety of skull base, cervical, and thoracic procedures. Historically, thyroid procedures have been the most common cause of iatrogenic paralyses; this may be changing as the anterior approach to cervical spine surgery becomes more widely performed.[1] This has also affected the "sidedness" of vocal paralysis due to the preference for right-sided approaches and the risk for paralysis in these cases.[2]

Despite appropriate evaluation (see below), a significant proportion of cases has continued to defy diagnosis. These are usually designated as "idiopathic" neuropathies. It has been suggested that viral neuritis may be responsible, based on analogies to other cranial palsies and occasional suggestive serologic associations.

Mechanical causes may be due to fixation of the joint from fibrosis or arthritis, posterior glottic stenosis, or neoplastic invasion of the vocal fold muscle. Arytenoid dislocation has been reported as a cause of immobility; the majority of laryngologists believe that this entity is rare, although the clinical history may be compelling in certain cases.[6]

Overall, however, the frequency of vocal fold paralysis by etiology varies considerably from study to study (Table 17–2).

TABLE 17–1. Causes of Vocal Fold Paralysis

1. TRAUMA

Iatrogenic Trauma
- Cervical surgery
  - eg, thyroidectomy, anterior approach to the cervical spine (ACD)
- Thoracic procedures
  - eg, repair of thoracic aortic anuerysm
- Skull base surgery
- Other medical procedures
  - Endotracheal intubation
  - Central venous catheterization
  - Forceps delivery

Noniatrogenic Trauma

2. TUMOR, MALIGNANT OR BENIGN

Brain or Skull Base

Cervical
- Thyroid
- Metastatic lymphadenopathy
- Parapharyngeal space masses
- Vagal neuroma

Thoracic
- Esophageal
- Mediastinal lymphadenopathy
- Thymoma

3. MEDICAL DISEASE

Cardiovascular Disease
- Left heart failure (Ortner's syndrome)
- Aortic arch aneurysm

Neurologic Disease
- Stroke—Wallenberg's syndrome
- Amyotrophic lateral sclerosis
- Postpolio syndrome
- Charcot-Marie-Tooth disease (hereditary peripheral nerve palsy)
- Bulbar palsies

Developmental Abnormalities
- Arnold-Chiari malformation

Drug Neurotoxicity
- Vinca alkaloids (vincristine/vinblastine)
- Organophosphates

Granulomatous disease
- Tuberculosis
- Sarcoid

4. IDIOPATHIC

TABLE 17–2. Etiology of Unilateral Vocal Fold Immobility

Etiology	Terris 1992[3]	Maisel 1974[4]	Benninger 1998[5]
Malignancy	40.5	25.2	24.7
Iatrogenic	34.5	15.7	23.9
Idiopathic	10.7	26.8	19.6
Trauma	1.2	10.2	11.1
Intubation	7.1	3.1	7.5
CNS tumors	2.4	7.9	7.9
Thoracic disease	—	6.3	5.4
Other	3.6	4.7	—

EVALUATION

The clinician evaluating the patient with vocal fold immobility is faced with two separate issues—the workup of the etiology of the vocal fold immobility and the management of the patient's symptoms related to the subsequent glottic insufficiency. It is paramount that the clinician conduct a rigorous search for the underlying etiology, such as malignancy, infection, or granulomatous disease, and not be distracted from the completion of this investigation by the management of the patient's voice or swallowing symptoms. Although the exact nature of the evaluation beyond history and physical examination is not widely agreed on, most practitioners routinely order computed tomography (CT) along the course of the recurrent laryngeal nerve. This is described in further detail below.

History

Patients with unilateral vocal fold immobility complain of a weak (asthenic), breathy, and hoarse voice, the severity of which is generally proportional to the gap between the vocal folds at adduction. Patients are particularly bothered by the increased *effort* of phonation and report progression of

Pathophysiology of Paralysis

"Paralysis" creates a mental image of a completely denervated, perfectly immobile vocal fold. The reality is considerably more complex and variable; vocal fold paralysis is not an all-or-none phenomenon as it has been commonly conceptualized. As the nervous system attempts to regenerate from a given nerve injury, reinnervation occurs at variable degrees and effectiveness. Nerve fibers must not only regenerate in sufficient number, but also return to their correct original target to enable recovery of meaningful motion. For the recurrent laryngeal nerve, both adductor and abductor fibers are intermingled and consequently varying degrees of dysfunctional (crossed or *synkinetic*) reinnervation is common. Such dysfunctional reinnervation may yield simultaneous excitation of adductor and abductor musculature resulting in minimal *net* vocal fold movement.

In the ideal scenario, presumably following neuropraxic lesions, there is appropriate and complete regeneration of neural input and resulting motor function. On the other end of the spectrum, some individuals appear to have little to no return of nervous inputs as evidenced by a flaccid and atrophied vocal fold. In most cases where there is persistent motion impairment, recovery probably occurs somewhere between the extremes, such that there is a certain degree of reinnervation but with variable adequacy and accuracy.

Both human and animal studies have shown that a paralyzed vocal fold is only sometimes a denervated fold,[7-9] and even in cases of deliberate recurrent nerve section for spasmodic dysphonia,[10] reinnervation is the rule. This robust tendency for the vocal musculature to become reinnervated over time may account for the return of acceptable voice in the absence of vocal fold motion in certain cases of paralysis, through restoration of muscular bulk and tone by nerve regrowth inadequate and/or inappropriate to restore motion.[11]

these symptoms over the day (vocal fatigue). Challenging acoustic situations, such as speaking over background noise or using a telephone, will exacerbate these complaints.

Complaints of mild or moderate dysphagia, particularly for liquids, are fairly common in cases of paralysis. Whatever degree of aspiration that may be present will be exacerbated by the attendant weak cough. Frank aspiration is rare with isolated recurrent nerve injury, but more common with so-called "high-vagal" injuries,

which impair both motor and sensory innervation to the larynx. Pooling of secretions in the piriform sinuses may be observed on the affected side. Because the recurrent laryngeal nerve also contributes to innervation of the cricopharyngeus muscle, delay in relaxation and opening of the upper esophageal sphincter may contribute to this problem.

Individuals may report breathlessness during speech due to rapid escape of air during phonation. Dyspnea with exertion may reflect different aspect of paralysis and requires careful consideration. Individuals at the extremes of fitness, such as the young athlete exercising to maximum capacity or the medically compromised aging patient, may symptomatically recognize partial obstruction of the glottis from failure of complete purposeful adduction. In most cases, however, the dyspnea represents a compromise of thoracic fixation during the Valsalva maneuver, which aids in a wide variety of everyday physical tasks like lifting objects, using the arms to assist in climbing stairs or rising from the sitting position, and defecation. Unfamiliarity with laryngeal biomechanics may lead the physician directly away from steps necessary to restore appropriate glottic competence.

In cases of paresis, the dysphonia may be subtle, particularly in the relatively quiet environment of the examination room, and the physician may have to rely on patient reports of fatigue, neck discomfort, and an intermittently poor voice.

Physical Examination

The clinician should assess the voice during both normal conversation and a variety of speech tasks. A breathy, diplophonic voice can occur because each vocal fold is at a different tension and will therefore vibrate at a different frequency for a given level of subglottic pressure. With a dense paralysis, patients will be unable to yell due to the flaccidity of the dysfunctional vocal fold. Simple bedside tests may approximately quantify the degree of glottic insufficiency, although they depend heavily on patient effort. Maximum phonation time (MPT) measures the duration that a patient can phonate the voiced vowel /i/. Normal values are greater than 21 seconds, although many individuals, especially singers, may have much longer phonation times.[12] The s/z ratio compares maximum phonation time between an unvoiced (/s/) and a voiced sound (/z/). In glottic insufficiency, this ratio increases as the phonation time for the voiced sound /z/ decreases (see chapter 8, Clinical and Instrumental Evaluation of the Voice Patient).

Prior to endoscopy, the patient should undergo a complete neurologic evaluation of the head and neck.[13] Signs such as a unilateral palatal weakness, tongue deviation, Horner's syndrome, and dysarthria may indicate the site of the lesion and suggest an underlying neurologic disease.

In most individuals, frank vocal paralysis will be readily detectable by flexible or rigid laryngoscopy. Slight vocal fold movement may occur due to cricothyroid, interarytenoid, and extralaryngeal muscle function, which may cause some diagnostic confusion. In such an individual, alternating sustained vowel phonation and sniffing (/i/-sniff) will highlight the inability of the paralyzed vocal fold to abduct.

The apex of the affected arytenoid may sag anteriomedially (Figure 17–1) due to a loss of active muscle stabilization (especially posterior cricoarytenoid) of the arytenoid cartilage on the crest of the cricoid. In this scenario, the vocal process is displaced caudally, and the paralyzed fold appears shortened and lower than its partner. Some patients may be able to approximate the vocal folds with low intensity phonation, but upon attempts to increase volume through raising subglottic pressure, a denervated fold tends to luff away from the midline due to flaccidity. Thus, one symptom that can differentiate a patient with paralysis from other causes of hoarseness is an inability to yell.

Often, the mobile arytenoid may "bump" the arytenoid on the denervated side and displace it laterally. The displacement of the muscular process of the paralyzed arytenoid under the mucosa of the piriform sinus is usually the most noticeable feature of this motion. This "jostle sign" was first described by Chevalier Jackson[14] and may serve as conclusive clinical evidence of a mobile arytenoid in cases where ankylosis or other fixation is suspected.

Ventricular fold hyperadduction may obscure the view of the vocal fold in some cases. This type of hyperfunction is in fact a common compensatory mechanism for glottic insufficiency[15] and should by itself direct the examiner's attention to glottal closure. In cases of paresis, it may be the only clue to the underlying problem (Figure 17–2).

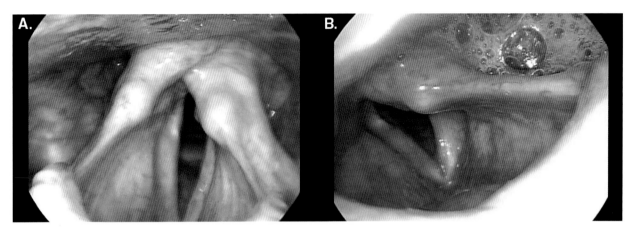

FIGURE 17–1. Left vocal fold paralysis. The individuals in both **A.** and **B.** have left vocal fold paralysis from metastatic mediastinal lymphadenopathy. They both have breathy diplophonic voices, and complain of extreme fatigue with prolonged speaking. The individual in **A.** has a fairly upright arytenoid with minimal flaccidity of the vocal fold, although atrophy is apparent. The individual in **B.** has an anteriorly prolapsed arytenoid, marked vocal fold flaccidity with bowing, and obvious pooling of secretions in the ipsilateral piriform sinus. These images illustrate the variability in presentation of vocal fold paralysis.

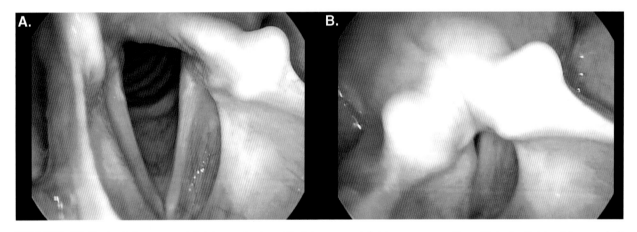

FIGURE 17–2. Left true vocal fold paralysis with false vocal fold compensation. This individual has a left vocal fold paralysis following a thoracic aneurysm repair. **A.** shows the vocal fold during abduction and **B.** during adduction. Note that the right hemilarynx attempts to compensate for the glottic insufficiency caused by paralysis of the left recurrent laryngeal nerve by recruiting the right false vocal (ventricular) fold during adduction to improve glottal closure. The reason for this behavior is obvious in this case, but false vocal fold hyperadduction may be the only clue to a subtle glottic insufficiency or paresis in other cases.

A detailed analysis of glottic configuration is important for planning surgical intervention. Vocal fold position must be assessed in both the coronal (rostral/caudal) and axial (abduction/adduction) planes. *Vertical height mismatches* are more likely to require an arytenoid procedure. Many studies also speak of posterior and anterior glottic closure. Posterior closure generally refers to contact at the vocal process, whereas

anterior closure refers to contact between the vibrating edge of the membranous vocal folds. This distinction is also important in the selection of medialization approaches.

Further Investigations

If the cause of the vocal fold mobility is not evident, such as immediately following neck surgery or other trauma, further workup should include a complete medical history to identify possible causes and imaging of the course of the vagus from skull base *through* the mediastinum. Although most practitioners obtain a CT scan, MRI of the brain and skull base should also be considered when high vagal or central lesions are suspected.

Several studies[16] have suggested that chest radiography (CXR) may be adequate, particularly if the paralysis is right-sided. This is in contrast to the findings from the CT literature. In one study,[17] 13 of 18 (72%) cases with *left*-sided aortopulmonary masses on CT scan had a *normal* appearing mediastinum on CXR; the mean size of these chest masses was 2.3 cm. The smallest mass detected in this paper by CXR group was 3.8 cm. This controversy has not been resolved scientifically, with equal percentages of practitioners in a recent national survey choosing CT and CXR.[13] An evidence-based medicine review of the existing literature failed to reveal any support for one over the other.[13] It is important to note that plain film will neither evaluate the skull base nor the cervical course of the vagus and recurrent laryngeal nerves.

Serologies are generally not revealing, and have no role unless there is strong suspicion based on clinical history.[3,13] Direct laryngoscopy, once considered a standard part of evaluation, has largely been supplanted by improved imaging and should be reserved for cases in which ankylosis or posterior glottic stenosis is considered. Laryngeal electromyography can also give important information regarding cause and prognosis of vocal fold immobility, as outlined in chapter 9. Coughing, "wet" voice quality, or other symptoms which suggest dysphagia should prompt a formal evaluation of swallowing.

MANAGEMENT

Decisions regarding treatment in cases of vocal fold paralysis are guided by the severity of voice, swallowing, and airway symptoms balanced against expectations for spontaneous recovery. In cases where there is potential for spontaneous return of movement, and the patient has an acceptable voice, minimal dysphagia, and an adequate cough, it may be reasonable to defer intervention. Alternatively, for the symptomatic patient in the same scenario, a temporary vocal fold augmentation procedure may provide immediate airway stabilization while awaiting recovery. In other cases where there is little hope of functional return, a permanent procedure can be considered.

Although poor voice may be the most obvious symptom to the casual observer, significant dysphagia, aspiration, and poor cough are the symptoms that clinically mandate early intervention. Aspiration has been identified in 18 to 38% of patients with unilateral vocal fold paralysis of all causes.[18-20] It is probably more likely in high vagal injuries[21] (lesion of the vagus proximal to the branching of the superior laryngeal nerve) and of more concern in the face of pulmonary dysfunction or additional cranial nerve deficits. For this reason, algorithms featuring prompt medialization have been proposed after skull base surgery[22-23] and thoracic surgery.[24-27] Although any type of vocal fold medialization (temporary or permanent) appears to be equally effective in improving swallowing dysfunction,[19] it is worth noting that a significant proportion of patients remain troubled by aspiration after medialization.[22,27]

There are no studies that provide clear information regarding the natural history of vocal fold paralysis, and existing clinical series offer variable data. Willatt and Stell[21] published a series in 1989 in which only idiopathic paralyses were followed prospectively; of the 42 patients, although half returned to normal or "near-normal" function, only a fraction of them had return of vocal fold motion. None returned after being immobile for 12 months. Despite the lack of data for all etiologies, a clinical consensus has arisen, which states that prognosis is poor for return of vocal fold movement after a prescribed time interval of 6 to 12 months. For symptomatic treatment before the paralysis has reached this watershed, temporary medialization, usually synonymous with injection augmentation, is recommended. After this time period, medialization thyroplasty (framework surgery) is preferred, as the vocal fold is felt to have reached a condition that will remain stable over the long term. It is important to understand that these practices should not be applied uniformly without regard to the specific clinical circumstance. Requiring a person vocally disabled by a paralysis of overwhelmingly poor prognosis, such as that due to mediastinal metastases, to wait 6 months for rehabilitation is suboptimal management. An additional note requires vigilance; Stell[28] and Ward[29] have independently noted the small but real incidence of delayed presentation of causative neoplasms in patients previously thought to have "idiopathic" vocal paralysis. As many as 10% of cases may eventually be discovered to be due to a vagal schwannoma or other indolent but treatable cause.

Many investigators have attempted to determine prognostic indicators in various cases of paralysis to allow more expeditious rehabilitation of these individuals. To date, laryngeal electromyography has provided the best, although imperfect, information in this regard, largely because reinnervation is not synonymous with recovery. Thus, the appearance of unambiguous signs of reinnervation does not always lead to return of motion. In cases of less than 6 months duration, accurate prediction of unilateral vocal fold motion recovery ranges from 13% to 80%.[30-35] As a general rule, the LEMG features that indicate a good prognosis are the same as those predicted by the basic electrophysiology of muscle: preservation of normal MUAP waveforms, activation during an appropriate voluntary task, preservation of brisk recruitment, and absence of spontaneous activity. Factors suggestive of poor outcome are the converse of these. It should be noted that LEMG is a more reliable predictor of poor prognosis (75% to 100%), which stands to reason, as there is little ambiguity regarding findings such as fibrillation potentials several months following injury. Time elapsed since injury is important, insofar as the earlier favorable signs are present, the more likely it is that spontaneous recovery will take place. An extremely early EMG assessment (3 weeks or less after injury) may exaggerate the degree of injury, and beyond 6 months, LEMG is of limited use, as prognosis is uniformly poor.[35]

SURGICAL OPTIONS

Injection Laryngoplasty (See Table 17–3)

Injection augmentation techniques improve glottic closure by augmentation of the paraglottic space with a biocompatible substance, thereby adding bulk to the vocal fold and medializing the free edge. Injection augmentation is usually considered a temporary measure because most available injection substances (autologous fat, Gelfoam, collagen preparations [Zyderm, Zyplast, others], micronized dermis [Cymetra], hyaluronic acid [Hylaform, Restylane, others]) are resorbed over time. As a general rule, the collagen preparations are felt to persist in the tissue approximately 3 to 6 months, and the hyaluronic acid probably lasts longer, although there is marked interpatient variability. The bovine collagen preparations (Zyderm, Zyplast) do require prior skin testing to ensure no allergic reaction to the injectate; human collagen preparations (Cymetra), hyaluronic acid, and the permanent injectables mentioned below do not require formal allergy testing although there are rare reports of adverse tissue reactions.

Polytetrafluoroethylene paste (Teflon, Polytef) and calcium hydroxylapatite paste (Radiesse) are permanent synthetic injectables. Teflon was used extensively in the past but has fallen out of favor due to the delayed formation of granulomas requiring surgical resection (see chapter 21). Calcium hydroxylapatite (Radiesse) paste has been shown effective in several preliminary studies,[37] but long-term data regarding safety and efficacy are not yet available at the time of this writing.

Injection augmentation may be performed perorally (Figure 17–3) or transcutaenously in the office under topical or local anesthetic, or by suspension laryngoscopy in the operative suite. Injection augmentation is generally felt to be more suitable in cases where the glottic closure is only mildly compromised and predominantly affecting the membranous vocal fold; it will not effectively reposition the arytenoid to rectify a

TABLE 17–3. Overview of Materials for Glottic Injection

Material	Ease of Use	Duration	Drawbacks
Fat	+	6 to 9 months	Requires donor site, general anesthesia
Teflon	+++	Permanent	Granuloma formation
Gelfoam	++	1 to 2 months	Difficult in the awake patient, large needle
Calcium Hydroxylapatite	+++	Permanent?	Irreversible
Collagen			
Bovine (*Zyplast, Zyderm*)	+++	4 to 6 months	Requires pretesting and waiting period
Human donor (*Cymetra*)	++	4 to 6 months	Preparation, short shelf life
Human tissue culture (*Cosmoplast*)	+++	Unknown	No track record in laryngology
Human autologous	+	Unknown	Requires skin harvest
Radiesse Voice Gel	+++	Unknown	No track record; made for vocal fold
Hyaluronic Acid	+++	6 to 12 months	Good rheology, supportive studies

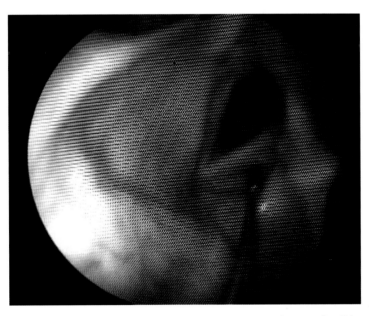

FIGURE 17–3. Injection augmentation. Image from a flexible nasolaryngoscope during a transoral injection laryngoplasty.

height discrepancy or close a posterior glottal gap. Most injection substances require overinjection to allow for resorption, rendering fine adjustments to vocal fold position virtually impossible. In addition, should the injectate infiltrate into an unintended site—typically and most distressingly, into the superficial layers of the vocal fold, impairing mucosal vibration—corrective intervention is challenging, and patients may have to await natural resolution over weeks to months. Some patients retain acceptable voice quality over time despite the use of a temporary injectable material, but it is not possible to definitively attribute these to injection alone (despite some assertions in the literature), given the tendency of paralytic dysphonia to improve over time.

Medialization Thyroplasty

Medialization thyroplasty is a precise, effective, permanent procedure that forms the mainstay of surgical management of vocal fold paralysis. This procedure involves creation of a window in the thyroid cartilage through which the paraglottic space can be accessed. An implant is then placed into the paraglottic space displacing the true vocal fold medially. Typically performed under local anesthesia, this procedure allows fine-tuning of the position, shape, and size of the implant guided by the immediate feedback of the patient's voice with each repositioning maneuver.

Initially introduced by Erwin Payr in 1915,[38] medialization thyroplasty was handicapped in its early iterations by the unpredictable durability of cartilage and bone used as medialization implants. This difficulty was solved with the introduction of the Silastic implant by Isshiki.[39] Since then, several additional medialization materials have been described. Solid prefabricated implants are available in a variety of materials (Silastic, hydroxyapatite, and bioimplantable metal). Due to ease of implant placement, many authors advocate the use of expanded polytetrafluoroethylene (Gore-Tex) ribbon, which can be layered into the paraglottic space through a small thyroplasty window until adequate voicing is achieved. Others prefer to hand carve individual implants out of Silastic

block, which allows custom variation of the height, depth, and width of each implant.

For the most part, the procedure is similar regardless of the implant used (Figure 17–4). Local anesthesia with epinephrine is injected into the skin and subcutaneous tissues of the anterior neck and along the thyroid cartilage. A modest incision just above the CT membrane extending just across the midline is created and subplatysmal flaps are elevated. The strap muscles are separated in the midline and retracted to expose the lateral aspect of the thyroid cartilage—some surgeons divide the medial 2 cm of the sternohyoid muscle to facilitate exposure.

The critical anatomic task is to identify the level of the vocal fold in relation to the thyroid lamina so that the thyroid cartilage window can be placed appropriately. In general, the vocal fold lies closer to the lower border of the thyroid cartilage than is generally believed. A lower cartilage strut is carefully preserved to stabilize the implant. The final dimensions and location of the window depend on the implant choice. The vocal fold is then medialized to yield a satisfactory voice (Figure 17–5). Visual feedback via a flexible fiberoptic laryngoscope intraoperatively is essential to ensure adequate medialization and accurate contact between the vibrating edges of the vocal folds.

During implant manipulation, some patients may not achieve optimal voicing due to persistence of hyperfunctional compensation. For this reason, some surgeons advocate preop voice therapy for "unloading" although others feel that these vocal patterns will "break" intraoperatively when physiologic vocal fold approximation is achieved.

When satisfactory placement has been achieved, and the surgeon is satisfied with the patient's voice and endoscopic view of the extent of medialization, the implant is secured with a permanent stitch, the strap muscles are reapproximated, and a small drain is placed. The patient is monitored overnight in the hospital for airway compromise. Voice rest is encouraged for 3 to 7 days and the patient is allowed to resume a regular diet although asked to refrain from heavy activity.

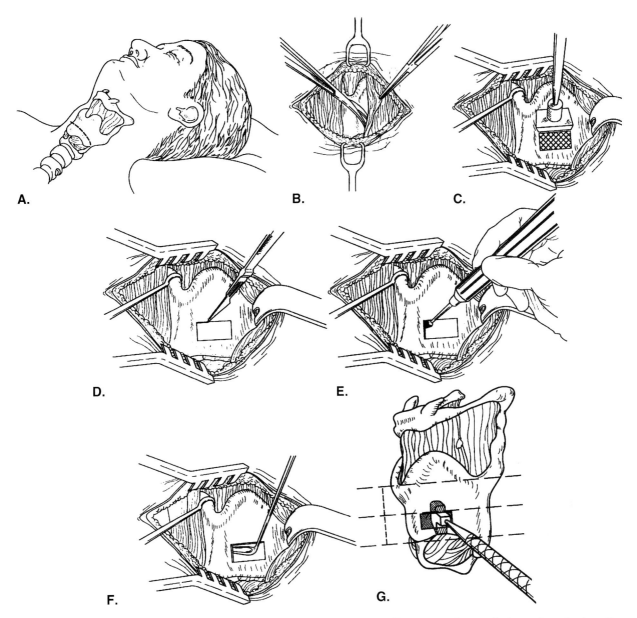

A.

B.

C.

D.

E.

F.

G.

FIGURE 17–4. Thyroplasty technique. This series of drawings illustrates the technique for placing the VoCoM thyroplasty implant. The basic principles are the same for any implant technique. **A.** A 5- to 6-cm skin incision is planned horizontally at the level of the cricoid cartilage. **B.** After elevation of subplatysmal flaps, the strap muscles are divided and retracted laterally. **C.** The larynx is rotated using a single hook and the location of the thyroplasty window is marked—this kit uses a specialized template tool. **D.** and **E.** The window can be fashioned using a scalpel, Kerrison punch, or an otologic drill. **F.** The paraglottic tissues are freed from the inner table of the thyroid cartilage. **G.** A series of trial implants are placed to determine the optimum implant size and position, after which the final implant is placed and secured. The position of the vocal fold relative to external landmarks is shown. (Images courtesy of Gyrus-ENT.)

Principal complications include airway obstruction and perforation into the laryngeal lumen. Necessarily, medialization narrows the airway, and in combination with postoperative edema and hematoma, this can cause airway obstruction. For this reason, many surgeons prefer

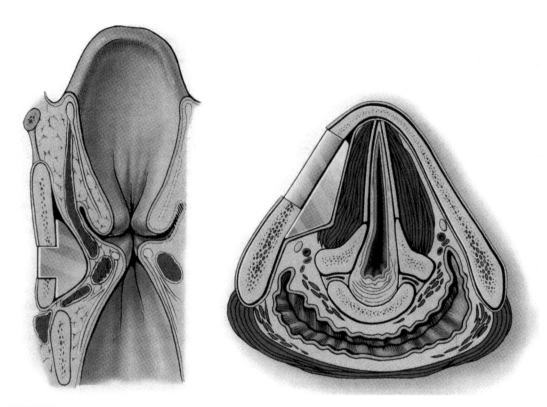

FIGURE 17–5. Coronal (*left*) and axial (*right*) views of final implant placement. (Reprinted from Ossoff R, *The Larynx.* Baltimore, Md: Lippincott Williams & Wilkins; 2003:292 with permission. Copyright 2003 Lippincott, Williams & Wilkins.)

to observe these patients in the hospital for one night following the procedure. Approximately 0.6% to 11% of patient undergoing medialization laryngoplasty, and 2.2% to 3.5% undergoing medialization plus arytenoid adduction, required intubation or tracheotomy in the immediate postoperative period.[40,41] The incidence of airway emergencies and implant extrusion have dropped in the years since the introduction of these procedures.

Violation of the laryngeal mucosa is significant because of the likelihood of infection and subsequent extrusion of implanted material. Perforation typically takes place in the delicate ventricular mucosa, which lies close to the thyroid lamina, or anteriorly, where there is little soft tissue cover; surgeons should use special care when undermining the paraglottic tissues in these areas. Mucosal tears are not always obvious, but any blood seen intralumenally via the endoscope should prompt a careful inspection. Flooding the operative field with irrigation and looking for

bubbles during a Valsalva maneuver is also useful, and may be performed in all cases prior to implant placement.

Dissatisfaction with the medialization procedure does not typically arise because of complications, but because of suboptimal voice results. These are typically due to technical factors, and revision rates have been reported to range from 5.4%[41] to 14%,[40] to as high as 33%[42] when adjunctive procedures such as fat injection are included. Certain causes of poor voice result occur with greater frequency, including a persistent posterior gap, undermedialization, and implant malposition, generally in too anterior or superior a position.

Persistent posterior glottic gap can account for as many as 50% of revisions in cases where arytenoid adduction has not been performed.[43] Revision medialization alone is generally ineffective in shifting arytenoid position. Even when the implant can displace the vocal process of the arytenoid medially, it cannot remedy a height mismatch, nor can it readily correct a mismatch in vocal fold tension, which is commonly found in cases of paralysis.

Undercorrection is another relatively frequent cause of poor results,[44] and may be especially likely to occur in cases that last longer than usual and allow the accumulation of intraoperative edema to mislead the surgeon regarding the degree of medialization required. In these cases, the initial voice result is satisfactory, but deteriorates with time as swelling resolves.

Netterville and Billante[45] have reported placing the implant too far superior as the most common cause for revision in their series, an error that probably arises from misconceptions regarding position of the vibratory margin of the fold in relation to the profile of the thyroid lamina. Too anterior an implant placement, on the other hand, likely arises from a poor appreciation of the overall length of the thyroid lamina and yields early mucosal contact during adduction, damping of phonatory oscillation, and a characteristic strained or pressed voice quality.

Arytenoid Repositioning Procedures

Although injection laryngoplasty and medialization thyroplasty provide excellent results and may be adequate treatment in many patients, some individuals require repositioning of the arytenoid to achieve optimal voicing. The typical clinical scenario involves an arytenoid that is tipped anteriorly into the airway and externally rotated, resulting in a flaccid foreshortened vocal fold with a lateralized vocal process. Despite successful medialization of the anterior membranous vocal fold, the vocal processes do not approximate, leaving a posterior gap and a vertical mismatch of the vocal fold level.

Several procedures to manipulate the arytenoid are described. The most common procedure is the placement of an *arytenoid adduction* suture (Figure 17-6). This suture theoretically mimics the action of the thyroarytenoid-lateral cricoarytenoid (TA-LCA) muscle complex and achieves glottal closure by internal rotation of the vocal process. Although some debate continues regarding the physiologic effect of arytenoid adduction, most surgeons agree that this procedure rotates the arytenoid cartilage medially, displaces the vocal process caudally and medially, and stabilizes the vocal process.[46,47] This effectively aids in closing a posterior gap and re-establishes vocal fold tension, which in turn improves glottic performance during phonation, particularly at increased vocal intensity.

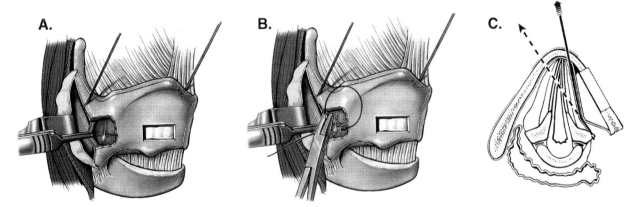

FIGURE 17–6. Arytenoid adduction suture. **A.** The arytenoid can be approached through exposure of the posterior edge of the thyroid lamina after the attachments of the inferior constrictor are dissected free. The mucosa of the piriform sinus is elevated from the internal surface of the cartilage, and a posterior fenestra can be created using a Kerrison punch. **B.** A stitch is placed through the muscular process of the arytenoid, mimicking the action of the lateral-cricoarytenoid muscle by bringing the free ends of the stitch through the thyroplasty window. **C.** An axial view showing the vector of pull of the arytenoid adduction stitch with a thyroplasty implant in place. (Reprinted from Ossoff R, *The Larynx.* Baltimore, Md: Lippincott Williams & Wilkins; 2003:296-297 with permission. Copyright, 2003 Lippincott, Williams & Wilkins.)

Exposure of the arytenoid requires approach around or through the posterior margin of the thyroid lamina, elevation of the piriform sinus mucosa, and identification of the muscular process. Most surgeons facilitate exposure by removing the posterior portion of the thyroid cartilage overlying the arytenoid and piriform with a rongeur. A nonabsorbable suture is passed through the muscular process of the arytenoid and tension placed anterolaterally to approximate the action of the thyroarytenoid-lateral cricoarytenoid (TA-LCA) muscle complex. Once rotation is judged adequate, the suture is secured to the thyroid cartilage. Very little tension is required on the arytenoid adduction suture.

Regardless of the exact technique chosen, arytenoid repositioning procedures are designed to internally rotate and/or suspend the arytenoid in the physiologic phonatory position. These procedures are technically challenging, time consuming, and have a higher rate of complications than simple medialization.[48] Elevation of the piriform sinus mucosa is a delicate task and presents an additional opportunity for perforation. Airway complications are more frequent due to additional manipulation and resultant edema. Despite these concerns, for the accomplished phonosurgeon, these procedures are an essential adjunct to medialization thyroplasty to achieve an optimal vocal outcome.

Laryngeal Reinnervation

Restoration of physiologic adductor and abductor function is the idealized goal of reinnervation procedures. Many methods of selective reinnervation have been described, including neuromuscular transfer, selective neural anastomosis, and direct nerve implantation, but reliable restoration of physiologic function has not been realized to date. Additionally there are no alternative donor nerves that will provide the complex respiratory and phonatory neural signals required. Thus, current reinnervation techniques restore neural input to the intrinsic laryngeal muscles to mimic the natural reinnervation process, thereby restoring the bulk and tone of the vocal fold and arytenoid musculature.

In cases of obvious nerve transection, primary nerve reanastomosis is probably worthwhile and beneficial, providing that sufficient length exists for tension-free approximation. When the procedure is performed for an intact nerve, the recurrent laryngeal nerve can be anastomosed to an alternative donor nerve, similar to facial reanimation techniques utilizing the XII to VII jump graft, in the hope that the number of functional axonal connections after reinnervation will exceed the existing quantity of functional axonal connections. Both the ansa cervicalis[49] and hypoglossal[50,51] have been proposed for this role, although in the second case, the surgeon must weigh carefully the added morbidity of hemitongue denervation.

The neuromuscular pedicle (NMP) technique involves transfer of a nerve with a small block of muscle (ansa cercicalis with omohyoid) into a denervated laryngeal muscle bed to encourage graft implantation with eventual arborization of the donor nerve into the host muscle. Again, the goal is to maintain bulk and tone of the thyroarytenoid muscle over time. These procedures can be combined with a medialization thyroplasty.

SPECIAL ISSUES IN PARALYSIS

Isolated SLN Paresis

Superior laryngeal nerve paresis manifests as sensory loss from the internal branch with motor weakness of the cricothyroideus muscle innervated from the external branch. Several authors have demonstrated a high association between SLN injury and dysfunction of the cricopharyngeus muscle, thus contributing to dysphagia.[52] This can occur independently of recurrent nerve injury and can be iatrogenic (thyroidectomy, neck dissection) or idiopathic. The sensory loss can cause throat clearing, coughing, and a globus sensation. Bilateral sensory loss can lead to aspiration. The vocal characteristics are due to loss of

Vocal Fold Position in Paralysis

Historically, it was felt that topographic information regarding the location of a neurologic insult along the course of the vagal nerve could be gained through evaluation of laryngeal and vocal fold position. Thus, a lesion of the recurrent nerve in isolation would theoretically give a vocal fold in the paramedian position, a lesion of the superior laryngeal nerve would be demonstrated by rotation of the laryngeal posterior commisure toward the side of nerve dysfunction, and a lesion of the vagal trunk would give a vocal fold in the cadaveric or lateral position. Theories such as the Wagner-Grossman hypothesis attempted to explain vocal fold position based on the presence or absence of cricothyroid muscle activity; Semon's law held that there was a differential vulnerability of nerve fibers to injury with the abductors affected first, followed by the adductors.[6] These theories, although prevalent in historical literature, have been successfully challenged by contemporary investigators. It is currently accepted that laryngeal and vocal fold position does not reliably correlate with the site of vagal nerve injury.[7,53,54]

symmetric cricothyroideus function. Although individuals without complicated vocal demands may not notice any vocal defect, singers will complain of a ceiling effect—inability to reach their highest registers. Additionally, individuals may complain of voice fatigue and diplophonia. On exam, pooling in the piriform on the affected side reflects the sensory defect, and rotation of the posterior commissure toward the side of the paralysis may occur during phonatory effort. The diagnosis can be confirmed by LEMG. Unfortunately, in the absence of spontaneous recovery, there are no unique medical or surgical interventions available for this process.

Bilateral Vocal Fold Immobility

Bilateral vocal fold immobility has a similar legion of etiologies, although with a differing incidence as compared to unilateral vocal fold immobility. Bilateral vocal fold paralysis is most often a result of surgical misadventure, with thyroidectomy accounting for the majority of cases. Fixation from posterior glottic stenosis after prolonged intubation, radiation-induced fibrosis, and infiltrative disorders (amyloid and granulomatous diseases) may mimic bilateral nerve injury. Esophageal malignancy extending to the tracheoesophageal groove may account for up to half of neoplastic causes.[5] The voice is usually close to normal, but patients may develop significant airway compromise from inability to abduct the vocal folds. Interestingly, even after bilateral injury, patients may tolerate the restricted airway for days to years before developing symptoms, which may then be misdiagnosed as asthma or bronchitis before the airway is examined. If the airway compromise is severe, an emergency tracheotomy may be required. This is best done awake as it may not be absolutely evident if the embarrassment is due to nerve injury or laryngeal fixation.

Once the nature and cause of the bilateral immobility is established, treatment should be determined by symptomatology. Although the best function is often obtained with tracheotomy, many patients are reluctant to accept this option. Vocal fold lateralization procedures for decannulation, such as a laser posterior cordotomy[55] and arytenoidectomy,[56] are destructive and irreversible. These procedures are designed to maintain approximation of the anterior membranous vocal folds for phonation but increase the posterior aperture for improved airflow. The Lichtenberger tech-nique of suture lateralization can be performed as a reversible or permanent method of opening the airway in these cases.[57,58] Bilateral vocal fold immobility is one of the greatest challenges in the treatment of benign laryngeal disorders.

Pediatric Laryngeal Nerve Paralysis

The symptoms and etiology of vocal fold immobility in children is different from adults and varies with the age of the patient population. Causes include surgical trauma (cardiac and thoracic), neurologic disease (Arnold-Chiari malformation and other neurologic defects), birth trauma, and idiopathic. Paralysis is the predominant cause of immobility, the second-most common cause of neonatal stridor (laryngomalacia being the first), and may account for 10% of congenital anomalies of the larynx.[59] Daya in 2000[60] reported a series from Great Ormond Street in which the percentage of bilateral immobility was approximately equal to that of unilateral immobility. As opposed to adults, unilateral immobility often causes stridor in addition to a weak cry, feeding difficulties, and aspiration. Also in contrast to adults, children with bilateral vocal fold paralysis may not require tracheotomy and may have a higher rate of spontaneous recovery.[60] Evaluation includes a complete neurologic exam, magnetic resonance imaging of the brain, neck, and mediastinum, fiberoptic laryngoscopy, and rigid endoscopy under anesthesia, as up to half of patients may have an associated upper airway anomaly. In the past, treatment is conservative as patients have shown a propensity to compensate over a number of years. The rate of actual vocal fold motion recovery is not known.

In most cases, vocal fold immobility or hypomobility is neurogenic, caused by disease of or traumatic insult to the laryngeal nerves. Mechanical factors may result in cricoarytenoid fixation,

usually after prolonged intubation or other trauma. Some cases of paralysis resolve, or at least improve symptomatically, without intervention; others require treatment. Distinguishing between these two groups remains a challenge, and many otolaryngologists consequently choose to delay treatment, sometimes despite considerable patient disability. In cases of unilateral paralysis, a broad armamentarium of procedures is available to alleviate symptoms including temporary and permanent injection laryngoplasty, medialization thyroplasty, arytenoid repositioning, and reinnervation procedures.

Review Questions

1. Describe in detail the types of laryngeal injectables, their duration, and potential complications.

2. Why do some individuals with a vocal fold paralysis have an adequate voice, and other individuals suffer extreme glottic insufficiency?

3. What findings on LEMG predict a favorable prognosis for return of function?
   a. Activation of motor unit potentials during an appropriate task, absence of fibrillation potentials, preservation of motor unit morphology
   b. Polyphasic motor unit potentials and decreased recruitment pattern
   c. Fibrillation potentials and positive sharp waves (spontaneous activity)
   d. Bilateral mildly diminished recruitment
   e. Electrical silence

4. Does reinnervation correlate with return of motion?

5. What are the treatment options for bilateral vocal fold immobility? What are the risks and benefits of each option?

6. A 45-year-old female undergoes a right thyroid lobectomy for benign disease and has a breathy voice postoperatively. Right vocal fold immobility is confirmed by endoscopy. LEMG at 1 month shows polyphasic potentials and absence of fibrillation potentials. She would like a better voice and has no swallowing complaints. What treatment option would you offer her?
   a. None as she has a good chance of spontaneous recovery
   b. Injection laryngoplasty with a permanent material
   c. Injection laryngoplasty with a temporary material with an option for future type I thyroplasty if there is inadequate return of function
   d. Type I thyroplasty and arytenoid adduction

REFERENCES

1. Merati AL, Shemirani N, Smith TL, Toohill RJ. Changing trends in the nature of vocal fold motion impairment. *Am J Otolaryngol.* 2006; 27(2):106-108.
2. Weisberg NK, Spengler DM, Netterville JL. Stretch-induced nerve injury as a cause of paralysis secondary to the anterior cervical approach. *Otolaryngol Head Neck Surg.* 1997;116(3):317-326.
3. Terris, DJ, Arnstein D, Nguyen HH, Contemporary evaluation of unilateral vocal cord paralysis. *Otolaryngol Head Neck Surg.* 1992;107(1):84-90.
4. Maisel RH, Ogura JH. Evaluation of vocal cord paralysis. *Laryngoscope.* 1974;84(2):302-316.
5. Benninger MS, Gillen JB, Altman JS. Changing etiology of vocal fold immobility. *Laryngoscope.* 1998;108(9):1346-1350.
6. Rubin AD, et al. Arytenoid cartilage dislocation: a 20-year experience. *J Voice.* 2005;19(4):687-701.
7. Blitzer A, Jahn AF, Keidar A, Semon's law revisited: an electromyographic analysis of laryngeal synki-

nesis. *Ann Otol Rhinol Laryngol.* 1996;105(10): 764-769.
8. Crumley RL, McCabe BF. Regeneration of the recurrent laryngeal nerve. *Otolaryngol Head Neck Surg.* 1982;90(4):442-447.
9. Zealear DL, Hamdan AL, Rainey CL, Effects of denervation on posterior cricoarytenoid muscle physiology and histochemistry. *Ann Otol Rhinol Laryngol.* 1994;103(10):780-788.
10. Netterville JL, Stone RE, Rainey C, Zealear DL, Ossoff RH. Recurrent laryngeal nerve avulsion for treatment of spastic dysphonia. *Ann Otol Rhinol Laryngol.* 1991;100(1):10-14.
11. Crumley RL, Laryngeal synkinesis revisited. *Ann Otol Rhinol Laryngol.* 2000;109(4):365-371.
12. Kent RD, Kent JF, Rosenbek JC, Maximum performance tests of speech production. *J Speech Hear Disord.* 1987;52(4):367-387.
13. Merati AL, Halum S, Smith TL. Diagnostic testing for vocal paralysis: A survey of contemporary practice and evidence-based medicine review. In press.
14. Jackson C. Jackson CL. *The Larynx and Its Diseases.* Philadelphia, Pa: WB Saunders; 1937.
15. Belafsky PC, Postma GN, Reulbach TR, Holland BW, Koufman JA. Muscle tension dysphonia as a sign of underlying glottal insufficiency. *Otolaryngol Head Neck Surg.* 2002;127(5):448-451.
16. Altman, JS, Benninger MS, The evaluation of unilateral vocal fold immobility: is chest X-ray enough? *J Voice.* 1997;11(3):364-367.
17. Glazer, H.S., et al., Extralaryngeal causes of vocal cord paralysis: CT evaluation. *Am J Roentgenol.* 1983;141(3):527-531.
18. Tabaee A, et al., Flexible endoscopic evaluation of swallowing with sensory testing in patients with unilateral vocal fold immobility: incidence and pathophysiology of aspiration. *Laryngoscope.* 2005;115(4):565-569.
19. Bhattacharyya N, Kotz T, and Shapiro J, Dysphagia and aspiration with unilateral vocal cord immobility: incidence, characterization, and response to surgical treatment. *Ann Otol Rhinol Laryngol.* 2002;111(8):672-679.
20. Heitmiller RF, Tseng E, Jones B. Prevalence of aspiration and laryngeal penetration in patients with unilateral vocal fold motion impairment. *Dysphagia.* 2000;15(4):184-187.
21. Flint, PW, Purcell LL, Cummings CW, Pathophysiology and indications for medialization thyroplasty in patients with dysphagia and aspiration. *Otolaryngol Head Neck Surg.* 1997;116(3):349-354.

22 Bielamowicz S. Gupta A, Sekhar LN, Early arytenoid adduction for vagal paralysis after skull base surgery. *Laryngoscope.* 2000;110(3 pt 1):346-351.

23. Netterville JL. Civantos FJ. Rehabilitation of cranial nerve deficits after neurotologic skull base surgery. *Laryngoscope.* 1993;103(11 pt 2 suppl 60): 45-54.

24. Bhattacharyya N, Batirel H, Swanson SJ, Improved outcomes with early vocal fold medialization for vocal fold paralysis after thoracic surgery. *Auris Nasus Larynx.* 2003;30(1):71-75.

25. Mom T., Filaire M, Advenier D, et al. Concomitant type I thyroplasty and thoracic operations for lung cancer: preventing respiratory complications associated with vagus or recurrent laryngeal nerve injury. *J Thorac Cardiovasc Surg.* 2001; 121(4): 642-648.

26. Abraham MT, Bains MS, Downey RJ, Korst RJ, Kraus DH. Type I thyroplasty for acute unilateral vocal fold paralysis following intrathoracic surgery. *Ann Otol Rhinol Laryngol.* 2002;111(8): 667-671.

27. Nayak VK, Bhattacharyya N, Kotz T, Shapiro J. Patterns of swallowing failure following medialization in unilateral vocal fold immobility. *Laryngoscope.* 2002;112(10):1840-1844.

28. Willatt DJ Stell PM. The prognosis and management of idiopathic vocal cord paralysis. *Clin Otolaryngol Allied Sci.* 1989;14(3):247-250.

29. Ward PH. Berci G. Observations on so-called idiopathic vocal cord paralysis. *Ann Otol Rhinol Laryngol.* 1982;91(6 pt 1):558-563.

30. Hirano M, et al. Electromyography for laryngeal paralysis. In: Hirano M, Kirchner JA, Bless DM, eds. *Neurolaryngology: Recent Advances.* San Diego, Calif: Singular Publishing; 1991:232-248.

31. Sittel C. et al. Prognostic value of laryngeal electromyography in vocal fold paralysis. *Arch Otolaryngol Head Neck Surg.* 2001;127(2):155-160.

32. Parnes SM, Satya-Murti S. Predictive value of laryngeal electromyography in patients with vocal cord paralysis of neurogenic origin. *Laryngoscope.* 1985;95(11):1323-1326.

33. Munin MC,Rosen CA, Zullo T. Utility of laryngeal electromyography in predicting recovery after vocal fold paralysis. *Arch Phys Med Rehabil.* 2003;84(8):1150-1153.

34. Mostafa BE, Gadallah NA, Nassar NM, Al Ibiary HM, Fahmy HA, Fouda NM. The role of laryngeal electromyography in vocal fold immobility. *J Otorhinolaryngol Relat Spec.* 2004;66(1):5-10.

35. Gupta SR, Bastian RW. Use of laryngeal electromyography in prediction of recovery after vocal cord paralysis. *Muscle Nerve.* 1993;16(9):977-978.

36. Hollinger LD, Hollinger PC, Hollinger PH. Etiology of bilateral abductor vocal cord parlaysis: a review of 389 cases. *Ann Otol Rhinol Laryngol.* 1976; 85(4 pt 1):428-436

37 Rosen CA, Thekdi AA. Vocal fold augmentation with injectable calcium hydroxylapatite: short-term results. *J Voice.* 2004;18(3):387-391.

38. Payr E. Plastik am Schildknorpel zur Behebung der Folgen einseitiger Stimmbandlähmung. *Deutsche Med Wochenshr.* 1915;41:1265.

39. Isshiki N, Morita H, Okamura H, Hiramoto M. Thyroplasty as a new phonosurgical technique. *Acta Otolaryngol.* 1974;78(5-6):451-477.

40. Weinman EC, Maragos NE, Airway compromise in thyroplasty surgery. *Laryngoscope.* 2000;110(7): 1082-1085.

41. Rosen CA. Complications of phonosurgery: results of a national survey. *Laryngoscope.* 1998; 108(11 pt 1):1697-1703.

42. Anderson TD, Spiegel JR, Sataloff RT. Thyroplasty revisions: frequency and predictive factors. *J Voice.* 2003;17(3): 442-448.

43. Woo P, et al. Failed medialization laryngoplasty: management by revision surgery. *Otolaryngol Head Neck Surg.* 2001;124(6):615-621.

44. Cohen JT, Bates DD, Postma GN. Revision Gore-Tex medialization laryngoplasty. *Otolaryngol Head Neck Surg.* 2004;131(3):236-240.

45. Netterville JL, Billante CR. The immobile vocal fold. In: Ossoff RH, Shapshay SM, Woodson GE, Netterville JL. eds. *The Larynx.* Philadelphia, Pa: Lippincott, Williams & Wilkins, 2004:269-305.

46. Woodson G. Cricopharyngeal myotomy and arytenoid adduction in the management of combined laryngeal and pharyngeal paralysis. *Otolaryngol Head Neck Surg.* 1997;116(3):339-343.

47. Woodson GE, et al. Arytenoid adduction: controlling vertical position. *Ann Otol Rhinol Laryngol.* 2000;109(4):360-364.

48. Abraham MT, Gonen M, Kraus DH. Complications of type I thyroplasty and arytenoid adduction. *Laryngoscope.* 2001;111(8):1322-1329.

49. Crumley RL, Update: ansa cervicalis to recurrent laryngeal nerve anastomosis for unilateral laryngeal paralysis. *Laryngoscope.* 1991;101(4 pt 1): 384-387. Discussion, 388.

50. Paniello RC. Lee P, Dahm JD. Hypoglossal nerve transfer for laryngeal reinnervation: a preliminary

study. *Ann Otol Rhinol Laryngol.* 1999. 108(3): 239-244.

51. Paniello RC, West SE, Lee P, Laryngeal reinnervation with the hypoglossal nerve. I. Physiology, histochemistry, electromyography, and retrograde labeling in a canine model. *Ann Otol Rhinol Laryngol.* 2001;110(6):532-542.

52. Halum S. et al. Electromyography findings of the cricopharyngeus in association with ipsilateral pharyngeal and laryngeal muscles. *Ann Otol Rhinol Laryngol.* In press.

53. Koufman JA, Walker FO, Joharji GM. The cricothyroid muscle does not influence vocal fold position in laryngeal paralysis. *Laryngoscope.* 1995; 105(4 pt 1):368-372.

54. Woodson GE. Configuration of the glottis in laryngeal paralysis. I: Clinical study. *Laryngoscope.* 1993;103(11 pt 1):1227-1234.

55. Kashima HK. Bilateral vocal fold motion impairment: pathophysiology and management by transverse cordotomy. *Ann Otol Rhinol Laryngol.* 1991;100(9 pt 1):717-721.

56. Ossoff RH, Sisson GA, Duncavage JA, Moselle HI, Andrews PE, McMillan WG. Endoscopic laser arytenoidectomy for the treatment of bilateral vocal cord paralysis. *Laryngoscope.* 1984;94(10): 1293-1297.

57. Lichtenberger G. Reversible lateralization of the paralyzed vocal cord without tracheostomy. *Ann Otol Rhinol Laryngol.* 2002;111(1):21-26.

58. Lichtenberger G. Comparison of endoscopic glottis-dilating operations. *Eur Arch Otorhinolaryngol.* 2003;260(2):57-61.

59. Holinger PH, Brown WT. Congenital webs, cysts, laryngoceles and other anomalies of the larynx. *Ann Otol Rhinol Laryngol* 1967; 76(4):744-752.

60. Daya H, Hosni A, Bejar-Solar I, Evans JN, Bailey CN. Pediatric vocal fold paralysis: a long-term retrospective study. *Arch Otolaryngol Head Neck Surg,* 2000;126(1):21-25.

61. Vilensky JA, Sinish PR. Semon and Semon's law. *Clin Anal.* 2004;17(8):605-606.

The Larynx in Parkinson's Disease

Mona M. Abaza, MD
Jennifer Spielman, MA, CCC-SLP

KEY POINTS

■ Parkinson's disease is a common progressive degenerative neurologic disorder in which significant dysphonia is present in at least 70% of cases.

■ A soft, breathy, monotone voice with or without a tremor is typical. The dysphonia can be associated with poor articulation, difficulty initiating speech, stutteringlike quality, and "flat" affect. Videostroboscopic examination of the larynx can provide helpful diagnostic characteristics such as glottal incompetence and decreased vocal fold vibration.

■ Parkinson's plus syndrome, a more severe and rapidly degenerating process, demonstrates more significant changes such as vocal fold paralysis and more significant tremor.

■ Systemic treatments of the disease, although often helping limb motion abnormalities, do not always help with vocal issues, whereas the Lee Silverman Voice Therapy (LSVT) has been shown to improve the dysphonia.

■ Dysphagia is a common complaint associated with the disorder and oropharyngeal abnormalities are present in almost all patients.

Parkinson's disease (PD), the most common movement disorder in patients over 55 years of age, affects an estimated 1.5 million people in the United States. It is a degenerative process of the brainstem nuclei significantly affecting the *substantia nigra*, creating decreased dopamine availability as the fundamental deficiency. Characteristic physical changes include resting tremors of the arms and legs, pill-rolling tremor movements at rest, overall rigidity, a festinating gait, reduced arm swing, and a slow initiation of movement. Approximately 70 to 89% of all patients demonstrate vocal difficulties with the disease, and over 30% of these patients find it the most disabling part of the disorder for them.[1] Dysphagia has been reported in most patients with oropharyngeal abnormalities seen on videofluoroscopy in almost all patients. Choking, piecemeal deglutition, regurgitation, and aspiration (silent and known) can all be present.[2] Postural abnormalities, olfactory dysfunction, depression, and micrographia are also reported as systemic components of PD.

The most characteristic voice in PD patients is soft, breathy, and monotonal. The voice is perceived by the patient as normal in loudness and quality, although it is not. A resting vocal tremor is also a common component, present in 55% of patients with idiopathic PD.[3] Vertical laryngeal movement secondary to tremor of the strap muscles is evident even at rest. The tremor occurs when the affected body part is at repose and completely supported. In general, it occurs at a rate of 4 to 10 Hz, whereas physiologic tremors occur at faster rates, 8 to 12 Hz, and cerebellar tremors are slower, 2 to 5 Hz.[4-6] Other components of the speech abnormalities include poor articulation, a variable rate speech, a stuttering-like voice quality, difficulty initiating speech, reduced facial expression, and overall "flat" affects. The speech of PD, although often breathy and of low intensity, does not always demonstrate the changes in a typical rhythmic fashion. Rather, the hypophonia is constant, with exacerbation by the articulatory difficulties and the cognitive problems associated with the disease.

The diagnosis of Parkinson's disease is often made by a neurologist, but dysphonia may be the first presentation, and the otolaryngologist may be the first to recognize the disorder. Assessing the fluidity of the voice, the quality of articulation, and the quality of the voice signal itself are easily accomplished by active listening during the patient history. As the differentiation of abnormal fluidity from poor articulation is important in differentiating PD from other movement disorders affecting the voice, such as essential tremors and stroke, an oral mechanism evaluation can be useful in these situations. Assessment of voice quality should include an assessment of the overall degree of dysphonia and the presence of raspiness, breathiness, and/or strain, which can be indications of other vocal pathology. Flexible fiberoptic and videostroboscopic examination findings are helpful in the diagnosis of PD. The examination of the larynx should be performed at rest and during a variety of phonatory tasks. Typically both a flexible fiberoptic scope and a rigid laryngoscope, each providing different information, are used in a complete exam. Whereas rigid stroboscopy allows one to assess the vibratory function and detailed anatomic structure of the vocal folds, portions of the neurolaryngeal examination are best performed with a flexible transnasal endoscope. Lingual traction, required for a transoral examinations, does not allow for connected speech evaluations, and the change in tongue position may suppress characteristic diagnostic signs.

Vocal fold bowing, midfold opening of the glottis during phonation, and a slowed vibration are considered characteristic of PD. Glottal incompetence is one of the most consistent findings described. Detected more commonly during rigid examination of the larynx, bowing may be over-called (due to distortion of the laryngeal anatomy by the rigid scoping procedure. The hypophonia of PD is considered a manifestation of incomplete glottic closure and poor breath support resulting from the chest wall rigidity. A paralyzed vocal fold can be a sign of Parkinson's plus syndromes. PPS includes multisystem degeneration,

Shy-Drager syndrome, basal ganglia degeneration, and progressive supranuclear palsy. These disorders show a more rapid progressive deterioration of motor functions, with significantly worse speech deficits. Vocal tremor is found in 55% of idiopathic Parkinson's patients, but 64% of Parkinson's plus patients. Stroboscopy findings of open phase closure and asymmetric vibration are more commonly found in general PD than in PPS.[2] Other findings on laryngeal exam include pooled hypopharyngeal secretions, decreased sensation, diminished cough reflex, and aspiration.

Diagnostic studies such as EMG and objective voice measures may provide some information in patients with PD. Single motor unit laryngeal EMG studies have been investigated in younger and older patients with PD of both sexes. A decreased firing rate and increased variability are seen in older patients and males only.[7] Objective instrumental measures of voice have revealed elevated jitter and shimmer and decreased harmonic-to-noise ratio, s/z ratio, and maximum phonation time in tremulous voices, abnormalities shared with other conditions of glottic insufficiency.[8] In addition, a brief generalized neurologic examination encompassing the upper extremities and gait can identify and reveal other characteristic signs of PD such as bradykinesia and cogwheeling.

TREATMENT

In addition to studying treatment of the overall disease process and its effect on communication, several treatments directed at the dysphonia of PD have been attempted, Collagen augmentation of the vocal folds has demonstrated temporary effectiveness (11/18 patients showing improvements lasting >2 months). No improvement of the articulatory function has been seen and often repeat procedures are required. It is also not as effective in severely affected patients.[9,10] Thalamic deep brain stimulation (DBS) by means of implanted electrodes, a neurosurgical intervention, is an evolving means of treating disabling, medication-resistant tremor and PD. Initial reports of postoperative dysarthria, particularly after bilateral procedures, created reservations about its utility in voice tremor, as speech and voice require a high degree of coordination. The procedure shows limited improvements to voice and speech function in PD, despite significant changes in limb movements.[11] Evidence does suggest DBS may be practical and useful in the treatment of the voice tremor component.[12-15] Standard Parkinson's treatment with L-dopa has had mixed results in PD dysphonia. Decreased jitter and increased fundamental frequency in a mildly affected population are shown by some, but not others.[16]

Despite the many forms of therapies tried, only behaviorally based intervention has been shown to have an effect on the voice and speech functions of patients with PD. Lee Silverman Voice Treatment (LSVT), an intensive rehabilitative program, is designed to increase intensity by increasing phonatory effort and maximum adductory vocal tasks. This approach depends on a behaviorally based system to generalize the increased effort by the patient toward audibly louder speech. LSVT should be administered by a speech pathologist certified in the therapy, as the program relies on carefully defined processes. Numerous studies have shown a sustained or improved vocal intensity over pretreatment levels.[17] Laryngeal examinations show a decrease in glottal incompetence without a significant change in supraglottal hyperfunctioning.[18] Swallowing function appears to be improved after treatment as well. Changes in tongue movement, both in the oral (lateral movement) and pharyngeal phase (tongue base retraction), are reduced post-therapy and appear to be a significant component of the noted decreased oral and pharyngeal transit time.[19] More research is underway to confirm and elaborate on these findings. Preliminary studies, using PET scans, show reduced activity in the globus pallidus, an effect similar to pallidotomy.[19] Initial data show that improvement in the overall affect and facial expression of the patient may be improved by this therapy as well.[20]

The Effects of the Lee Silverman Voice Therapy (LSVT) on Emotional Expression in PD

Impaired emotional expression is a common consequence of PD, marked by reduction of both vocal[21] and facial[22] mobility and variability. Despite the potentially serious social and medical consequences of decreased expressivity[24] efforts to improve expression in PD have been few, and the success limited.[24-26]

As described in this chapter, the LSVT was developed to specifically treat the speech and voice deficits associated with PD[28] and is considered among the most efficacious speech treatments for PD.[28,29] It is showing unexpected and far-reaching effects beyond the improvement of voice and speech. One such improvement appears to be an increase in facial expressivity. In a recent prospective, randomized pilot study,[30] 36 individuals with PD received either respiratory therapy (n = 14) or LSVT (n = 22) and were videotaped before and after treatment. Twenty-second video samples were judged by inexperienced observers on "expressivity," defined as *meaningful* and *communicative* facial movement. The data revealed a positive trend ($p = 0.067$) in the direction of the LSVT group.

A more detailed study using the same group of subjects was done with six trained female raters[31] These raters were trained to examine multiple variables for facial expression, including *mobility*, *engagement*, and *positive emotion*. Results indicate that members of the LSVT group were perceived as having increased their facial *mobility* ($p = 0.036$) and *engagement* ($p = 0.056$) following treatment relative to members of the respiratory group. Additionally, the LSVT group demonstrated a greater extent of change for facial *mobility* after treatment compared to the respiratory group ($p = 0.05$) (see Figure 18-1)

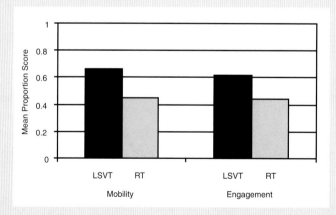

FIGURE 18–1. Mean ratings for facial mobility and engagement

Ongoing research is underway to examine facial expression using more detailed protocols, and to evaluate the effects of the LSVT on specific areas of vocal expressivity. A quick look at the speech of one subject receiving LSVT shows the extent of change in voice variability and quality during spontaneous speech that is typical following treatment (Figure 18–2).

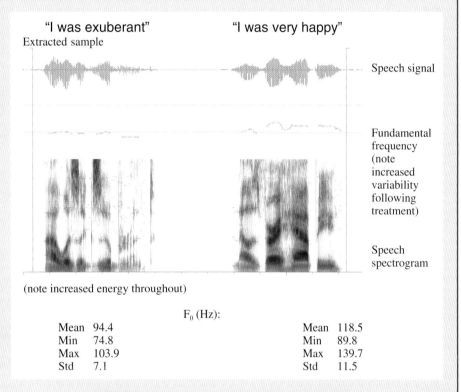

"I was exuberant"
Extracted sample

"I was very happy"

Speech signal

Fundamental frequency (note increased variability following treatment)

Speech spectrogram

(note increased energy throughout)

F_0 (Hz):

Mean	94.4		Mean	118.5
Min	74.8		Min	89.8
Max	103.9		Max	139.7
Std	7.1		Std	11.5

FIGURE 18–2. Pre- versus post-LSVT therapy.

Further evaluation is necessary to quantify the type and extent of change, and determine whether these quantitative results reflect functional improvements in expression and communication for individuals with PD. Ideally, this programmatic approach to the study of communicative disorders will yield benefit beyond the voice and speech

Parkinson's disease is a very common motor disorder with significant voice and speech, and swallowing components. The otolaryngologist and trained speech pathologist, particularly through the Lee Silverman Voice Treatment, can play a large role in the rehabilitation of these patients by both identification of the disorder in its early stages and in provision of treatment.

Review Questions

1. Vocal complaints are present in approximately what percentage of Parkinson's disease patients?
   a. 20%
   b. 40%
   c. 60%
   d. 80%
   e. 100%

2. Parkinson's tremor occurs at which frequency range?
   a. 1 to 2 Hz
   b. 4 to 10 Hz
   c. 10 to 20 Hz
   d. It cannot be measured

3. The best established treatment for patients with dysphonia related to Parkinson's disease is:
   a. Vocal resonance therapy
   b. Lee Silverman Voice Treatment
   c. Collagen injection laryngoplasty
   d. Deep brain stimulation
   e. Pallidotomy

4. According to estimates, Parkinson's affects approximately what number of persons in the United States?
   a. 500,000
   b. 1,000,000
   c. 1,500,000
   d. 2,000,000
   e. 2,500,000

REFERENCES

1. Hartelius L, Svensson P. Speech and swallowing symptoms associated with Parkinson's disease and multiple sclerosis: a survey. *Folia Phoniatr Logoped*. 1994;46:9–17.

2. Monte FS, da Silva-Junior FP, Braga-Neto P, Nobre e Souza MA, Sales de Bruin VM. Swallowing abnor-malities and dyskinesia in Parkinson's disease. *Mov Disord*. 2005;20(4):457–462.

3. Perez KS, Ramig LO, Smith ME, Dromey C. The Parkinson larynx: tremor and videostroboscopic findings. *J Voice*. 1996;10:354–361.

4. Elble RJ. Diagnostic criteria for essential tremor and differential diagnosis. *Neurology*. 2000;54 (suppl 4):S2–S6.

5. Fahn S, Greene PE, Ford B, Bressman SB. *Handbook of Movement Disorders*. Philadelphia, Pa; Current Medicine, Inc, 1998.

6. Findley LJ. Epidemiology and genetics of essential tremor. *Neurology*. 2000;54(suppl 4):S8–S13.

7. Luschei ES, Ramig LO, Baker KL, et al. Discharge characteristics of laryngeal single motor units during phonation in younger and older adults and in persons with Parkinson's disease. *J Neurophysiol*. 1999;81:2131–2139.

8. Gamboa J, Jimenez-Jimenez FJ, Nieto A, et al. Acoustic voice analysis in patients with essential tremor. *J Voice*. 1998;12:444–452.

9. Kim SH, Kearney JJ, Atkins JP. Percutaneous laryngeal augmentation for treatment of Parkinsonian hypophonia. *Otolaryngol Head Neck Surg*. 2002;126:653–656.

10. Berke GS, Gerratt B, Kreiman J, et al. Treatment of Parkinson's hypophonia with percutaneous collagen augmentation. *Laryngoscope*. 1999;109:1295–1299.

11. Gentil M, Chauvin P, Pinto S, et al. Effect of bilateral stimulation of the subthalamic nucleus on Parkinsonian voice. *Brain Lang.*. 2001;78:233–240.

12. Carpenter MA, Pahwa R, Miyawaki KL, Wilkinson SB, Send JP, Koller WC. Reduction in voice tremor under thalamic stimulation. *Neurology*. 1998;50:796–798.

13. Yoon MS, Munz M, Sataloff RT, Spiegel JR, Heuer RJ. Vocal tremor reduction with deep brain stimulation. *Stereotact Funct Neurosurg*. 1999;72:241–244.

14. Pahwa R, Lyons K, Koller WC. Surgical treatment of essential tremor. *Neurology*. 2000;54 (suppl 4):S39–S44.

15. Taha JM, Janszen MA, Favre J. Thalamic deep brain stimulation for the treatment of head, voice and bilateral limb tremor. *J Neurosurg*. 1999;91:68–72.

16. Dedo HH. Recurrent laryngeal nerve section for spastic dysphonia. *Ann Otol Rhinol Laryngol*. 1976;85:451–459.

17. Poluha PC, Euling HL, Brookshire RH. Handwriting and speech changes across the levodopa cycle

in Parkinson's disease. *Acta Psychol.* 1998;100: 71-84.

18. Ramig LO, Sapir S, Countryman S, et al. Intensive voice treatment (LSVT) for patients with Parkinson's disease: a two year follow up. *J Neurol.* 2001;71:493-498.

19. Liotti M, Ramig LO, Vogel D, et al. Hypophonia in Parkinson's patients:neural correlates of voice treatment revealed by PET. *Neurology.* 2003;60: 432-440.

20. Sharkawi AE, Ramig LO, Logemann JA, et al. Swallowing and voice effects of Lee Silverman Voice Treatment (LSVT): a pilot study. *J Neurology Neurosurg Psychiatry.* 2002;72:31-36.

21. Stewart C, Winfield L, Hunt A. Bressman S. Fahn, S. Blitzer A. Brin M. Speech dysfunction in early Parkinson's disease. *Mov Disord.* 1995;10(5):1995: 562-565.

22. Madeley P, Ellis A, Mindham R. Facial expressions and Parkinson's disease. *Behav Neurol.* 1995;8: 115-119.

23. Pentland B, Gray, JM, Riddle, WJR, Pitcairn, TK. The effects of reduced nonverbal communication in Parkinson's disease. *Br J Disord Commun.* 1988;23:31-34.

24. Katsikitis, M, Pilowsky I.. A controlled study of facial mobility treatment in Parkinson's disease. *J Psychosom Res.* 1996;40(4):387-396.

25. Scott S, Caird FI, Williams BO. *Communication in Parkinson's Disease.* Rockville, Md: Aspen; 1985.

26. Robertson S, Thomson F. Speech therapy in Parkinson's disease: a study of the efficacy and long term effects of intensive treatment. *Br J Disord Commun.* 1984;19:213-224.

27. Ramig LO, Countryman S, Thompson LL, Horii Y. Comparison of two forms of intensive speech treatment for Parkinson disease. *J Speech Hear Res.* 1995;38:1232-1251.

28. Schulz G. The effects of speech therapy and pharmacological treatments on voice and speech in Parkinson s disease: a review of the literature. *Curr Med Chem.* 2002;9(14):1359-1366.

29. Yorkston K, Spencer K, and Duffy J. Behavioral management of respiratory/phonatory dysfunction from dysarthria: a systematic review of the evidence. *J Med Speech Lang Pathol.* 2003;11(2): xiii-xxxviii.

30. Spielman J, Ramig LO, Borod J. Preliminary effects of voice therapy on facial expression in Parkinson's disease. *J Int Neuropsycholog Assn.* 2001; 7(2):244.

31. Spielman J, Borod J, Ramig L. The effects of intensive voice treatment on facial expressiveness in Parkinson disease: preliminary data. *Cog Behav Neurol.* 2003;16(3):177-188.

Essential Voice Tremor

Lucian Sulica, MD
Elan Louis, MD, MS

KEY POINTS

■ Essential tremor is an age-related disease of involuntary movement. Voice is affected in some 25 to 30% of patients.

■ Essential voice tremor usually affects pharyngeal, palatal, and extrinsic laryngeal muscles in addition to intrinsic laryngeal muscles.

■ Essential voice tremor usually produces rhythmic oscillatory motion of both vocal folds, and may be present during quiet breathing in addition to phonation.

■ There are no pharmacologic agents of documented benefit in essential voice tremor.

■ Botulinum toxin injections may be helpful in carefully selected patients with essential voice tremor.

The phonatory apparatus may be involved in 25 to 30% of patients with essential tremor.[1,2] Voice tremor may be the only manifestation of essential tremor,[3] but usually it is associated with tremor in other parts of the body, including the upper extremities or head. In order to recognize and treat the symptoms of essential voice tremor, an understanding of essential tremor as a diagnostic entity must be combined with knowledge of phonatory biomechanics.

ESSENTIAL TREMOR

Essential tremor is an age-related disease of involuntary movement. Although generally acknowledged to be the most common adult-onset movement disorder, it is difficult to fix a precise incidence because essential tremor may be mild enough to go unnoticed in 50% or more of affected people.[4,5] In many instances, the disease is familial and can be inherited in an autosomal dominant fashion; the remainder of cases appear to be sporadic.[1,4-6] Absence of a family history of tremor does not preclude a diagnosis of essential tremor.

The diagnosis of essential tremor, like that of most movement disorders, is clinical—that is, there are no pathognomonic laboratory or radio-logical abnormalities. The most characteristic feature of the disease is tremor, which is further described below. The tremor begins insidiously and progresses at a variable rate,[7] although generally slowly. Most commonly, the tremor begins in the upper extremities, and it is usually mildly asymmetric.[8] Tremors are classified according to the circumstances in which they occur. Broadly, these can be divided into rest and action tremors. Tremor at rest occurs when the affected body part is at repose and completely supported against gravity, and is typical of Parkinson's disease (PD). Action tremors are further subdivided into posture-holding tremors, which occur when a limb is held outstretched against gravity; kinetic tremors, which occur with voluntary movement (eg, writing, pouring); and task-specific tremors, which occur only during a specific activity. For instance, enhanced physiologic tremor (ie, the tremor that occurs in most normal individuals) occurs with voluntary movement and posture holding, whereas dystonic tremor may be task-specific. Essential tremor is an action tremor that occurs during voluntary movement and posture-holding, without task-specific characteristics.[9] Much has been written about tremor frequencies. In general, essential tremor occurs at a rate of 4 to 10 Hz (Figure 19-1), whereas enhanced physiologic tremor occurs at a rate of 8 to 12 Hz.

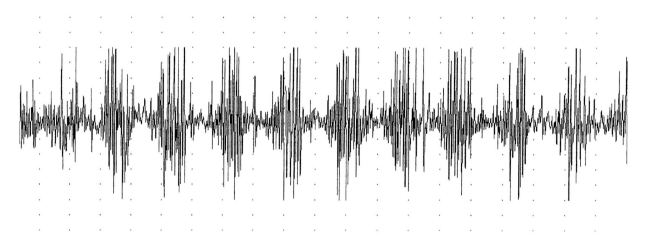

FIGURE 19–1. This EMG recording of the thyroarytenoid muscle of a patient with essential voice tremor during sustained /i/ phonation clearly reveals the rhythmic waxing and waning activation of the muscle typical of tremor, in this case at a rate of 5 Hz. Normally, muscle activation should be continuous during this activity (each horizontal division = 100 msec; each vertical division = 100 μvolts).

Intention ("cerebellar") tremor is slower, occurring at a rate of 2 to 5 Hz.[4,9] As is evident, there is considerable overlap in the frequencies of different tremors and, as a result, clinical circumstance (resting versus action) is a more useful diagnostic feature than is tremor frequency.

ESSENTIAL VOICE TREMOR

Essential tremor, when it affects the voice, is usually not restricted to the intrinsic muscles of the larynx. Other muscles of the phonatory apparatus that are often variably involved include extrinsic laryngeal muscles, pharyngeal and palatal muscles, the muscles of articulatory structures, as well as muscles of the diaphragm, chest wall, and abdomen, which affect phonatory expiration.[10-12] The term "essential voice tremor" thus describes the clinical situation better and is more apt than "essential laryngeal tremor."

Because of this broad involvement of different muscle groups, a given patient with essential voice tremor may present with variability in frequency as well as (or in place of) intensity. Most often, though, patients complain of intensity fluctuations associated with a perception of increased phonatory effort. Muscular discomfort and fatigue may result from efforts to stabilize the vocal tract. Symptoms are usually present across all phonatory activity, although they may be difficult to perceive during whispering in which variable glottic aperture may have relatively little acoustic impact. For this reason, patients with severe vocal tremor may adopt whispering as their customary mode of phonation, rendering the diagnosis obscure until revealed by louder sustained vowel phonation or endoscopic examination. Usually there is no dysphagia or dyspnea. Occasional patients complain of dyspnea; however, this represents breathlessness during voicing from glottic insufficiency, similar to that experienced by patients with unilateral vocal fold paralysis, rather than true difficulty breathing. Precise questioning will usually reveal the difference.

Patients with essential glottic tremor generally report slowly worsening symptoms over months to years. Voicing worsens with anxiety or stress[13] and is especially troublesome under more demanding acoustic conditions, such as speaking against background noise, addressing a classroom or conference, or using the telephone. In common with other manifestations of essential tremor, alcohol may effect a voice improvement. That these features are also found in spasmodic dysphonia is a source of diagnostic confusion.

Brief reflection on the overall prevalence of essential tremor and of laryngeal involvement discussed above suggests that only a small proportion of patients with vocal tremor present for evaluation by the otolaryngologist. Were it otherwise, essential vocal tremor would certainly form a greater proportion of our caseload than, say, spasmodic dysphonia. This in turn suggests a relatively low prevalence of severe or incapacitating vocal symptoms, although effective pharmacologic treatment (prescribed by neurologists) or simply a lack of information about appropriate specialty care may also contribute to this phenomenon.

A brief neurologic examination encompassing the upper extremities and gait in addition to the head and neck will serve to identify and distinguish among associated action and rest tremors and reveal signs of PD such as bradykinesia and cogwheel rigidity in the limbs. Laryngeal examination is best performed with a flexible transnasal endoscope, as the lingual traction necessary for transoral examination prevents connected speech, and the required posture may suppress characteristic signs. Rhythmic, oscillatory motion of the palate, pharynx, and/or vocal folds is diagnostic. Vocal fold tremor is bilateral and grossly symmetric. Tremor may be present across all laryngeal tasks, including quiet respiration as well as phonation; the traditional distinction between rest and activity appears unhelpful in the larynx. In fact, neither during breathing nor during phonation is the larynx truly at rest. Its activity is probably better defined as posture-holding during both of these tasks, which renders the clinical finding of tremor during "rest" more intelligible. Instrumental measures of voice have revealed (1) elevated jitter and shimmer and (2) decreased harmonic-to-noise ratio, s/z ratio, and maximum phonation time, which are abnormalities shared with other conditions of glottic insufficiency.[14]

If both history and examination are characteristic, further investigation is unnecessary. If findings are atypical or ambiguous, and especially if onset of symptoms is rapid, it is prudent to consult a neurologist. Ruling out thyrotoxicosis and drug-induced tremor—in the otolaryngologic pharmacopeia, adrenergic decongestants are the most common source—will prevent an unnecessary referral.

DIFFERENTIAL DIAGNOSIS

Asymptomatic Tremor

Occasionally, the examiner will incidentally note several cycles of vocal fold tremor during respiration or as the larynx assumes phonatory posture during laryngeal exam. In the absence of associated findings or complaints, the nature of this is an academic question. There is no evidence that this is a reflection of underlying neural dysfunction.

Parkinsonian Tremor

Tremor, most commonly involving the strap muscles and producing vertical laryngeal movement, is present in 55% of patients with idiopathic PD.[15] However, both associated physical findings and speech characteristics differ. Examination may reveal lack of facial affect and upper extremity rigidity with cogwheeling, shuffling gait, and other manifestations of bradykinesia. Any tremor present will tend to be more evident at rest rather than during activity. Most important, the speech of PD, although often breathy and of low intensity, does not demonstrate these characteristics in a rhythmic fashion. Rather, the characteristic hypophonia of PD is relatively constant, a

manifestation of incomplete glottic closure and poor breath support resulting from chest wall rigidity, often exacerbated by articulatory difficulties and sometimes by cognitive problems associated with the disease. These issues are discussed in detail in the previous chapter.

Myoclonus and Tics

The vocal characteristics of myoclonus and tics will occasionally resemble the cyclic phonatory changes of tremor. However, the rhythmic and oscillatory nature of the motion of essential tremor usually serves to distinguish it from these entities. Myoclonus, which can affect the same variety of muscles as tremor, resembles a sudden jerk, usually followed by a slower return to the null position. Hiccough is a common form of myoclonus, and serves to illustrate the essential quality of myoclonic movement. Tic disorders, including Gilles de la Tourette syndrome, are heterogeneous and may involve the larynx. In general, tics are suppressible for a time. Patients usually describe associated sensory phenomena as well as an urge to perform the tic motion, features absent from essential tremor. It is not often that tic or myoclonic activity is truly rhythmic.

Spasmodic Dysphonia and Tremor

Sometimes, the involuntary vocal fold adduction or abduction of spasmodic dysphonia will occur with rhythmic or near-rhythmic regularity, creating a pattern of phonatory breaks nearly indistinguishable from that of severe essential tremor.[16,17] Dystonic tremor has been noted in up to one-third of spasmodic dysphonia patients,[18] a feature spasmodic dysphonia shares with other focal or segmental dystonias, such as torticollis and writer's cramp.[1,9] Like dystonic activity as a whole and unlike essential tremor, dystonic tremor is often task-specific and may decrease with a sensory trick (a method of touching an affected body part to reduce the severity of the involuntary motion).[9] In the larynx, a dystonic tremor may be more evident during connected speech than during singing or sustained-vowel phonation and may be suppressed by insertion of a flexible fiberoptic laryngoscope. Dystonic tremor is usually somewhat aperiodic, although this may be extremely hard to appreciate. Ultimately, a therapeutic trial may be required to distinguish essential voice tremor from laryngeal dystonia. In the author's experience, botulinum toxin treatment of spasmodic dysphonia that is consistently followed by prolonged (greater than 10 days) and severe breathiness should raise the possibility of essential tremor. See chapter 20 for further details regarding spasmodic dysphonia.

TREATMENT

First-line treatment of essential tremor is pharmacologic. Propranolol and primidone are mainstays of treatment, with proven efficacy in controlled clinical trials. Their utility in treating voice tremor is less well documented. Propranolol is a beta-adrenergic blocker that reduces tremor amplitude by means of peripheral modulation of beta-adrenergic receptors in skeletal muscle, resulting in symptomatic relief in up to 50% of patients.[19] Primidone is an anticonvulsant that is effective in the control of tremor symptoms in about 50% of patients; the mechanism is not fully understood but it may involve enhancement of gamma-aminobutyric acid neurotransmission in the central nervous system.[19] Neither primidone[20] nor propranolol[21] has been shown to improve voice tremor in studies of small numbers of patients. Methazolamide, a carbonic-anhydrase inhibitor, appeared to improve vocal symptoms in more than half of patients (16 of 28) treated in an open trial,[22] results not supported by a subsequent blinded investigation.[23] A case of effective treatment with gabapentin has been reported.[24] These few reports notwithstanding, pharmacologic treatment of voice tremor has been sparsely studied; further investigation is called for.

Botulinum toxin treatment of essential voice tremor is predicated on the assumption that vocal fold tremor and resulting inappropriate glottal aperture account for the greater part of the symptoms of essential tremor of the phonatory tract. Generally, botulinum toxin is injected into one[27] or both thyroarytenoid muscles[19,25-28] in the manner of treatment of adductor spasmodic dysphonia and in comparable doses. According to patient self-perception of vocal quality, botulinum toxin injections were useful to 67 to 80% of cases. Acoustic measures documented benefit less often, leading investigators to hypothesize that much of the perceived improvement resulted from decreased phonatory effort. The reader is referred to the primary reports for details of treatment and results (Table 19–1).

Botulinum Toxin Treatment: Essential Voice Tremor Versus Spasmodic Dysphonia

Botulinum toxin treatment of essential voice tremor yields qualitatively different results than the treatment of spasmodic dysphonia, and personal experience with such treatment has not been entirely consistent with the sanguine reports in the literature. Botulinum toxin does not eliminate the tremor, but rather decreases tremor amplitude. However, this does not always translate reliably into acoustic improvement or greater voice functionality. Not infrequently, treatment of adductor muscles yields prolonged and troublesome breathy dysphonia. Neither injecting abductor muscles nor limiting treatment to one side has yielded reliably better results. Such results are also typical of botulinum toxin treatment of hand and head tremor, in which muscle chemodenervation has not offered consistent and predictable functional benefit.[5,34] Many patients with essential voice tremor do not elect to continue long-term botulinum toxin treatment for essential voice tremor, in sharp contrast to those with spasmodic dysphonia.

This striking difference may be due to distinctions in the pathophysiology of essential tremor and dystonia. There is some evidence to suggest that an afferent signal plays some role in dystonia, and that botulinum toxin may achieve part of its therapeutic effect by altering feedback to the central nervous system.[29,30] On the other hand, essential tremor is likely the result of abnormalities in cerebellar-thalamic outflow pathways without an afferent component, potentially compromising an important part of the effect of botulinum toxin.

TABLE 19–1. Botulinum Toxin Treatment of Essential Voice Tremor: Summary of Studies

Study	Type of Study	Number of Subjects	Muscles Injected	Dose Used	Outcome		
					Patient Subjective Evaluation	Blinded Perceptual Evaluation	Acoustic Analysis
Hertegard et al[25]	Open trial	15	Bilateral TA, occasionally thyrohyoid & cricothyroid	0.6 to 5U per side (TA)	10 of 15 (67%) reported benefit	Significant mean improvement on VAS	Significant decrease of F_0 & F_0 variation
Warrick et al[27]	Open trial with crossover (unilateral vs. bilateral injection)	10	Bilateral TA<hr>Unilateral TA	2.5U per side<hr>15U	8 of 10 (80%) wished to be treated again	No statistically significant improvement	No statistically significant change
Koller et al[19]	Open trial	?	Bilateral TA	1.0 to 2.5U per side	Significant mean improvement on 0–100 scale of function	Not reported	Not reported
Adler et al[28]	Dose-randomized open trial	13	Bilateral TA	1.25U, 2.5U or 3.75U per side	Significant mean improvement on 5-point tremor severity scale	Significant mean improvement on 5-point tremor severity scale	Significant mean improvement in F_0 variation

U = Units of botulinum toxin type A; TA = Thyroarytenoid; VAS = 100 mm visual analog scale; F_0 = fundamental frequency

Extralaryngeal muscles are commonly involved in essential voice tremor, and extending botulinum toxin treatment to these may offer improved results,[25] although swallowing difficulties are likely to impose limits on such treatment. Because essential voice tremor is a clinically heterogeneous disorder, it may also be possible to select patients who are more likely to benefit from botulinum toxin treatment based on differences in muscle involvement seen in the clinical examination; these studies remain to be performed.

Thalamic deep brain stimulation (DBS) by means of implanted electrodes is an evolving method of treating disabling, medication-resistant essential tremor and PD. This method is increasingly taking the place of thalamotomy. Initial reports of postoperative dysarthria, particularly after bilateral procedures, created reservations regarding the utility of DBS in the treatment of essential voice tremor, as both speech and voice are tightly time-gated activities requiring a high degree of coordination. However, mounting evidence suggests that DBS may be efficacious in the treatment of voice tremor.[31-36]

Essential voice tremor is a clinically heterogeneous disorder that may involve a variety of muscles of the phonatory apparatus, both laryngeal and extralaryngeal. It is probably more common than is generally suspected. Diagnosis as well as differentiation from similar disorders affecting the larynx depends on thorough clinical examination. Its salient feature is kinetic (action-induced) tremor, which produces rhythmic fluctuation in voice intensity and/or pitch, and an absence of rigidity, bradykinesia, and spasms typical of other disorders of involuntary motion.

Despite limited evidence of efficacy, it seems reasonable to begin with pharmacologic treatment, particularly when patients with essential voice tremor have other troublesome manifestations of the disease (eg, tremor of the upper extremities) that may benefit from such treatment (Figure 19-2). Patients whose only complaint is voice tremor, on the other hand, may choose between pharmacologic treatment and botulinum toxin injections as initial treatment. Benefit is by no means universal, and functional

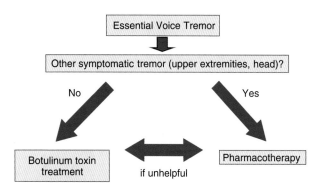

FIGURE 19–2. Management algorithm for essential voice tremor.

voice improvement often remains. The effect of combined chemodenervation and medical treatment remains to be determined. Voice tremor alone has yet to become an indication for deep brain stimulation, although the possibility exists in truly crippling cases. As in most voice disorders due to benign pathology, a well-informed and well-advised patient is usually the person best suited to weigh treatment options.

Review Questions

1. Which features are typical of essential tremor?
   a. More common with age
   b. Autosomal recessive inheritance
   c. Slow progression
   d. The voice is affected in half of patients
   e. The tremor improved with alcohol intake

2. Which clinical characteristics are typical of essential tremor?
   a. Asymmetric.
   b. Resting tremor
   c. Cogwheeling
   d. Bradykinesia
   e. Action-induced

3. What features of connected speech suggest essential voice tremor?
   a. Weak, breathy voice with poor articulation
   b. Strangled voice breaks
   c. Rhythmic fluctuation in intensity and/or pitch.
   d. Irregular breathy voice breaks
   e. "Scanning speech"

4. Which method of examining the larynx is least likely to obscure the typical signs of essential tremor?

5. Which medications have a documented benefit in essential voice tremor?
   a. Propranolol
   b. Primidone
   c. Methazolamide
   d. None of the above

REFERENCES

1. Factor SA, Weiner WJ. Hyperkinetic movement disorders. In: Weiner WJ, Goetz CG, eds. *Neurology for the Non-Neurologist*. Philadelphia, Pa: Lippincott, Williams & Wilkins; 1999:143-177.

2. Koller WC, Busenbark K, Miner K. The relationship of essential tremor to other movement disorders: report on 678 patients. *Ann Neurol*. 1994;35:717-723.

3. Findley LJ, Gresty M. Head, facial and voice tremor. *Adv Neurol*. 1988;49:239-253.

4. Elble RJ. Diagnostic criteria for essential tremor and differential diagnosis. *Neurology*. 2000;54 (suppl 4):S2-S6.

5. Louis ED. Essential tremor. *Lancet Neurol*. 2005;4:100-110.

6. Louis ED, Ottman R. How familial is familial tremor? The genetric epidemiology of essential tremor. *Neurology*. 1996;46:1200-1205.

7. Louis ED, Ford B, Barnes LF. Clinical subtypes of essential tremor. *Arch Neurol*. 2000;57:1194-1198.

8. Jankovic J. Essential tremor: Clinical characteristics. *Neurology*. 2000;54 (suppl 4):S21-S25.

9. Fahn S, Greene PE, Ford B, Bressman SB. *Handbook of Movement Disorders*. Philadelphia, Pa: Current Medicine, Inc; 1998.

10. Tomoda H, Shibasaki H, Kuroda Y, Shin T. Voice tremor: dysregulation of voluntary expiratory muscles. *Neurology*. 1987;37:117-122.

11. Koda J, Ludlow CL. An evaluation of laryngeal muscle activation in patients with voice tremor. *Otolaryngol Head Neck Surg*. 1992;107:684-696.

12. Finnegan EM, Luschei ES, Barkmeier JM, Hoffman HT. Synchrony of laryngeal muscle activity in persons with vocal tremor. *Arch Otolaryngol Head Neck Surg*. 2003;129:313-318.

13. Mendoza E, Carballo G. Vocal tremor and psychological stress. *J Voice*. 1999;13:105-112.

14. Gamboa J, Jimenez-Jimenez FJ, Nieto A, et al. Acoustic voice analysis in patients with essential tremor. *J Voice*. 1998;12:444-452.

15. Perez KS, Ramig LO, Smith ME, Dromey C. The Parkinson larynx: tremor and videostroboscopic findings. *J Voice*. 1996;10:354-361.

16. Aronson AE, Hartman DE. Adductor spastic dysphonia as a sign of essential voice tremor. *J Speech Hear Disord*. 1981;46:52-58.

17. Barkmeier JM, Case JL, Ludlow CL. Identification of symptoms for spasmodic dysphonia and vocal tremor: a comparison of expert and nonexpert judges. *J Commun Disord*. 2001;34:21-37.

18. Blitzer A, Brin MF, Stewart CF. Botulinum toxin management of spasmodic dysphonia (laryngeal dystonia): a 12-year experience in more than 900 patients. *Laryngoscope*. 1998;108:1435-1441.

19. Koller WC, Hristova A, Brin M. Pharmacologic treatment of essential tremor. *Neurology*. 2000;54 (suppl 4):S30-S38.

20. Hartman DE, Vishwanat B. Spastic dysphonia and essential (voice) tremor treated with primidone. *Arch Otolaryngol*. 1984;110:394-397.

21. Koller WC, Graner D, Micoch A. Essential voice tremor: treatment with propranolol. *Neurology*. 1985;35:106-108.

22. Muenter MD, Daube JR, Caviness JN, Miller PM. Treatment of essential tremor with methazolamide. *Mayo Clin Proc*. 1991;66:991-997.

23. Busenbark K, Ramig L, Dromey C, Koller WC. Methazolamide for essential voice tremor. *Neurology*. 1996;47:1331-1332.

24. Padilla F, Berthier ML, Campos-Arillo VM. Temblor essencial de la voz y tratamiento con gabapentina. *Rev Neurol*. 2000;31:798.

25. Hertegard S, Granqvist S, Lindestad PA. Botulinum toxin injections for essential voice tremor. *Ann Otol Rhinol Laryngol.* 2000;109:204-209.

26. Warrick P, Dromey C, Irish J, Durkin. The treatment of essential voice tremor with botulinum toxin A: a longitudinal case report. *J Voice.* 2000; 14:410-412.

27. Warrick P, Dromey C, Irish JC, Durkin L, Pakiam A, Lang A. Botulinum toxin for essential tremor of the voice with multiple anatomical sites of tremor: a crossover design study of unilateral versus bilateral injection. *Laryngoscope.* 2000a;110: 1366-1374.

28. Adler CH, Bansberg SF, Hentz JG, et al. Botulinum toxin type A for treating voice tremor. *Arch Neurol.* 2004;61:1416-1420.

29. Hallett M. How does botulinum toxin work? *Ann Neurol.* 2000;48:7-8.

30. Sulica L. Contemporary management of spasmodic dysphonia. *Curr Opin Otolaryngol Head Neck Surg.* 2004;12:543-548.

31. Carpenter MA, Pahwa R, Miyawaki KL, Wilkinson SB, Send JP, Koller WC. Reduction in voice tremor under thalamic stimulation. *Neurology.* 1998;50: 796-798.

32. Yoon MS, Munz M, Sataloff RT, Spiegel JR, Heuer RJ. Vocal tremor reduction with deep brain stimulation. *Stereotact Funct Neurosurg.* 1999;72: 241-244.

33. Taha JM, Janszen MA, Favre J. Thalamic deep brain stimulation for the treatment of head, voice and bilateral limb tremor. *J Neurosurg.* 1999;91: 68-72.

34. Pahwa R, Lyons K, Koller WC. Surgical treatment of essential tremor. *Neurology.* 2000;54(suppl 4): S39-S44.

35. Lyons KE, Pahwa R. Deep brain stimulation and essential tremor. *J Clin Neurophysiol.* 2004;21:2-5.

36. Lyons KE, Pahwa R, Comella CL, et al. Benefits and risks of pharmacologic treatment for essential tremor. *Drug Safety.* 2003;26:461-481.

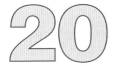

20

Spasmodic Dysphonia

Joel H. Blumin, MD, FACS
Gerald S. Berke, MD, FACS

KEY POINTS

■ Spasmodic dysphonia is a neurologic voice disorder that affects the fluency of connected speech.

■ The majority of patients with adductor spasmodic dysphonia have a stereotypical staccato, strangled speech quality.

■ The diagnosis of muscle tension dysphonia should be considered in the differential diagnosis and ruled out before entering the patient into treatment.

■ Botulinum toxin remains the mainstay of treatment, although many patients have been successfully treated by a surgical approach.

Spasmodic dysphonia is an idiopathic focal dystonia of the larynx. A *dystonia* is a neuromuscular disorder characterized by involuntary, sporadic, and irregularly occurring muscle contractions. Dystonias can be generalized or focal, affecting the entire body or only a specific muscle group. Certain dystonias, like spasmodic dysphonia, tend to be task-specific and do not affect the muscle group during vegetative function or at rest. Dystonias are chronic conditions and, like other movement disorders, are not typically associated with dementia or other cognitive deficits.

HISTORY, ETIOLOGY, AND DEMOGRAPHICS

Traube is credited with first writing about the condition we know today as spasmodic dysphonia.[1] In 1871, he coined the term "spastic dysphonia" to describe a patient with a nervous hoarseness. Others have noted the stereotypical speech patterns and described them as a "vocal fold stutter" or talking "while being choked."[2,3] For almost a century, it was assumed that the disorder was of a psychiatric etiology[4] and only recently was it identified as a neurologic disorder similar to other dystonias. The terms "spasmodic dysphonia" and "laryngeal dystonia" were recommended by Brin and Blitzer to specifically associate the disorder with other dystonias.[5] Many patients with spasmodic dysphonia have a high incidence of other neurological disorders including other dystonias.[6,7] Abnormalities have been shown in the brainstem reflexes and other aspects of central processing in those with spasmodic dysphonia.[8] A subset of patients with dystonia demonstrate a familial and genetic origin for their disorder.[5,9-11] Diagnostically, spasmodic dysphonia and muscle tension dysphonia should be considered in patients with a characteristic strained-strangled voice quality.[12] Muscle tension dysphonia is a term that describes a voice disorder that stems from behavioral misuse of laryngeal tension during voicing.[13] Estimates from the National Spasmodic Dysphonia Association suggest that spasmodic dysphonia affects approximately 35,000 to 50,000 Americans. These estimates are rough and were derived from extrapolations of populations with dystonia in general. No formal population study on the incidence of spasmodic dysphonia has been performed, but, in general, this is a rare disease.

The etiology of spasmodic dysphonia is considered to be idiopathic. Several studies have looked for commonalities in those patients with spasmodic dysphonia.[5,14] This disease affects women two to three times as often as men. The mean age of onset is in the 5th to 6th decade with a wide range of onset, from teenager to octogenarian. Ten to 20% of patients associate a blunt trauma (such as motor vehicle accident) or an upper respiratory infection with the time of onset. Whether this is causative or happenstance is unknown. Childhood measles or mumps infections have been noted in 45 to 65% of patients and, although this incidence may reflect a bias of the studied cohorts, the numbers are greater than the general population and may suggest a viral association.[14] Other neurologic diseases, such as herpes zoster, have been associated with latent viral infections.

PATHOPHYSIOLOGY, SYMPTOMOLOGY, AND DIAGNOSIS

Spasmodic dysphonia affects a patient's ability to produce fluent connected speech. It is a task-specific dystonia: the affected task is voice production, and the specific muscles affected are those that control movement of the vocal folds. In general, spasmodic dysphonia does not affect the muscles associated with resonance (pharynx, palate) or articulation (tongue, lips). However, some patients have dystonias in other muscle groups. It is not uncommon to have multiple focal dystonias clustered in a given patient. Meige's syndrome, for example, is a dystonia of the face, tongue, jaw, and lips as well as larynx and can affect a patient's ability to articulate.[15]

A specific pathologic finding that leads to the development of spasmodic dysphonia has not been demonstrated. Spasmodic dysphonia is thought to be a disorder of central nervous system processing, although the exact mechanism has not been elucidated. Research has suggested an abnormality of motor responses to sensory input and feedback from the larynx, possibly by disinhibition of laryngeal motor responses.[8,16] Changes in laryngeal muscle and nerve histology have been demonstrated but likely suggest an end result of central remodeling rather than a peripheral injury or myositis.[17]

Spasmodic dysphonia is subcategorized into multiple subtypes depending on a patient's predominate symptomatology and clinical findings.[7] Approximately 80 to 90% of patients with spasmodic dysphonia have the adductor type. These patients have involuntary spasms of the laryngeal adductors, namely, the thyroarytenoid and the lateral cricoarytenoid. Some patients also have spasms of the intra-arytenoid muscles.[18] Patients with adductor spasmodic dysphonia tend to have a stereotypical strained-strangled quality of speech. More specifically, these patients exhibit vocal breaks or stops when attempting to produce a speech task loaded with voiced consonants (b, d, g, z, v, j, m, n). The symptoms are less pronounced when the task is loaded with voiceless consonants (p, t, k, s, f, ch) or when phonating a less complicated utterance, such as the production of a continuous vowel sound.[6,19,20]

Abductor spasmodic dysphonia affects up to 17% of patients who have spasmodic dysphonia.[4] In this disorder, the spasms are primarily noted in the laryngeal abductor, the large posterior cricoarytenoid muscles. Patients with this disorder have spasms that produce inappropriate loss of laryngeal resistance resulting in a perceptual quality of intermittent breathiness. They also have difficulty during connected speech tasks, but their problem is more noted when the task is loaded with voiceless consonants and utterances with softer attacks (eg, "how hard did he hit him?").

Although the majority of patients have a spasmodic dysphonia that falls into one of the major subcategories, some may have a mixed disorder characterized by both abductor and adductor phonatory breaks. Some authors believe that all spasmodic dysphonia patients have both types of disorder but are more dominant for a certain subtype at a given point in time, and the dominant symptoms can change over the course of a patient's life.[21,22] Many patients also consciously and unconsciously alter laryngeal resistance as a strategy for coping with these disorders. This can result in perceptual voice qualities that deviate significantly from the stereotypical disorder where they lose some of the task specificity, and sound strained or breathy all the time, or change their fundamental frequency.[23,24]

Many patients with spasmodic dysphonia also have vocal tremor.[25,26] Vocal tremor typically affects muscle groups outside the larynx including strap and pharyngeal musculature. The auditory perception of this disorder is characterized by a tremulous, shaky, or quavering voice quality that occurs with all speech tasks. This tremor tends to be more resistant to treatment then the dystonia. Treatment of the spasmodic dysphonia can make a coexisting underlying tremor more noticeable.

The task specificity of spasmodic dysphonia goes beyond the consonant and vowel sounds within a given speech task. Many patients experience differences in voice difficulty depending on environment. For instance, almost all patients have more difficulty with telephone conversations then face-to-face conversations. They will also note that their voice is worse when reading a new passage aloud over reciting a memorized passage. Singing may be normal, as well as spontaneous emotional speech such as laughing or crying. The reason for these phenomena is unknown, but thought to be associated with differences in central nervous system processing of the different speech tasks. These features were noted by practitioners long ago and resulted in the incorrect consideration of spasmodic dysphonia as a psychiatric or psychological disorder.[21]

The diagnosis of spasmodic dysphonia can be difficult as there is no pathognomonic sign or specific test that will provide the diagnosis. In the past, the diagnosis was often delayed for years after the patient developed symptoms and sought medical care. Other more common voice and laryngeal disorders are often attributed to the patient before he or she finds an experienced practitioner who correctly recognizes their disorder.

The experienced clinician spends most of the interview *listening* to the patient's voice quality, especially during specific tasks, and the majority of the physical exam is spent ruling out other voice disorders. Although specific diagnostic tests and procedures can be helpful in supporting or discounting the disorder, the final diagnosis is usually associated with a clinical history and auditory perceptual findings that support the diagnosis. Imaging and laboratory testing are not routinely recommended; however, they can be helpful in ruling out other neurologic diagnoses, if suspected. Laryngeal electromyography is of limited diagnostic benefit[27]; however, in some patients with treatment-resistant spasmodic dysphonia, fine-wire electromyography of all intrinsic muscles has shown spasm in the intra-arytenoid muscle, an uncommon finding which may otherwise be overlooked.[18,25,28] Measurement of acoustic and aerodynamic perturbations may support the diagnosis, but are not diagnostic.

TREATMENT

All treatment for spasmodic dysphonia is aimed at reducing symptomatology and the impact of the voice disorder on a patient's daily function. No treatment is aimed at the source of disease and therefore cannot be considered truly curative. Four basic approaches exist and can be used singularly or in combination: speech therapy, pharmacologic agents, intramuscular injections of botulinum toxin, and surgical treatment (Figure 20-1).

Speech Therapy

Although some have reported speech therapy as a successful adjunct to botulinum toxin injection,[29] speech therapy as a sole treatment has a very limited role and often serves only to frustrate the patient with spasmodic dysphonia. Most

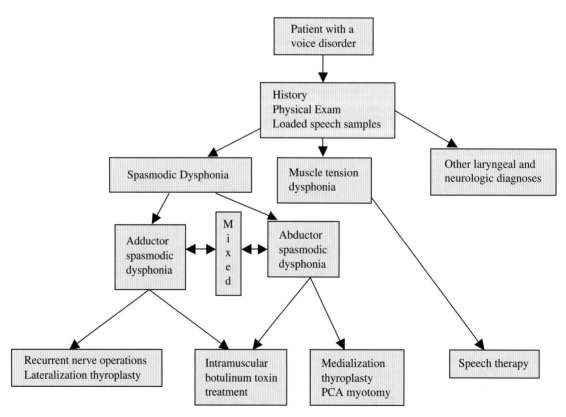

FIGURE 20–1. Management algorithm for spasmodic dysphonia.

believe that speech therapy with a goal for cure is an unreasonable expectation. Speech therapy is often used to distinguish patients with diagnostic difficulties, as those with spasmodic dysphonia, from patients with muscle tension dysphonia.[12,30]

Medical Therapy

Oral medical therapy has no proven benefit for patients with spasmodic dysphonia. There is no specific antidystonia agent, and although benzodiazepines, anticholinergics, dopamine depleters, and gabapentin are dosed empirically, they are often limited by central nervous system side effects including sedation.[31] Interestingly, many patients with spasmodic dysphonia note a diminution of symptoms with alcohol intake.

Botulinum Toxin Therapy

Fermentation of *Clostridium botulinum* produces a group of seven antigenically distinct exotoxin compounds that block neurotransmitter transmission at the mammalian neuromuscular junction.[32] Subtypes A, B, C, D, E, F, and G have been identified, but only A, B, E, F, and G have been known to cause the disease botulism. Botulinum toxin subtypes A and B are commercially available for clinical use, although they are not specifically the U.S. Food and Drug Administration approved for use in spasmodic dysphonia. Nonetheless, a large body of literature supports the use of intramuscular injections of botulinum toxin for treatment of spasmodic dysphonia[33] and its use is considered to be at the standard of care for this group of patients. Botulinum toxin type A has been used clinically to treat spasmodic dysphonia since 1984.[34] Type B has only become clinically available since 2000.[35] Type A is manufactured and distributed by a number of companies worldwide with Botox (Allergan, Inc, Irvine, Calif) dominating the commercial market. Type B is manufactured and distributed by Solstice Neurosciences, Inc. (South San Francisco, Calif) as Myobloc.

After being injected intramuscularly, botulinum toxin causes a flaccid paralysis by blocking presynaptic release of acetylcholine at the neuromuscular junction.[34] A dose-dependent effect and side-effect period are seen in patients with spasmodic dysphonia. Initially, patients will develop a breathy voice quality followed by a more fluent, less spastic voice quality. As the neuromuscular junctions recover, the patient gradually redevelops spastic voice.[36, 37] With toxin type A, the effect lasts about 3 months and once stable dosing is achieved, a given patient's response to injection is often quite reproducible. Toxin type B lasts a shorter period of time (approximately 6 weeks) and the conversion factor for type B is 50 to 80 times the dose of toxin A for similar effect.[35]

A variety of injection methods and dosing strategies are utilized by practitioners. No strategy has been shown to be superior to another. Most preferentially inject the thyroarytenoid muscle as the target for patients with adductor spasmodic dysphonia, although some recommend the lateral cricoarytenoid (the strongest laryngeal adductor) or the intra-arytenoid (when spastic activity has been identified on fine-wire electromyography).[7,24,28,38] The posterior cricoarytenoid muscle is the target for patients with abductor spasmodic dysphonia.[39] Injection technique is also highly variable from physician to physician and none has been demonstrated superior to another.[31] The toxin can be delivered to the muscle via a percutaneous[5] or permucosal approach,[40] with or without optical guidance, with[27] or without[41] electromyographic guidance. The posterior cricoarytenoid muscles can be approached from either a posteriolateral or a transcricothyroid membrane, transtracheal approach.[42] Dosages of toxin to muscle are typically low-dose with the majority of patients receiving about 3 units of type A toxin per muscle.[7] Others have recommended larger doses, even entering double digits per muscle, for longer effect. Unilateral or bilateral injections can be done.[43,44] Dosing strategies aim at maximizing the fluent voice, while minimizing the breathiness at the onset of toxin activity. These strategies vary from patient to patient depending on an individual's desires and level of voice use. As an example, a speaking professional performing radio voiceovers may come in for unilateral ½-unit doses every month, trading the frequency of dosing for minimal breathy side effect, whereas an elderly homemaker may come in every 6 months for a 5-unit bilateral dose, trading a few weeks of breathy voice for the inconvenience of the physician visit.

Although widely used as primary therapy for spasmodic dysphonia, botulinum toxin therapy does have its limitations. Many patients do not like the relative "roller-coaster effect" of the medicine, which produces a poor breathy voice shortly after injection, followed by a fluent voice, followed again by a dysphonic voice. Even though the toxin effect lasts a few months, a patient may state that his or her best voice only existed for several weeks in the middle of dosing. Other patients find traveling to a treating physician inconvenient, as treating patients with spasmodic dysphonia is not commonly practiced by the majority of otolaryngologists or neurologists. Some patients find erratic responses after each injection, thus never achieving a stable dose.

Botulinum toxin treatment of abductor spasmodic dysphonia seems to be less effective then treatment of adductor spasmodic dysphonia.[7,39] This may be related to the dual role of the abductor muscles as the most important laryngeal muscle of breathing. The belly of the muscle is larger than the other intrinsic laryngeal muscles and probably requires a larger dose for ultimate efficacy; however, the practitioner must treat at a lower dose to avoid total paralysis and airway obstruction.

Surgery

Adductor Spasmodic Dysphonia

An operative approach to spasmodic dysphonia predates the use of botulinum toxin. Dedo, in 1976, is credited for recognizing spasmodic dysphonia as a neurologic dysphonia with abnormal feedback between the end organ (larynx) and the central nervous system.[45,46] He proposed a procedure in which one recurrent laryngeal nerve is severed, thus interrupting the aberrant central-peripheral nervous system interaction.[45,47] The initial reports of the recurrent laryngeal

nerve section were exciting; however, several manuscripts over the ensuing decade suggested that cure of spasticity was evident in about one-third.[48-50] The majority of patients traded the dysphonia of spasmodic dysphonia for that of a vocal fold paralysis with a breathy harsh sound. Electromyographic data showed that spontaneous reinnervation of the treated hemilarynx occurred despite nerve transaction.[51] Modifications of the original procedure were suggested; however, the patients developed either a breathy dysphonia or recurrence of spasm.[52-54]

Selective laryngeal adductor denervation and reinnervation represents a more extensive modification of the original nerve severing procedure.[55-57] Four significant modifications of the original recurrent laryngeal nerve section were instituted. First, a bilateral recurrent laryngeal nerve operation should be more effective than a unilateral procedure; however, severing both recurrent nerves would put the patient at significant risk for dyspnea or airway obstruction. Second, the denervation should be specific to the adductors while preserving the innervation to the abductors of the larynx. Third, a method to prevent muscle atrphy associated with recurrent nerve transection was proposed. Lastly, late reinnervation from the "diseased" recurrent laryngeal nerve should be avoided. In the selective laryngeal adductor denervation and reinnervation procedure large windows are made into the thyroid cartilage bilaterally to widely expose the paraglottic space, revealing the intrinsic adductor muscles and the terminal portion of the recurrent laryngeal nerve. The anterior branch of the recurrent laryngeal nerve is identified under magnification and branches to the thyroarytenoid and the lateral cricoarytenoid muscles are severed and physically transposed outside the laryngeal cartilage to prevent reinnervation. A microneurorrhaphy is made between the proximal cut end of the sternohyoid branch of the ansa cervicalis to the distal branch of the recurrent laryngeal nerve just before it terminates in the thyroarytenoid muscle (Figure 20–2). This final step reinnervates the muscle providing thyroarytenoid muscle tone and, most importantly, prevents reinnervation from the proximal transected end of the recurrent laryngeal nerve. As a

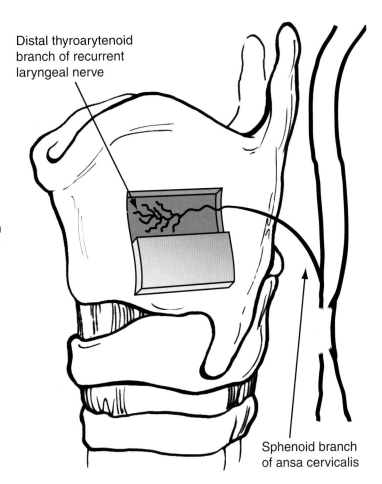

Distal thyroarytenoid
branch of recurrent
laryngeal nerve

Sphenoid branch
of ansa cervicalis

FIGURE 20–2. Microneurorrhapy between the proximal cut end of the ansa cervicalis to the distal branch of the recurrent laryngeal nerve.

part of the selective laryngeal adductor denervation and reinnervation procedure, the lateral cricoarytenoid is partially transected to weaken it because the terminal branch to the lateral cricoarytenoid is too small to be amenable to reliable reinnervation.[17,56]

Initial reports of this procedure are very promising with only a handful of treated patients failing therapy.[56] Although a degree of breathiness is noted from blinded observers, patients self-report a very high satisfaction rate in both voice quality and loss of spasticity.[58] This procedure has been repeated and further reported in the literature.[57] Long-term results on additional patients are quite enthusiastic.[58]

Another approach to spasmodic dysphonia is aimed at altering laryngeal biomechanics through framework surgery rather then by altering neuromuscular tensions. Isshiki and others have performed and modified this type II thyroplasty in which the vocal folds are lateralized away from each other.[59-62] The procedure is per-formed under local anesthesia and the patient is allowed to talk, as in other phonosurgical procedures. A midline thyrotomy is made with care not to enter the mucosa. The cartilage halves of the thyroid ala are separated and then secured in position with a shim when the desired voice effect is heard. In this approach, the spasms of spasmodic dysphonia may still occur, but because the vocal folds are held apart, the audible quality of these spasms are lessened. Long-term results have been poor,[63] but this technique seems to have little morbidity and is a reasonable alternative for some patients.

Myotomy or myectomy alone of the thyroarytenoid has been proposed experimentally but has had limited success in clinical treatment of patients.[17,63] This can be performed through an open approach, or alternatively, via an endoscopic approach where a laser can be used to selectively vaporize and coagulate thyroarytenoid fibers. A cited advantage of the open approach is that it can be performed in the

Alternative Therapies

As a rare disease with an unknown etiology, discussions of diagnosis and treatment of spasmodic dysphonia often spark debate in both medical and lay communities. Although therapies offered by traditional allopathic medicine such as botulinum toxin and the different operations have defined track records with reasonable science behind them, other nontraditional treatments for spasmodic dysphonia are constantly being offered to patients. Herbal supplements, hypnotherapy, psychotherapy, and voice therapy for cure are offered to this vulnerable population of patients, often in exchange for significant cash outlays. Although some patients have been helped by such treatments, the data are anecdotal at best. It is likely hat many of the patients successfully treated did not actually have spasmodic dysphonia (a dystonia) but in reality had a nonorganic dysphonia such as muscle tension dysphonia. These nonorganic dysphonias often respond to psychological interventions including relaxation, motivation, and antidepressive techniques.

Other alternative therapies have been looked at by more credible sources. Some patients have seen improvements with acupuncture and a group of medical acupuncturists have reported on their data. Unfortunately, in their 2003 manuscript, Lee et al[64] were unable to show convincing evidence of success to blinded observers. Seven of ten patients reported improvements in voice symptoms, but only four of them continued with treatment. The National Institutes of Health is conducting an ongoing study on the effects of dextromethorphan, a commonly used over-the-counter cough suppressant, on voice disorders including spasmodic dysphonia. This medicine can inhibit laryngeal reflexes and decrease laryngeal tension.

With the expansion of the Internet, a person with a voice disorder is exposed to a veritable information overload before seeking professional medical care. Because voice disorders are not life-threatening, a patient may not even go to a physician or speech pathologist to seek an accurate diagnosis. Patients with nonorganic dysphonia can inaccurately diagnose themselves with spasmodic dysphonia and then report success after taking an herbal supplement, adding further confusion to a treatment decision made by those with the real diagnosis.

awake phonating patient, thus allowing the surgeon to titrate the extent of operation to voice quality.[65] Although the endoscopic approach avoids an apparent neck incision, one should weigh the negative effect of inducing mucosal scar and producing a harsh voice quality that is difficult to further remedy. Care should be made to keep the mucosal incisions lateral on the ventricular surface of the vocal folds. As a part of the selective laryngeal adductor denervation and reinnervation procedure, the lateral cricoarytenoid is partially transected to weaken it as the terminal branch of the recurrent laryngeal nerve is too small to be amenable to reliable reinnervation.[17,66]

Abductor Spasmodic Dysphonia

Because botulinum toxin treatment of abductor spasmodic dysphonia is less beneficial than in patients with adductor spasmodic dysphonia, alternative treatments have been developed. Some of the limitations to the treatment of abductor spasmodic dysphonia are related to difficulties associated with severe weakening of the posterior cricoarytenoid muscle, especially bilaterally. Both muscle-specific and framework procedures have been performed with limited success. Shaw and others reported on three cases treated by selective trimming (myoplasty) of the posterior cricoarytenoid muscle.[67] Others[68] have recommended permucosal selective electrocautery of the posterior cricoarytenoid muscle via the postcricoid area during a direct laryngoscopy approach. Some have reported limited success with medialization type I thyroplasty in these patients, using a concept similar to treating the adductor patients with a lateralization framework approach.[7,39] By moving the vocal folds together, the effect and auditory perception of the breathy voice break is lessened. This approach may be used as a supplement to botulinum toxin injection of the posterior cricoarytenoid muscle.

FUTURE DIRECTIONS

Although we continue to treat patients' symptomology, the true cure for spasmodic dysphonia and other dystonias probably lies in the central nervous system. In reality, we do not know if all patients with the symptoms of spasmodic dysphonia even have the same disease. Could there be multiple central disorders with a common end product of a spasmodic voice? The dystonia literature has pointed toward genetics as a possible source of disease. Familial segregation of dystonias has led toward identification of a number of dystonia genes and their protein products; however, none of these have been specifically implicated as the defect in spasmodic dysphonia. Further identification of the effects of gene mutation may yield better disease identification and, one hopes, a cure.

Our colleagues in neurosurgery are working with implantable devices capable of modifying in vivo neurologic communication in the basal ganglia.[68] Implantation of these deep brain stimulators has shown success in treating other movement disorders including Parkinson's disease, tremor, and generalized dystonia. As the electronics and programming of these products become more refined, a role in treating all centrally mediated motor disorders may develop.

Review Questions

1. You have diagnosed a patient with adductor spasmodic dysphonia and both you and she decide on treatment with botulinum toxin type A injections. Approximately how many units of toxin would you deliver to each thyroarytenoid muscle?
   a. 2 units
   b. 20 units
   c. 200 units
   d. 2000 units
   e. 20000 units

2. Spasmodic dysphonia is a psychiatric illness.
   a. True
   b. False

3. Abductor spasmodic dysphonia is characterized by:
   a. Vocal fold spasms most apparent while speaking passages weighted with voiced consonants
   b. Vocal fold spasms most apparent while speaking passages weighted with voiceless consonants

c. Vocal fold tremor without spasm most apparent while speaking prolonged vowel sounds like "a" in ah

d. Vocal fold spasms most apparent while speaking prolonged vowel sounds like "a" in ah

e. b and d

4. Diagnosis of adductor spasmodic dysphonia is substantiated
   a. By findings of thalamic injury seen on magnetic resonance imaging
   b. By demonstration of a high titers of anti-cytomegalovirus IgG on plasma chemistry
   c. By listening for specific speech breaks during loaded sentences
   d. By demonstration of high vocal tract airflow during utterance of prolonged vowel sounds

5. Speech therapy with intent to cure is a reliable primary method of treating patients with spasmodic dysphonia.
   a. True
   b. False

REFERENCES

1. Traube L. *Gesammelte Beitrge Zur Pathologie Und Physiologie*. 2nd ed. Berlin: Verlag von August Hirschwald; 1871.

2. Critchley M. Spastic dysphonia ("inspiratory speech") *Brain*. 1939;62:96-103.

3. Bellussi G. Le disfonie impercinetiche. *Atti Labor Fonet Univ Padova*. 1952;3:1.

4. Bloch P. Neuro-psychiatric aspects of spastic dysphonia. *Folia Phoniatr (Basel)*. 1965;17:310-364.

5. Brin MF, Blitzer A, Stewart C. Laryngeal dystonia (spasmodic dysphonia): observations of 901 patients and treatment with botulinum toxin. *Adv Neurol*. 1998;78:237-252.

6. Aminoff MJ, Dedo HH, Izdebski K. Clinical aspects of spasmodic dysphonia. *J Neurol Neurosurg Psychiatry*. 1978;41:361-365.

7. Blitzer A, Brin MF, Stewart CF. Botulinum toxin management of spasmodic dysphonia (laryngeal dystonia): a 12-year experience in more than 900 patients. *Laryngoscope*. 1998;108:1435-1441.

8. Deleyiannis FW, Gillespie M, Bielamowicz S, Yamashita T, Ludlow CL. Laryngeal long latency re-sponse conditioning in abductor spasmodic dysphonia. *Ann Otol Rhinol Laryngol*. 1999;108: 612-619.

9. Bressman SB. Dystonia genotypes, phenotypes, and classification. *Adv Neurol*. 2004;94:101-107.

10. Saunders-Pullman R, Shriberg J, Shanker V, Bressman SB. Penetrance and expression of dystonia genes. *Adv Neurol*. 2004;94:121-125.

11. Bressman SB. Dystonia: phenotypes and genotypes. *Rev Neurol (Paris)*. 2003;159:849-856.

12. Roy N, Ford CN, Bless DM. Muscle tension dysphonia and spasmodic dysphonia: the role of manual laryngeal tension reduction in diagnosis and management. *Ann Otol Rhinol Laryngol*. 1996;105: 851-856.

13. Morrison M. Pattern recognition in muscle misuse voice disorders: How I do it. *J Voice*. 1997;11:108-114.

14. Schweinfurth JM, Billante M, Courey MS. Risk factors and demographics in patients with spasmodic dysphonia. *Laryngoscope*. 2002;112:220-223.

15. Tolosa E, Marti MJ. Blepharospasm–oromandibular dystonia syndrome (Meige's syndrome): clinical aspects. *Adv Neurol*. 1988;49:73-84.

16. Bielamowicz S, Ludlow CL. Effects of botulinum toxin on pathophysiology in spasmodic dysphonia. *Ann Otol Rhinol Laryngol*. 2000;109:194-203.

17. Chhetri DK, Blumin JH, Vinters HV, Berke GS. Histology of nerves and muscles in adductor spasmodic dysphonia. *Ann Otol Rhinol Laryngol*. 2003;112:334-341.

18. Hillel AD. The study of laryngeal muscle activity in normal human subjects and in patients with laryngeal dystonia using multiple fine-wire electromyography. *Laryngoscope*. 2001;111:1-47.

19. Sapienza CM, Walton S, Murry T. Adductor spasmodic dysphonia and muscular tension dysphonia: acoustic analysis of sustained phonation and reading. *J Voice*. 2000;14:502-520.

20. Roy N, Gouse M, Mauszycki SC, Merrill RM, Smith ME. Task specificity in adductor spasmodic dysphonia versus muscle tension dysphonia. *Laryngoscope*. 2005;115:311-316.

21. Cannito MP, Johnson JP. Spastic dysphonia: a continuum disorder. *J Commun Disord.* 1981;14:215-233.

22. Cyrus CB, Bielamowicz S, Evans FJ, Ludlow CL. Adductor muscle activity abnormalities in abductor spasmodic dysphonia. *Otolaryngol Head Neck Surg.* 2001;124:23-30.

23. Blitzer A, Brin MF, Fahn S, Lovelace RE. Clinical and laboratory characteristics of focal laryngeal dystonia: study of 110 cases. *Laryngoscope.* 1988; 98:636-640.

24. Blitzer A, Brin MF. Laryngeal dystonia: a series with botulinum toxin therapy. *Ann Otol Rhinol Laryngol.* 1991;100:85-89.

25. Klotz DA, Maronian NC, Waugh PF, Shahinfar A, Robinson L, Hillel AD. Findings of multiple muscle involvement in a study of 214 patients with laryngeal dystonia using fine-wire electromyography. *Ann Otol Rhinol Laryngol.* 2004;113:602-612.

26. Barkmeier JM, Case JL, Ludlow CL. Identification of symptoms for spasmodic dysphonia and vocal tremor: a comparison of expert and nonexpert judges. *J Commun Disord.* 2001;34:21-37.

27. Sataloff RT, Mandel S, Mann EA, Ludlow CL. Laryngeal electromyography: an evidence-based review. *Muscle Nerve.* 2003;28:767-772.

28. Hillel AD, Maronian NC, Waugh PF, Robinson L, Klotz DA. Treatment of the interarytenoid muscle with botulinum toxin for laryngeal dystonia. *Ann Otol Rhinol Laryngol.* 2004;113:341-348.

29. Murry T, Woodson GE. Combined-modality treatment of adductor spasmodic dysphonia with botulinum toxin and voice therapy. *J Voice.* 1995;9: 460-465.

30. Morrison MD, Rammage LA, Belisle GM, Pullan CB, Nichol H. Muscular tension dysphonia. *J Otolaryngol.* 1983;12:302-306.

31. Sulica L. Contemporary management of spasmodic dysphonia. *Curr Op Otolaryngol Head Neck Surg.* 2004;12:543-548.

32. Blitzer A, Sulica L. Botulinum toxin: basic science and clinical uses in otolaryngology. *Laryngoscope.* 2001;111:218-226.

33. American Academy of Otolaryngology-Head and Neck Surgery Foundation Policy Statements. Botulinum toxin treatment. Available at: http://www.entlink.net/practice/rules/botox_treatment.cfm. Accessed July 20, 1990.

34. Blitzer A, Brin MF, Fahn S, Lange D, Lovelace RE. Botulinum toxin (Botox) for the treatment of "spastic dysphonia" as part of a trial of toxin injections for the treatment of other cranial dystonias. *Laryngoscope.* 1986;96:1300-1301.

35. Adler CH, Bansberg SF, Krein-Jones K, Hentz JG. Safety and efficacy of botulinum toxin type B (myobloc) in adductor spasmodic dysphonia. *Mov Disord.* 2004;19:1075-1079.

36. Brin MF, Blitzer A, Fahn S, Gould W, Lovelace RE. Adductor laryngeal dystonia (spastic dysphonia): treatment with local injections of botulinum toxin (Botox). *Mov Disord.* 1989;4:287-296.

37. Ludlow CL, Naunton RF, Fujita M, Sedory SE. Spasmodic dysphonia: botulinum toxin injection after recurrent nerve surgery. *Otolaryngol Head Neck Surg.* 1990;102:122-131.

38. Grillone GA, Blitzer A, Brin MF, Annino DJ, Jr, Saint-Hilaire MH. Treatment of adductor laryngeal breathing dystonia with botulinum toxin type A. *Laryngoscope.* 1994;104:30-32.

39. Blitzer A, Brin MF, Stewart C, Aviv JE, Fahn S. Abductor laryngeal dystonia: a series treated with botulinum toxin. *Laryngoscope.* 1992;102: 163-167.

40. Ford CN, Bless DM, Lowery JD. Indirect laryngoscopic approach for injection of botulinum toxin in spasmodic dysphonia. *Otolaryngol Head Neck Surg.* 1990;103:752-758.

41. Green DC, Berke GS, Ward PH, Gerratt BR. Point-touch technique of botulinum toxin injection for the treatment of spasmodic dysphonia. *Ann Otol Rhinol Laryngol.* 1992;101:883-887.

42. Bielamowicz S, Squire S, Bidus K, Ludlow CL. Assessment of posterior cricoarytenoid botulinum toxin injections in patients with abductor spasmodic dysphonia. *Ann Otol Rhinol Laryngol.* 2001;110:406-412.

43. Zwirner P, Murry T, Woodson GE. A comparison of bilateral and unilateral botulinum toxin treatments for spasmodic dysphonia. *Eur Arch Otorhinolaryngol.* 1993;250:271-276.

44. Bielamowicz S, Stager SV, Badillo A, Godlewski A. Unilateral versus bilateral injections of botulinum toxin in patients with adductor spasmodic dysphonia. *J Voice.* 2002;16:117-123.

45. Dedo HH. Recurrent laryngeal nerve section for spastic dysphonia. *Ann Otol Rhinol Laryngol.* 1976;85:451-459.

46. Dedo HH, Townsend JJ, Izdebski K. Current evidence for the organic etiology of spastic dysphonia. *Otolaryngology.* 1978;86:875-880.

47. Dedo HH, Behlau MS. Recurrent laryngeal nerve section for spastic dysphonia: 5- to 14-year preliminary results in the first 300 patients. *Ann Otol Rhinol Laryngol.* 1991;100:274-279.

48. Aronson AE, DeSanto LW. Adductor spastic dysphonia: 1½ years after recurrent laryngeal nerve resection. *Ann Otol Rhinol Laryngol.* 1981;90:2-6.

49. Aronson AE, De Santo LW. Adductor spastic dysphonia: three years after recurrent laryngeal nerve resection. *Laryngoscope.* 1983;93:1-8.

50. Dedo HH, Izdebski K. Problems with surgical (RLN section) treatment of spastic dysphonia. *Laryngoscope.* 1983;93:268-271.

51. Sulica L, Blitzer A, Brin MF, Stewart CF. Botulinum toxin management of adductor spasmodic dysphonia after failed recurrent laryngeal nerve section. *Ann Otol Rhinol Laryngol.* 2003;112:499-505.

52. Biller HF, Som ML, Lawson W. Laryngeal nerve crush for spastic dysphonia. *Ann Otol Rhinol Laryngol.* 1983;92:469.

53. Netterville JL, Stone RE, Rainey C, Zealear DL, Ossoff RH. Recurrent laryngeal nerve avulsion for treatment of spastic dysphonia. *Ann Otol Rhinol Laryngol.* 1991;100:10-14.

54. Weed DT, Jewett BS, Rainey C, et al. Long-term follow-up of recurrent laryngeal nerve avulsion for the treatment of spastic dysphonia. *Ann Otol Rhinol Laryngol.* 1996;105:592-601.

55. Sercarz JA, Berke GS, Ming Y, Rothschiller J, Graves MC. Bilateral thyroarytenoid denervation: a new treatment for laryngeal hyperadduction disorders studied in the canine. *Otolaryngol Head Neck Surg.* 1992;107:657-668.

56. Berke GS, Blackwell KE, Gerratt BR, Verneil A, Jackson KS, Sercarz JA. Selective laryngeal adductor denervation-reinnervation: a new surgical treatment for adductor spasmodic dysphonia. *Ann Otol Rhinol Laryngol.* 1999;108:227-231.

57. Allegretto M, Morrison M, Rammage L, Lau DP. Selective denervation: reinnervation for the control of adductor spasmodic dysphonia. *J Otolaryngol.* 2003;32:185-189.

58. Chhetri DK, Mendelsohn A, Blumin JH, Berke GS. Long-term follow-up results of the selective laryngeal adductor denervation-reinnervation surgery for adductor spasmodic dysphonia. *Laryngoscope.* 2006;116:635-642.

59. Isshiki N, Tsuji DH, Yamamoto Y, Iizuka Y. Midline lateralization thyroplasty for adductor spasmodic dysphonia. *Ann Otol Rhinol Laryngol.* 2000;109: 187-193.

60. Isshiki N, Haji T, Yamamoto Y, Mahieu HF. Thyroplasty for adductor spasmodic dysphonia: further experiences. *Laryngoscope.* 2001;111:615-621.

61. Tucker HM. Laryngeal framework surgery in the management of spasmodic dysphonia. Preliminary report. *Ann Otol Rhinol Laryngol.* 1989;98:52-54.

62. Tucker HM. Anterior commissure laryngoplasty for adjustment of vocal fold tension. *Ann Otol Rhinol Laryngol.* 1985;94:547-549.

63. Chan SW, Baxter M, Oates J, Yorston A. Long-term results of type II thyroplasty for adductor spasmodic dysphonia. Laryngoscope. 2004;114(9): 1604-1608.

64. Lee L, Daughton S, Scheer S, et al. Use of acupuncture for the treatment of adductor spasmodic dysphonia: a preliminary investigation. *J Voice.* 2003;17:411-424.

65. Genack SH, Woo P, Colton RH, Goyette D. Partial thyroarytenoid myectomy: an animal study investigating a proposed new treatment for adductor spasmodic dysphonia. *Otolaryngol Head Neck Surg.* 1993; 08:256-264.

66. Koufman JA, Rees CJ, Halum SL, Blalock D. Treatment of adductor-type spasmodic dysphonia by surgical myectomy: a preliminary report. Ann Otol Rhinol Laryngol. 2006;115(2):97-102.

67. Shaw GY, Sechtem PR, Rideout B. Posterior cricoarytenoid myoplasty with medialization thyroplasty in the management of refractory abductor spasmodic dysphonia. *Ann Otol Rhinol Laryngol.* 2003;112:303-306.

68. Koufman JA. Management of abductor spasmodic dysphonia by endoscopic partial posterior cricoarytenoid (partial) myectomy. *Phonoscope.* 1999;2:159-166.

69. Marks WJ. Deep brain stimulation for dystonia. *Curr Treat Options Neurol.* 2005;7:237-243.

B. Inflammatory and Structural Disorders

21

Localized Inflammatory Disorders of the Larynx

Natasha Mirza, MD, FACS

KEY POINTS

■ Most acute laryngeal inflammation is self-limiting; whereas viral laryngitis may result in secondary bacterial infections, empiric antibiotic therapy has not been shown to be beneficial.

■ Severe infections of the upper airway, such as *supraglottitis* and *bacterial tracheitis*, must be aggressively treated with antibiotics and supportive care; management of the airway is the paramount concern.

■ Laryngeal *candidiasis* occurs in immune-compromised persons.

■ A persistent lesion of the larynx must always be considered to be a possible malignancy; although rarely indicated in the acutely inflamed larynx at the first visit, biopsy should be considered for persistent lesions.

■ Posterior laryngeal granuloma has a high rate of recurrence following excision. Treatment involves antireflux medication and possibly speech therapy.

Local laryngeal inflammatory conditions cover a spectrum of infectious and irritative lesions. They also include immune mediated conditions whereby the laryngeal tissues mount a response to an exogenous or endogenous insult. They are all characterized by a local reaction to an insult with changes in the laryngeal tissues that can either be localized to one site, involve several subsites, or involve the entire larynx. Many of the systemic disorders affecting the larynx are reviewed in detail in chapter 22 immediately following. There is some overlap, however, between the two chapters.

The management of inflammatory conditions of the larynx depends to a great extent on the etiology of the condition. This is, however, not often easily apparent when the patient first presents. The clinical course can be variable and the symptoms and signs nonspecific. Several of these disorders, such as acute viral laryngitis, are among the most common conditions affecting the upper aerodigestive tract. Recognition and knowledge of the more elusive conditions is necessary so that the appropriate tests are ordered, cultures and biopsies are taken, and eventually the appropriate management instituted.

Most cases where there is laryngeal involvement present with dysphonia, odynophonia, and occasionally cough and dyspnea. Complaints related to swallowing problems and odynophagia are rarer and may represent advanced infection or inflammation.

Biopsy may be required in cases that are not self-limiting. For most patients, this means a trip to the operating room for direct laryngoscopy and an evaluation of the trachea and bronchi if possible. All suspicious lesions should be biopsied to help make a conclusive diagnosis and also to rule out malignancy, a constant concern. Cultures of the surface of the lesions and also of the biopsied material are also helpful in some situations.

In this chapter, we review some of the laryngeal lesions with an infectious, immune, or irritative etiology, their typical presentation, laryngeal findings, and management (Figures 22–1 and 22–2). These will be distinguished by whether or not they typically involve the entire larynx at the time of presentation.

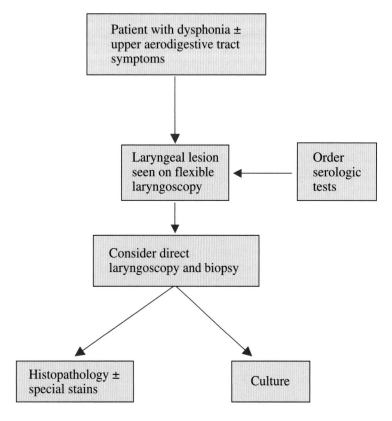

FIGURE 21–1. Clinical approach to a patient with a suspected inflammatory laryngeal lesion.

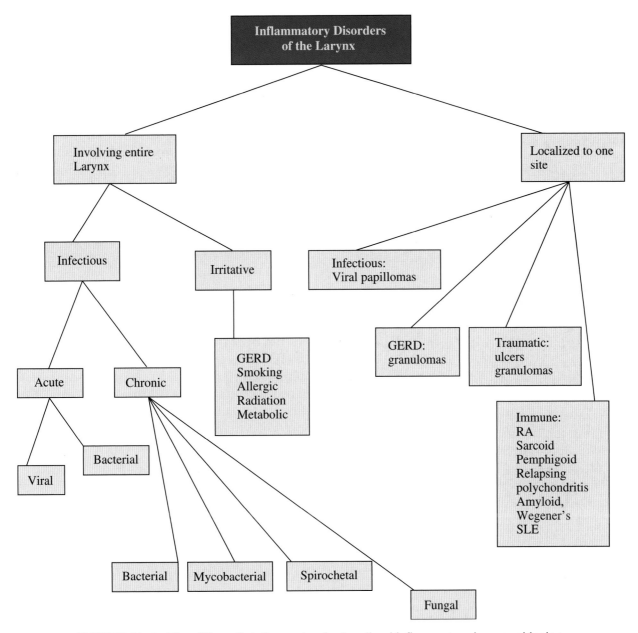

FIGURE 21–2. The differential diagnosis of a localized inflammatory laryngeal lesion.

LESIONS INVOLVING ENTIRE LARYNX

Acute Infections: Viral

The most common cause of laryngeal symptoms is acute viral laryngitis related to an upper respiratory tract infection. Presenting symptoms include dysphonia and even loss of voice, cough, fever, and often symptoms of rhinitis. Laryngoscopic findings include erythema and edema which involves the vocal folds and often the supraglottis as well. Treatment includes voice rest and hydration. Most conditions are self-limited and resolve in about 1 week.

In more advanced cases, *viral* laryngotracheitis can result in more profound illness with airway obstruction. In children and adults *parainfluenza* or *influenza*[1,2] viruses are leading causes of croup. In addition to general supportive measures, dexamethasone appears to be beneficial in reducing the overall severity of advanced cases of laryngotracheitis during the first 24 hours after infection.[3] Further airway issues in children are discussed in Chapter 28, Pediatric Laryngology.

Acute Infections: Bacterial

Bacterial laryngitis is not common, although when it does occur, it can be quite severe. Two clinical entities, epiglottitis and bacterial laryngotracheitis, are discussed below. When the larynx appears to be infected and purulent debris is present on the laryngeal mucosa, it is tempting to treat the patient with antibiotics If the patient does not exhibit signs of toxicity, as in the more severe forms, this is not likely to be beneficial. Two studies, both from Sweden, compared penicillin and erythromycin, respectively, to placebo in patients with suspected bacterial superinfection involving the larynx.[4,5] The local symptoms and voice quality were felt to be equivalent between the two groups.

Bacterial tracheitis, a severe disorder, remains rare. The agent responsible is typically *Staphylococcus*, although *Hemophilus influenzae* and Group A *streptococcus* have also been implicated (among others). The characteristic patient will present with a high fever, dyspnea progressing to stridor, dysphonia, and cough. The diagnosis is made on the basis of thick purulence and crusts in the airway, erythema, and laryngeal edema. Blood cultures are often positive for the infectious agent. The mainstay of management is high vigilance; if the condition does not improve on antibiotics, hydration, and humidification, it is necessary to take the patient to the operating room and perform laryngotracheal toilet and suctioning. A tracheostomy is very rarely needed. The condition can be particularly dangerous in children due to the relatively small size of the central airways. One recent report has described an increase in the incidence of positive viral cultures (for influenza) and a lessening morbidity to the disease.[6]

Acute Supraglottitis/Epiglottitis

The infectious agent in adult supraglottitis (also known as *epiglottitis*, a less precise name) is usually *Hemophilus influenzae*. Although historically thought of as a children's disease, it has become relatively more common in adults. This is particularly true with the advent and widespread use of the *H. influenzae B* vaccine in children.[7] Presenting symptoms range from fever and odynophagia to stridor and drooling in the severe forms. Diagnosis in children is based on clinical suspicion and often a lateral neck film showing the "thumb sign" of epiglottic edema. In most adults, flexible laryngoscopy can be performed safely; this examination will reveal diffuse edema and erythema of the supraglottis. The diagnosis is based on clinical grounds and may be confirmed by blood cultures. Viral supraglottitis has also been described.[8] Surface cultures may be obtained if the patient has been taken to the operating room for airway management. The mainstay of management is to secure the airway. In children this involves an intubation in the OR whereas, in adults observation in the ICU, intubation, or even a tracheotomy may be necessary, though not common. A recent review of 23 adult cases from one institution in Ireland revealed that only three of the 23 required intubation or tracheotomy; indeed, all three had presented with rapidly progressing symptoms.[9] Although antibiotic therapy is critical, the concurrent use of antibiotics and steroids is a poorly defined but common practice.[10]

Chronic Infectious Conditions

1. Bacterial: Klebsiella (Rhinoscleroma)
2. Spirochetal: Syphilis, Lyme
3. Fungal: Candida
   Blastomycosis
   Histoplasmosis
   Coccidiomycosis
   Aspergillosis
4. Tuberculosis

Bacterial: Klebsiella

Respiratory scleroma is a rare, chronic progressive granulomatous disease that usually begins in

---

Symptomatic Relief of "Sore Throat"

Most patients do not present to the otolaryngologist for the evaluation and management of self-limiting benign inflammatory disorders of the upper aerodigestive tract. Nonetheless, the symptomatic treatment of patients with viral respiratory tract illness is a major over-the-counter industry and these problems represent a significant source of patient morbidity. Although many patients may receive temporary relief with alcohol/phenol based analgesia, prolonged use will exacerbate the problem. The term "pharyngitis medicamentosa" was coined for this clinical situation.[11]

Other than the sensible recommendations of hydration and the avoidance of irritants, what can reasonably be done for these patients once bacterial disease and its complications have been excluded? There has been significant interest in zinc preparations in the past decade, with mixed results.[12,13] Principal concerns with zinc studies include difficulties associated performing blinded studies with zinc products due their strong taste. In one double-blind placebo-controlled study, flurbiprofen, an anti-inflammatory, was given in lozenge form to patients complaining of sore throat. The treatment group had significant relief compared with placebo.[14]

---

the nose and then affects the upper and lower respiratory tract in approximately 40% of cases. The causative organism is *Klebsiella rhinoscleromatis* which is a gram-negative coccobacillus. The disease has three stages: catarrhal, granulomatous, and sclerotic. Patients initially present with dysphonia but airway obstruction generally occurs in the last stage of the disease. Patients rarely present with isolated laryngeal lesions, and there is usually a continuum of rhinologic and airway involvement. Laryngoscopic findings vary from isolated granulomas and nodules to stenosis at the glottic and subglottic levels. Management is based on first establishing a diagnosis with biopsies, which may show the specific Mikulicz cells which are large macrophages containing the bacilli and on cultures of the causative organism. Early cases may be successfully treated with oral tetracycline and the use of fluoroquinolones is being studied. In the more advanced cases it is important to secure the airway either with a tracheotomy or with endoscopic procedures such as dilatations and serial laser incisions and in some situations with a laryngosfissure and open excision of the lesions. In a report of 22 patients, Shindo noted that 13 had laryngotracheal involvement, three of whom required emergency tracheotomy at some point for obstruction.[15]

Spirochetal

While laryngeal involvement can occur at any stage, Stage I and II syphilis may present with laryngeal ulcers and cervical lymphadenopathy. In the tertiary stage, the larynx may develop fibrosis and stenosis. Diagnosis can be made on the basis of serologic testing but, to prove that laryngeal lesions are associated with the syphilitic conditions, biopsies of lesions and identification of spirochetes are necessary. Treatment is with long-term antibiotics. This disorder is exceedingly rare today, but represented a significant source of chronic disease in the past.[16]

Fungal

Most of these infections occur in the endemic geographic areas in individuals who are also immunocompromised. Typical symptoms are vague and flulike with dysphonia and cough if there is laryngeal involvement. The diagnosis is made generally on the generalized symptoms but a biopsy of the laryngeal lesions is necessary to clinch the diagnosis.[17] Fungal stains are generally positive. Granulomas are found and the epithelium may show changes known as pseudoepitheliomatous hyperplasia, which can be mistaken for a malignancy. The main factor differentiating these conditions is the endemic region in which the individual resides. Treatment with long-term amphotericin-B is still the best modality; however, ketoconazole has also been tried for periods of 6 months or more. These are discussed in great detail in the following chapter, Systemic Inflammatory Disorders Affecting the Larynx.

Laryngeal candidiasis, in contrast to the disorders listed above, is a commonly seen fungal infection due to *Candida albicans*. This disease can occur in both immunocompromised patients and healthy patients with predisposing factors such as the use of corticosteroids, particularly inhaled steroids in asthmatics, broad-spectrum antibiotics, diabetes, burns, alcoholism, endotracheal intubation, and recent laryngitis. Sulica has published a recent review of this clinical entity.[18] Two forms of laryngeal candidiasis have been described. One is the benign, isolated laryngeal candidiasis commonly seen in asthmatics with chronic use of steroid inhalers (Figure 21–3). These otherwise healthy patients present with isolated hoarseness and typically no other symptoms. The clinical exam shows diffuse laryngeal erythema with an irregular, superficial white exudate usually involving the true vocal folds. The second form is invasive laryngeal candidiasis seen in the immunocompromised patient, which is typically more serious and can be life-threatening. In these patients, the infection is rarely limited to the larynx and may involve the esophagus, oropharynx, and lower airway. Invasive candidiasis presents with symptoms of hoarseness, odyno-

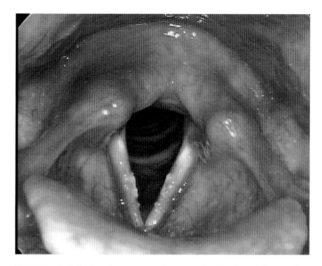

FIGURE 21–3. Laryngeal candiadasis. Note the bilateral white irregularities of the membranous vocal folds.

phagia, and dysphagia. Laryngoscopy typically shows mucosal edema, ulceration, and possibly tissue necrosis. Significant airway obstruction can occur.

The diagnosis is confirmed with staining (fungal prep), culture, and/or biopsy. Further workup for immunosuppression is necessary in a patient with no known predisposing factors. This would include an HIV test as laryngeal candidiasis can be a presenting manifestation. For isolated laryngeal candidiasis, treatment usually consists of either topical antifungal gargles or troches versus systemic antifungals (ketoconazole or fluconazole) for 10 days to 2 weeks. Retreatment may be necessary due to the underlying predisposing factors. For invasive candidiasis, IV amphotericin-B is recommended and airway support as needed.

LOCALIZED INFLAMMATORY LESIONS OF THE LARYNX

Immune-Mediated

Many of the inflammatory disorders with local laryngeal manifestations are immune-mediated.

They are discussed in detail in the following chapter, including rheumatoid arthritis and relapsing polychondritis. Other disorders are also presented, such as amyloidosis, sarcoidosis, and Wegener's granulomatosis. Loehrl and Smith have published an excellent review of these issues.[19]

Pemphigus Vulgaris and Pemphigoid

These two autoimmune disorders involve epithelial disease. Pemphigus vulgaris represents *intraepithelial* antibodies resulting in bleb for[20] Pemphigoid, on the other hand, is a *subepithelial* process, although many of the laryngeal presentations are similar. The patient may manifest local signs of inflammation with hoarseness or throat pain (Figure 21-4). In a recent review of *pemphigus* patients, 21/53 (40%) had laryngeal complaints, many of whom responded to an increase in systemic steroid therapy.[21] Cicatricial pemphigoid may affect the larynx; this subtype has a propensity for mucosa, most commonly affecting the oral cavity.[22] Advanced cases may result in laryngeal stenosis. The acute management of the patient, once the disorder is considered, is to rule out a superimposed fungal infection (see above) which may mimic the local lesions in the

larynx. With the cooperation of the patient's internist or dermatologist, the systemic immunosuppresion may be guided by the status of the laryngeal inflammation. Systemic therapy may also include more toxic agents such as dapsone, methotrexate, and cyclophosphamide.

Irritative and Inflammatory Lesions

Laryngeal Granuloma

These characteristic posterior laryngeal lesions are benign growths of hypertrophic granulation tissue; they most commonly occur at the vocal process of the arytenoid. They likely begin as ulcerations of the larynx (contact ulcers). Repeated trauma and inflammation then produce granulation tissue (Figures 21-5A and 21-5B). Although patients who develop these after intubation may be different, the typical patient with a spontaneous posterior granuloma suffers from laryngopharyngeal reflux (see chapter 23 for more on reflux and the larynx). Ylitalo and others have demonstrated a high incidence of positive pH probe studies in these patients.[23] They have a high incidence of recurrence following surgical therapy and should only be excised for airway obstruction or concern over possible malignancy.

Patients present with odynophagia, odynophonia, and dysphonia. Whereas 24-hour pH probe monitoring may be helpful, empiric therapy with a proton-pump inhibitor is reasonable. Speech therapy, although controversial as a meaningful treatment for granuloma, may be beneficial.[24] Another option for patients is the use of botulinum toxin to create a chemical "voice rest."[25] The injection of botulinum toxin works by preventing the forceful adduction of the arytenoids which contributes to the local phonotrauma and high recurrence/persistence rates. In fact, Nasri et al have reported on the efficacious effect of Botox injections alone without excision of the granulomas by preventing mucosal damage caused by adduction of the arytenoids.[25] Studies are underway regarding the use of inhaled steroids for the treatment of posterior laryngeal granuloma.

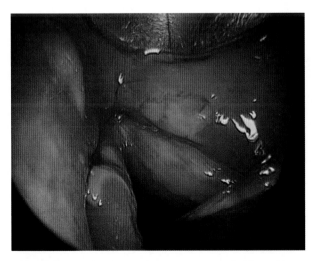

FIGURE 21–4. Direct laryngoscopy findings in a patient with active pemphigus vulgaris involving the larynx. A 70-degree telescope was used for this image.

A.

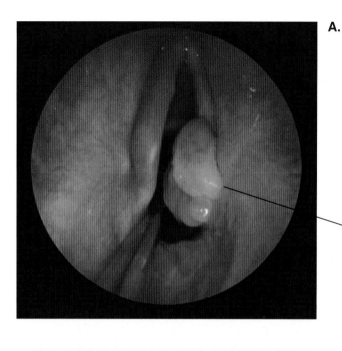

Multilobulated
granuloma of the
vocal process of
the arytenoid

B.

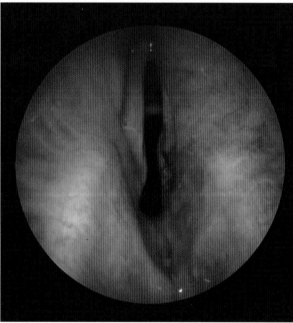

FIGURE 21–5. Posterior laryngeal granuloma before **A.** and after **B.** excision. This large granuloma was causing obstructive symptoms. Note the characteristic location centered at the vocal process of the arytenoids.

Teflon Granuloma

Teflon augmentation of the vocal folds was a popular and well-established technique for achieving medialization of a paralyzed vocal fold for most of the 1970s and 1980s. As laryngeal framework surgery became more popular, Teflon injection fell out of favor, particularly in light of the development of local reaction to the injected material over time. While the incidence of histo-

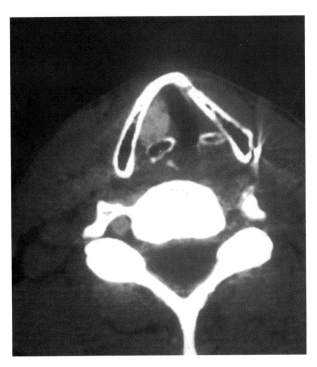

FIGURE 21–6. CT image of a right-sided Teflon granuloma.

logic reaction to Teflon is common, the clinical manifestations of this local inflammation are estimated to occur in 2 to 10% of patients; it is thought to be associated with over injection or misplaced Teflon.[26] The enlarging mass of Teflon/inflammation leads to dysphonia and airway compromise (Figure 21–6). Surgical removal may be required but must be considered carefully; advocates for endoscopic[27] and open[28] removal caution against the further disruption of normal tissue which may occur with surgical resection. A conservative endoscopic "contouring" of the involved vocal fold to create a straight edge for the working fold to vibrate against may be the best option in patients whose granuloma is intimately involved with the vocal ligament, as so many are.

This chapter has briefly outlined the clinical presentation and management of some of the inflammatory conditions of the larynx. While basic supportive treatment is appropriate for common self-limiting conditions such as acute viral laryngitis, serious disorders such as bacterial tracheitis and supraglottitis must be considered in the sick patient.

Biopsy may be considered for patients in whom malignancy is suspected or in the face of failure of medical management. Specific conditions, such as posterior granuloma and Teflon granuloma, must be handled with full knowledge of the natural history of these local processes.

Review Questions

1. An adult presents to your Emergency Room with progressive throat pain and dyspnea over a 24-hour period. His temperature is 102 degrees F. He has some stridor but is not in acute distress. You will most likely need to perform:
   a. Cricothyrotomy
   b. Elective endotracheal intubation
   c. Tracheotomy
   d. Transtracheal jet ventilation
   e. None of the above

2. A healthy, nondiabetic female has 2 weeks of sore throat following a sinus infection. Her rhinologic symptoms have resolved but she is hoarse and clearing her throat a great deal. Laryngeal examination reveals diffuse white specks on the vocal folds, which themselves are reddened. She:
   a. Has candidiasis; treat with antifungals
   b. Cannot have candidiasis without being diabetic or otherwise immunocompromised
   c. Should not be treated without cultures of the vocal folds
   d. This is a manifestation of reflux
   e. Should resume antibiotics for her sinusitis, now involving the larynx

3. A 45-year-old homeless man is admitted for shortness of breath. His chest x-ray is clear but the admitting medical service notes sinusitis and laryngotracheitis. He is coughing and appears ill. His sputum reveals gram-negative coccobacillary organisms. Biopsy of his respiratory mucosa reveals Mikulicz cells. He has:
   a. Wegener's
   b. Amyloidosis
   c. Sarcoidosis
   d. Rhinoscleroma
   e. Teflon granuloma

4. A 55-year-old female is now 25 years s/p left thyroid lobectomy. She was treated for a vocal paralysis shortly after her surgery. After years of getting by with modest hoarseness and no dysphagia, she is now complaining of a globus sensation and her voice is more tense. Examination reveals:
   a. A bilobed granuloma at her vocal process on the nonparalyzed side
   b. A bilobed granuloma at her vocal process on the paralyzed side
   c. A Teflon granuloma in the paraglottic space on the nonparalyzed side
   d. A Teflon granuloma in the paraglottic space on the paralyzed side
   e. Gelfoam extruding from an old injection laryngoplasty site

5. A 65-year-old banker has chronic throat clearing. Examination reveals a smooth 5 mm bilobed granuloma at the vocal process on the left side. He is a nonsmoker. You:
   a. Reassure him that this is not cancer
   b. Recommend immediate biopsy
   c. Recommend antireflux treatment
   d. Inject botulinum toxin into the right vocal fold
   e. Inject botulinum toxin into the left vocal fold

REFERENCES

1. Cherry JD. State of the evidence for standard-of-care treatments for croup: are we where we need to be? *Pediatr Infect Dis J.* 2005;24(11 suppl):S198–S202.

2. Woo PC, Young K, Tsang KW, Ooi CG, Peiris M, Yuen K. Adult croup: a rare but more severe condition. *Respiration.* 2000;67(6):684–688.

3. Super DM, Cartelli NA, Brooks LJ, Lembo RM, Kumar ML. A prospective randomized double-blind study to evaluate the effect of dexamethasone in acute laryngotracheitis. *J Pediatr.* 1989;115(2):323–329.

4. Schalen L, Eliasson I, Kamme C, Schalen C. Erythromycin in acute laryngitis in adults. *Ann Otol Rhinol Laryngol.* 1993;102(3 pt 1):209–214.

5. Schalen L, Christensen P, Eliasson I, Fex S, Kamme C, Schalen C. Inefficacy of penicillin V in acute laryngitis in adults. Evaluation from results of double-blind study. *Ann Otol Rhinol Laryngol.* 1985;94(1 pt 1):14–17.

6. Bernstein T, Brilli R, Jacobs B. Is bacterial tracheitis changing? A 14-month experience in a pediatric intensive care unit. *Clin Infect Dis.* 1998;27(3):458–462.

7. Gorelick MH, Baker MD. Epiglottitis in children, 1979 through 1992. Effects of *Haemophilus influenzae type b* immunization. *Arch Pediatr Adolesc Med.* 1994;148(1):47–50.

8. D'Angelo AJ Jr, Zwillenberg S, Olekszyk JP, Marlowe FI, Mobini J. Adult supraglottitis due to herpes simplex virus. *J Otolaryngol.* 1990;19(3):179–181.

9. Madhotra D, Fenton JE, Makura ZG, Charters P, Roland NJ. Airway intervention in adult supraglottitis. *Ir J Med Sci.* 2004;173(4):197–199.

10. Shah RK, Roberson DW, Jones DT. Epiglottitis in the *Hemophilus influenzae type B* vaccine era: changing trends. *Laryngoscope.* 2004;114(3):557–560.

11. Halwell R. Pharyngitis medicamentosa. *Arch Otolaryngol Head Neck Surg.* 1989;115(8):995.

12. Mossad SB, Macknin ML, Medendorp SV, Mason P. Zinc gluconate lozenges for treating the common cold.in children: a randomized double-blind, placebo-controlled study. *Ann Intern Med.* 1996;125(2):81–88.

13. Macknin ML, Piedmonte M, Calendine C, Janosky J, Wald E. Zinc gluconate lozgenges for treating

the common cold in children: a randomized controlled trial. *JAMA*. 1998;279(24):1962-1967.

14 Blagden M, Christian J, Miller K, Charlesworth A. Multidose flurbiprofen 8.75 mg lozenges in the treatment of sore throat: a randomized, double-blind, placebo-controlled study in UK general practice centres. *Int J Clin Prac*. 2002;56(2): 95-100.15. Amoils CP, Shindo ML. Laryngotracheal manifestations of rhinoscleroma. *Ann Otol Rhinol Laryngol*. 1996;105(5): 336-340

15. Amoils CP, Shindo ML. Laryngotracheal manifestations of rhinoscleroma. *Ann Otol Rhinol Laryngol*. 1996;105(5):336-340.

16. Grunwald E. *Diseases of the Larynx*. Philadelphia, Pa: WB Saunders, 1900:64.

17. Makitie AA, Back L, Aaltonen LM, Leivo I, Valtonen M. fungal infection of the epiglottis simulating a clinical malignancy. *Arch Otolaryngol Head Neck Surg*. 2003;129(1):124-126.

18. Sulica L. Laryngeal thrush. *Ann Otol Rhinol Laryngol*. 2005;114(5):369-375

19. Loehrl TA, Smith TL. Inflammatory and granulomatous lesions of the larynx and pharynx. *Am J Med*. 2001;111(suppl 8A):113S-S117.

20. Pathak PN. Pemphigus of the larynx. *J Laryngol Otol*. 1971;85(1):81-82.

21. Hale EK, Bystryn JC. Laryngeal and nasal involvement in pemphigus vulgaris. *J Am Acad Dermatol*. 2001;44(4):609-611

22. Hanson RD, Olsen KD, Rogers RS 3rd. Upper aerodigestive tract manifestations of cicatricial pemphigoid. *Ann Otol Rhinol Laryngol*. 1988; 97(5 pt 1):493-499.

23. Ylitalo R, Ramel S. Extraesophageal reflux in patients with contact granuloma: a prospective controlled study. *Ann Otol Rhinol Laryngol*. 2002;111(5 pt 1):441-446.

24. Ylitalo R. Hammarberg B. Voice characteristics, effects of voice therapy, and long-term follow-up of contact granuloma patients. *J Voice*. 2000; 14(4):557-566.

25. Nasri S, Sercarz JA, McAlpin T, Berke GS. Treatment of vocal fold granuloma using Botulinum toxin type A. *Laryngoscope*. 1995;105:585-588.

26. Kasperbauer JL, Slavit DH, Maragos NE. Teflon granulomas and overinjection of Teflon: a therapeutic challenge for the otolaryngologist. *Ann Otol Rhinol Laryngol*. 1993;102(10):748-751.

27. Nakayama M, Ford CN, Bless DM. Teflon vocal fold augmentation: failures and management in 28 cases. *Otolaryngol Head Neck Surg*. 1993;109(3 pt 1): 493-498.

28. Netterville JL, Coleman JR Jr, Chang S, Rainey CL, Reinisch L, Ossoff RH. Lateral laryngotomy for the removal of Teflon granuloma. *Ann Otol Rhinol Laryngol*. 1998;107(9 pt 1):735-744.

22

Systemic Inflammatory Disorders Affecting the Larynx

Felicia L. Johnson, MD
James W. Ragland, MD

KEY POINTS

- Laryngeal inflammation is a nonspecific finding that has many etiologies; not all laryngeal inflammation is due to laryngopharyngeal reflux.

- The larynx may be the first area affected in many of these systemic inflammatory diseases with no other organ system involvement.

- Direct laryngoscopy with biopsy and histopathologic examination is warranted and may be necessary to make the diagnosis in many of these conditions.

- The incidence of laryngeal tuberculosis may be increasing; systemic mycobacterial disease is present in a minority of these patients.

- Directed surgical therapy in the larynx is beneficial in the management of some systemic inflammatory diseases in combination with medical therapy.

TUBERCULOSIS

Epidemiology/Pathogenesis

Laryngeal tuberculosis (TB) is a chronic often indolent bacterial infection caused by *Mycobacterium tuberculosis*. Previously, TB was one of the most common granulomatous diseases affecting the larynx. But with the development of antibiotics, laryngeal TB has become more uncommon, especially in developed countries. However, recently there has been a noted increase in the incidence of this disease in both developing and developed countries. This is thought to be due to the increasing number of patients with human immunodeficiency virus (HIV) infection and the emergence of multi-drug resistant mycobacterium. Also, in developed countries there has been a decrease in immunization for TB and an increasing immigration from countries with a high incidence of TB. A recent study by Shin et al[1] reported a changing trend in the patient population presenting with laryngeal TB. Their results show that the average age at the time of presentation is 42 years, older than that previously reported in the 1950s during which time the typical patient with laryngeal TB was 20 to 30 years old. They also reported a 2:1 male predominance in their patient population. The other significant finding in the Shin paper was the surprisingly low prevalence of active pulmonary TB in their patients with only 7 of 22 having active disease. This differs significantly with previous reports where laryngeal TB was almost always associated with advanced pulmonary disease.

The true pathogenesis of laryngeal TB is debated in the literature. There is a primary infection of the larynx in which the mycobacterial organisms directly infect the laryngeal mucosa in the absence of pulmonary disease. A secondary infection of the larynx may occur in several ways. The classically described pathway involves a patient with advanced pulmonary disease who subsequently inoculates the posterior larynx with infected sputum, resulting in laryngeal disease. Another mechanism is hematogenous or lymphatic drainage from affected tissues may seed the larynx. Most recent reports tend to favor the latter theory of pathogenesis in the current era of laryngeal TB, although primary cases of laryngeal disease have been reported. Shin et al[1] reported a 40% (9/22) incidence of primary laryngeal TB.

Clinical Presentation

Tuberculosis is often referred to as a masquerader as it can mimic carcinoma. The presenting symptoms can be identical to laryngeal carcinoma including hoarseness, odynophagia, dysphagia, cough, and weight loss. Indirect laryngoscopy can show a variety of lesions and can affect the supraglottis and glottis. The classically described posterior interarytenoid mucosal involvement seems to be less common as noted in the current literature. Instead, the most common sites of involvement include the true vocal folds, false vocal folds, and epiglottis. Shin et al[1] classified the types of lesions seen into four categories: nonspecific inflammatory, polypoid, white/ulcerative, and "ulcerofungative" lesions. Interestingly, they found that patients with active pulmonary disease tended to present with multiple lesions that were ulcerative in nature. Those patients without pulmonary disease typically presented with a single lesion that was nonspecific inflammatory in nature. This is a strong reminder to consider TB in the differential diagnosis of a patient presenting with what appears to be an early laryngeal carcinoma.

Evaluation and Testing

These cases rely on direct laryngoscopy and biopsy of affected tissues with appropriate staining for acid-fast bacilli. The specimen is also obtained to evaluate for the presence or absence of carcinoma. Other important tests needed when laryngeal TB is suspected include PPD testing, chest x-ray, and sputum cultures. Laryngeal histology is diagnostic showing caseating granulomas surrounded by pallisading epithelioid histocytes with lymphocytic infiltration and multinucleated giant cells. The differential diagnosis includes syphilis, sarcoidosis, Wegener's granulomatosis, cat-scratch disease, carcinoma, and fungal laryngitis. CT scans of the neck may also by helpful. The CT findings that are characteristic of laryngeal TB are bilateral involvement, thickening of the free margin of the epiglottis, and preservation of the pre-epiglottic/paraglottic spaces even in the presence of extensive mucosal involvement.[2,3]

Treatment

The standard treatment for laryngeal TB is long-term administration of multiple antituberculous medications with a general good prognosis. In Shin et al[1] the average time until resolution of laryngeal symptoms was 5.6 months, although several patients symptomatically improved within 1 to 2 months. The full scope of medical treatment for mycobacterial disease is beyond the scope of this chapter; the need for multiple drug therapy and the world-wide concern over emerging resistance should be noted.

BLASTOMYCOSIS

Epidemiology/Pathogenesis

Blastomycosis is a chronic pulmonary infection caused by the fungus *Blastomyces dermatitidis*. This organism is found in damp wooded areas and is endemic in the United States around the Great Lakes and the Mississippi and Ohio River valleys. Laryngeal involvement occurs in 2 to 5% of all cases.

Clinical Presentation

Patients may complain of severe hoarseness, cough, dysphagia, and dyspnea that has been present for many months. Typical laryngoscopy findings include erythematous granulomatous masses and/or exophytic bulky lesions with irregular borders involving the true vocal folds and occasionally the supraglottis. (see Figure 22–1). Advanced disease can present with vocal fold fixation. Like laryngeal TB, blastomycosis may also mimic carcinoma.

Evaluation and Testing

The diagnosis is made through direct laryngoscopy and biopsy of the tissue. Histopathologic examination will show caseating necrosis with an acute inflammatory infiltration and microabscesses. *Pseudoepitheliomatous hyperplasia* is characteristically seen in the laryngeal epithelium which can lead to a misdiagnosis of squamous cell carcinoma. Periodic acid-Schiff (PAS) and Gomori silver stains will show large broad-based budding yeast near the region of microabscesses. The chest x-ray is often normal and not helpful with the diagnosis.

Treatment

Blastomycosis is treated with either IV amphotericin-B or itraconazole for an average time of 6 months with good response. Surgical intervention is limited to biopsy or drainage of microabscesses as needed.

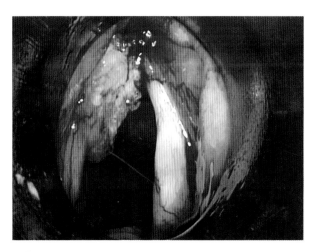

FIGURE 22–1. Blastomycosis affecting the larynx. The left membranous true vocal fold is the main site of involvement.

HISTOPLASMOSIS

Epidemiology/Pathogenesis

Histoplasmosis is caused by the dimorphic fungus *Histoplasma capsulatum* which is endemic to the Mississippi and Ohio River valleys. The mode of dissemination is via inhalation of spores from bird and bat feces. Symptoms at the time of the initial inoculation may be general and resemble a vague, flulike illness. Chronic pulmonary histoplasmosis can result in a disseminated form of the disease with hematogenous spread of the fungus which can ultimately involve the oral cavity, oropharynx, and larynx.

Clinical Presentation

The typical patient with laryngeal histoplasmosis is over 40 years of age and presents with symptoms of hoarseness, dysphagia, odynophagia, dyspnea, and hemoptysis. Patients may also present with painful oral cavity or oropharyngeal ulcerations. Indirect laryngoscopy may reveal a variety of lesions ranging from flat, white plaques to nodular granulomas that can eventually become ulcerative resulting in significant pain. The typical areas affected in the larynx with histoplasmosis include the true vocal folds, epiglottis, and false vocal folds.

Evaluation and Testing

Direct laryngoscopy with biopsy is necessary for diagnosis. Histopathology shows caseating granulomas with giant cells, lymphocytes, and large numbers of macrophages with intracellular yeast buds seen on PAS or Gomori methenamine silver stain. Chest x-ray may demonstrate pulmonary calcifications. Serology for *Histoplasma* antigen is generally not recommended for laryngeal histoplasmosis due to reported low sensitivities.

The sensitivity varies with the severity and extent of the infection, with the greatest sensitivity seen in disseminated or acute diffuse pulmonary disease. Antigen detection is less useful in cases of subacute or chronic pulmonary disease and other manifestations of self-limited histoplasmosis, such as focal laryngeal histoplasmosis. The reported sensitivity in chronic pulmonary histoplasmosis ranges from 6 to14%.[4,5]

Treatment

The treatment for laryngeal histoplasmosis is oral itraconazole for 2 to 6 months with some protocols adding initial treatment with IV amphotericin-B. In general, the prognosis is good with complete resolution of the laryngeal disease.

SARCOIDOSIS

Epidemiology/Pathogenesis

Sarcoidosis is a chronic systemic granulomatous disease of unknown etiology. It is more prevalent in women and typically presents between the ages of 20 and 40. In the United States, it occurs more commonly in African-Americans and Hispanics. Various reports estimate the incidence of laryngeal involvement in sarcoidosis to be between 1 and 5%.[6-8] The pathogenesis of sarcoidosis is still unclear but it appears to be a host response to an unknown stimulus such as an infectious agent (*Mycobacteria* or *Propionibacteria* are two current putative causes) or in response to an environmental agent. Recently, several studies have shown a heightened T helper-1 immune response in patients with sarcoidosis.[9,10] It is unclear at this point whether this is a form of autoimmunity or rather an immunologic response to a previously described or undescribed stimulus.

Clinical Presentation

The most common presenting symptoms of laryngeal sarcoidosis are hoarseness, dysphagia, dyspnea, cough, and globus sensation. Typical laryngeal findings include pale, edematous mucosa with diffuse enlargement of the supraglottis particularly the epiglottis, aryepiglottic folds, arytenoids, and false vocal folds (see Figure 22–2). The true vocal folds are usually spared but the subglottis can be involved. Other head and neck signs of sarcoidosis may be present including parotid swelling and lymphoid hypertrophy. Vocal fold paralysis may be present, but always in association with mediastinal disease.

Evaluation and Testing

The diagnosis of laryngeal sarcoidosis is based on the typical supraglottic appearance and biopsy of the tissue. Histopathology demonstrates non-caseating granulomas and negative stains for fungus or acid-fast bacilli. The differential diagnosis includes tuberculosis, carcinoma, fungal laryngitis, amyloidosis, and radiation fibrosis. Other ancillary tests for systemic sarcoidosis include a chest x-ray, CBC, sedimentation rate, urine/serum calcium, protein electrophoresis, gallium-67 scan, and serum angiotensin-converting enzyme (ACE) levels. Abnormalities seen in systemic sarcoidosis include hilar lymphadenopathy on the chest x-ray, hypercalcemia, hypercalciuria, elevated gamma globulin, and inflammation in salivary and lacrimal tissue on gallium scanning. Serum ACE levels are not useful for diagnostic purposes due to their low sensitivity; however, they can be useful to monitor the progression of the disease. Laryngeal sarcoidosis can occur in isolation with no systemic involvement and in one series occurred in 27% of the cases.[11]

Treatment

If the patient is currently asymptomatic or only mildly symptomatic, then close observation is reasonable. The mainstay of treatment for symptomatic laryngeal involvement is either systemic or intralesional steroids. In a review by Bower et al,[11] systemic steroids were very effective in the treatment of laryngeal sarcoidosis. In addition, intralesional steroid injections were found to be successful in selected patients with focal disease and no impending airway obstruction. A combination of both systemic and intralesional steroids were needed in a minority of patients. The precise indications for each of these treatments have yet to be defined. Other treatment options include tracheotomy for acute airway management, limited surgical resection, other cytotoxic medications, and low-dose external beam radiation. It is difficult to truly evaluate the efficacy of various treatments in laryngeal sarcoidosis because of the frequent spontaneous remissions that occur with this disease.

WEGENER'S GRANULOMATOSIS

Epidemiology/Pathogenesis

Wegener's granulomatosis (WG) is a systemic granulomatous disease of unknown etiology characterized by necrotizing granuloma and vasculitis involving the upper respiratory tract, lungs, and kidneys. Laryngeal involvement may occur in up to 23% of cases. Other areas of the head and neck, most notably the paranasal sinuses and the middle ear, are much more likely to be affected in WG.

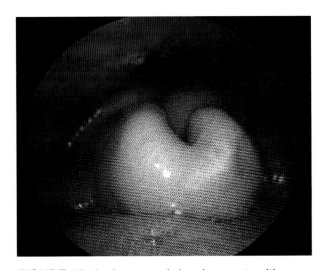

FIGURE 22–2. Laryngeal involvement with sarcoidosis; note the enlargement of the supraglottic structures.

Clinical Presentation

Patients with laryngeal involvement present with dyspnea and hoarseness. The main subsite of the larynx affected is the subglottis often resulting in severe subglottic stenosis. The clinical exam resembles that of idiopathic subglottic stenosis with no distinguishing characteristics. Other head and neck manifestations include recurrent sinusitis, septal perforation, saddle-nose deformity, and chronic serous otitis media.

Evaluation and Testing

Subglottic tissue biopsy is usually negative and not helpful in making the diagnosis. Patients should undergo direct microlaryngoscopy more for treatment than for diagnostic purposes. CT scans of the larynx and trachea may be helpful to determine the extent of the subglottic stenosis and the degree of cartilage involvement. Serology testing for antinuclear cytoplasmic antibodies (ANCA) is often helpful in making the diagnosis. There is a high specificity (more than 90%) with c-ANCA testing in Wegener's granulomatosis.[12] However, the sensitivity of c-ANCA depends on the extent of involvement and the current activity of the disease process. When a patient is in the granulomatous phase of this disease rather than the vasculitic phase, the sensitivity of this test is significantly lower. Also, p-ANCA testing can be positive in up to 20% of patients with WG.[13]

Treatment

If the patient is symptomatic from the subglottic stenosis, then treatment with surgical intervention is warranted. CO_2 laser incision with dilation and topical application of mitomycin-C and corticosteroids is the standard of care. It has been estimated that nearly 50% of all patients with WG will require a tracheotomy at some point in their disease process. Laryngotracheal reconstruction for those who fail endoscopic management is another option for treatment. Medical therapy is also warranted especially in patients with multiorgan involvement. Corticosteroids combined with cyclosporine or methotrexate are the only two regimens that have thus far been shown to induce remission of active WG affecting a major organ. Once remission has been induced, azathioprine and methotrexate have been used to maintain remission.

AMYLOIDOSIS

Epidemiology/Pathogenesis

Amyloidosis is an idiopathic dysproteinemia resulting in extracellular deposition of fibrillar proteins. It is not an inflammatory disorder in the traditional sense, but is included here as the clinical evaluation and decision-making are similar to

---

What if a Patient Doesn't Respond to Empiric Therapy?

Always consider other etiologies of laryngeal inflammation especially when a patient does not respond to empiric treatment. Many of these inflammatory diseases cannot be diagnosed without direct laryngeal examination and biopsy of the affected tissue. When something does not make sense, think of other less common etiologies in the differential diagnosis.

the other disorders presented in this chapter. This disease process may affect multiple organ systems; approximately 300 cases of laryngeal amyloidosis have been reported. Patients who present with laryngeal involvement often have no systemic signs of amyloidosis. There is equal distribution between males and females and the average age at the time of presentation is between the ages of 40 and 50.

Clinical Presentation

Patients with laryngeal amyloidosis present with symptoms of hoarseness, diplophonia, dyspnea, cough, hemoptysis, dysphagia, and globus sensation. Laryngoscopy reveals smooth although sometimes granular, pink/gray submucosal lesions. The lesions may even take on an orange hue. The site of laryngeal involvement varies with the most common site being the infraglottic aspect of the true vocal fold (Figure 22–3). Other sites of involvement include the ventricle, false vocal fold, aryepiglottic fold, and anterior subglottis.

Evaluation and Testing

Direct laryngoscopy with biopsy is necessary for diagnosis. The Congo red stain is diagnostic for

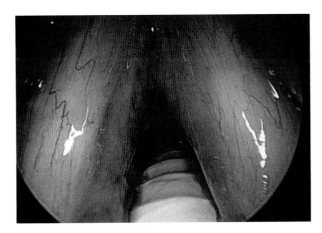

FIGURE 22–3. Laryngeal amyloidosis. The medial and infraglottic surfaces of the vocal folds are often involved.

amyloidosis showing apple-green birefringence with polarized light. Although the majority of patients with laryngeal amyloidosis do not have systemic disease, many authors still recommend a systemic workup to rule out other collagen vascular diseases, tuberculosis, and multiple myeloma. The differential diagnosis includes metastatic medullary thyroid cancer, laryngeal sarcoidosis, benign laryngeal polyps, carcinoma, benign minor salivary tumors, chondromas, neuroendocrine tumors, and lipoid proteinosis.

Treatment

Nondestructive surgical removal of amyloid deposits to restore laryngeal function is generally recommended in the literature. Dedo et al[14] showed that CO_2 laser excision of laryngeal amyloid deposits was effective in restoring vocal quality in a series of 10 patients with an average follow up of 6.5 years. There is no documented medical therapy which has been shown to be effective in isolated laryngeal amyloidosis.

OTHER SYSTEMIC INFLAMMATORY DISORDERS

Systemic lupus erythematosus (SLE) is an autoimmune collagen vascular disease that can present with laryngeal manifestations. The most commonly reported symptoms are hoarseness and dyspnea. Typical laryngoscopy findings include generalized vocal fold edema and/or ulcerations. Vocal fold paralysis and fixation have also been commonly reported. The histopathology is nonspecific. Urgent airway intervention such as a tracheotomy has been reported in some patients. Primary treatment of this disease is with medications such as steroids.

Rheumatoid arthritis (RA) is an autoimmune disorder resulting in polyarthropathy. Laryngeal involvement is not uncommon. The most common laryngeal finding is cricoarytenoid joint fixation, which may be present in as many as 25% of patients with generalized disease.[15] Other findings include rheumatoid nodules, which occur submucosally in the true vocal folds and result in decreased vibration of the vocal folds and dysphonia. Surgical removal of the nodules may be accomplished via a microflap approach, although this is controversial. One compelling recent publication has shed light on another clinical presentation in which the larynx is affected by RA, although not at the level of the larynx itself. Thompson reported on a series of patients with RA and vocal fold paralysis (some bilateral) due to cervicomedullary compression.[16] The site of compression was at the atlantoaxial joint and the skull base. All three patients in this paper had a long-standing history of RA and this did not represent a new diagnosis of the disease.

Relapsing polychondritis is a rare idiopathic autoimmune disease that causes cartilage inflammation. Laryngeal symptoms may include hoarseness, dyspnea, cough, stridor, pain, and sometimes hemoptysis. Laryngeal examination often reveals severe glottic and subglottic edema but no pathognomonic signs. Treatment is airway intervention as needed along with steroids and/or dapsone.

Review Questions

1. The following are true regarding patients with laryngeal amyloidosis:
   a. mean age at presentation is over 70 years of age
   b. predominantly female
   c. roughly 1 in 4 has systemic amyloidosis
   d. responds to medical therapy
   e. has a predilection for the subglottis

2. Laryngeal tuberculosis:
   a. occurs predominantly in young adults and the very old
   b. occurs predominantly in association with active pulmonary TB
   c. is becoming rarer
   d. is responsive to medication within several months
   e. none of the above

3. The most characteristic site of laryngotracheal involvement in sarcoidosis is:
   a. supraglottis
   b. anterior glottis
   c. posterior glottis
   d. subglottis
   e. trachea

4. A 45-year-old woman with a history of generalized rheumatoid arthritis presents with hoarseness of 4 months' duration. She is a nonsmoker. Her clinical examination reveals no stridor but she is moderately dysphonic. Videostroboscopy reveals a yellowish intracordal mass in the left vocal fold. It is transversely oriented. You also detect sluggish vocal fold motion on that side. Her skull base/neck/chest CT scan is unremarkable. You recommend:
   a. intralesional steroid injection
   b. microdirect laryngoscopy with excision of intracordal cyst and injection laryngoplasty at the same setting
   c. injection laryngoplasty
   d. laryngofissure with cyst excision
   e. trial of speech therapy followed by microdirect laryngoscopy with excision of intracordal cyst

5. A microbiological specimen taken from a larynx during direct laryngoscopy reveals several areas suspicious for cancer, though there is no definitive malignancy; special stains demonstrate broad-based budding yeast. The chest radiograph is negative. You suspect:
   a. carcinoma with bacterial superinfection
   b. carcinoma with fungal colonization
   c. disseminated Aspergillosis
   d. Blastomycosis of the larynx
   e. Sarcoidosis

REFERENCES

1. Shin JE, Nam SY, Yoo SY, et al. Changing trends in clinical manifestations of laryngeal tuberculosis. *Laryngoscope.* 2000;110:1950-1953.
2. Moon WK, Han MH, Chang KH, et al. Laryngeal tuberculosis: CT findings. *Am J Roentgenol.* 1996;166:445-449.
3. Kim MD, Kim DI, Yune HY, et al. CT findings of laryngeal TB: comparison to laryngeal carcinoma. *J Comput Assist Tomogr.* 1997;21:29-34.
4. Wheat LJ, Kohler RB, Tewari RP. Diagnosis of disseminated histoplasmosis by detection of *Histoplasma capsulatum* antigen in serum and urine specimens. *N Engl J Med.* 1986;314:83-88.
5. Williams B, Fojtasek M, Connolly-Stringfield P, et al. Diagnosis of histoplasmosis by antigen detection during an outbreak in Indianapolis, Ind. *Arch Path Lab Med.* 1994;118:1205-1208.
6. Devine KD. Sarcoidosis and sarcoidosis of the larynx. *Laryngoscope* 1965;75:533-569.
7. Krespi YP, Mitrani M, Husains S, et al. Treatment of laryngeal sarcoidosis with intralesional steroid injection. *Ann Otol Rhinol Laryngol.* 1987;96:713-715.
8. Ellison DE, Canalis RF. Sarcoidosis of head and neck. *Clin Dermatol.* 1986;44:136-141.
9. Robinson BW, McLemore TL, Crystal RG. Gamma interferon is spontaneously released by alveolar macrophages and lung T lymphocytes in patients with pulmonary sarcoidosis. *J Clin Invest.* 1985; 75:1488-1495.
10. Moller DR, Forman JD, Liu MC, et al. Enhanced expression of IL-12 associated with Th1 cytokine profiles in active pulmonary sarcoidosis. *J Immunol.* 1996;156:4952-4960.
11. Bower JS, Belen JE, Weg JG, et al. Manifestations and treatment of laryngeal sarcoidosis. *Am Rev Respir Dis.* 1980;122:325-332.
12. Specks U, Wheatley CL, McDonald TJ. ANCA in the diagnosis and follow-up of Wegener's. *Mayo Clinic Proc.* 1989;64:28-39.
13. Gluth MB. Subglottic stenosis associated with Wegener's granulomatosis. *Laryngoscope.* 2003; 113:1304-1307.
14. Dedo HH, Izdebski K. Laryngeal amyloidosis in 10 patients. *Laryngoscope.* 2004;114:1742-1746.
15. Montgomery WW. Cricoarytenoid arthritis. *Laryngoscope.* 1963;73:801-836.
16. Thompson-Link D, McCaffrey T V, Krauss WE, Link MJ, Ferguson MT. Cervicomedullary compression: an unrecognized cause of vocal cord paralysis in rheumatoid arthritis. *Ann Otol Rhinol Laryngol.* 1998;107(6):462-471.

23

Reflux and Its Impact on Laryngology

Riitta Ylitalo, MD, PhD

KEY POINTS

- Detailed history and laryngoscopic examination constitute the basis for diagnosis of laryngeal and pharyngeal reflux (LPR). Fewer than 50% of patients with LPR will complain of heartburn.

- Laryngoscopic examination will most commonly demonstrate findings in the posterior glottis and vocal folds.

- Laboratory investigations include barium esophagography and ambulatory 24-hour pH probe; esophagoscopy is used to screen for complications related to GERD as well as for possible malignancy.

- Acid suppression with proton pump inhibitors (PPI) on a long-term basis is the mainstay of treatment; a trial of PPIs may also be useful as a diagnostic maneuver.

Gastroesophageal reflux (GER) can be a normal physiologic phenomenon that occurs in most people, particularly after meals. Gastroesophageal reflux disease (GERD) develops when the reflux causes symptoms like heartburn and acid regurgitation, with or without esophagitis. Laryngopharyngeal reflux (LPR) happens when gastric contents pass the upper esophageal sphincter (UES) causing symptoms and tissue damage in the upper airway. All episodes of GER are not necessarily associated with LPR. Furthermore, the pattern of reflux is also different between LPR and GER patients. LPR occurs predominantly during the daytime in the upright position whereas GERD takes place more often in the, supine position. In fact, the patients may be quite different in terms of body habitus as well. Within the GI literature, reports have described the association[1,2] between obesity and GERD. In contrast, in a group of patients with laryngeal and pharyngeal symptoms, those with abnormal *pharyngeal* reflux events did not have a higher mean body-mass index (BMI) than those with normal studies.[3] A significantly higher percentage of *esophageal* reflux events was, however, seen in obese versus nonobese participants. The authors concluded that abnormal esophageal reflux (GERD) is associated with increasing BMI and obesity, although this was not true for patients with pharyngeal reflux.

It is estimated that up to 10% of patients visiting otolaryngology clinics have reflux-related disease, and up to 55% of patients with hoarseness have LPR.[4-6] Thus, LPR is considered one of the most important and common factors causing inflammation in the upper airways. The tissue damage—demonstrated in both animals and human beings—may be caused by direct exposure to acid, pepsin and bile, by vagally mediated reflexes,[7,8] or perhaps factors yet to be defined. The variance between esophageal symptoms/findings and upper aerodigestive tract disease may reflect the relative susceptibility of the laryngeal epithelium of the larynx and trachea/bronchi to reflux-related injury. LPR also occurs in healthy individuals without symptoms or laryngeal pathology but less frequently than in patients with reflux laryngitis.[9,10] Additionally, reflux-related laryngeal findings have been shown to have a slower resolution pattern and require higher medication levels than uncomplicated esophagitis. Reflux has been implicated in the pathogenesis of nearly all major categories of laryngeal disease, including stenosis, malignancy, benign lesions, dysphagia, and functional disorders.[4]

DIAGNOSIS

For the majority of otolaryngologists, the diagnosis of LPR begins with the history. It is then confirmed by laryngoscopy and subsequently validated by response to a trial of proton pump inhibitor therapy. Although some institutions do perform routine pH testing, for the majority of cases this testing is reserved for refractory or complicated cases.

Symptoms

In addition to hoarseness, the most common symptoms associated with LPR are cough, throat clearing, sore throat, globus, excess throat mucus, choking, and asthma. However, these entities have a multifactorial etiology and may be caused by recent sinusitis or other respiratory infections, smoking, voice abuse, and allergy, making the accurate diagnosis based on history a challenge. Belafsky et al developed the Reflux Symptom Index (RSI), a self-administered nine-item questionnaire to help categorize the severity of LPR (see Table 23–1). An RSI of greater than 13 is considered abnormal. Symptoms of GERD, which include heartburn, chest pain, indigestion or a regurgitation of acid, are important, but it should be noted that 50 to 80% of patients with LPR do not have these classic GERD symptoms.[11]

Laryngeal Examination

The most frequent laryngeal finding related to LPR is posterior laryngitis (PL) that occurs in up

TABLE 23–1. Reflux Symptom Index (RSI)[12] (A total score of 13 is thought to be clinically significant.)

Within the last month, how did the following problem affect you?	0—No Problem 5—Severe Problem					
1. Hoarseness or a problem with your voice	0	1	2	3	4	5
2. Clearing your throat	0	1	2	3	4	5
3. Excess throat mucus or postnasal drip	0	1	2	3	4	5
4. Difficulty swallowing food, liquid, or pills	0	1	2	3	4	5
5. Coughing after you eat or after lying down	0	1	2	3	4	5
6. Breathing difficulties or choking episodes	0	1	2	3	4	5
7. Troublesome or annoying cough	0	1	2	3	4	5
8. Sensations of something sticking in your throat or a lump in your throat	0	1	2	3	4	5
9. Heartburn, chest pain, indigestion, or stomach acid coming up	0	1	2	3	4	5

to 70% of LPR patients. It is characterized by edema or hypertrophy, and sometimes erythema and hyperemia on the posterior wall of the glottis. Occasionally the inflammation reaches up to the medial surface of the arytenoid cartilages and aryepiglottic folds. Most authors use the terms posterior laryngitis and reflux laryngitis synonymously, although this is not accurate. Furthermore, diffuse vocal fold edema, infraglottic edema reaching from the anterior commissure to the posterior wall, also referred to as *pseudosulcus*, and vocal fold granuloma are strongly associated with LPR (Figure 23-1). Of patients with pseudosulcus, 60 to 90% have LPR whereas 65% of granuloma patients are LPR positive. The nature of endolaryngeal mucus if it is thick and tenacious will also point to PL. Any or all of these findings can occur.[4] The difficulty in making a PL diagnosis is that the findings are sometimes quite subtle signs of inflammation and irritation and patients may display a quite normal looking larynx. Furthermore, it has been difficult to show any correlation between a sole laryngeal finding and the occurrence of hypopharyngeal reflux episodes.[10] As none of these findings alone is

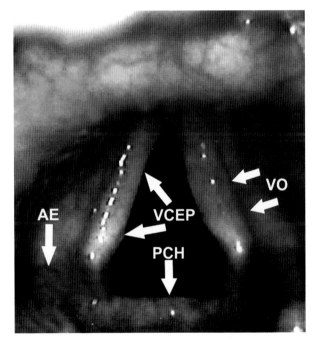

FIGURE 23–1. Magnified laryngoscopy showing some of the findings of reflux laryngitis with diffuse laryngeal edema, ventricular obliteration (*VO*), vocal fold edema and polypoid changes (*VCEP*), posterior wall hypertrophy (*PCH*), and arytenoid erythema (*AE*).

pathognomonic for LPR, a recently developed Reflux Finding Score (RFS) may be quite useful in categorizing the severity of the mucosal injury[13] (Table 23-2). Indeed, later work reported by Oelschlager described laryngoscopy as "complementary" to pH probe testing.[14] Patients both with significant scores on the RFS as well as positive pH probes were more likely to be responders to treatment than those with a low RFS.

In all suspected cases, endoscopic examination should include flexible or rigid laryngoscopy. As normal mucosa of the posterior glottis may look thickened during adduction, especially when the vocal folds are in the paramedian position, care should be taken to evaluate this part in full abduction. The evaluation of erythema is very dependent on the technical equipment, and should be limited to the estimation of color compared to that of the surrounding tissue.

On balance, findings on laryngoscopy are quite important and in fact predictive of clinical outcome in patients with the clinical diagnosis of LPR. A recent medical trial was published that reinforced the findings of Hanson et al years earlier[15]; in a prospective, double-blind-randomized, placebo-controlled study, two laryngeal findings—interarytenoid mucosal erythema and vocal fold abnormalities—were found to be predictive of symptomatic improvement following medical therapy.[16]

Empiric Trial of Acid Suppression as a Diagnostic Test

An empiric trial of PPI therapy over a prolonged period has been proposed as a valid diagnostic test for LPR. The typical regime is twice-a-day proton pump inhibitor (PPI) therapy for a duration of 1 to 4 months. This recommendation is based on the fact that we have not identified the specific symptom combination, or combination of symptoms and laryngeal signs, pathognomonic to LPR. Besides, ambulatory 24-hour double-probe pH measurement still has imperfect sensitivity and specificity, and is not available in all clinics. The prinicipal disadvantage of PPI therapy trial

TABLE 23–2. Reflux Finding Score (RFS)[13] (A total score of 7 is thought to be clinically significant.)

Subglottic Edema	2 = present 0 = absent
Ventricular Obliteration	2 = partial 4 = complete
Erythema/Hyperemia	2 = arytenoids only 4 = diffuse
Vocal Cord Edema	1 = mild 2 = moderate 3 = severe 4 = polypoid
Diffuse Laryngeal Edema	1 = mild 2 = moderate 3 = severe 4 = obstructing
Posterior Commissure Hypertrophy	1 = mild 2 = moderate 3 = severe 4 = obstructing
Granuloma/Granulation	2 = present 0 = absent
Thick Endolaryngeal Mucus	2 = present 0 = absent
	TOTAL

is its high cost, making some patients unwilling to engage in such a treatment trial, and possible placebo effect. However, the symptoms that do not improve after aggressive acid reduction therapy are unlikely to be caused by acid-related reflux.

DIAGNOSTIC STUDIES

pH Probe Testing

Although not perfect, at the present time pH probe testing is the best method of testing the presence of gastric refluxate in the area of the hypopharynx and larynx. The upper probe must be placed in a consistent zone at or above (2 cm) the functional upper esophageal sphincter (UES). This allows the lower probe to be placed

Controversy: Laryngoscopy in the Diagnosis of Reflux

Concerns have been raised by many authors regarding the significance of laryngoscopy and laryngeal findings in the support of the clinical diagnosis of reflux. Branski and colleagues[17] reported on a series of patients in whom reflux findings were scrutinized by five observers reviewing videotaped examinations. The conclusions of the paper were that significant variability exists in describing reflux-attributable findings. This paper has been cited while criticizing the assertion that physical examination of the larynx is an unpredictable diagnostic tool for the clinical evaluation of LPR. The study's limitations are important to note, however. First of all, the patients mostly complained of dysphonia—in fact, half of the subjects had vocal lesions on examination. It should not be surprising that a great deal of variability was found in assessment of reflux findings; this was not the primary source of laryngeal abnormality in most of these patients.

Perhaps the most cited paper in this arena came from Hicks and colleagues at the Cleveland Clinic.[30] In this important study, 100 "normal" subjects underwent laryngoscopy; their examinations were then reviewed by otolaryngologists and speech-language pathologists to estimate the presence of "reflux-attributable" lesions in these healthy volunteers. The key finding in this study, that nearly 80% of "normals" were found to have an interarytenoid bar or posterior commissure hypertrophy—helped to shed light on the possible insignificance of this one finding. Unfortunately, this revelation has been taken by many to be an indication that laryngoscopy in general is not useful in the clinical evaluation of reflux disease. Important findings, such as arytenoid erythema and vocal fold changes, continue to be valuable in the evaluation and treatment of LPR.

approximately 5 cm above the lower esophageal sphincter (LES). Normal pH values for the distal esophagus have been well established in the gastroenterology literature although there is still disagreement regarding pH values for the hypopharynx. A reflux *event* is currently defined as a fall in hypopharyngeal pH to less than 4.0 with a simultaneous drop to 4 or below in the distal esophagus. Acid exposure time (AET, percentage of time pH <4) is calculated as the frac- tion of time below this level at a given probe site. At the upper probe, an AET greater than 0.01% total, 0.02% upright, or 0% supine has been reported to be pathologic. This limit may be reached during one reflux event in the 24-hour period[17] (Table 23-3). One area of controversy, however, stems from the activity of pepsin at different pH levels. Pepsin has been shown to retain activity at a pH of 5.0, suggesting that a threshold at pH 5.0 may be more valid[5] when assessing

TABLE 23–3. Ambulatory pH Measurements at Upper Probe in Patients with LPR Involved in Controlled Studies (n = 529)*

Authors	Year	Probe Level	No. of Patients and Sex	Reflux Events			Acid Exposure Time		
				No. Positive	Range	Mean	Range (s)	Range (min)	Mean %
Koufman[4]	1991	2 cm above UES	88 (NR)	44/88	NR	NR	NR	NR	NR
Shaker et al[9]	1995	2 cm above UES	14 (NR)	12/14	0–27	4.36	0–1,296	0–12.97	0.24
Toohill et al[19] and Ulualp et al[20]	1998 & 1999	2 cm above UES	12 (7M, 5F)	8/12	0–12	2.42	0–104	0–1.74	0.009
Kuhn et al[21]	1998	2 cm above UES	11 (2M, 9F)	7/11	0–9	2.30	0–216	0–3.6	0.07
Ulualp et al[22]	1999	2 cm above UES	20 (13M, 7F)	15/20	0–12	2.65	0–536	0–8.9	0.13
Ulualp et al[23]	1999	2 cm above UES	11 (NR)	7/11	0–12	2.64	0–605	0–10.1	0.01
Ylitalo et al[10]	2001	1 cm above UES	26 (14M, 12F)	18/26	0–26	1.50	0–1,050	0–17.5	0.034
Eubanks et al[24]	2001	1.5–2 cm above UES	222 (86M, 136F)	90/222	0–36	NR	NR	NR	NR
Oelschlager et al[25]	2002	1.5–2 cm above UES	76 (NR)	32/76	NR	3.4	NR	NR	NR
Loehrl et al[26]	2002	2 cm above UES	12 (NR)	9/12	NR	NR	NR	NR	NR
Powitzky et al[27]	2003	2 cm above UES	37 (NR)	29/37	0–47	6.9	NR	NR	NR

NR: sex not recorded by author, UES: upper esophageal sphincter
*Reprinted with permission from Merati et al.[18]

the clinical presence or absence of pathologic reflux. A patient with a pH above 4 at times during the study may have a "negative" or normal study, though the pepsin in that patient's refluxate maintains noxious and damaging activity in their pharynx, larynx, and esophagus. Indeed, up to 20 to 30% of patients with PL may have a negative pH study, but this also does not rule out reflux as the causative factor. Esophageal single-probe pH monitoring does not identify patients with pharyngeal reflux, but patients with abnormal esophageal acid exposure are three times more likely to have LPR than those with normal esophageal monitoring.

Esophageal Manometry

Esophageal manometry is particularly important for the accurate placement of pH probes. Another indication in reflux patients is preoperative assessment of those being considered for antireflux surgery if there is any question of alternative or confounding esophageal disease, especially achalasia or profound dysmotility. As a solitary test for the presence or absence of reflux, it is not accurate enough. It may be important in the postoperative assessment of lower esophageal function following antireflux surgery, particularly in combination with radiographic studies and endoscopy.

Esophagoscopy

Endoscopic examination of the esophagus, either by traditional sedated or nonsedated transnasal techniques (TNE, see chapter 11), is generally used to screen complications related to GERD, or to exclude other diseases. Thus, it is performed to diagnose esophagitis or hiatal hernia, to screen for Barrett's esophagus, and to exclude other diseases or complications (esophageal cancer, peptic strictures) that may be detected on endoscopy. Indications for endoscopy may include dysphagia, bleeding, and weight loss, especially when patient history reveals smoking and alcohol abuse. Esophagoscopy alone, however, does not diagnose LPR. Esophagitis occurs in fewer than 20% of patients with LPR, whereas Barrett's esophagus is rare (<10%). It is the minority of patients with LPR, therefore, that have abnormal esophagoscopy.

Radiographic Imaging: Esophagography

The esophagram is an inexpensive and convenient technique used to detect significant deglutition or esophageal abnormalities that may otherwise be overlooked. It may be used to evaluate GERD patients with hiatal hernia, strictures, and esophageal rings. However, this examination is relatively insensitive in the evaluation of reflux. It is a short procedure that is noninvasive, requires no more than 30 minutes to perform and available in most clinical units.[28]

TREATMENT

The therapeutic approaches for LPR include lifestyle modifications, acid suppressive medications, and surgical therapy. Lifestyle modifications include elevation of the head of the bed, decreased intake of fat, citrus, tomato, chocolate, caffeine, and alcohol, cessation of smoking, and avoiding

recumbancy and further eating 3 hours before bedtime. These measures are helpful if there is associated abnormal esophageal acid exposure. If only LPR is present these measures may be less meaningful because pharyngeal reflux occurs most often in upright position during the daytime. Although Hanson described a 50% response rate to these measures alone in patients with chronic laryngitis,[29] there is minimal supportive data on the efficacy of these measures in LPR.

Medical acid suppression is the most important and common method of treatment. Proton-pump inhibitors are the most widely used drugs for the treatment of reflux. They maintain a potent and consistent effect on gastric acid secretion with few adverse effects. Comparisons between the five available compounds (omeprazole, rabeprazole, lansoprazole, esomeprazole, and pantoprazole) show that they have a similar antisecretory potency on a milligram basis. Treatment recommendation at present is twice-daily dosing of PPIs for at least 3 to 4 months. Symptoms frequently improve before the laryngoscopic findings resolve. It should be kept in mind that, even if the pH is elevated with antireflux medication, reflux itself continues, meaning pharynx and larynx are still exposed to bile, pepsin, and other gastric contents. All available H2 receptor antagonists (H$_2$RA)—cimetidine, ranitidine, famotidine, and nizatidine—all inhibit acid secretion equally when taken in equipotent doses. They have a low incidence of side effects and are less expensive as compared to proton pump inhibitors (PPI). There has been some renewed interest in the H2 blockers as an adjunct to PPI treatment. A recent study by Park et al, however, failed to show any added benefit to the addition of H2 blockers to a regime of twice-daily PPIs in patients with laryngeal and pharyngeal complaints.[16]

Surgical Treatment

A complete description of the surgical management of reflux is beyond the scope of this chapter. The dominant procedure for the operative management of reflux disease continues to be the Nissen fundoplication. In this procedure, the fundus of the stomach is wrapped around the LES to provide a snug, mechanical antireflux barrier. It is most commonly performed laparascopically, and is referred to as a "laparoscopic Nissen fundoplication" (LNF). It should be considered in patients who obtain only partial relief from medications, or in those who prefer operative management to the possibility of long-term or even a lifetime of PPI treatment. Prior to embarking on a surgical intervention, the reasons for failure of medical acid suppression in some patients should be considered. In patients with good control of classic GER or LPR symptoms, fundoplication may be an option. In patients who do not respond to medication, their ongoing inflammation may be due to volume reflux of nonacidic entities, as noted above. These include pepsin and bile reflux. This group of patients may indeed respond to a laproscopic Nissen fundoplication, with reported success rates as high as 90%.[30] Operative management of LPR has not, however, been widely accepted.

The reflux of gastric and duodenal contents into the upper aerodigestive tract is common and is an important source of laryngeal disease. Fewer than 50% of patients present with heartburn; symptoms such as dysphonia, dysphagia, throat clearing, and even globus sensation are more typical. Laryngeal findings on examination are important and may be predictive of treatment outcome.

The variability of patient presentations and response to treatment may reflect the differences in cellular tissue response to injury as well as the presence of nonacidic injurious agents such as bile.

Empiric therapy with twice-daily proton-pump inhibitors is a reasonable initial step in the management of suspected laryngopharyngeal reflux. Long-term PPI treatment appears to be safe for the vast majority of patients. Nissen fundoplication has no role in the initial treatment of LPR although it may be highly beneficial in selected patients.

Review Questions

1. A 45-year-old male has been on PPI for 1 month with little clinical response; he stops taking his medication following a "negative" pH probe study. His LPR symptoms worsen. You ask the patient to resume the medical regime because:
   a. pH probe testing is not reliable
   b. the patient has not had an adequate length of treatment
   c. it will sterilize his oral flora
   d. surgery is not an option for a 45-year-old male.

2. The patient with a diagnosis of reflux laryngitis will:
   a. Not have an associated problem with gastroesophageal reflux disease (GERD)
   b. Have associated GERD in 20% of cases
   c. Have associated GERD in 50% of cases
   d. Have associated GERD in 95% of cases

3. When 24-hour ambulatory pH probe testing is preformed in patients with reflux laryngitis a positive result is:
   a. At least 10 hypopharyngeal events at pH 6 or below
   b. Acid exposure time of greater than 60 seconds per 24 hours
   c. A single drop in the pH below 5
   d. Acid exposure time (AET) of more than 0.01% at the upper probe.

4. Successful treatment for most LPR patients consists of:
   a. Proton-pump inhibitors
   b. Lifestyle modifications
   c. H2 blockers
   d. endoscopic cricopharyngeal myotomy
   e. a and b

REFERENCES

1. Smith KJ, O'Brien SM, Smithers BM, et al. Interactions among smoking, obesity, and symptoms of acid reflux in Barrett's esophagus. *Cancer Epidemiol Biomarkers Prev.* 2005;14(11 pt 1): 2481-2486.
2. Stein DJ, El-Serag HB, Kuczynski J, Kramer JR, Sampliner RE. The association of body mass index with Barrett's oesophagus. *Aliment Pharmacol Ther.* 2005;22(10):1005-1010.
3. Halum SL, Postma GN, Johnston C, Belafsky PC, Koufman JA. Patients with isolated laryngopharyngeal reflux are not obese. *Laryngoscope.* 2005; 115(6):1042-1045.
4. Koufman JA. The otolaryngologic manifestations of gastroesophageal reflux disease (GERD): a clinical investigation of 225 patients using ambulatory 24-hour pH monitoring and an experimental investigation of the role of acid and pepsin in the development of laryngeal injury. *Laryngoscope.* 1991;101:1-78.
5. Koufman JA. Aviv JE, Casiano RR, Shaw GY. Laryngopharyngeal reflux: position statement of the committee on speech, voice, and swallowing disorders of the American Academy of Otolaryngology-Head and Neck Surgery. *Otolaryngol Head Neck Surg.* 2002;127:32-35.
6. Ulualp SO, Toohill RJ. Laryngopharyngeal reflux, state of the art diagnosis and treatment. *Otolaryngol Clin North Am.* 2000;33(4):785-801.
7. Shaker R, Hogan WJ, Normal physiology of the aerodigestive tract and its effect on the upper gut. *Am J Med.* 2003;115(suppl 3A):2S-9S.
8. Shaker R, Dodds WJ, Ren J, Hogan WJ, Arndorfer RC. Esophagoglottal closure reflex: a mechanism of airway protection. *Gastroenterology.* 1992; 102(3):857-861.
9. Shaker R, Milbrath M, Ren J, et al. Esophagopharyngeal distribution of refluxed gastric acid in patients with reflux laryngitis. *Gastroenterology.* 1995;109:1575-1582.
10. Ylitalo R, Lindestad PA, Ramel S. Symptoms, laryngeal findings, and 24-hour pH monitoring in patients with suspected gastroesophago-pharyngeal reflux. *Laryngoscope.* 2001;111:1735-1741.
11. Belafsky PC, Postma GN, Koufman JA. Laryngopharyngeal reflux symptoms improve before changes in physical findings. *Laryngoscope.* 2001;111:979-981.
12. Belafsky PC, Postma GN, Koufman JA. Validity and reliability of the reflux symptom index (RSI). *J Voice.* 2002;16(2):274-277.
13. Belafsky PC, Postma GN, Koufman JA. The validity and reliability of the Reflux Finding Score (RFS). *Laryngoscope.* 2001;111:1313-1317.
14. Oelschlager BK, Eubanks TR, Maronian N, et al. Laryngoscopy and pharyngeal pH are complementary in the diagnosis of gastroesophageal-laryngeal reflux. *J Gastrointest Surg.* 2002;6(2): 189-194.
15. Hanson DG, Jiang J, Chi W. Quantitative color analysis of laryngeal erythema in chronic posterior laryngitis. *J Voice.* 1998;12(1):78-83.
16. Park W. Hicks DM, Khandwala F, et al. Laryngopharyngeal reflux: prospective cohort study evaluating optimal dose of proton-pump inhibitor therapy and pretherapy predictors of response. *Laryngoscope.* 2005;115(7):1230-1238.
17. Branski RC, Bhattacharyya N, Shapiro J. The reliability of the assessment of endoscopic laryngeal findings associated with laryngopharyngeal reflux disease. *Laryngoscope.* 2002;112(6):1019-1024.
18. Merati AL, Lim HJ, Ulualp SO, Toohill RJ. Meta-analysis of upper probe measurements in normal subjects and patients with laryngopharyngeal reflux. *Ann Otol Rhinol Laryngol.* 2005;114: 177-182.
19. Toohill RJ, Ulualp SO, Shaker R. Evaluation of gastroesophageal reflux in patients with laryngotracheal stenosis. *Ann Otol Rhinol Laryngol.* 1998; 107:1010-1014.
20. Ulualp SO, Toohill RJ, Shaker R. Pharyngeal acid reflux in patients with single and multiple otolaryngologic disorders. *Otolaryngol Head Neck Surg.* 1999;121:725-730.
21. Kuhn, J, Toohill, RJ, Ulualp SO, et al. Pharyngeal acid reflux events in patients with vocal cord nodules. *Laryngoscope.* 1998;108:1146-1149.
22. Ulualp SO, Toohill RJ, Hoffmann R, Shaker R. Pharyngeal pH monitoring in patients with posterior laryngitis. *Otolaryngol Head Neck Surg.* 1999; 120:672-677.
23. Ulualp SO, Toohill RJ, Hoffmann R, Shaker R. Possible relationship of gastroesophagopharyngeal acid reflux with pathogenesis of chronic sinusitis. *Am J Rhinol.* 1999;13:197-202.
24. Eubanks TR, Omelanczuk PE, Maronian N, Hillel A, Pope CE 2nd, Pellegrini CA. Pharyngeal pH monitoring in 222 patients with suspected laryngeal reflux. *J Gastrointest Surg.* 2001;5(2): 183-190.

25. Oelschlager BK, Eubanks TR, Maronian N, et al. Laryngoscopy and pharyngeal pH are complementary in the diagnosis of gastroesophageal-laryngeal reflux. *J Gastrointest Surg.* 2002;6(2): 189-194.

26. Loehrl TA, Smith TL, Darling RJ, et al. Autonomic dysfunction, vasomotor rhinitis, and extraesophageal manifestations of gastroesophageal reflux. *Otolaryngol Head Neck Surg.* 2002;126(4): 382-387.

27. Powitzky ES, Khaitan L, Garrett CG, Richards WO, Courey M. Symptoms, quality of life, videolaryngoscopy, and twenty-four-hour triple-probe pH monitoring in patients with typical and extraesophageal reflux. *Ann Otol Rhinol Laryngol.* 2003;112(10):859-865.

28. Kuhn JC, Massick D, Toohill RJ. *Role of the Esophagram in the Management of Dysphonia.* Presented at the Middle Section Triological Society; Kansas City, Missouri; January 24-26, 1997.

29. Hanson DG, Kamel PL, Kahrilas PJ. Outcomes of antireflux therapy for the treatment of chronic laryngitis. *Ann Otol Rhinol Laryngol.* 1995; 104(7):550-555.

30. Lindstrom DR, Wallace J, Loehrl TA, Merati AL, Toohill RJ. Nissen fundoplication surgery for extraesophageal manifestations of gastroesophageal reflux (EER). *Laryngoscope.* 2002;112:1762-1765.

31. Hicks DM, Ours TM, Abelson TI, Vaezi MF, Richter JE. The prevalence of hypopharynx findings associated with gastroesophageal reflux in normal volunteers. *J Voice.* 2002;16(4):564-579.

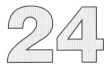

24

Benign Lesions of the Larynx

Timothy D. Anderson, MD

KEY POINTS

■ As terminology of laryngeal lesions is inconsistent, a detailed description of the lesion is generally more informative than a diagnostic term with different meanings to various clinicians.

■ Diagnosis and management of benign laryngeal lesions require assessment of the underlying cause, the patients' vocal habits and needs, as well as laryngeal mechanics and structure.

■ Most patients with benign vocal fold lesions should undergo evaluation and treatment by a speech therapist prior to contemplation of surgical therapy.

■ Vocal fold scar currently has no reliability effective treatment. In patients who require microlaryngeal surgery, vocal fold scarring can be avoided by minimizing operative trauma and pursuing preoperative speech therapy to prevent abusive voice behaviors postoperatively.

■ Videostroboscopy can be extremely useful in the diagnosis and documentation of vocal fold lesions. Some diagnoses, most notably vocal fold scar, can only be made with the aid of stroboscopy. Documentation of the preoperative vibratory status of the vocal fold is important for guiding expectations of surgical results.

Benign laryngeal lesions are common problems. Most are evaluated due to voice changes; an accurate diagnosis and appropriate management are required to restore the voice. Many patients can be successfully managed without operative intervention. The most important step in successful management is to determine why the patient developed a voice problem in the first place. Without a clear understanding of the underlying factors contributing to the development of a benign laryngeal lesion, recurrence, poor surgical results, persistent voice problems are common. The general principles of evaluation and management of benign laryngeal growths are discussed first, followed by specific information regarding the most common lesions.

VOCAL TRAUMA

Vocal trauma is the most common cause of benign laryngeal lesions.[1] *Vocal fold nodules* are the most obvious example. Virtually all vocal nodules will resolve with changes in vocal use patterns. If the traumatic voice behaviors are not addressed prior to surgery, the patient will continue to abuse the voice in the postoperative period. At best, the nodules will recur. At worst, the patient will develop dense vocal fold scar and be permanently hoarse.

Given the high incidence of traumatic vocal behaviors in patients with benign vocal fold lesions, most patients with these problems should undergo evaluation and management by a speech-language therapist before surgery is contemplated.[2,3] Many patients will have adequate voice improvement with speech therapy alone and will not require surgery.[4,5] Patients who still require surgery will be better prepared for the postoperative recovery process and their surgical results will be better due to less trauma during the delicate early healing process.

DIAGNOSIS

Although visualization of the larynx is important in the diagnosis of laryngeal pathology, the history and complete otolaryngologic examination should be considered an essential part of the diagnostic process. Careful attention to voice use patterns, the sound of the voice, the history of the voice problem, and other symptoms or medical problems almost always reveals the diagnosis before examination of the larynx. Laryngeal examination then confirms the clinical suspicion. Laryngeal examination should not be confined to anatomy, but must also take into account voice use patterns and evaluate for the presence and severity of hyperfunctional voice disorders, reflux, and so forth. Video recording of the examination is helpful for patient counseling and medicolegal documentation and allows detailed review of the examination in challenging cases. Stroboscopy is the only widely available technique to evaluate the vibratory function of the vocal folds and is therefore extremely useful. Some diagnoses, such as diffuse vocal fold scar, can only be accurately diagnosed by stroboscopic examination. In many cases of benign vocal fold masses, determination of the degree of vocal fold stiffness can have important prognostic significance (see chapter 6, Videostroboscopy).

CLASSIFICATION

Diagnosis and treatment of benign laryngeal lesions depends on a detailed knowledge of vocal fold anatomy, as well as a clear understanding of the implications of the layered microstructure of the vocal folds. Hirano's description of the layered structure of the vocal fold is central to the surgical techniques of modern laryngology.[6] The relative paucity of fibroblasts in the superficial layer of the lamina propria (SLP) is thought to allow surgical disruption of this plane with relatively little postoperative scarring. Interwoven collagen fibrils and copious fibroblasts make the vocal ligament (deep layers of the lamina propria) a source of dense scar when surgically injured. Surgical results for lesions of the superficial layer of the lamina propria are generally excellent (polyps and nodules), as these do not result in a severe disruption or loss of SLP. Surgery for pathology that results in great disruption of the SLP (cysts and Reinke's edema) is less likely to produce perfect voices. Lesions involving the deep layer (sulcus vocalis) or all layers (vocal fold scar, invasive carcinoma) are surgical challenges and should be approached with trepidation given the risks of permanent vocal fold scar and impaired voice.

Several categorization schemes have been used to classify benign laryngeal lesions, all of which have some merit.[7-9] Anatomic descriptors have the advantage of clear pathologic correlations and knowledge of the location of lesions in the vocal fold microstructure has important surgical implications. Unfortunately, anatomic descriptions alone fail to consider causative factors that can be essential in proper management of benign laryngeal lesions. Anatomy also fails to consider the time course and differential expression of a single process—pathology of an acute hemorrhage, posthemorrhagic polyp, dilated ectatic vessel, and resolved hemorrhage with scar will all obviously be quite different, although they are all different aspects of a single pathophysiologic process. Categorization by cause of lesion is similarly flawed, as many "causes" are unproven or speculative and groupings are often arbitrary.

Nomenclature of Laryngeal Lesions

Unfortunately, a universally accepted terminology for benign laryngeal masses does not exist. Several attempts have been made to standardize the terminology by using videostroboscopic, pathologic, anatomic, or clinical behavior, but all have suffered from limitations that have prevented widespread acceptance.[7-9] When communicating with other otolaryngologists, adjectives describing the location and appearance of a lesion are generally preferred over arbitrary and frequently misunderstood labels. Similarly, published papers must be carefully read to determine what definitions are being used in order to properly evaluate techniques and results.

Terminology of Benign Laryngeal Lesions

Generally Accepted Terms	Terms with Varying Definitions
Sulcus vocalis	Nodule
Vocal fold scar	Polyp
Acute hemorrhage	Mass
Mucus retention cyst	Pseudocyst
Epithelial cyst	Granuloma
Papilloma	Varix
Reinke's edema	Edema
Polypoid degeneration	
Vascular ectasia	

Vascular Abnormalities

Acute Hemorrhage

Acute hemorrhage is an uncommon, but potentially devastating, problem that occurs due to trauma and rupture of a submucosal vessel. Bright red blood accumulates in the lamina propria, causing deformations of vocal fold shape, decreasing vibratory wave propagation, and leading to rapid hoarseness (Figure 24-1). Vocal trauma is frequently cited as the inciting cause, with singing, crying, screaming, and coughing most often reported.[10,11] Singers will often report that their voice becomes hoarse between notes. If the time to evaluation is delayed, the initial bright red color will often fade to shades of yellow and green as the hemoglobin is broken down, similar to bruising in other locations. At the time of acute hemorrhage, vocal fold vasculature is generally obscured by the submucosal blood and can only be seen after the hemorrhage begins to resolve.

Acute vocal fold hemorrhage seems to be more common in women than men and has been reported to be more common in the premenstrual period, although supporting data are weak. Use of blood thinners, including aspirin and ibuprofen, has also been implicated.[11,12] Some patients will suffer recurrent hemorrhage and may present with evidence of both acute and chronic

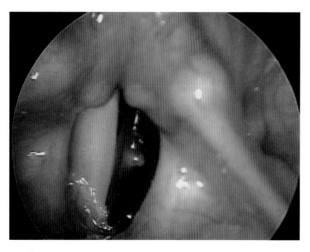

FIGURE 24–1. Acute left vocal fold hemorrhage.

areas of hemorrhage. Many of these patients will have an abnormal appearance of the vocal fold vascularity. This can take the form of dilated capillaries (ectasia) or blebs in the vessels. Weak vessel walls may rupture more easily, while vessels that are not in the longitudinal axis of the vocal fold are exposed to massive shearing forces during vibration. Normal vessels in the vocal fold run predominately along the length of the vocal fold and are generally quite narrow.

Acute vocal fold hemorrhage is generally treated conservatively. Patients are generally kept on complete voice rest (no talking or singing for any reason) for at least a week. Cough should be treated aggressively with suppressants and use of anticoagulant medications minimized.[11,12] Many over-the-counter cold medications contain salicylates, and patients should be warned about these medications as well. Herbal remedies, including ginko and garlic, have blood-thinning properties and should be avoided.[13,14] The value of voice rest in subacute hemorrhage is unclear. High-level voice professionals should probably be advised to pursue a course of voice rest to maximize the chances of full recovery. Patients with less demanding voice requirements can frequently be observed, especially if they are already improving and have no evidence of incipient complications. Except in very unusual cases, there is no role for surgery in acute hemorrhage.

Posthemorrhagic Masses

Posthemorrhagic masses are red-brown masses that can occur anywhere on the vocal fold. They range from very small, sessile swellings (Figures 24-2 and 24-3) to huge, pedunculated masses. The pedunculated masses frequently ball-valve into the larynx during inspiration, causing intermittent periods of severe hoarseness when the mass is between the vocal folds alternating with periods of relatively normal voice when they move laterally above the vibratory edge of the vocal fold. There is almost always stiffness of the affected vocal fold, although preoperative stroboscopy is frequently difficult to interpret due to the damping effect of the masses and their interference with glottic closure and vocal fold

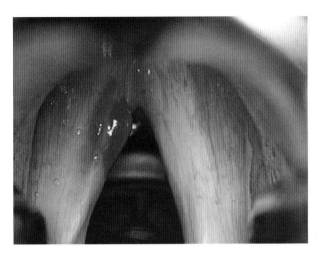

FIGURE 24–2. Small, broad-based, posthemorrhagic mass.

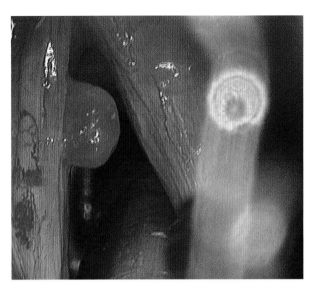

FIGURE 24–4. Posthemorrhagic mass with multiple vascular ectasias on superior surface of vocal fold.

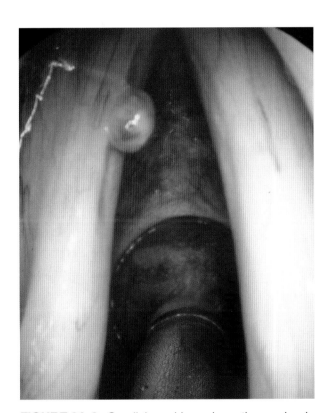

FIGURE 24–3. Small, broad-based, posthemorrhagic mass with underlying sulcus vocalis.

entrainment. With large masses, it is sometimes difficult to see any part of the vocal fold or even to determine which side is affected. Occasionally, posthemorrhagic masses can appear to be a

purplish submucosal cyst with surrounding edema. Abnormal vessels can frequently be seen in the region of the masses (Figure 24-4).

Posthemorrhagic masses likely form due to coalescence of clot from acute hemorrhage due to continued vocal fold use. Clot consolidation and contraction, damage of the gel-like lamina propria, inflammation from the clotting cascade, and macrophage activation all contribute to both scar formation and development of vocal fold masses. Once mature, these masses rarely involute, even with aggressive nonoperative therapy.

Treatment of posthemorrhagic masses is generally surgical. Preoperative speech therapy is helpful to minimize postoperative vocal trauma, but rarely results in significant voice improvement. Unfortunately, posthemorrhagic masses are generally associated with other vocal fold trauma, stiffness, and scarring, so surgery rarely results in perfect voice. However, as most patients have a severely disordered voice preoperatively, marked postoperative voice improvement is usually seen. Many surgeons advocate treating the abnormal vessels at the time of surgery to prevent recurrent hemorrhage.[15,16] Many techniques have been proposed, including CO_2 laser ablation, pulsed dye laser treatment, and resection of abnormal vessels. No randomized studies have evaluated any of these practices, but expert opinion supports their approaches.[15,16] Treatment of abnormal vascularity has also been recommended for patients with recurrent acute hemorrhages, with anecdotal supporting evidence.

Vascular Tumors

Occasional vascular tumors have been reported in the larynx, and generally have a very similar appearance to posthemorrhagic masses (Figure 24-5). Onset is generally chronic, although they can occasionally be associated with hemoptysis or airway obstruction. Erythematous masses involving the supraglottis or subglottis, or evidence of deep vocal fold involvement, should be approached cautiously, as the visible portion may be only a small portion of the entire mass. Workup for

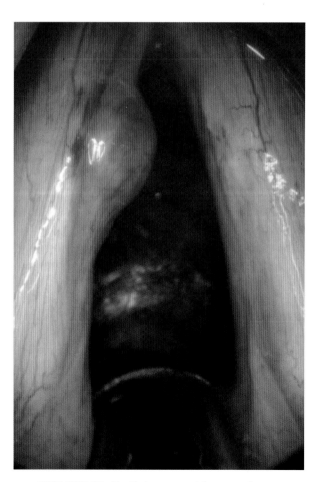

FIGURE 24–5. Submucosal hemangioma.

suspected vascular tumors should include a computed tomography (CT) and/or magnetic resonance imaging (MRI) to define the extent and vascularity of the lesion. Most vascular tumors are benign and can generally be cured if completely resected. Biopsy can result in massive hemorrhage and should be conducted under controlled circumstances.

Lesions Resulting from Overuse, Misuse, or Vocal Trauma

Transient, Mild Edema

Patients will frequently develop complaints of mild hoarseness that persists for several hours to days after vigorous voice use. Symptoms generally slowly abate with voice rest, but recur after the next performance, presentation, or conversation in a loud, smoky bar. When patients are examined while symptomatic, they generally give an impression of redundant contact of the vocal folds in the midportion during vibration. Rapid inspiration may result in subtle rounding of the vocal folds, suggesting mild increase in the volume of the lamina propria. Muscle tension dysphonia is almost always present, although singers will occasionally manifest mild postperformance edema despite excellent technique. Treatment generally includes reassurance and speech therapy to decrease hyperfunctional voice behaviors and improve vocal hygiene. In addition, reasonable voice use duration should be discussed with the patient. Some adults expect to sing for 1.5 hours for 2 sessions on a Friday, 3 sessions on a Saturday, followed by 3 sessions on a Sunday. Some patients cannot endure this grueling activity level and must learn reasonable voice expectations.

Vocal Nodules

Vocal nodules are symmetric masses that occur at the junction between the anterior and middle thirds of the vocal folds; this corresponds roughly to the midpoint of the musculomembranous vocal fold. They will frequently be the only area of contact between the vocal folds during soft phonation (Figure 24-6). There is generally little stiffness underlying these lesions, yet they do interfere with vibration. Nodules form at the region of maximal excursion of the vocal fold epithelium during vibration. These lesions generally involve the superficial lamina propria and epithelium, but do not involve the deeper layers. If aggressive vocal trauma persists, these lesions can evolve into relatively symmetric, firm large vocal fold nodules (Figure 24-7).

Patients with vocal fold nodules are characterized as outgoing, loud talkers with aggressive

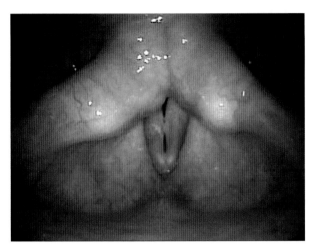

FIGURE 24–6. Subtle vocal nodules exhibiting premature contact during soft phonation.

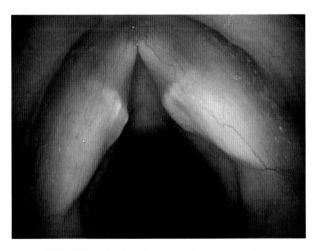

FIGURE 24–7. Firm vocal fold nodules.

glottal attacks. The typical nodule patient is irrepressibly talkative with loud, pressed phonation.[17] The voice ranges from coarse and raspy to fuzzy. Singers with vocal fold nodules frequently complain of breaks in the passagio. Fibrotic masses, cysts, and other lesions are commonly misdiagnosed as nodules. Vocal fold nodules are bilateral; unilateral nodules, by definition, do not occur.

Vocal nodules almost always resolve with reduction in the underlying hyperkinetic voice behaviors.[18,19] In addition, vocal fold nodules are often associated with a clinical diagnosis of laryngopharyngeal reflux. Chronic throat clearing and the laryngeal inflammation may represent a secondary causative factor for the development of vocal fold nodules. Aggressive management with antireflux therapy is indicated in these patients. Chronic nodules occasionally require surgery after a prolonged trial of speech therapy fails to result in complete resolution. Although relative voice rest can be helpful early in the course of speech therapy, absolute voice rest is rarely necessary. Surgical intervention should be limited to the area of visible abnormality. Vocal fold stripping is never indicated for nodules due to the potential for widespread postoperative scarring and poor voice results. With modern phonomicrosurgical techniques, surgical success rates are generally excellent due to the superficial nature of these lesions.

Granulomas

Granulomas are exophytic lesions that occur most commonly on the medial surface of the vocal process of the arytenoid. Postintubation granulomas tend to be larger, pedunculated and more obvious (Figures 24-8 and 24-9) than granulomas resulting from hyperfunctional voice (Figure 24-10). Hyperfunctional granulomas are more sessile, frequently have an erythematous rim, and often present with pain on speaking or swallowing. In the earliest form, these hyperfunctional lesions are ulcerative (Figure 24-11). Because they are located on the posterior aspect of the cartilaginous vocal fold, granulomas cause few voice complaints. However, large granulomas can result in intermittent airway obstruction symptoms.

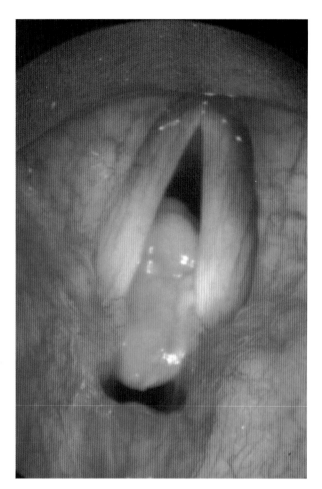

FIGURE 24–8. Intraoperative photo of a large post-intubation granuloma filling the interarytenoid region.

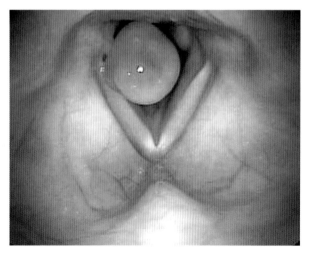

FIGURE 24–9. Postintubation pedunculated granuloma.

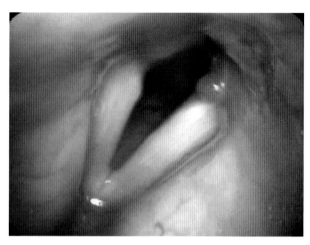

FIGURE 24–10. Granuloma secondary to hyperfunctional use.

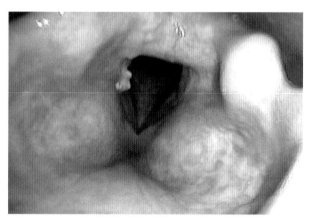

FIGURE 24–11. Small healing ulcer on the vocal process of the arytenoid due to trauma from hyperfunctional voice behaviors.

Granulomas are exuberant reparative processes that develop as the result of injury and inflammation. Ulceration is felt to form due to local trauma (throat clearing, coughing, hyperfunctional voice use, or intubation) as well as inflammation from laryngopharyngeal reflux. Granulomas can occasionally form at other sites on the vocal folds due to other sources of trauma and inflammation.

Granulomas are often quite frustrating to treat. Identification and elimination of underlying causes is paramount, with surgical resection reserved for refractory cases or large granulomas once the causative factors are controlled. As granulomas form in response to injury, surgical resection (with a resulting surgical injury) almost invariably leads to recurrence if any source of inflammation persists. Proton pump inhibitors are frequently helpful in the gradual control and elimination of granulomas, and antibiotics, inhaled steroids, and other medications may occasionally be useful.[20-23] Control of hyperfunctional voice behaviors is important to avoid further injury.[24] Botox injections are occasionally used to temporarily paralyze the affected vocal fold and thus reduce adductory forces.[25] Preliminary reports suggest that the pulsed dye laser may have a role in the treatment of granuloma.[26]

Vocal Fold Injury

Mucosal Tears

Violent vocal fold trauma can occasionally cause small mucosal tears rather than acute hemorrhage. These tears are generally quite subtle on examination and heal quickly, so a high index of suspicion is required to make an accurate diagnosis. Small linear areas of mucosal disruption with associated underlying stiffness are the most common finding. Patients most often report severe retching, persistent hard coughing, or similar trauma with abrupt change in voice. Hoarseness is frequently severe, especially when compared to the subtle findings on examination. The underlying cause of the trauma must be addressed to prevent further injury and voice rest is generally recommended.

Sulcus Vocalis

Sulcus vocalis is a narrow, linear depression in the surface of the vocal fold running longitudinally along the vocal fold (Figure 24-12). It must be distinguished from pseudosulcus vocalis, a wider furrow below the vocal fold that extends posterior to the vocal process of the arytenoid (Figure 24-13). Sulcus is a deficiency in the lamina propria of the vocal fold, and must therefore end at the tip of the vocal process of the arytenoid

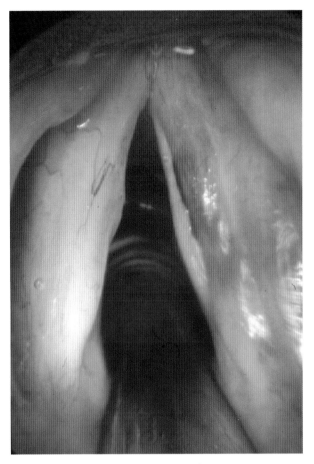

FIGURE 24–12. Extensive sulcus vocalis running the entire length of the right vocal fold.

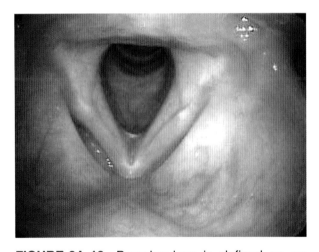

FIGURE 24–13. Pseudosulcus is defined as an apparent "groove" running the length of the vocal fold extending into the cartilaginous vocal fold. This "groove" represents subglottic edema.

as the layered structure of the vocal fold ends there as well. Pseudosulcus represents infraglottic edema. Sulcus vocalis frequently disrupts normal vibration of the vocal fold, especially if the sulcus extends to the vocal ligament. It may occur in the striking zone of the vocal fold and is not visible at all points of the vibratory cycle. Sulcus vocalis may occur in conjunction with unilateral vocal fold bowing or scar.

The pathogenesis of sulcus vocalis is debatable.[27] Theories include a response to injury with resultant loss of portions of the lamina propria with adherence of the epithelium to the vocal ligament. Some cases are clearly a congenital malformation of the vocal fold. Lastly, some speculate that some sulcus vocalis lesions develop due to rupture of a vocal fold cyst, with focal loss of SLP and adherence of the deep cyst epithelium to the vocal ligament.

Sulcus vocalis is extremely difficult to treat successfully. Multiple surgical options have been described, but the involvement of the vocal ligament and frequent associated scarring make surgical success a difficult proposition.[27-30] Occasionally, treatment of associated factors such as vocal fold bowing will result in marked voice improvements.[31]

Fibrotic Masses:

Fibrotic masses are dense, firm, white frequently unilateral masses. They often have dilated, ectatic vessels toward their base (Figure 24-14). They tend to be broad based and appear to be densely adherent to the vocal ligament. A contact lesion is often seen on the opposite vocal fold, centered at the point of contact with the fibrotic mass. The contact lesion is usually smaller than the primary lesion (Figure 24-15). Fibrotic masses with associated reactive swelling are frequently misdiagnosed as vocal nodules, but only the reactive mass will improve with speech therapy. Vocal fold vibration is generally severely disordered. The voice quality is variable, ranging from breathy to harsh depending on the dimensions of the mass and stiffness of the vocal fold.

Fibrotic masses may occur due to prior surgery, focal vocal fold trauma, or chronic vocal

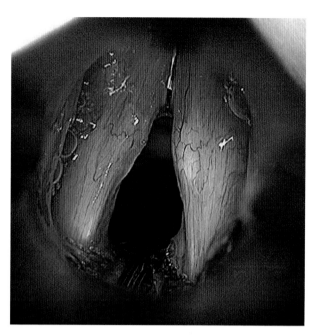

FIGURE 24–14. Bilateral fibrotic masses with abnormal vascularity.

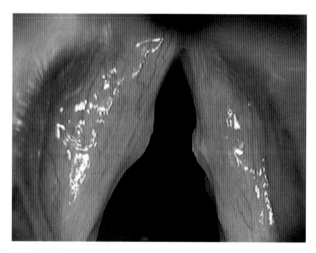

FIGURE 24–15. Irregular fibrotic mass of the right vocal fold with a smoother, softer left-sided reactive mass.

fold abuse. Often, the cause is unclear. These masses are associated with scar throughout the lamina propria, and clear demarcations between the fibrotic mass and scar is uncommon. Sulcus vocalis is occasionally noted at the time of surgery.

Speech therapy is worthwhile as an initial treatment as it will frequently reduce the size of a reactive mass. This occasionally results in marked voice improvement. Surgery is generally required, however. Surgery on fibrotic masses is difficult as the margins of the mass are generally unclear and frequently will extend to the vocal ligament and be densely adherent to the epithelium. If the contralateral vocal fold has good vibratory function, reasonable postoperative voice can be attained by simply resecting the mass and providing a smooth surface to allow good glottic closure.

Diffuse Vocal Fold Scar

Diffuse vocal fold scar is difficult to diagnose without stroboscopy. Scarred vocal folds will often look normal with conventional endoscopy, but stroboscopy will show absence of the mucosal wave or severely disordered and vibration. Some patients have dilated, abnormal vessels visible on the superior surface of the vocal fold. In severe scarring, marked compensatory hyperfunctional voice behaviors are frequently present and many

---

Parsing Hoarseness

Seth Dailey, MD

Patients with vocal problems will often use the term "hoarseness." Although indicative of an anatomic problem, this term does not aid the physician in detailing the specific nature of patients' concerns. The voice clinician may find it useful to distinguish if the voice issue is principally *aerodynamic* or *acoustic* in nature. It is important to note that a patient may have both types of complaints; they are not exclusive of one another.

Aerodynamic symptoms relate to the glottis as a valve—when the laryngeal valve mechanism is functioning properly, the valve is functioning efficiently. Any pathology (scar, polyp, nodules) that contributes to inefficient valving will produce effortful voicing, vocal fatigue, and difficulties with projection. These symptoms are generally speaking *aerodynamic* symptoms. Problems related to how the patient or other people perceive the sound of their voice can be termed *acoustic* symptoms.

Understanding which symptom category is of concern to the patient is important in evaluating potential treatment success. For example, a procedure for vocal fold scarring, if successful, is likely to significantly improve aerodynamic symptoms by improving the glottal gap; it is unlikely, however, to improve vocal quality (the acoustic symptoms). Conversely, a simple vocal polyp presents a case where acoustic and aerodynamic improvement is highly likely, and the patient can be counseled accordingly. As most patients who pursue medical attention for their vocal problems care a great deal about their phonatory function this mental tool for expectation management may aid in the counseling process and not set the patient and surgeon up for "failure" even if the operation is executed without error.

patients rely on false vocal fold vibration to produce a gravelly, low-pitched voice. Patients with dense scar will frequently complain more about the effort involved in producing voice, than the strained or breathy voice quality.

Vocal fold scar forms due to injury. The depth and severity of injury frequently correlates with the density of scarring. In addition to surgical injury, dense scar can result from infection, radiation therapy, chronic voice abuse, recurrent vocal fold hemorrhage, and other causes.

Treatment of vocal fold scar is generally unsatisfying. It is essential that the patient have reasonable expectations of any treatment that is contemplated. Treatments may improve voice stamina and ease of use, but improvements in voice quality are limited. Some authors feel that collagen injection into the scarred vocal folds may create some softening of scar due to collagenase activity.[32] Temporary closure of glottic gaps provides immediate benefit. However, in cases of severe scarring, closure of a glottic gap occasionally increases, rather than reduces, the effort required to produce voice. A variety of procedures have been described to reconstitute the lamina propria, including fat implantation, mucosal grafting, hyaluronic acid injection, and others.[33-36] Results have been mixed, with no procedure emerging as the cure for vocal fold scarring. Many patients will be best served by speech therapy to improve voice efficiency.

Structural Lesions

Cysts

Vocal fold cysts generally occur in the deeper layers of the SLP and may abut the vocal ligament. These lesions may represent either a mucus retention cyst or a squamous epithelial cyst. Epithelial cysts generally have a white color, are football shaped, and the edges of the cyst can be clearly distinguished from surrounding edematous lamina propria (Figure 24–16). Mucus retention cysts are often yellow in color. These lesions usually deform the surface of the affected vocal fold and may cause a contralateral reactive mass.

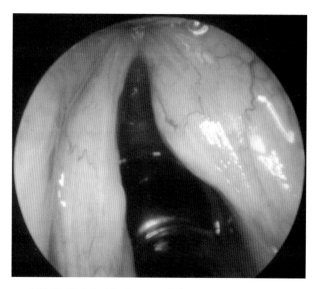

FIGURE 24–16. Large right epidermoid cyst.

Over time, cysts occasionally change in size, and may produce waxing and waning symptoms. Hoarse, pressed phonation is common, especially with larger cysts.

Epithelial-filled cysts may be congenital or traumatic in origin.[37] Mucus retention cysts are thought to be due to obstruction of a laryngeal mucous gland with gradual accumulation of material and do not have an epithelial lining (Figure 24–17). Ruptured cysts may generate vocal fold pits, sulcus vocalis, or mucosal bridges.[38]

Surgery is generally required for symptomatic cysts, although occasional patients will have adequate improvement with speech therapy alone.[38-39] As the cysts generally span the intermediate layer of the lamina propria, postoperative stiffness is common, even with meticulous surgical technique.

Polyps

Localized, soft masses on the medial surface of the vocal fold filled with clear fluid are common findings. When large and pedunculated, they are generally termed polyps; when sessile and smaller, they may be called polyps, nodules (if bilateral and symmetrical) or pseudocysts (Figure 24–18). If a polyp has recently hemorrhaged, it is usually referred to as a hemorrhagic polyp. For the

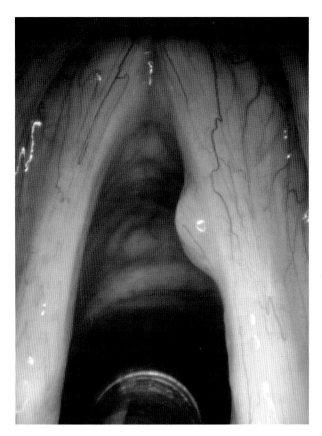

FIGURE 24–17. Small submucosal mucous retention cyst.

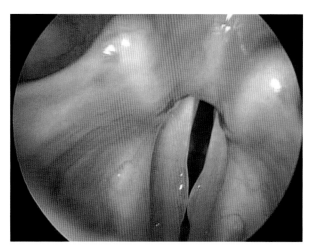

FIGURE 24–18. Bilateral pseudocysts.

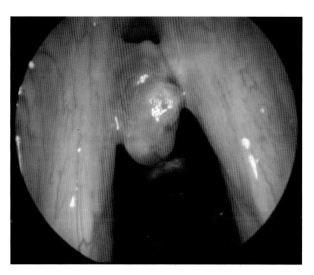

FIGURE 24–19. Polyp composed of granulation tissue and distended epithelium.

smaller lesions, a cyst wall is not identified during microsurgical exploration and a gel-like excess lamina propria is often found that is similar in consistency to that found in Reinke's edema. On examination, lucent areas are often seen just under the epithelium, suggesting the diagnosis. Larger superficial polyps can be located anywhere along the free edge or superior or inferior surface of the vocal fold and can cause intermittent voice complaints. Surgical exploration often reveals either granulation tissue or a myxomatous matrix with overlying distended epithelium. (Figure 24-19). Small polyps are soft and deformable on contact and generally exhibit normal or increased amplitude of the mucosal wave during voicing. Voices are generally lowered by the increased mass of the vocal fold.

Small and large polyps probably represent a final common pathway rather than being distinct pathologic entities.[40] Over time, some posthem-orrhagic polyps may reabsorb all clot and hemoglobin and take on a softer, whitish appearance. Small polyps may form in response to injury or be localized areas of edema. Some cases may be focal areas of Reinke's edema. These lesions are often associated with a diagnosis of paresis. Generally, pathologic examination of the excised material will show a bland, virtually acellular matrix similar to normal lamina propria.

Treatment of small and large polyps must be individualized according to the patients' vocal demands and expectations, the size and location of the mass, and the severity of the voice changes. Larger masses, severely disordered voices, and high vocal demands all increase the likelihood that surgical resection will be required.

Lesions Associated with Smoking

Reinke's Edema

Reinke's edema (also called polypoid degeneration) occurs almost exclusively in heavy cigarette smokers and is much more noticeable in women, who complain of a masculinized voice. The increased mass of the vocal fold results in a lowered vibration frequency and a lower fundamental frequency. Physical examination reveals severely edematous, rounded vocal folds with increased mucosal wave amplitude and redundant contact. On inspiration, the vocal folds round out toward the posterior portion of the vocal fold (Figure 24-20). The vocal fold color becomes somewhat yellow or even yellow-green. Severe signs of laryngopharyngeal reflux are commonly present. Although voice quality is generally poor, the voice requires very little effort and hyperfunctional voice behaviors are rare.

Although polypoid degeneration of the vocal folds can be seen with severe hypothyroidism, most patients have normal thyroid function.[41] Formation of excess lamina propria probably occurs as a reaction and defense against chronic irritation from cigarette smoke and acid reflux.

Smoking cessation is an essential first step in the treatment of Reinke's edema. Many patients with mild Reinke's edema will have normalization of the voice within 6 to 12 months after stopping cigarettes. Surgical removal of excess lamina propria and mucosa is occasionally required.[42] Many surgeons prefer to only operate on one side at a time to reduce the risk of bilateral scarring, mucosal bridges, and other unusual complications.

Lesions Associated with Infections

Papilloma

In the adult, laryngeal papillomatosis can present as a solitary mass (Figure 24-21), diffuse vocal fold thickening and erythema (Figure 24-22), or as extensive glottic and supraglottic disease (Figure 24-23). Careful rigid stroboscopic examination will often reveal the typical punctate erythema with a grapelike surface typical of papilloma. Unfortunately, granuloma, squamous cell carcinoma, and other unusual tumors can have an identical appearance, so accurate diagnosis requires biopsy and pathologic examination.

Adult presentation of laryngeal papillomatosis is generally less severe than that seen in children, possibly due to maturity of the adult immune system. Human papilloma virus is the causative agent. Laryngeal papillomatosis is not thought to be easily transmittable and is associated with squamous cell cancer development.

Although adults generally have less severe disease, serial surgical excision is generally required. Many agents are used to modify the dis-

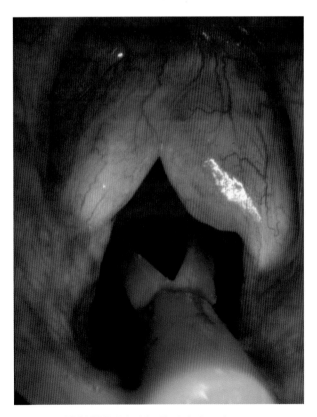

FIGURE 24–20. Reinke's edema.

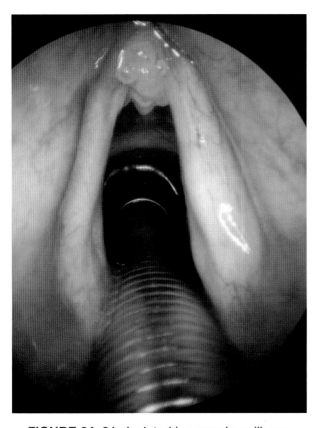

FIGURE 24–21. Isolated laryngeal papilloma.

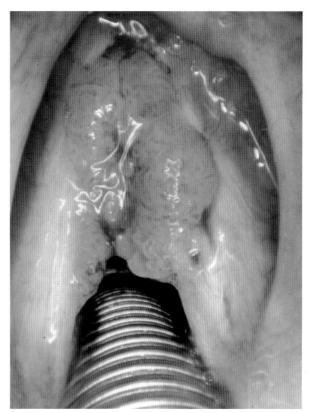

FIGURE 24–22. Diffuse laryngeal papilloma.

ease course, none of which results in complete control of disease while preserving laryngeal function. Currently, intralesional cidofovir injections seem to have promise, but not all patients seem to respond and optimal dosing and injection intervals are still unclear.[43] Because multiple procedures are generally required over time, each surgical procedure should cause minimal trauma to normal structures and minimize scarring and other complications. Powered instrumentation and the pulsed dye laser are currently being investigated as less traumatic methods for surgical papilloma control.[44-45]

Fungal Infections

Vocal fold fungal infections may present with hoarseness, coughing, or pain. Examination reveals glistening white lesions with rounded edges on the vocal folds with surrounding erythema and dilated vessels (Figure 24-24). Although originally

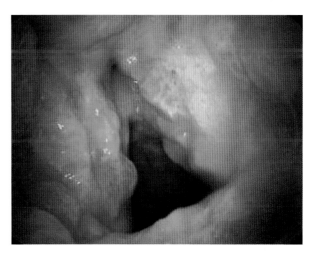

FIGURE 24–23. Extensive glottic and supraglottic papilloma.

described as a disease of immunocompromised patients, it is now known to occur in patients with local immunocompromise due to topical

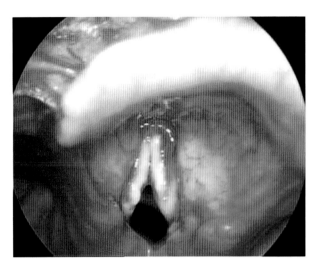

FIGURE 24–24. Fungal laryngitis. Note the rounded edges and the white lesions are not confluent at the anterior commissure.

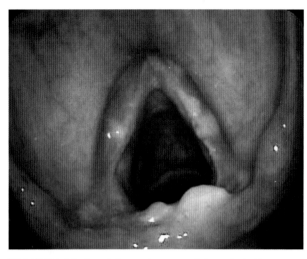

FIGURE 24–25. Ulcerative candida mimicking erythroleukoplakia.

steroid inhalers or after changes in the normal microbial environment.[46] In some cases, laryngeal *Candida* may appear as diffuse leukoplakia or mimic invasive carcinoma (Figure 24-25).[47-48]

In patients with risk factors for fungal overgrowth and a typical laryngeal appearance, it may be worthwhile to pursue empiric treatment with antifungal therapy prior to proceeding with an operative biopsy. Alternatively, in-office brush biopsy can be performed to confirm the diagnosis with minimal trauma. For further information, see chapter 21, Localized Inflammatory Disorders of the Larynx.

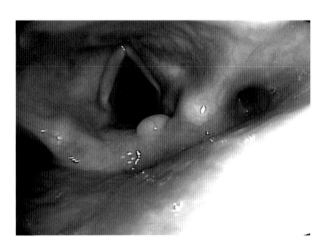

FIGURE 24–26. Neurofibroma.

Neoplasia

Benign laryngeal neoplasms are rare, require biopsy for diagnosis, and can generally be treated with complete surgical excision. Neurofibromas are the most common benign laryngeal tumors. They are generally small, rarely cause symptoms, and appear very similar to inclusion cysts (Figure 24-26). When grasped with forceps, they are much firmer than inclusion cysts, and obviously cannot be unroofed. Asymptomatic laryngeal masses with a benign appearance can be observed without biopsy in most cases.

Benign laryngeal lesions are commonly seen in general otolaryngology practice and usually are accurately diagnosed without a tissue biopsy. Stroboscopy is extremely helpful and necessary in some cases. Knowledge of the natural history and anatomic location of these lesions guides therapy and can have prognostic value. As terminology of many of these lesions changes over time, a precise description of the lesion aids communication between health care providers and avoids misunderstandings.

Review Questions

1. A 36-year-old woman complains of hoarseness for 6 months. She has been placed on voice rest and proton-pump inhibitors with little benefit. She is a nonsmoker and has no other symptoms. She eventually undergoes microdirect laryngoscopy, from which the following picture is obtained. Your clinical diagnosis is:

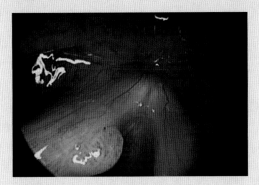

a. Vocal nodule, unilateral
b. Laryngeal papilloma
c. Granuloma
d. Hemorrhagic polyp
e. Pseudopolyp

2. A 16-year-old aspiring singer has had 10 bouts of acute tonsillitis in the past 2 years. She is undergoing tonsillectomy and microdirect laryngoscopy. You note the findings seen below. Both vocal folds are soft on palpation. Your assessment and plan based on these findings is:

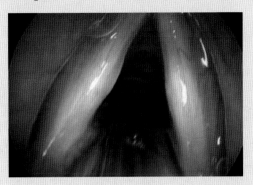

a. Chronic laryngitis with normal vocal folds; no operative intervention on vocal folds at this time
b. Bilateral intracordal cysts; bilateral microflap excision of vocal masses
c. Bilateral intracordal cysts: no operative intervention on vocal folds at this time
d. Vocal nodules: no operative intervention on vocal folds at this time
e. Vocal nodules; staged micro-excision to avoid contamination from tonsillectomy

3. A 55-year-old banker has complained of vocal fatigue and hoarseness for 2 years. She has been on voice rest and speech therapy with no benefit. Her laryngeal hygiene is immaculate. At microlaryngoscopy, you note firmness in the left true vocal fold; the right is soft to palpation (see below). Your diagnosis is:

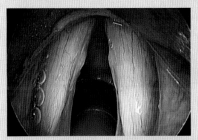

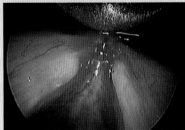

a. T1 SCCA left true vocal fold (TVF)
b. Intracordal cyst, left TVF
c. Vocal nodules, bilateral
d. Vocal nodule, left TVF with companion lesion on the right
e. Sulcus vocalis

4. After deciding on a surgical plan, your surgical decision is to perform a microflap excision of the left true vocal fold mass. The mass is easily dissected at first, but eventually pops. You have removed the superficial aspect of the mass but you are not confident that the attachments to the vocal ligament are cleanly dissected (see below). At this point, you:

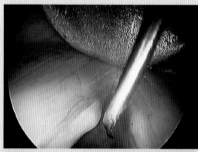

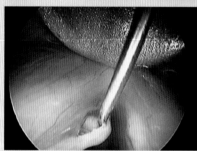

a. Open the vocal fold more widely, and attempt to regain the plane of dissection in previously uninvolved mucosa
b. Meticulously dissect the remnant from the ligament through the same incision
c. Use the laser to avoid any chance of scarring
d. Advance mucosa from nearby vocal fold to cover the defect
e. Abandon the procedure

5. Sulcus vocalis:
a. Requires surgical treatment
b. Represents a loss of the superficial layer of lamina propria
c. Represents a loss of middle layer of the lamina propria
d. Represents a loss of the deep layer of lamina propria
e. Responds to systemic steroid treatment

REFERENCES

1. Andrade DF, Heuer R, Hockstein NE, Castro E, Spiegel JR, Sataloff RT. The frequency of hard glottal attacks in patients with muscle tension dysphonia, unilateral benign masses and bilateral benign masses. *J Voice.* 2000;4(2):240-246.
2. Altman KW, Atkinson C, Lazarus C. Current and emerging concepts in muscle tension dysphonia: a 30-month review. *J Voice.* 2005;19(2):261-267.
3. Pedersen M, Beranova A, Moller S. Dysphonia: medical treatment and a medical voice hygiene advice approach. A prospective randomised pilot study. *Eur Arch Otorhinolaryngol.* 2004;261(6): 312-315.
4. MacKenzie K, Millar A, Wilson JA, Sellars C, Deary IJ. Is voice therapy an effective treatment for dysphonia? A randomised controlled trial. *Br Med J.* 200122;323(7314):658-661.
5. Carding PN, Horsley IA, Docherty GJ. A study of the effectiveness of voice therapy in the treatment of 45 patients with nonorganic dysphonia. *J Voice.* 1999;13(1):72-104
6. Hirano M. Morphological structure of the vocal cord as a vibrator and its variations. *Folia Phoniatr (Basel).* 1974;26(2):89-94
7. Rosen CA, Murray T. Nomenclature of voice disorders and vocal pathology. *Otolaryngol Clin North Am.* 2000;33(5):1035-1046.
8. Milutinovic Z. Classification of voice pathology. *Folia Phoniatr Logop.* 1996;48(6):301-308.
9. Zeitels S, et al. Voice and Swallowing Committee, American Academy of Otolaryngology-Head and Neck Surgery. Management of common voice problems: Committee report. *Otolaryngol Head Neck Surg.* 2002;126(4):333-348.
10. Rosen CA, Murray T. Phonotrauma associated with crying. *J Voice.* 2000;14(4):575-580.

11. Kerr HD, Kwaselow A. Vocal cord hematomas complicating anticoagulant therapy. *Ann Emerg Med.* 1984:552-553.

12. Neely JL, Rosen C. Vocal fold hemorrhage associated with coumadin therapy in an opera singer. *J Voice.* 2000;14(2):272-277.

13. Koch E. Inhibition of platelet activating factor (PAF)-induced aggregation of human thrombocytes by ginkgolides: considerations on possible bleeding complications after oral intake of *Ginkgo biloba* extracts. *Phytomedicine.* 2005;12(1-2):10-16.

14. Hodges PJ, Kam PC. The peri-operative implications of herbal medicines. *Anaesthesia.* 2002;57(9):889-899.

15. Hochman I, Sataloff RT, Hillman RE, Zeitels SM. Ectasias and varices of the vocal fold: clearing the striking zone. *Ann Otol Rhinol Laryngol.* 1999;108(1):10-16.

16. Postma GN, Courey MS, Ossoff RH. Microvascular lesions of the true vocal fold. *Ann Otol Rhinol Laryngol.* 1998;107(6):472-426.

17. Hogikyan ND, Appel S, Guinn LW, Haxer MJ. Vocal fold nodules in adult singers: regional opinions about etiologic factors, career impact, and treatment. A survey of otolaryngologists, speech pathologists, and teachers of singing. *J Voice.* 1999;13(1):128-142.

18. McCrory E. Voice therapy outcomes in vocal fold nodules: a retrospective audit. *Int J Lang Commun Disord.* 2001;36(suppl):19-24.

19. Holmberg EB, Hillman RE, Hammarberg B, Sodersten M, Doyle P. Efficacy of a behaviorally based voice therapy protocol for vocal nodules. *J Voice.* 2001;15(3):395-412.

20. Hoffman HT, Overholt E, Karnell M, McCulloch TM. Vocal process granuloma. *Head Neck.* 2001;23(12):1061-1074.

21. Scheid SC, Anderson TD, Sataloff RT. Nonoperative treatment of laryngeal granuloma. *Ear Nose Throat J.* 2003;82(4):244-245.

22. Roh HJ, Goh EK, Chon KM, Wang SG. Topical inhalant steroid (budesonide, Pulmicort nasal) therapy in intubation granuloma. *J Laryngol Otol.* 1999;113(5):427-432.

23. Mitchell G, Pearson CR, Henk JM, Rhys-Evans P. Excision and low-dose radiotherapy for refractory laryngeal granuloma. *J Laryngol Otol.* 1998;112(5):491-493.

24. Leonard R, Kendall K. Effects of voice therapy on vocal process granuloma: a phonoscopic approach. *Am J Otolaryngol.* 2005;26(2):101-107.

25. Nasri S, Sercarz JA, McAlpin T, Berke GS. Treatment of vocal fold granuloma using botulinum toxin type A. *Laryngoscope.* 1995;105(6):585-588.

26. Clyne SB, Halum SL, Koufman JA, Postma GN. Pulsed dye laser treatment of laryngeal granulomas. *Ann Otol Rhinol Laryngol.* 2005;114(3):198-201

27. Ford CN, Inagi K, Khidr A, Bless DM, Gilchrist KW. Sulcus vocalis: a rational analytical approach to diagnosis and management. *Ann Otol Rhinol Laryngol.* 1996;105(3):189-200.

28. Welham NV, Rousseau B, Ford CN, Bless DM. Tracking outcomes after phonosurgery for sulcus vocalis: a case report. *J Voice.* 2003;17(4):571-578.

29. Hsiung MW, Kang BH, Pai L, Su WF, Lin YH. Combination of fascia transplantation and fat injection into the vocal fold for sulcus vocalis: long-term results. *Ann Otol Rhinol Laryngol.* 2004;113(5):359-366

30. Pontes P, Behlau M. Treatment of sulcus vocalis: auditory perceptual and acoustical analysis of the slicing mucosa surgical technique. *J Voice.* 1993;7(4):365-376.

31. Su CY, Tsai SS, Chiu JF, Cheng CA. Medialization laryngoplasty with strap muscle transposition for vocal fold atrophy with or without sulcus vocalis. *Laryngoscope.* 2004;114(6):1106-1112.

32. Bjorck G, D'Agata L, Hertegard S. Vibratory capacity and voice outcome in patients with scarred vocal folds treated with collagen injections—case studies. *Logoped Phoniatr Vocol.* 2002;27(1):4-11.

33. Benninger MS, Alessi D, Archer S, et al. Vocal fold scarring: current concepts and management. *Otolaryngol Head Neck Surg.* 1996;115(5):474-482.

34. Neuenschwander MC, Sataloff RT, Abaza MM, Hawkshaw MJ, Reiter D, Spiegel JR. Management of vocal fold scar with autologous fat implantation: perceptual results. *J Voice.* 2001;15(2):295-304.

35. Rosen CA. Vocal fold scar: evaluation and treatment. *Otolaryngol Clin North Am.* 2000;33(5):1081-1086.

36. Hirano S. Current treatment of vocal fold scarring. *Curr Opin Otolaryngol Head Neck Surg.* 2005;13(3):143-147.

37. Milutinovic Z, Vasiljevic J. Contribution to the understanding of the etiology of vocal fold cysts: a functional and histologic study. *Laryngoscope.* 1992;102(5):568-571.

38. Bouchayer M, Cornut G, Witzig E, Loire R, Roch JB, Bastian RW. Epidermoid cysts, sulci, and

mucosal bridges of the true vocal cord: a report of 157 cases. *Laryngoscope.* 1985;95(9 pt 1): 1087–1094.

39. Monday LA, Cornut G, Bouchayer M, Roch JB. Epidermoid cysts of the vocal cords. *Ann Otol Rhinol Laryngol.* 1983;92(2 pt 1):124–127.

40. Wallis L, Jackson-Menaldi C, Holland W, Giraldo A. Vocal fold nodule vs. vocal fold polyp: answer from surgical pathologist and voice pathologist point of view. *J Voice.* 2004;18(1):125–129.

41. White A, Sim DW, Maran AG. Reinke's oedema and thyroid function. *J Laryngol Otol.* 1991;105(4): 291–292.

42. Lumpkin SM, Bennett S, Bishop SG. Postsurgical follow-up study of patients with severe polypoid degeneration. *Laryngoscope.* 1990;100(4):399–402.

43. Shehab N, Sweet BV, Hogikyan ND. Cidofovir for the treatment of recurrent respiratory papillomatosis: a review of the literature. *Pharmacotherapy.* 2005;25(7):977–989.

44. Zeitels SM, Franco RA Jr, Dailey SH, Burns JA, Hillman RE, Anderson RR. Office-based treatment of glottal dysplasia and papillomatosis with the 585-nm pulsed dye laser and local anesthesia. *Ann Otol Rhinol Laryngol.* 2004;113(4):265–276.

45. El-Bitar MA, Zalzal GH. Powered instrumentation in the treatment of recurrent respiratory papillomatosis: an alternative to the carbon dioxide laser. *Arch Otolaryngol Head Neck Surg.* 2002;128(4): 425–428.

46. Mehanna HM, Kuo T, Chaplin J, Taylor G, Morton RP. Fungal laryngitis in immunocompetent patients. *J Laryngol Otol.* 2004;118(5):379–381.

47. Scheid SC, Anderson TD, Sataloff RT. Ulcerative fungal laryngitis. *Ear Nose Throat J.* 2003;82(3): 168–169.

48. Hanson JM, Spector G, El-Mofty SK. Laryngeal blastomycosis: a commonly missed diagnosis. Report of two cases and review of the literature. *Ann Otol Rhinol Laryngol.* 2000;109(3):281–286.

25

Malignant Neoplasms of the Larynx

Jason P. Hunt, MD
Andrew J. McWhorter, MD

KEY POINTS

■ Squamous cell carcinoma makes up over 90% of malignant laryngeal neoplasms. Supraglottic tumors usually present late with associated symptoms, glottic tumors usually present early with voice change, and subglottic tumors present late with airway obstruction.

■ Complete endoscopic evaluation for staging requires a plan for airway management, examination of all at-risk mucosal surfaces, and an assessment of cricoarytenoid joint mobility. The neck must be examined and second primaries must be ruled out.

■ Pretreatment evaluation of voice and swallowing is of significant benefit. The treatment of laryngeal malignancy must strive to eliminate the cancer but maintain at least one competent laryngeal valve, if possible, to preserve airway protection and phonation.

■ Following treatment, ongoing surveillance must be performed to detect possible recurrence and the development of any second primary tumors.

Laryngeal cancer affects 10,000 people annually and accounts for 3,000 deaths per year. It is among the most common head and neck malignancies in the United States.[1] If detected early, it can be effectively treated; however, over 40% of laryngeal cancers present with advanced-stage disease.[2] The larynx is integral in respiration, phonation, and deglutition, and malignancies may disrupt any or all of these functions. Treatment of these malignancies must consider preservation of these functions, which are vital to a patient's quality of life. When determining treatment, the clinician must balance these quality of life issues with the survival advantage of the therapy. Advances in technology have expanded treatment paradigms with an increased utilization of chemotherapy and radiation therapy. Recently, conservation laryngeal surgery options are being re-examined with the increased acceptance of endoscopic resections. The numerous treatment choices now available can create complex decision making. A multidisciplinary approach provides the opportunity for evaluating all treatment options and should be utilized in the management of these patients.

PATHOGENESIS AND RISK FACTORS

The larynx is lined with stratified squamous epithelium down to the level of the true vocal folds. This transitions to pseudostratified respiratory epithelium toward the central airways. There is normally an ordered array of maturation from the basement membrane to the surface. When the epidermis suffers an insult, the area may become thickened and abnormal. The pathologic correlate for these changes may appear as *hyperkeratosis*. This may appear as a white, raised lesion. Clinically, this finding is termed *leukoplakia* (Figure 25–1) and, if not treated, has an approximately 3% chance of progressing to invasive carcinoma.[3] *Erythroplakia* represents a different response of the epithelium. These lesions are red due to increased vascularity and are thought to carry an even greater risk of progression to carcinoma.[4] When the normal epithelial maturation is disrupted from the basement membrane to the surface, it is termed dysplasia. Dysplasia is graded from mild to severe. When it fills the entire epithelium, it is termed carcinoma-in-situ (CIS). CIS progresses to

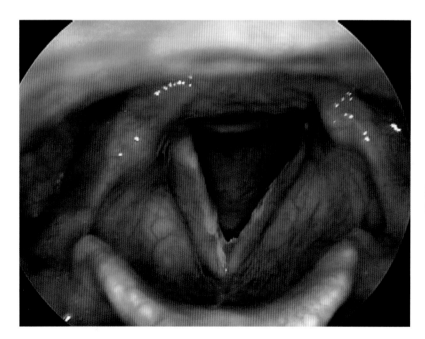

FIGURE 25–1. Bilateral true vocal fold leukoplakia.

invasive carcinoma as the basement membrane is invaded. This continuum of disease is currently being investigated to better understand the molecular basis of this tumor progression model.[5]

Malignancies of the larynx, like most malignancies of the head and neck, are heavily linked to cigarette use. More than 90% of patients with laryngeal cancer have a significant history of tobacco use. There is a positive relationship between the quantity of cigarettes smoked and the increase in risk of developing laryngeal cancer.[6] When tobacco is combined with alcohol use, the effect is synergistic with even higher rates of malignancy. Alcohol use by itself may be a risk factor as well, but this role is less well defined.

Other risk factors have also been implicated in the development of laryngeal cancer (Figure 25-2). Human papilloma virus (HPV), especially subtypes 16 and 18, is known to predispose a patient to squamous cell carcinoma.[7-9] Viral evidence of HPV infection has been found in 40% of laryngeal cancer specimens.[10] Gastroesophageal reflux disease (GERD) has been long suspected as a risk factor and recent evidence has shown support for GERD as a risk factor for laryngeal cancer.[11] Other pathogens such as asbestos, radiation exposure, and wood dust are environmental factors that pose a higher risk for the development of laryngeal cancer.[12] In contrast, some compounds may provide a protective effect such as fruits and dark green vegetables.

As with most cancers, there is an intricate interplay between the host and various environmental factors. Immunocompromised individuals are believed to be more susceptible to malignant transformation. A great amount of research is being invested into the effects of various carcinogens as well as the host's defense against malignant transformation. Elimination of known common carcinogens, such as tobacco and alcohol, should be a primary concern to prevent recurrence and the development of second primaries.

EPIDEMIOLOGY

Laryngeal cancer accounts for 1% of all cancer-related deaths. There were over 10,000 new laryngeal cancers in 2004.[13] Despite efforts to improve treatment outcomes, the 5-year survival has remained around 65% for the past 25 years. Malignancy can occur in all three divisions of the larynx: supraglottis, glottis, and subglottis. Although subglottic malignancies are universally rare, the relative occurrence at the other two sites varies by global region. Glottic malignancies are the most common laryngeal malignancy in the United States with an incidence of 56% (Figure 25-3).[2] Other countries have a higher incidence of supraglottic cancers.[13] This variable presentation may be related to both environmental factors (tobacco, alcohol use, etc) as well as genetic predisposition in certain populations.

Laryngeal cancer primarily affects persons in the fifth, sixth, and seventh decades of life with the highest incidence in the sixth decade. Men are more commonly affected than women

◆ Tobacco

◆ Tobacco and Alcohol, synergistically

◆ Human Papilloma Virus (HPV)

◆ Gastroesophageal reflux disease

FIGURE 25–2. Known and suspected risk factors associated with laryngeal cancer.

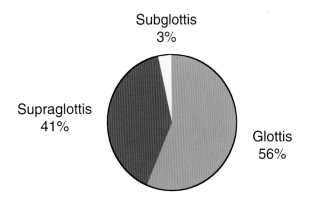

FIGURE 25–3. Incidence of laryngeal cancer in the United States by site.

with a male to female ratio of 3.6:1.[14] This ratio of males to females has been decreasing from a previous high of 5.6:1 in 1973 to 1974. It is postulated that this change is due to the increased use of cigarettes in females.

In the United States, there are differences in survival between whites and African-Americans diagnosed with laryngeal cancer. Five-year survival among African-Americans was 60% versus 66% for whites in the years of 1974 to 1976. This gap has continued to widen over the past two decades. Currently, there is a 14% difference in 5-year survival between the groups. Figure 25–4 shows representative 5-year survival rates over the past three decades.[13]

ANATOMY AND PATTERNS OF SPREAD

The larynx is the gatekeeper of the airway. Three valves are contained within the larynx that enable phonation, respiration, and deglutition. The valves from inferior to superior are the (1) true vocal folds, (2) false vocal folds, and (3) epiglottis to arytenoids, aryepiglottic folds. Dysfunction of these valves may lead to voice changes, aspiration, and or airway obstruction. The patient's symptoms related to pathologic function of these valves allows lesions to be localized to the affected region.

The spread of laryngeal cancer may be anticipated by the site of the lesion and the anatomic compartments of the larynx (Figure 25–5). These patterns of spread are better understood by considering the embryologic origin and the fibroelastic membranes and ligaments that divide the larynx into its various compartments. The *supraglottis* is derived from the midline buccopharyngeal primordium and branchial arches 3 and 4. It is richly supplied by lymphatics. In contrast, the glottis is derived from the tracheobronchial primordium and arches 4, 5, and 6 with relatively few lymphatics in this location. These differences are likely the basis of a low incidence of lymphatic spread for glottic cancer versus supraglottic cancer. Furthermore, the rich lymphatic network of the supraglottis predisposes for bilateral lymph node metastasis from supraglottic cancer compared to unilateral spread in glottic lesions.

The fibroelastic membranes and ligaments divide the larynx into compartments that are potential conduits for the spread of tumor. At the level of the *glottis*, the vocalis tendon attaches to the thyroid cartilage via Broyle's ligament. This is an ineffective barrier and allows spread of cancer into the thyroid cartilage. Other compart-

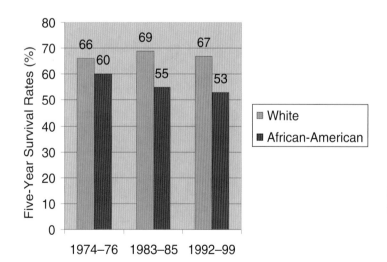

FIGURE 25–4. Comparison of survival differences by ethnicity.

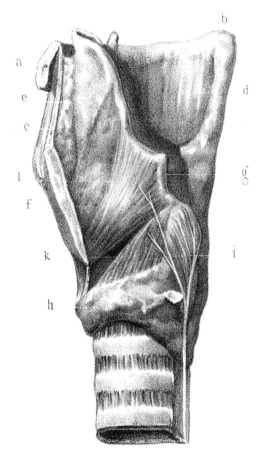

FIGURE 25–5. Bougery and Jacob's published this illustration in 1831 of the paraglotic and pre-epiglottic spaces with the lateral border of the thyroid cartilage removed. **a.** split midline of hyoid bone. **b.** greater horn of the hyoid bone. **c.** pre-epiglottic space. **d.** thyrohyoid membrane. **e.** epiglottis. **f.** midline split thyroid cartilage. **g.** posterior body of the aryetnoid cartilage. **h.** cricoid cartilage. **i.** posterior cricoarytenoid cartilage muscle. **k.** lateral cricoarytenoid muscle. **l.** thryoarytenoid muscle.

ments to consider are the pre-epiglottic and the paraglottic spaces. The pre-epiglottic space is contained by the following boundaries: thyroepiglottic ligament inferiorly, hyoepiglottic ligament superiorly, the thyrohyoid membrane anteriorly, and the epiglottis posteriorly. At this level, the thyroepiglottic ligament is an ineffective barrier to the spread of tumor. From the laryngeal surface of the epiglottis, tumor may spread directly into the pre-epiglottic space via perforations in the carti-

lage of the epiglottis called lacunae. The paraglottic space is a potential space that is bounded medially by the quadrangular membrane above the ventricle and the conus elasticus below the ventricle. The anterior and lateral boundaries are the thyroid cartilage and the mucosa of the medial wall of the piriform sinus forms the posterior boundary. This space allows tumor to spread transglottically and impair the movement of the true vocal fold. The paraglottic space and pre-epiglottic space communicate with one another. Once in the paraglottic space, the tumor may extend outside the larynx by erosion of the thyroid cartilage or extension between the inferior aspect of the thyroid cartilage and the cricoid cartilage.

Lymphatic spread of the tumor occurs in a predictable fashion and has allowed surgeons to limit neck dissections to include only the lymph node basins at risk. Lindberg first showed these patterns in 1972 by mapping out affected lymph nodes by primary site of tumor.[15] His studies demonstrated that laryngeal cancer most commonly spreads to levels II to V. It also showed a high prevalence of contralateral neck involvement in supraglottic tumors. Shah confirmed which lymph node basins were at risk in 1990.[16]

STAGING

Staging systems allow for better prediction of outcomes and comparison of data between institutions. A universal staging system is helpful in counseling patients and in treatment planning. The scheme currently employed in the United States is the TNM staging system of the American Joint Committee on Cancer.[17] This staging system was last revised in 2002; it is dependent on anatomic descriptors and is based on characteristics of the primary tumor, cervical lymph node status, and distant metastases. Data are obtained through physical examination as well as imaging. Confirmation is obtained from surgical pathology for resected tumors. The staging system is outlined below (Figure 25-6).

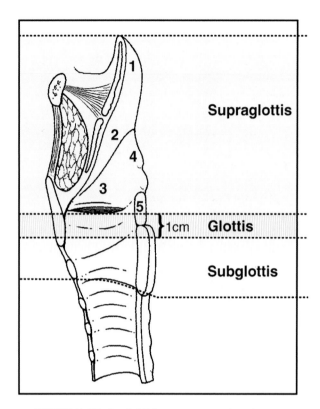

FIGURE 25–6. AJCC cancer staging: larynx.

Supraglottis: From the tip of the epiglottis to a lateral plane through the ventricle at the superior surface of the true vocal fold. *Supraglottic Subsites:* 1. Suprahyoid epiglottis; 2. Infrahyoid epiglottis; 3. False vocal fold; 4. Aryepiglottic fold; 5. Arytenoid.

Glottis: True vocal folds including the superior and inferior surfaces as well as the anterior and posterior commissure.

Subglottis: Zone from 1 cm below the plane defining the separation of the glottis from supraglottis to the bottom of the cricoid cartilage.

Laryngeal Cancer Staging by TNM (Adapted from The American Joint Committee on Cancer (AJCC) TNM Classification: Larynx)[17]

Primary tumor (T): TX: Primary tumor cannot be assessed, T0: No evidence of primary tumor, Tis: Carcinoma in situ.

Supraglottis

T1: Tumor limited to one subsite* of supraglottis with normal vocal cord mobility.

T2: Tumor invades mucosa of more than one adjacent subsite* of supraglottis or glottis or region outside the supraglottis (eg, mucosa of base of tongue, vallecula, medial wall of piriform sinus) without fixation of the larynx.

T3: Tumor limited to larynx with vocal cord fixation and/or invades any of the following: postcricoid area, pre-epiglottic tissues, paraglottic space, and/or minor thyroid cartilage erosion (eg, inner cortex).

T4a: Tumor invades through the thyroid cartilage, and/or invades tissues beyond the larynx (eg, trachea, soft tissues of the neck including deep extrinsic muscle of the tongue, strap muscles, thyroid, or esophagus).

T4b: Tumor invades prevertebral space, encases carotid artery, or invades mediastinal structures.

*Subsites include the following: suprahyoid epiglottis, infrahyoid epiglottis, vestibular folds (false vocal cords), aryepiglottic folds, arytenoids.

Glottis

T1: Tumor limited to the vocal cord(s) (may involve anterior or posterior commissure) with normal mobility.

T1a: Tumor limited to one vocal cord.

T1b: Tumor involves both vocal cords.

T2: Tumor extends to supraglottis and/or subglottis, and/or with impaired vocal cord mobility.

T3: Tumor limited to the larynx with vocal cord fixation and/or invades paraglottic space, and/or minor thyroid cartilage erosion (eg, inner cortex).

T4a: Tumor invades through the thyroid cartilage and/or invades tissues beyond the larynx (eg, trachea, soft tissues of neck, including deep extrinsic muscle of the tongue, strap muscles, thyroid, or esophagus).

T4b: Tumor invades prevertebral space, encases carotid artery, or invades mediastinal structures.

Subglottis

T1: Tumor limited to the subglottis.

T2: Tumor extends to vocal cord(s) with normal or impaired mobility.

T3: Tumor limited to larynx with vocal cord fixation.

T4a: Tumor invades cricoid or thyroid cartilage and/or invades tissues beyond the larynx (eg, trachea, soft tissues of neck, including deep extrinsic muscles of the tongue, strap muscles, thyroid, or esophagus).

T4b: Tumor invades prevertebral space, encases carotid artery, or invades mediastinal structures.

Regional lymph nodes (N): NX: Regional lymph nodes cannot be assessed; N0: No regional lymph node metastasis.

N1: Metastasis in a single ipsilateral lymph node, 3 cm or less in greatest dimension.

N2a: Metastasis in a single ipsilateral lymph node more than 3 cm but not more than 6 cm in greatest dimension.

N2b: Metastasis in multiple ipsilateral lymph nodes, none more than 6 cm in greatest dimension.

N2c: Metastasis in bilateral or contralateral lymph nodes, none more than 6 cm in greatest dimension.

N3: Metastasis in a lymph node more than 6 cm in greatest dimension.

Distant metastasis (M):

MX: Distant metastasis cannot be assessed.

M0: No distant metastasis.

M1: Distant metastasis.

Stage

Stage 0: Tis, N0, M0

Stage I: T1, N0, M0

Stage II: T2, N0, M0

Stage III: T3, N0, M0 or T1, N1, M0 or T2, N1, M0 or T3, N1, M0

Stage IVA: T1, N2, M0 or T2, N2, M0 or T3, N2, M0 or T4a, N2 or less, M0

Stage IVB: T4b, any N, M0 or any T, N3, M0

Stage IVC: Any T, any N, M1

A commonly accepted and useful addition to the AJCC staging system is that proposed by Harwood and DeBoer.[18] They found that patients with mobile but impaired motion of the vocal fold had a 12% decrease in 5-year survival compared to those with full mobility. This finding has been substantiated in multiple series. On this basis, they proposed subdividing T2 glottic tumors into T2a-normal mobility and T2b-impaired mobility.

TABLE 25–1. Survival by Stage and Laryngeal Site*

Stage	Supraglottic	Glottic
I	53–82%	74–100%
II	50–64%	64–76%
III	50–60%	50–60%
IV	<50%	30–57%

*Compiled from Shah and Eckel[2,19]

On review of outcomes of patients with T2 carcinomas, they noted a 12% decrease in survival when there was motion impairment but not fixation of vocal cord mobility. Table 25-1 above outlines survival by stage and site.

Although the AJCC staging system categorizes tumors based on size and extent of disease, it does not look at other factors that may predict prognosis. Certain histologic characteristics of the tumor indicate poorer prognosis, such as extracapsular spread of nodal metastases, angiolymphatic spread, perineural invasion, and histologic grade. Current investigation is directed toward chromosomal and molecular markers that may also have prognostic value. Other research is focused on evaluating comorbidity as it relates to outcomes.[20]

PATIENT EVALUATION

History and Physical Examination

As with many laryngeal conditions, the history and physical exam will lead the physician to the diagnosis in the vast majority of cases. The symptoms encountered depend largely on the location of the lesion and the stage of the tumor. These symptoms include dysphonia, dyspnea, dysphagia, and otalgia. The presence of ear pain is a common complaint of patients with laryngeal carcinomas, especially supraglottic lesions. This phenomenon is referred pain from cranial nerve X that innervates both the laryngopharynx and

the ear. This highlights the importance of examining the laryngopharynx when ear findings do not reveal a cause of otalgia. In addition to laryngeal-related symptoms, constitutional symptoms such as weight loss must also be noted. The weight loss may occur due to advanced-stage cancer or the patient's decreased ability to eat as well as tumor biology and humoral effects in advanced cases. Past medical history is important in assessing general functional status and comorbidities. These assessments in the history will aid in determining appropriate therapy. Tobacco and alcohol history should also be obtained and quantified.

Glottic cancers, as compared to supraglottic lesions, may be noted at earlier stages due to the changes in voice. Changes in voice occur with subtle disruptions in the vocal fold vibrations. Changes in voice unresolved after 2 weeks require visualization. Supraglottic cancers present with fewer symptoms in the early stages. This delay of symptoms allows supraglottic lesions to grow until advanced-stage symptoms appear: dysphagia, otalgia, neck pain, hemoptysis, and airway obstruction. Also, the presence of a cervical mass may be the first sign of a supraglottic malignancy. Subglottic malignancies which originate in the confines of the cricoid cartilage present with airway obstructive symptoms.

After a detailed history, a thorough head and neck examination takes place to assess the extent of tumor involvement and overall health status of the patient. The larynx is examined with a mirror or with the aid of a flexible endoscope. The extent of the lesion and functional status of the vocal folds are noted. The adequacy of the airway is assessed as well as a careful examination for cervical lymphatic involvement. Videostroboscopy (Figure 25–7) may also be used to note subtle changes in vocal fold vibration in the assessment of early glottic lesions (see chapter 6, Videolaryngostroboscopy).

Imaging

Physical exam is often limited in the evaluation of the depth of tumor penetration. Radiographic

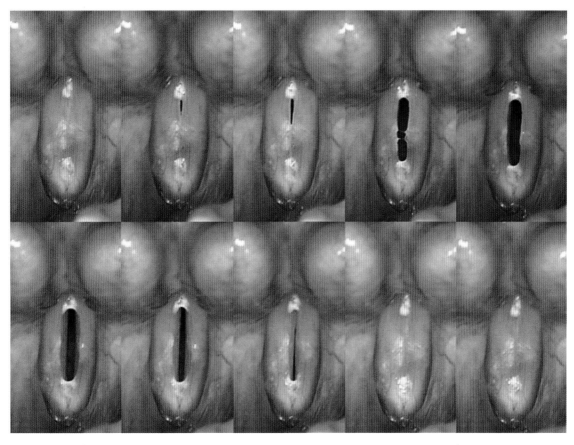

FIGURE 25–7. Montage of vibratory cycle as visualized on videostroboscopy.

imaging allows evaluation of the deep laryngeal spaces, involvement of the thyroid cartilage, and extrinsic muscles of the neck. These characteristics influence treatment options and are essential in proper treatment planning. Thyroid cartilage invasion is an important but difficult radiographic determination. Both computed tomography (CT) and magnetic resonance imaging (MRI) are useful radiographic modalities in this assessment. MRI is a more sensitive measure of cartilage invasion, but lacks specificity and can overestimate cartilage invasion. CT is less sensitive, but more specific for cartilage invasion.[21] Currently, at most centers, CT is considered the standard in the evaluation of advanced laryngeal cancers (Figure 25-8).

Positron emission tomography (PET) is becoming increasingly common in the evaluation of malignancies including laryngeal cancer. PET scanning utilizes fluorescence-tagged glucose

molecules and measurement of their preferential uptake by the hypermetabolic state of cancer. The utility of this tool has yet to be fully determined, but is currently being evaluated for determination of occult nodal disease, unknown primary tumors, and distant metastatic spread (Figure 25-9). Early studies have had promising results showing a high sensitivity and specificity for detecting lymph node and distant metastasis as well as recurrent disease and second primaries.[22,23] Although the data are promising, work is continuing in regard to the best timing of PET scan, the effects of chemotherapy and radiation therapy, and cost and availability.

Ultrasound is the preferred technique for evaluation of nodal disease in Europe. This low-cost and noninvasive technique is gaining prevalence in the United States as well. Evaluation of the larynx is problematic due to the limitations

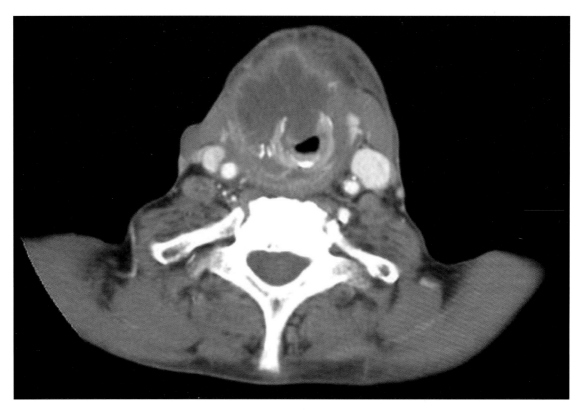

FIGURE 25–8. Axial CT scan through the laryrnx demonstrating massive extralaryngeal spread with cartilage destruction.

of the cartilage framework of the larynx and ultrasound penetration. Current studies are evaluating the use of endoscopic ultrasound, developed for esophageal and lung cancer, in the evaluation of laryngeal lesions (Figure 25-10). Chapter 10 reviews radiology of the larynx.

Operative Endoscopy and Biopsy

Panendoscopy is a term that is often used to describe complete endoscopic evaluation of the upper aerodigestive tract. It involves laryngoscopy, esophagoscopy, and tracheobronchoscopy. Its purpose is twofold: evaluation of the primary malignancy and evaluation for second primaries. It is estimated that the incidence of second primaries of the upper aerodigestive tract is 1% for synchronous lesions and 5 to 10% for metachronous lesions.

Direct laryngoscopy allows direct visualization of the tumor under general anesthesia (Figure 25-11). A map of tumor involvement can be created to assist in staging, treatment planning, and in following treatment response. All sites of involvement are noted, with telescopic examination helping to better assess the extent of involvement particularly in the ventricle and subglottis. Palpation of the true vocal fold, vocal process, and arytenoid is important to differentiate vocal cord paralysis from vocal cord fixation. The pre-epiglottic space can be evaluated by bimanual palpation.

Historically, endoscopy of the esophagus has been performed with rigid esophagoscopes. Flexible esophagoscopy has great advantage in complete mucosal assessment and distal evaluation into the stomach. Bronchoscopy may be performed with rigid or flexible bronchoscopes. The yield of bronchoscopy in the asymptomatic

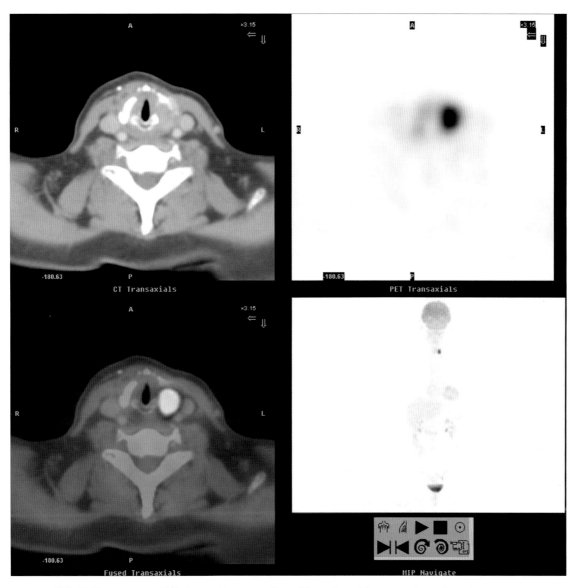

FIGURE 25–9. PET/CT axial image of papillary thyroid cancer invading the larynx.

patient is low due to the limitation of only visualizing endobronchial lesions. Imaging is often substituted for bronchoscopy.

Transnasalesophagoscopy (TNE) is a procedure developed for endoscopic esophageal evaluation in the office setting with only topical anesthesia. TNE has been adapted for panendoscopy in select patients with head and neck malignancies to evaluate and biopsy the nasopharynx, oropharynx, hypopharynx, larynx, and esophagus without the need for operative evaluation. TNE does not allow for palpation of the vocal cords and assessment cricoarytenoid joint mobility. This emerging technology is discussed in chapter 11.

Evaluation of Distant Disease

In addition to the thorough evaluation and staging of the larynx and neck, the clinician must evaluate the patient for distant metastases. Laryngeal

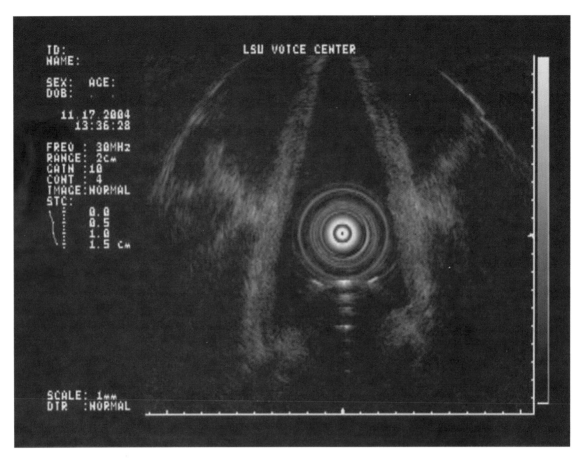

FIGURE 25–10. 30-MHz endoscopic ultrasound image of the larynx at the level of the true vocal folds.

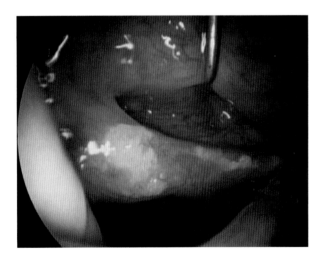

FIGURE 25–11. 70° telescopic evaluation of the ventricle during direct microlaryngoscopy with blunt tip, right-angle assistance.

cancer is very unlikely to be cured when there are distant metastases; treatment typically becomes palliative. The primary sites of metastases are the lungs, liver, and bone with an overall incidence of less than 10%. Distant metastasis is very unlikely to occur without regional nodal disease.

The lungs may be evaluated by bronchoscopy or imaging. Bronchoscopy may detect endobronchial lesions, but has a poor yield for metastatic lesions which are usually located peripherally in the lung. Bronchial washings are used to improve the rate of detection for metastases or second primaries. There is a low yield, however, from this method and a false positive may be obtained if tumor from the larynx is accidentally dislodged and picked up with the washings. Imaging is the modality of choice. This is accomplished with chest radiograph, computed tomography (CT), or PET scan. Chest radiographs are inexpensive and readily available as a screening tool, but may miss small lesions. Chest CT has a higher sensitivity, but also detects small lesions that are unable to be classified. It is often not necessary for early stage lesions, but for recurrent lesions and extensive cervical nodal disease, it is warranted due to the higher incidence of distant metastases. PET scanning, especially when combined with CT, is highly sensitive but again with a higher rate of false positives. As cost decreases and availability increases, its utility will likely improve.

The liver is rarely involved by tumor if the lung is not involved. Therefore, the yield in primary-imaging the liver and the abdomen in general is low. Liver function tests should be obtained as an inexpensive screening evaluation. If abnormal, a CT of the abdomen is then obtained with or without PET scanning. Bone metastases are also very rare in the absence of lung metastasis. Alkaline phosphatase and calcium levels are used as screening tools for bony involvement. Bone scans and PET are utilized when there are abnormal lab values.

DIFFERENTIAL DIAGNOSIS

Squamous cell carcinoma comprises 95 to 99% of laryngeal malignancies. These tumors follow a linear progression of dedifferentiation into invasive carcinoma. As previously described, leukoplakia and erythroplakia can represent premalignant lesions. A tumor progression model has been proposed in the pathway to carcinogenesis (Figure 25-12).

Squamous Cell Carcinoma Subtypes

A small percentage of squamous cell carcinomas can be further subdivided into the following subtypes. Basaloid squamous cell carcinoma represents a very small subset of laryngeal squamous cell carcinoma with less than 100 cases reported in the literature. They have a predilection for the supraglottis and reportedly have a more aggressive clinical course.[24-26] Adenosquamous carcinoma is another rare subset of squamous cell carcinoma and has a very aggressive course with frequent lymph node metastasis and a high rate of local recurrence.[27,28] Spindle cell carcinoma is a variant of squamous cell carcinoma that has been assigned different nomenclature but is frequently referred to as carcinosarcoma. It is a fleshy, polypoid tumor that exhibits a dedifferentiation toward a sarcomalike component and is associated with a higher rate of radiation resistance and local recurrence.[29]

Verrucous carcinoma (Figure 25-13) is the most common histologic variant of squamous cell carcinoma representing 1 to 3% of all laryngeal malignancies. It has a high rate of HPV infection when analyzed. The tumor has "pushing borders" with a propensity for local recurrence but an extremely low rate of metastasis. Its typical exophytic gray-white fronds are very distinctive. Controversy still exists regarding anaplastic transformation following radiation therapy; despite conclusive evidence, surgery remains the treatment of choice.[30,31] Papillosquamous carcinoma is an entity distinct from verrucous carcinoma with greater cellular pleomorphism. It has a more aggressive clinical course similar to squamous cell carcinoma.

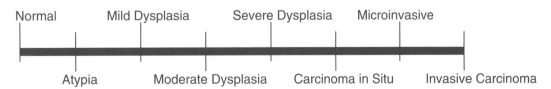

FIGURE 25–12. Tumor progression model for squamous cell carcinoma.

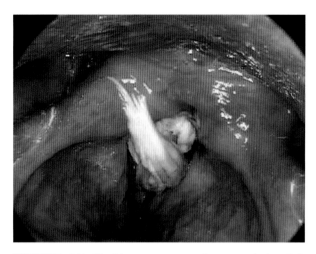

FIGURE 25–13. Verrucous carcinoma of the left true vocal fold.

Nonsquamous Malignancies

Nonsquamous malignant tumors of the larynx form a large catchall group with the majority being sarcomas, minor salivary gland tumors, and neuroendocrine tumors.

Sarcomas

Multiple sarcomas have been described in the larynx: chondrosarcoma, osteosarcoma, malignant fibrous histiocytoma, fibrosarcoma, liposarcoma, angiosarcoma, synovial cell sarcoma, Kaposi's sarcoma, and rhabdomyosarcoma. In this unusual subset of laryngeal malignancies, it is difficult to make broad generalizations as they individually behave differently. As an example, angiosarcoma is an extremely aggressive tumor whereas chondrosarcoma can be difficult to differentiate from a benign chondroma.

Chondrosarcoma, however, is the most prevalent of this tumor class and one of the more common nonsquamous malignancies of the larynx. The majority of these tumors arise from the cricoid cartilage and present with airway obstructive symptoms. They are divided into low, medium, and high grades based on their histology which helps determine their treatment approach (Figures 25–14A and 25–14B). Overall, these tumors do extremely well and low-grade malignancies have good outcomes with conservative resection.[32,33]

Minor Salivary Gland Tumors

There are a variety of minor salivary malignancies that occur in the larynx, including adenoid cystic carcinoma, mucoepidermoid carcinoma, acinic cell carcinoma, adenocarcinoma, and malignant mixed carcinoma. They are typically found in the supraglottic larynx but can present in the subglottis with a predilection of adenoid cystic carcinoma for this region. They behave like typical minor salivary neoplasms in other head and neck sites. Adenocarcinomas have the least favorable prognosis. Mucoepidermoid carcinomas are graded based on their degree of differentiation with high-grade tumors being more aggressive. Adenoid cystic carcinomas have their traditional propensity for neural invasion with high local recurrence rates and submucosal spread into the trachea.[34-36]

Neuroendocrine

Neuroendocrine malignancies are composed of paragangliomas, atypical carcinoids, large cell tumors, and small cell tumors. This apparently similar group of tumors behave very differently and correct diagnosis through immunohistochemistry is essential in formulating an appropriate treatment plan. Paragangliomas are relatively indolent tumors usually found in the supraglottis. These vascular masses are managed through surgical excision. Atypical carcinoids are the most common neuroendocrine tumor and are also usually found in the supraglottis. They are aggressive tumors and require surgical excision, as they are relatively chemoradiation resistant. Atypical carcinoids carry a poor prognosis and should be followed with calcitonin levels. Small cell tumors are the most aggressive of the neuroendocrine tumors and behave similarly to other anatomic sites. Treatment is typically nonsurgical with chemoradiation therapy.[37-42]

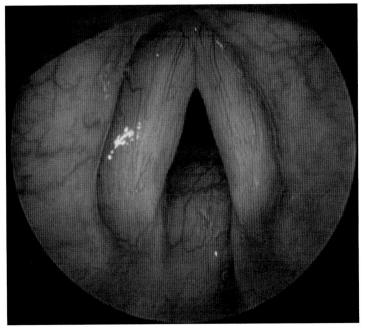

A.

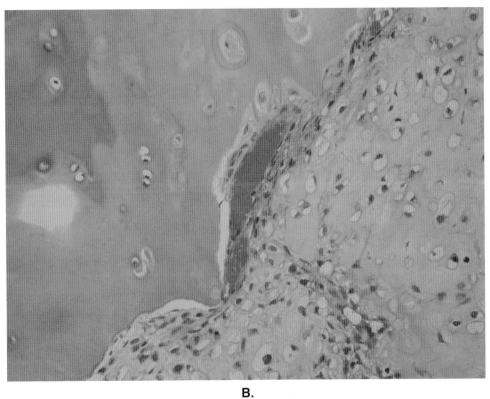

B.

FIGURE 25–14. A. Low-grade chondrosarcoma of the cricoid cartilage that presented with airway obstruction symptoms. **B.** Histologic section showing low-grade chondrosarcoma (*lower right*) abutting normal cartilage of the larynx (*upper left*). Note increased cellularity in the chondrosarcoma.

Other Malignancies

Lymphoproliferative lesions in the larynx usually occur in the supraglottis. Mucosal associated lymphoid tissue (MALT) lymphomas are a subtype of non-Hodgkin's lymphoma. These tumors are usually low-grade and respond to radiation with chemotherapy used for advanced-stage tumors. Newer chemotherapy and monoclonal antibody therapies may change this paradigm. Extramedullary plasmacytomas can be treated with surgery or radiation but require workup to rule out multiple myeloma.[43-45]

Melanoma of the larynx can be a laryngeal primary but is more commonly a metastasis. Metastatic lesions are usually adenocarcinomas from common sites such as breast and colon. Renal cell carcinoma, however, is the most common laryngeal metastasis. Nonlaryngeal malignancies can also invade the larynx by direct extension. Frequently large tumors can extend into the larynx from the hypopharynx or base of tongue. Nonaerodigestive cancers such as thyroid can also invade the cartilaginous larynx by direct extension.[46]

TREATMENT

Treatment of laryngeal cancer can be broken down into early stage versus advanced stage tumors as well as by glottic versus supraglottic tumors. Early stage tumors should be treated with *single modality therapy* in most cases (ie, surgery or radiation). Advanced staged lesions often require multimodality treatment with surgery followed by radiation or radiation with the addition of chemotherapy. There is considerable debate over the therapeutic choices and differences among institutions in their treatment philosophies. These differences underscore the need for a multidisciplinary approach with consideration of each case on an individual basis.

Precancerous Lesions

As previously described, leukoplakia and erythroplakia can histologically vary from benign to pre-malignant to malignant disease. Dysplastic lesions and carcinoma-in-situ (CIS) are premalignant lesions that may proceed to invasive cancer if not properly managed. The spectrum of management includes observation, serial excision, radiation, and laser treatment. The aggressiveness of the treatment takes into account patient risk factors, the feasibility of surveillance, and the morbidity of treatment. Serial excision has been shown to be effective in preventing the progression of premalignant lesions to invasive carcinoma.[47] Zeitels et al have shown effective treatment of dysplastic lesions in the office setting using a pulsed dye laser.[48] Any treatment plan must include counseling on avoiding risk factors such as tobacco, alcohol, and acid reflux which may promote tumor progression.

Early Stage Laryngeal Carcinoma

Stage I and II laryngeal cancers have similar survival with surgical therapy or radiation therapy. An advantage of surgery is a shorter and less costly course of treatment compared to the 6 to 7 weeks of radiation therapy. Surgery also reserves radiation for loco-regional recurrence or second primary. The disadvantage of surgery is the potential detrimental effect on voice and swallowing. The surgical options for early laryngeal cancer include open partial laryngectomy or transoral endoscopic excision. These procedures usually have very acceptable voice and swallowing outcomes with equivalent survival, while avoiding radiation. Voice and swallowing outcomes depend on the ability to reconstruct the resected larynx and maintain valvular competence. Specific surgical procedures with their indications are discussed below.

Radiation therapy as a single modality is another option and the most commonly employed therapy. The advantage is the potential preservation of voice; surgery will still be available for salvage of recurrence. The potential disadvantages of radiation therapy are a longer course of therapy and radiation changes and late tissue effects. The early risks of radiation include mucositis, odynophagia, and edema. The long-term effects of radiation include fibrosis, chondroradionecrosis, xerostomia, hypothyroidism, and esophageal stricture.

The choice of treatment is controversial and there are proponents for each therapy. As no definitive prospective randomized trials exist for early stage lesions, the treatment decisions must be tailored to each patient taking into account survival, toxicities, surgeon's experience, and the patient's goals.

Advanced Laryngeal Cancers

With rare exception, advanced laryngeal tumors require multimodality treatment. Surgery followed by radiation is commonly used for large T3 and T4 lesions. The surgical options include total laryngectomy and open partial laryngectomy when possible. Some T3 and T4 lesions are amenable to transoral laser excision, although this requires special expertise of the surgeon. This is discussed later in the chapter. T3 lesions may be treated with an organ preservation approach that involves the combination of chemotherapy and radiation therapy. The choice of treatment again depends on the characteristics of the tumor, comorbidities of the patient, and the expertise of the treating surgeon. Each treatment is discussed in more detail in this chapter.

Treatment of the Neck

In the management of laryngeal cancer, the treatment of the neck must be considered along with that of the primary tumor. The decision whether or not to treat the neck takes into account the likelihood of regional spread of disease to the cervical lymphatics. When there is palpable or radiographic evidence of nodal disease, the neck should be treated. This decision is more difficult when there is not evidence of cervical nodal disease (N0). Generally accepted guidelines suggest treatment of the neck if there is a 20 to 30% chance of spread of disease to the neck. The two factors that help the clinician in this treatment decision include: (1) site, and (2) the T stage. The supraglottis with its rich lymphatics has a high rate of metastatic spread and all supraglottic lesions warrant consideration of treatment for the nodal basins at risk, that is, levels 2 to 4 and the central nodal compartment 6. The glottis with its paucity of lymphatics is unlikely to have regional involvement until stage T3 or greater when tumor has spread beyond the limits of the glottis. Table 25–2 below shows the likelihood of cervical metastases based on T stage and subsite.

The treatment of the N0 neck at risk for nodal metastasis can be either radiation therapy or surgery. The decision will depend on the treatment of the primary. If the primary tumor is to be treated with radiation, then the fields should be extended to include the nodal basins at risk. If the neck is to be incised to remove the tumor, then a selective neck dissection can be done with limited morbidity. N1 necks can be treated with radiation or selective neck dissection as well. For N2 and N3 neck disease, the neck is best treated with multimodality therapy including surgery and radiation. Advanced nodal stage often requires a more extensive neck dissection including levels I to V, either modified radical neck dissection or radical neck dissection depending on structures involved. See Table 25–3 for treatment guidelines.

TABLE 25–2. Incidence of Cervical Metastases Based on Site and T Stage*

	T1	T2	T3	T4
Glottis	<5%	5–10%	10–20%	25–40%
Supraglottis	6–40%	30–70%	50–65%	>65%

*Compiled from data in references 49–53.

TABLE 25–3. Recommended Treatment of the Neck by Stage and Site

N Stage	T Stage	Neck Treatment
N0	**Glottis:** T1 or T2	Observation
N0	**Glottis:** T3 or T4 **Supraglottis:** Any T Stage	Radiation or Selective Neck Dissection
N1	**Glottis:** Any T Stage **Supraglottis:** Any T Stage	Radiation or Selective Neck Dissection
N2 and N3	**Glottis:** Any T Stage **Supraglottis:** Any T Stage	Modified vs. Radical Neck Dissection Plus Radiation

Surgical Treatment of Laryngeal Cancer

The surgical options for laryngeal cancer are numerous. The spectrum ranges from the less invasive microlaryngeal techniques to the most familiar, total laryngectomy. Treatment has come full circle from the earliest transoral procedures in the 1800s to open procedures and now is trending back toward transoral resection. The 5-year survival rates for surgical intervention are comparable to radiation outcomes and, in some cases, better than those achieved with radiation. The key is choosing the correct candidate for the correct procedure. This choice must consider the characteristics of the tumor, the patient's desires and comorbidities, as well as the expertise of the surgeon. Not all tumors can be resected while maintaining both a sound oncologic surgery and limiting the impact on the patient's quality of life.

Endoscopic Resection

The technique of direct laryngoscopy with resection of a lesion followed the development of indirect laryngoscopy and the development of cocaine anesthesia. The early techniques have been revised over the past century and dramatically expanded after the introduction of the laser through the laryngoscope by Strong and Jako in 1972.[54] The work of pioneers in this field such as Steiner and Rudert has created a new concept of transoral laser microsurgery for tumors of the upper aerodigestive tract. First described for

small T1 and T2 tumors, the indications have expanded with improvements in technology to include select T1 to T4 tumors of the glottis and supraglottis. This technique utilizes endoscopes, carbon dioxide laser, and microscope to resect both glottic and supraglottic cancers by following the path of the tumor and transecting the tumor to aid in determination of depth of penetration (Figures 25–15A and 15B). Local control rates and survival are similar to open-partial laryngectomies. Ambrosch et al found 5-year local control rates for T1 and T2 supraglottic lesions to be 100% and 89%, respectively.[55] Voice outcomes were excellent with 97% local control rate and voice preservation for T2 lesions. The major advantage over the open procedures is not deconstructing the laryngeal suspension and the avoidance of a tracheotomy. The limitations of this procedure are the requirement for special instrumentation and training.

Partial Laryngectomy Procedures

Laryngofissure and Cordectomy. This procedure is an open approach to removing a tumor of the true vocal fold. Splitting the thyroid cartilage for endolaryngeal access was first developed for foreign body removal in the late 1700s, but the first curative procedure for carcinoma was not until 1867 by Solis-Cohen of Philadelphia. The skin is incised horizontally and the strap muscles are divided in the midline to expose the thyroid cartilage. A midline thyrotomy then takes place where the thyroid cartilage is incised vertically in

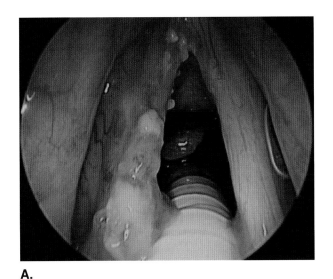

A.

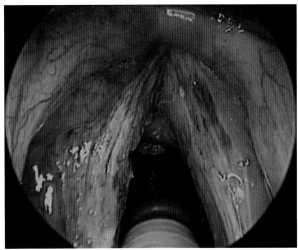

B.

FIGURE 25–15. A. Zero-degree telescope view of an early T1b squamous cell carcinoma during direct laryngoscopy. **B.** Zero-degree telescope view following resection of carcinoma.

the midline to access the glottis. The tumor is visualized and resected. After full-tumor resection is confirmed with frozen sections, a neocord may be reconstructed and the thyroid cartilage is reapproximated. Only T1 glottic lesions are amenable to this procedure with greater than 90% cure rates in these individuals.

Vertical Hemilaryngectomy

The *vertical hemilaryngectomy* (VH) is an organ-sparing procedure for more advanced glottic lesions with en bloc resection of the vocal fold and a portion of the thyroid cartilage (Figure 25-16). Contraindications to hemilaryngectomy are the following: (1) subglottic extension greater than 1 cm; (2) nonmobile cricoarytenoid unit; (3) cartilage involvement; (4) extralaryngeal soft-tissue involvement. In addition to the above criteria, the patient's overall health status must be considered. It is contraindicated in debilitated patients who cannot tolerate temporary aspiration and in those with poor pulmonary reserve. First, the skin is incised horizontally separate from the tracheotomy site. Inferior and superior skin flaps are then raised. The strap muscles are retracted to expose the larynx. The external perichondrium and musculature are elevated.

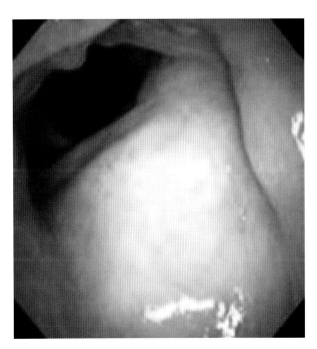

FIGURE 25–16. One-year postoperative flexible laryngoscopy image of larynx following right vertical hemilaryngectomy.

A midline thyrotomy incision is then made along with a cricothyroidotomy and a superior incision along the petiole to expose the tumor. The raised perichondrium and sometimes strap muscles previously raised are then used to reconstruct the neoglottis. Candidates for vertical hemilaryngectomy include T1, T2, selected T3, and rare T4 lesions. Contraindications include the following: arytenoid fixation, interarytenoid involvement, thyroid cartilage invasion, pre-epiglottic space involvement, subglottic extension that extends to the cricoid cartilage, and extralaryngeal spread. Poor medical condition, as with many laryngeal conservation surgeries, is a relative contraindication. Survival is similar between radiation and open surgical techniques. The voice results are generally considered inferior to primary radiotherapy and VH is often considered as a salvage surgery in radiation failures.

Extended Vertical Hemilaryngectomy

The extended vertical hemilaryngectomy can be subdivided into the frontolateral vertical hemilaryngectomy and the posterolateral vertical hemilaryngectomy. A frontolateral hemilaryngectomy is for glottic lesions involving the anterior commissure and can include up to the anterior one-third of the contralateral true vocal fold. The posterolateral vertical hemilaryngectomy is for lesions involving the ipsilateral arytenoid without fixation.

Supraglottic Laryngectomy

The supraglottic laryngectomy (Figure 25-17), also known as the horizontal hemilaryngectomy, is treatment for supraglottic disease. It was popularized by Alonzo in 1947 as a two-stage procedure. It was subsequently refined and modified by Ogura in 1958 and Som in 1959 to a one-stage procedure.[56] This procedure involves resection of the supraglottic structures above the true vocal folds. The larynx is exposed with an apron incision and retraction of the strap muscles for exposure of the larynx. After elevating the thyroid cartilage perichondrium, a transverse incision in the thyroid cartilage is made at the junction of the superior one-third and inferior two-thirds. The supraglottic larynx to the hyoid

bone is resected. The perichondrium is then sutured to the base of tongue. This procedure may be considered in supraglottic cancers staged as T1, T2, or T3 with limited pre-epiglottic space invasion. Lesions of the epiglottis, aryepiglottic folds, and false vocal folds may be treated with this procedure. Selection of lesions amenable to resection with this procedure must have the following characteristics: (1) mobile vocal folds, (2) no cartilage involvement, (3) good pulmonary status, (4) limited base of tongue extension, (5) no involvement of the apex of the piriform sinus. A temporary tracheotomy tube is required for pulmonary toilet and *all* patients will aspirate temporarily. Thus, patients must have an adequate cardiopulmonary reserve to undergo this procedure. Return of safe swallowing function can be prolonged and may require extensive rehabilitation. Local control rates with a supraglottic laryngectomy are better than those achieved with radiation. Voice results are also excellent for supraglottic laryngectomy. However, supraglottic laryngectomy is only indicated for specific lesions with patients in good medical condition who are committed to their rehabilitation of swallowing. This procedure may be used for radiation failure, but is considerably more difficult due to fibrosis of tissues and decreased elevation of the larynx.

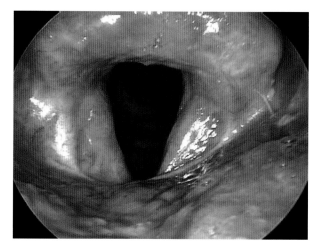

FIGURE 25–17. 70° rigid endoscopic view of larynx 4 years after open supraglottic laryngectomy.

Supracricoid Partial Laryngectomy (SCPL)

This technique is an expansion from the classic supraglottic laryngectomy that also removes the thyroid cartilage and true vocal folds in addition to the supraglottis. Majer and Rieder first described the procedure in 1959 as an alternative to total laryngectomy for selected patients.[57] Laccourreye et al have shown SCPL to have similar local control rates and survival to total laryngectomy.[58,59] The procedure preserves the cricoid cartilage and at least one arytenoid cartilage. It is combined with a cricohyoidopexy (CHP) or a cricohyoidoepiglottopexy (CHEP) for reconstruction depending on the presence or absence of an epiglottic remnant (Figure 25–18). It is indicated for T1b, T2, T3, and T4 cancers of the supraglottis and glottis.[58,59] It has the same limitations in patient selection as the traditional supraglottic laryngectomy. Patients must be selected for appropriate wound healing, pulmonary function, and general medical health. It has been successfully utilized as salvage therapy after radiation failure but with extended time of rehabilitation.[60]

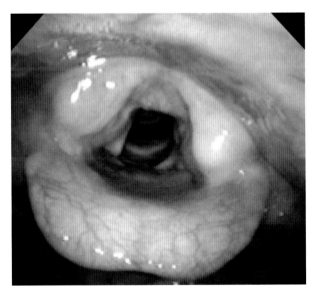

FIGURE 25–18. Flexible laryngoscopy view of larynx 4 months after supracricoid partial laryngectomy with cricohyoidoepiglottopexy for rT2b squamous cell carcinoma of the left true vocal fold with sacrifice of the left vocal process.

Voice is recreated by an aryepiglottic or arytenoid to tongue base closure and is expectedly rough but serviceable.

Near-Total Laryngectomy

Near-total laryngectomy is a voice preservation surgery used for advanced cancers of the unilateral larynx. Also called the subtotal laryngectomy, this procedure was developed by Pearson in the early 1980s.[61,62] The procedure involves the resection of one hemilarynx with the anterior portion of the contralateral cord. The resection includes the ipsilateral cricoid and can be extended to include a portion of the proximal trachea. A dynamic tracheoesophageal shunt is created for voice while a permanent tracheostoma is created for respirations. Some have described this procedure as a "three-quarter laryngectomy" with the remaining arytenoid valving the tracheoesophageal fistula for voice. It is indicated in unilateral T3 and T4 laryngeal carcinomas and piriform sinus carcinomas. Contraindications to the procedure include interarytenoid involvement, postcricoid involvement, and the inability to preserve two thirds of the contralateral vocal fold. The alternatives to near-total laryngectomy include combined chemoradiation therapy or total laryngectomy.

Total Laryngectomy

Total laryngectomy represents the gold standard for treatment of laryngeal cancer and all partial laryngeal procedures should strive to match its oncologic outcomes. It was first successfully performed by Billroth in 1873 but refined by Gluck and Sorenson to the procedure we recognize today. A total laryngectomy includes resection of the hyoid bone through the thyroid and cricoid cartilages to the upper tracheal rings inferiorly. The resection may be combined with variable resection of the tongue base or pharynx if indicated. The remaining pharyngeal mucosa is reapproximated to separate the pharyngoesophagus from the trachea and provide the digestive conduit. The remaining trachea is sutured to the lower anterior neck to create a permanent tracheal stoma. It is indicated for advanced-stage, T3 and T4, laryngeal cancers. Radiation failures as well as conservative resection failures are often salvaged with total laryngectomy. Total laryngectomy provides excellent local control rates but at the expense of the patient's natural voice. Voice rehabilitation is accomplished with prosthetic enabled tracheoesophageal speech, esophageal speech, or the artificial electrolarynx. Tracheoesophageal speech usually provides the best voice for the alaryngeal patient. However, this requires correct patient selection and a close working relationship with the speech therapist to learn and maintain this prosthetic enabled speech. Alaryngeal speech is reviewed in chapter 29.

Radiation Therapy

External beam radiation therapy uses ionizing radiation to generate free radicals within cell nuclei creating DNA and cellular damage that results in cell death. Radiation has evolved with different dosing strategies and fractionation schemes to achieve better outcomes while limiting untoward effects on the remaining tissues. Most recently, intensity-modulated radiation therapy (IMRT) is being used to focus radiation on tumor sites while limiting effects on surrounding tissues. IMRT uses computerized tomography to calculate radiation doses to the tumor from multiple angles of delivery.

Radiation therapy is commonly used as a primary treatment modality for laryngeal cancer. Treatment typically involves an external beam approach that delivers daily doses of radiation 5 days per week for 6 to 7 weeks. The total dose of radiation delivered to the tumor site is 6000 to 7000 cGy. Primary radiation therapy as single-modality therapy is indicated for T1, T2, and some T3 lesions. More advanced-stage tumors benefit from the addition of chemotherapy. Radiation is also used for palliation in unresectable tumors and in those individuals who are poor surgical candidates. Prior radiation to the same site is considered a relative contraindication. The fields for radiation include the cervical lymphatics if there is N+ disease or if the risk of cervical lymphatic spread is greater than 20 to 30%. Radiation therapy may also be given in the postoperative period. The indications for postoperative radiation are: (1) advanced-stage disease, (2) positive margins, (3) extracapsular spread of tumor in a lymph node, (4) perineural or angiolymphatic spread of tumor, (5) involvement of multiple lymph nodes in the neck, and (6) subglottic extension of tumor.

Prerequisites for radiation include a thorough dental examination. The radiation fields are evaluated by the dentist and carious teeth that will be included in the fields of radiation are extracted to prevent further tooth decay from xerostomia and osteoradionecrosis. The side effects of radiation can be divided into early and late side effects. The early side effects include mucositis, odynophagia, dysphagia, skin breakdown, loss of taste, and edema. These effects last up to 6 weeks after completion of radiation therapy. The long-term effects include fibrosis, xerostomia, edema, loss of taste, hypothyroidism, and radionecrosis.

Chemotherapy

Chemotherapy is most commonly used in conjunction with radiation to treat laryngeal cancer. Cisplatin and 5-fluorouracil are most often employed. The two most common methods include concurrent and induction chemotherapy. Chemotherapy is also used as a palliative measure in patients where radiation is not an option. Chemotherapy has not traditionally been used as primary therapy for laryngeal cancer. Some studies have shown, however, that induction chemotherapy does have a small percentage of complete responders with only chemotherapy. These results have led to investigation of this paradigm and work is continuing in this field. (See the box on Induction Chemotherapy for further discussion of this experimental therapy.)

The utility of multimodality therapy in laryngeal cancer has been well documented by several studies, including the Veteran's Affairs (VA) Study Group.[63] Patients in the experimental

---

Emerging Concept: Induction Chemotherapy

Chemotherapy is traditionally thought of as adjuvant therapy in the treatment of laryngeal carcinoma. Laccourreye and colleagues in Paris have written multiple papers regarding a subset of patients who were complete clinical responders following induction chemotherapy for laryngeal cancers. Although this group was a minority, they had excellent 5-year survival and local control rates.[64-67] In further investigation of this concept, investigators at MD Anderson presented their data at the American Society of Clinical Oncology Meeting in 2004. Kies et al examined 29 patients with T2–T4 laryngeal carcinomas felt to be resectable by conservation laryngeal surgery and treated them with 3 cycles of paclitaxel, ifosfamide, and cisplatin; 34% of these patients had a complete response.[68] Although all of this work remains experimental, it remains a promising frontier of investigation.

---

arm were treated with 2 cycles of cisplatin and 5-fluorouracil and reassessed. If there was a partial response, a third round was given followed by radiation. Poor responders after 2 cycles of chemotherapy were treated with surgery. This experimental arm was compared to standard therapy of surgery followed by postoperative radiation. Patients treated with induction chemotherapy and radiation had similar survival to those treated with total laryngectomy and postoperative radiation (68% at 5 years). Also, 64% of those in the radiation group retained their larynx at 5 years. An equally important study in evaluating the benefits of radiation therapy in laryngeal cancer is the RTOG 91-11 study.[69] This study evaluated the benefit of chemotherapy given concomitantly with radiation and found higher local control rates but no increase in long-term survival.

Surgical Complications

Complications of laryngeal surgery are similar to other major ablative head and neck surgeries with bleeding, infection, and flap necrosis. There are other complications more related to laryngeal surgeries that deal with voice and swallowing.

Pharyngocutaneous fistulas connecting the pharynx to the skin are a major concern. They result from a failure of the surgical closure of the pharynx or larynx to seal its contents from entering the neck and eventually reaching the skin. Once a fistula has developed, the patient must have oral feedings withheld and local wound care for a few to several weeks. If the fistula fails to close after local wound care, regional or microvascular clamps may be required. The risks of fistulas increase with poor nutrition and previous radiation surgery. If fistulas occur late or do not respond to conservative and flap reinforcement, residual cancer must be considered.

Swallowing dysfunction is another problem encountered with laryngeal surgery. There are several reasons why patients may have swallowing difficulties. Partial laryngeal surgeries have a risk of aspiration. Aspiration may persist and put the patient at risk for recurrent aspiration pneumonia. Recurrent aspiration pneumonia is treated with nonoral feeding and may even require total laryngectomy to prevent aspiration. Esophageal stricture can also occur following laryngectomy. This may require periodic esophageal dilation. Swallowing may also be complicated by postradiation xerostomia.

Thought Box: Second Laryngeal Cancers in Previously Treated Patients

McGuirt and colleagues published a comprehensive review from Wake Forest in which 377 survivors of laryngeal cancer (855 treated database patients overall, with 532 not undergoing laryngectomy) were characterized in terms of their incidence of metachronous lesions and the maintenance of laryngeal speech.[70] Nineteen of 377 (5.1%) patients who had survived more then 3 years developed second primary tumors in the larynx. The likelihood of a new laryngeal cancer was lower in the patients who were originally treated with radiotherapy (4.3%) compared to the rate seen in surgical patients (9.2%), although there was a much higher rate of laryngeal voicing in patients in the surgical group. The authors concluded that the preservation of laryngeal voicing in these circumstances supported the choice of surgical treatment of laryngeal cancer, despite the higher incidence of metachronous lesions in this group; for these surgical patients, all treatment options, that is, surgery, chemotherapy, and radiation were still available. Another interesting finding was that second primary tumors were equally distributed between those patients who stopped smoking after their original diagnosis and those who continued to abuse tobacco.

Airway problems following treatment are divided into airway protection problems leading to aspiration and dysphagia as above and the less common airway obstructive complications. Obstructive symptoms can occur following surgical therapy but are seen more typically after nonsurgical therapy with resultant decreased motion of the bilateral true vocal folds. This complication can occur as a late effect and has been reported over 10 years after completion of radiation therapy. Airway obstructive complications after surgical therapy are atypical but can develop following vertical conservation procedures.

Loss of taste and smell is a well-recognized but frequently overlooked complication of total laryngectomy that is not an infrequent complaint of the alaryngeal patient. Preoperative counseling with speech pathology is a valuable service for these patients and their families to help them prepare for the postoperative consequences of total laryngectomy.

Hypothyroidism is a potential complication of both surgical and radiation therapy and is higher in patients treated with both modalities. Serial thyroid stimulating hormone testing is indicated to prevent the consequences of this very treatable complication.

Laryngeal neoplasms are challenging tumors in head and neck oncology. They vary in their presentation and outcomes by only incrementally changing their anatomic location within the same organ. As in other head and neck cancers, our field has made very little progress in improving survival in laryngeal cancer patients. The essential functions of respiration, deglutition, and phonation frequently remain difficult to maintain following treatment without usually compromising one function or another. The future will be brighter, however, as technology and molecular and immunologic therapies advance. Look for a continued movement toward less invasive but more effective surgery, earlier detection methods through improved screening, and better targeted molecular therapies.

Review Questions

1. A patient presents with an exophytic tumor extending from the left aryepiglottic fold back to the arytenoid mucosa and down to and involving the left true vocal fold. The left vocal fold is mobile but its motion is impaired. The patient has no piriform sinus involvement but has a 2-cm level III lymph node on palpation of the left neck. The lymph node has features of concern on the CT scan. There is no further information for staging from the CT of the neck or chest. You stage this patient's tumor as:
   a   T3 N2 M0
   b. T3 N1 M0
   c. T2 N2 M0
   d. T2 N1 M0
   e. T1 N1 M0

2. A 60-year-old minister presents with 6 months of hoarseness and the following lesion at direct microlaryngoscopy (see below). The rest of his preoperative evaluation, including endoscopy and chest radiography, are negative. Your biopsy reveals squamous cell carcinoma. All of the following are reasonable treatment options except:

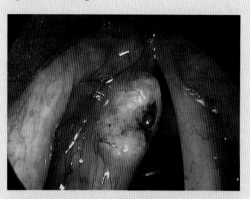

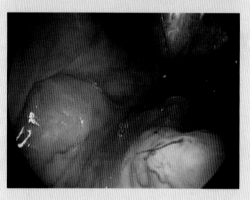

   a. Endoscopic resection of the left true vocal fold cancer
   b. Radiotherapy
   c. Laryngofissure with cordectomy
   d. Supracricoid laryngectomy
   e. Vertical hemilaryngectomy

3. The same patient from question 2 is noted on subsequent chest radiography (9 months later) to have a 2-cm pulmonary mass. His neck is negative to palpation and his vocal fold has healed well. The new chest finding is most likely to be:
   a. Incidental finding
   b. Primary lung cancer
   c. Metastasis from laryngeal cancer
   d. Reactivation of tuberculosis
   e. None of the above

4. The overall survival for malignancy of which organ has *declined* in the past 10 years?
   a. Pancreas
   b. Esophagus
   c. Lung
   d. Larynx
   e. Colon

5. Which of the following correctly ranks the incidence of laryngeal cancer by subsite (from most common to least common)?
   a. Supraglottic, subglottic, glottic
   b. Subglottic, glottic, supraglottic
   c. Supraglottic, glottic, subglottic
   d. Glottic, subglottic, supraglottic
   e. Glottic, supraglottic, subglottic

REFERENCES

1. Hoffman HT, Karnell LH, Funk GF. The National Cancer Database report on cancer of the head and neck. *Arch Otolaryngol Head Neck Surg.* 1998;124:951-962.

2. Shah JP, Karnell LH, Hoffman HT, et al. Patterns of care for cancer of the larynx in the United States. *Arch Otolaryngol Head Neck Surg.* 1997;123: 475-483.

3. Sllamniku B, Bauer W, Painter C, et al. The transformation of laryngeal keratosis into invasive carcinoma. *Am J Otolaryngol.* 1989;10:42-54.

4. Helquist H, Lundgren J, Olofsson J. Hyperplasia, keratosis, dysplasia and carcinoma in situ of the vocal cords: a follow-up study. *Clin Otolaryngol.* 1982;7:11-27.

5. Califano J, van der Riet P, Westra W, et al. Genetic progression model for head and neck cancer: implications for field cancerization. *Cancer Res.* 1996;56:2488-2492.

6. Falk RT, Pickle LW, Brown LM, et al. Effect of smoking and alcohol consumption on laryngeal cancer risk in coastal Texas. *Cancer Res.* 1989;49:4024.

7. McKaig RG, Baric RS, Olshan AF. Human papilloma virus and head and neck cancer: epidemiol-ogy and molecular biology. *Head Neck.* 1998;20: 250.

8. Venuti A, Manni V, Morello R, et al. Physical state and expression of human papilloma virus in laryngeal carcinoma and surrounding normal mucosa. *J Med Virology.* 2000;60:396.

9. Brandwein MS, Nuovo GJ, Biller H. Analysis of prevalence of human papilloma virus in laryngeal carcinomas. Study of 40 cases using PCR and consensus primers. *Ann Oto Rhinol Laryng.* 1993; 102:309.

10. Kiyabu MT, Shibata D, Arnheim N, et al. Detection of human papilloma virus in formalin-fixed, invasive squamous cell carcinoma using polymerase chain reaction. *Am J Surg Pathol.* 1989;13: 221-224.

11. El-Serag HB, Hepworth EJ, Lee P, et al. Gastroesophageal reflux disease is a risk factor for laryngeal and pharyngeal cancer. *Am J Gastroenterol.* 2001;96:2013.

12. Whortley P, Vaughan TL, Davis S, et al. A case-controlled study of occupational risk factors for laryngeal cancer. *Br J Indust Med.* 1992;49:37.

13. Jemal A, Tiwani RC, Murray T, et al. Cancer statistics, 2004. *CA Cancer J Clin* 2004;54:8-29.

14. DeRienzo DP, Greenberg SD, Fraire AE. Carcinoma in the larynx. Changing incidence in women. *Arch Otolaryngol Head Neck Surg.* 1991;117:681.

15. Lindberg R. Distribution of cervical lymph node metastases from squamous cell carcinoma of the upper respiratory and digestive tracts. *Cancer.* 1972;29(6):1446-1449.

16. Shah JP. Patterns of cervical lymph node metastasis from squamous cell carcinoma of the upper aerodigestive tract. *Am J Surg.* 1990;160:282-286.

17. Greene, et al. *American Joint Committee on Cancer: AJCC Cancer Staging Manual.* 6th ed. New York, Berlin, Heidelberg: Springer-Verlag; 2002:47-57.

18. Harwood AR, DeBoer G. Prognostic factors in T2 glottic cancer. *Cancer.* 1980;45(5):991-995.

19. Eckel HE. Local recurrences following transoral laser surgery for early glottic carcinoma: frequency, management, and outcome. *Ann Otol Rhinol Laryngol.* 2001;110(1):7.

20. Piccirillo JF. Importance of comorbidity in head and neck cancer. *Laryngoscope.* 2000;110(4): 593.

21. Zbaren P, Becker M, Lang H. Staging of laryngeal cancer: endoscopy, computed tomography and magnetic resonance versus histopathology. *Eur Arch Otorhinolaryngol.* 1997;254(suppl 1):117.

22. Kresnick E, Mikosch P, Gallowitsch HJ, et al. Evaluation of head and neck cancer with 18F-FDG PET: a comparison with conventional methods. *Eur J Nucl Med*. 2001;28:816.

23. Stokkel MP, ten Broek FW, Hordijk GJ, et al. Preoperative evaluation of patients with primary head and neck cancer using dual-head 18-fluorodeoxyglucose positron emission tomography. *Ann Surg*. 2000;231:229.

24. Erisen LM, Coskun H, Ozuysal S, et al. Basaloid squamous cell carcinoma of the larynx: a report of four new cases. *Laryngoscope*. 2004;114(7): 1179-1183.

25. Bahar G, Feinmesser R, Popovtzer A, et al. Basaloid squamous carcinoma of the larynx. *Am J Otolaryngol*. 2003;24(3):204-208.

26. Ferlito A, Altavilla G, Rinaldo A, Doglioni C. Basaloid squamous cell carcinoma of the larynx and hypopharynx. *Ann Otol Rhinol Laryngol*. 1997;106(12):1024-1035.

27. Keelawat S, Liu CZ, Roehm PC, Barnes L. Adenosquamous carcinoma of the upper aerodigestive tract: a clinicopathologic study of 12 cases and review of the literature. *Am J Otolaryngol*. 2002;23(3):160-168.

28. Ferlito A, Devaney KO, Rinaldo A, Milroy CM, Carbone A. Mucosal adenoid squamous cell carcinoma of the head and neck. *Ann Otol Rhinol Laryngol*. 1996;105(5):409-413.

29. Lewis JE, Olsen KD, Sebo TJ. Spindle cell carcinoma of the larynx: review of 26 cases including DNA content and immunohistochemistry. *Hum Pathol*. 1997;28(6):664-673.

30. McCaffrey TV, Witte M, Ferguson MT. Verrucous carcinoma of the larynx. *Ann Otol Rhinol Laryngol*. 1998;107(5 pt 1):391-395.

31. Maurizi M, Cadoni G, Ottaviani F, Rabitti C, Almadori G. Verrucous squamous cell carcinoma of the larynx: diagnostic and therapeutic considerations. *Eur Arch Otorhinolaryngol*. 1996; 253(3):130-135.

32. Baatenburg de Jong RJ, van Lent S, Hogendoorn PC. Chondroma and chondrosarcoma of the larynx. *Curr Opin Otolaryngol Head Neck Surg*. 2004;12(2):98-105.

33. Thome R, Thome DC, de la Cortina RA. Long-term follow-up of cartilaginous tumors of the larynx. *Otolaryngol Head Neck Surg*. 2001;124(6): 634-640.

34. Donovan DT, Conley J. Adenoid cystic carcinoma of the subglottic region. *Ann Otol Rhinol Laryngol*. 1983;92(5 pt 1):491-495.

35. Mahlstedt K, Ussmuller J, Donath K. Malignant sialogenic tumours of the larynx. *J Laryngol Otol*. 2002;116(2):119-122.

36. Cohen J, Guillamondegui OM, Batsakis JG, Medina JE. Cancer of the minor salivary glands of the larynx. *Am J Surg*. 1985;150(4):513-518.

37. Milroy CM, Ferlito A. Immunohistochemical markers in the diagnosis of neuroendocrine neoplasms of the head and neck. *Ann Otol Rhinol Laryngol*. 1995;104(5):413-418.

38. Myssiorek D, Rinaldo A, Barnes L, Ferlito A. Laryngeal paraganglioma: an updated critical review. *Acta Otolaryngol*. 2004;124(9):995-999.

39. Overholt SM, Donovan DT, Schwartz MR, Laucirica R, Green LK, Alford BR. Neuroendocrine neoplasms of the larynx. *Laryngoscope*. 1995;105 (8 pt 1):789-794.

40. Gripp FM, Risse EK, Leverstein H, Snow GB, Meijer CJ. Neuroendocrine neoplasms of the larynx. Importance of the correct diagnosis and differences between atypical carcinoid tumors and small-cell neuroendocrine carcinoma. *Eur Arch Otorhinolaryngol*. 1995;252(5):280-286.

41. Rinaldo A, Devaney KO, Ferlito A. Immunohistochemical studies in support of a diagnosis of small cell neuroendocrine carcinoma of the larynx. *Acta Otolaryngol*. 2004;124(5):638-641.

42. Batsakis JG, el-Naggar AK, Luna MA. Neuroendocrine tumors of larynx. *Ann Otol Rhinol Laryngol*. 1992;101(8):710-714.

43. Nayak JV, Cook JR, Molina JT, et al. Primary lymphoma of the larynx: new diagnostic and therapeutic approaches. *J Otorhinolaryngol Relat Spec*. 2003;65(6):321-326.

44. Kania RE, Hartl DM, Badoual C, Le Maignan C, Brasnu DF. Primary mucosa-associated lymphoid tissue (MALT) lymphoma of the larynx. *Head Neck*. 2005;27(3):258-262.

45. Nofsinger YC, Mirza N, Rowan PT, Lanza D, Weinstein G. Head and neck manifestations of plasma cell neoplasms. *Laryngoscope*. 1997;107(6):741-746.

46. Batsakis JG, Luna MA, Byers RM. Metastases to the larynx. *Head Neck Surg*. 1985;7(6):458-460.

47. Schweinfurth JM, Powitzky E, Ossoff RH. Regression of laryngeal dysplasia after serial microflap excision. *Ann Otol Rhinol Laryngol*. 2001;110: 811-814.

48. Zeitels SM, Franco RA Jr, Dailey SH, Burns JA, et al. Office-based treatment of glottal dysplasia and papillomatosis with the 585-nm pulsed dye laser and local anesthesia. *Ann Otol Rhinol Laryngol*. 2004;113:265-276.

49. Redaelli de Zinis LO, Nicolai P, Barezzani MG, et al. Incidence and distribution of lymph node metastases in supraglottic squamous cell carcinoma: therapeutic implications [in Italian]. *Acta Otorhinolaryngol Ital.* 1994;14(1):19-27.

50. Bocca E, Pignataro O, Odini C. Supraglottic laryngectomy: 30 years of experience. *Ann Otol Rhinol Laryngol.* 1983;92(1 pt 1):14-18.

51. Johnson JT, Myers EN: Cervical lymph Node disease in laryngeal cancer. In: Silver CE , ed. Laryngeal Cancer. New York, NY: Thieme; 1991.

52. Daly CJ, Strong EW: Carcinoma of the glottic larynx. *Am J Surg.* 1975;130:489.

53. Jesse RH. The evaluation and treatment of patients with extensive squamous cancer of the vocal cords. *Laryngoscope.* 1975;85:1424.

54. Strong MS, Jako GJ. Laser surgery in the larynx: early experience with continuous CO_2 laser. *Ann Otol Rhinol Laryngol.* 1972;81:791-798.

55. Ambrosch P, Kron M, Steiner W. Carbon dioxide laser microsurgery for early supraglottic carcinoma. *Ann Otol Rhinol Laryngol.* 1998;107(8):680-688.

56. Zeitels SM. Surgical management of early supraglottic cancer. *Otolaryngol Clin North Am.* 1997;30(1):59-78.

57. Majer EH, Rieder W. Technic of laryngectomy permitting the conservation of respiratory permeability (cricohyoidopexy). *Ann Otolaryngol Chir Cervicofac.* 1959;76:677-681.

58. Laccourreye H, Lacau St Guily J, Brasnu D, Fabre A, Menard M. Supracricoid hemilaryngopharyngectomy. Analysis of 240 cases. *Ann Otol Rhinol Laryngol.* 987;96(2 pt 1):217-221.

59. Laccourreye H, Laccourreye O, Weinstein G, Menard M, Brasnur D. Supracricoid laryngectomy with cricohyoidoepiglottopexy: a partial laryngeal procedure for glottic carcinoma. *Ann Otol Rhinol Laryngol.* 1990;99(6 pt 1):421-426.

60. Laccourreye O, Weinstein G, Naudo P, Cauchois R, Laccourreye H, Brasnu D. Supracricoid partial laryngectomy after failed laryngeal radiation therapy. *Laryngoscope.* 1996;106(4):495-498.

61. Pearson BW, Woods RD, Hartman DE. Extended hemilaryngectomy for T3 glottic carcinoma with preservation of speech and swallowing. *Laryngoscope.* 1980;90:1950-1961.

62. Pearson BW. Subtotal laryngectomy. *Laryngoscope.* 1981; 91:1904-1912.

63. The Department of Veterans Affairs Laryngeal Cancer Study Group. Induction chemotherapy plus radiation compared with surgery plus radiation in patients with advanced laryngeal cancer. *N Engl J Med.* 1991;324(24):1685-1690.

64. Vachin F, Hans S, Atlan D, Brasnu D, Menard M, Laccourreye O. [Long-term results of exclusive chemotherapy for glottic squamous cell carcinoma complete clinical responders after induction chemotherapy.] *Ann Otolaryngol Chir Cervicofac.* 2004;121(3):140-147.

65. Laccourreye O, Veivers D, Bassot V, Menard M, Brasnu D, Laccourreye H. Analysis of local recurrence in patients with selected $T_{1-3}N_0M_0$ squamous cell carcinoma of the true vocal cord managed with a platinum-based chemotherapy-alone regimen for cure. *Ann Otol Rhinol Laryngol.* 2002;111(4):315-321.

66. Laccourreye O, Veivers D, Hans S, Menard M, Brasnu D, Laccourreye H. Chemotherapy alone with curative intent in patients with invasive squamous cell carcinoma of the pharyngolarynx classified as $T_{1-3}T_4N_0M_0$ complete clinical responders. *Cancer.* 2001;92(6):1504-1511.

67. Laccourreye O, Brasnu D, Bassot V, Menard M, Khayat D, Laccourreye H. Cisplatin-fluorouracil exclusive chemotherapy for T1-T3N0 glottic squamous cell carcinoma complete clinical responders: five-year results. *J Clin Oncol.* 1996;14(8):2331-2336.

68. Kies MS, Lewin JS, Diaz EM, et al. Definitive treatment of intermediate stage laryngeal squamous cell (SCC/L) cancer with chemotherapy (CT). Abstract No. 5533. American Society of Clinical Oncology. Annual Meeting; New Orleans, La; 2004.

69. Forastiere AA, Goepfert H, Maor M, Pajak TF, Weber R, Morrison W, Glisson B, Trotti A, Ridge JA, Chao C, Peters G, Lee DJ, Leaf A, Ensley J, Cooper J. Concurrent chemotherapy and radiotherapy for organ preservation in advanced laryngeal cancer. *N Engl J Med.* 2003;349(22):2091-2098.

70. McGuirt WF, Ray M. Second laryngeal cancers in previously treated larynges. *Laryngoscope.* 1999; 109(9):1406-1408.

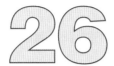

Laryngotracheal Stenosis

Michael Pitman, MD
Robert H. Ossoff, DMD, MD

KEY POINTS

■ Endotracheal intubation continues to be the dominant cause of airway stenosis; over 10% of patients will develop stenosis after just 10 days of intubation.

■ Many patients with airway obstruction will initially be misdiagnosed with asthma or other pulmonary conditions.

■ Although controversy exists with regard to the ideal treatment of laryngotracheal stenosis, the majority of cases are managed endoscopically. Mitomycin-C is a promising but unproven adjunct to endoscopic surgery.

■ Decision-making in airway surgery depends on many factors, including the patient's underlying medical condition, and ease of access to the airway (jaw, neck, obesity, difficult laryngoscopy). These factors are just as critical as the nature of the stenosis itself.

■ Bypassing the obstructed airway with a tracheotomy tube is a reasonable option for many patients, particularly those with multilevel stenoses or significant medical comorbidities.

Laryngotracheal stenosis (LTS) is a devastating problem for patients and a difficult disease for physicians to treat. When the airway is impaired, respiratory function is limited and the quality of life suffers. The patient's phonation may also be affected by the initial injury or the subsequent treatment. Many patients undergo multiple procedures, often following a prolonged critical illness during which the stenosis developed. For the physician, there is not a clearly defined treatment algorithm which applies to all patients or ensures excellent results. Stenoses range in severity from minimal to complete; they may affect the supraglottis, glottis, subglottis, trachea, or a combination of the above. The wide array of surgical techniques that have evolved and are currently employed is a testament to the complexity of this problem. Many patients do not have a reasonable treatment option and are appropriately managed with a tracheotomy tube.

ETIOLOGY

Intubation Injury

There are multiple causes of LTS, but the majority are due to complications of endotracheal intubation or tracheotomy.[1,2] Mechanical trauma from the endotracheal tube cuff or the tube itself are inciting factors. The endotracheal tube rests in the posterior aspect of the larynx and is in contact with the posterior commissure. Pressure from the tube is exerted on the vocal processes of the arytenoids, interarytenoid area, and the posterior cricoid plate. If the pressure of the tube or cuff exceeds mucosal perfusion pressure, blood flow to the mucosa will be limited, leading to ischemic ulceration of the mucosa. In more severe cases, ischemic necrosis of the cartilage will also occur.[3] This insult may then result in soft tissue scar and contracture as well as possible cartilaginous collapse resulting in airway stenosis. The phenomenon occurs more often when a patient is intubated with a tube that is too large and the pressure caused by the endo-

tracheal tube is increased. A similar phenomenon occurs at the site of the endotracheal tube cuff. The low-pressure high-volume cuffs used today can be overinflated causing circumferential mucosal injury and necrosis (Figure 26–1) These injuries are the basis for the recommendations against prolonged intubation and for conversion to tracheotomy at approximately the 7th day of endotracheal intubation. Approximately 12% of patients intubated for longer than 10 days will develop a laryngotracheal stenosis.[5]

Tracheotomy tubes and cuffs can cause ischemic injury by the same mechanisms as described for endotracheal tubes. In addition, the performance of a tracheotomy itself may lead to airway stenosis. If a tracheotomy is performed too high or through the cricothyroid membrane, it may result in cricoid erosion. In a well-placed tracheotomy the anterior tracheal wall superior to the stoma site may be forced posteriorly narrowing the tracheal lumen. Percutaneous tracheotomy may result in an increased number of

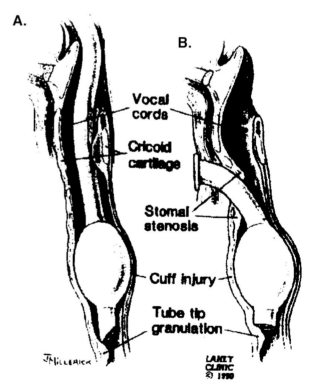

FIGURE 26–1. Airway injury from **A.** endotracheal intubation and **B.** tracheotomy tube.[4]

stenoses due to this phenomenon but this is still controversial.[6,7] Copious granulation at the stoma site as well as infection can lead to contracture as the site heals after decannulation, leading to collapse of the lateral tracheal wall. Ischemic injury due to direct pressure of the tracheotomy tube against the tracheal wall when it is not correctly supported during mechanical ventilation will cause ischemic necrosis and stenosis similar to that from an endotracheal tube. Again, as the injured site heals by secondary intention, granulation tissue, scar, and ultimately stenosis form. If the cartilage is involved it may weaken and collapse causing an additional airway compromise.

Airway Stenosis Unrelated to Intubation

Although complications of endotracheal intubation and tracheotomy are the leading cause of LTS, there are many other etiologies of LTS (see Table 26–1). Those of particular interest are highlighted below.

External Trauma

Blunt trauma to the neck may not result in acute airway compromise, yet there may be a laryngeal fracture, mucosal laceration, or hematoma. As these injuries heal there may be cartilaginous necrosis and tissues may contract resulting in a delayed airway stenosis.[8] It is imperative that these injuries are noted at the time of the trauma and repaired in an expeditious fashion so that a devastating and unnecessary airway stenosis can be avoided.

Wegener's Granulomatosis

Although many granulomatous diseases can result in airway compromise, Wegener's granulomatosis (WG) is the most common. WG is a multisystem inflammatory disease characterized by necrotizing granulomatous inflammation and vasculitis of unknown etiology. It generally affects the upper airway, lungs, and kidneys. Subglottic stenosis has been found to occur in 16 to 23% of patients

TABLE 26-1. Causes of Laryngotracheal Stenosis

Trauma
  Endotracheal Intubation
  Tracheotomy
  External Laryngotracheal Injury
  Endotracheal Burn

Infectious
  Diphtheria
  Syphilis
  Fungal
  Tuberculosis
  Klebsiella

Systemic
  Wegener's Granulomatosis
  Sarcoidosis
  Amyloidosis
  Laryngopharyngeal Reflux
  Relapsing Polychondritis
  Pemphigoid

Neoplastic Lesions
Congenital Lesions
Idiopathic

with WG.[9,10] Isolated subglottic stenosis with dyspnea on exertion may be the sole presenting feature in up to 37% of patients with WG who have subglottic stenosis.[11] Often a biopsy of the subglottis will be negative and the diagnosis of WG will not be made without pursuing serum testing. As a result, c-ANCA and p-ANCA should be tested in all patients with subglottic stenosis of an unknown origin. If c-ANCA is positive, it is quite specific for WG with rare false positives. The p-ANCA test is much less specific. If only p-ANCA is positive then a diagnosis of WG can only be made with confirmative histopathology and a corroborative clinical scenario. This is also reviewed in chapter 22.

Idiopathic Subglottic Stenosis

Idiopathic subglottic stenosis (ISS) is a rare, slowly progressive, nonspecific inflammatory process that results in stenosis of the subglottis and proximal trachea. It is a diagnosis of exclusion that can be made only after all other known causes of LTS have been ruled out by history, physical exam, histopathology, tissue culture, and serologic testing. ISS occurs *predominantly in women* age 30 to 50 years of age. There are rare cases of ISS in males with a ratio of approximately 1:35.[12-14] Despite this disparity, biopsies of the subglottis have failed to provide evidence of estrogen receptors.[12,13,15] Laryngopharyngeal reflux (LPR) has been suggested as a cause of ISS but this has not been clearly demonstrated.[16,17] Some investigators have suggested that LPR is not a contributing factor, citing the lack of vocal fold inflammation at surgery and the lack of recurrence of the stenosis after laryngotracheal resection despite absence of treatment for LPR.[14]

Iatrogenic Glottic Stenosis

The most common cause of anterior glottic stenosis is scarring following vocal fold surgery. If the anterior commissure is denuded bilaterally, the anterior vocal folds will heal together forming an anterior glottic web and stenosis. This can be avoided by taking care to leave the anterior vocal fold epithelium intact on one of the vocal folds. If surgery is necessary on the anterior aspect of both vocal folds, then the surgery must be staged so that the operated vocal fold will have a chance to heal prior to denuding the epithelium of the opposite vocal fold.

PRESENTATION

Patients with airway stenosis complain of dyspnea on exertion and even at rest. Patients with post-intubation injuries will begin to develop symptoms approximately 6 weeks after the inciting injury, reflecting the time it takes for scar tissue to form. As the scar tissue begins to mature and contract there is a resultant decrease in the area of the airway and stenosis formation. Symptoms usually occur as the area of the lumen approaches 50% of normal. Because of the delay in the onset of symptoms, patients will often be incorrectly

diagnosed with new-onset asthma. They are then sent for an otolaryngology consultation when the patient's symptoms are unresponsive to medication. The patient may have voice complaints related to the original injury (intubation, external trauma). Patients with mild to moderate airway obstruction may also complain of dysphagia or "slowing down" to eat as the obligatory respiratory pause related to swallowing compounds the restriction from the stenosis.

DIAGNOSIS/WORKUP

History

As with any medical problem the history and physical examination are essential to a correct diagnosis and treatment plan. The severity of the patient's stenosis is determined by these clinical histories. Does the patient have dyspnea at rest or only on exertion? What is the exercise tolerance? Does an upper respiratory infection increase symptom severity? If a tracheotomy is in place, can the patient tolerate capping? If so, for how long? Are there any voice problems that may indicate glottal involvement?

When did the patient's symptoms begin? Is there a history of intubation or tracheotomy? Has the patient had any treatment for this problem, medical or surgical? Are there symptoms of laryngopharyngeal reflux?

In addition, a general review of symptoms and medical history is significant. This may help one assess a patient's anesthetic risk and chances of a successful surgical repair as well as uncover systemic causes of the disease. The nature of patients with airway stenosis (ie, often with a history of prolonged intubation and survival of a profound critical illness) compounds the challenges of managing these cases.

Physical Examination

The first priority of the clinical evaluation is to determine the level of the patient's respiratory distress and determine if there is urgency or emergency to the required management. If the patient is stable, a thorough physical exam is performed. Examination of the neck will give clues of prior surgery or trauma. If a tracheotomy tube is in place, its position relative to the cricoid should be noted, in addition to the tracheotomy tube characteristics (inner and outer diameter, fenestration, cuff). Also note the size of the stoma and any irregularities. Fenestrated tracheotomy tubes are notorious for their aggravation of intratracheal and subglottic granulation tissue; they should be avoided if at all possible.

Flexible laryngoscopy, or mirror laryngoscopy, should be performed to evaluate the supraglottis and glottis. The integrity of the supraglottic structures should be noted. Is there scarring or stenosis in this area? Is there prolapse of the supraglottis that may be causing obstruction on inspiration? When evaluating the glottis, vocal fold mobility should be assessed; the larynx should be inspected for any sign of scar tissue that may be preventing abduction. The subglottis can often be visualized by passing a flexible laryngoscope. through the vocal folds. The view may not be optimal as this often elicits a cough reflex if topical anesthesia is not used. If a tracheotomy is in place, the subglottis may be viewed from below. The best assessment of the subglottis and trachea can be achieved following topical application of local anesthesia; this is often performed with a transnasal esophagoscope[18] although any adequate length flexible scope will do. The trachea and glottis are anesthetized by dripping 3 to 4 ml of 4% lidocaine through the working channel on the vocal folds as the patient phonates. The total recommended maximum dose is 4.5 mg/kg, though this amount should never be required for this procedure. After time is allowed for anesthesia, the esophagoscope is passed through the vocal folds to the mainstem bronchi. The acquired images can be reviewed with the patient following the examination. The dynamic stability of the trachea during respiration can also be evaluated. This is important in the evaluation of the contribution of tracheal malacia to the airway obstruction. When a patient inspires, negative pressure is created in the cervical trachea. Areas of tracheal

malacia will collapse, causing a dynamic airway compromise. This is in contrast to the airway evaluation under general anesthesia, during which the trachea is not subject to the negative intraluminal pressure. Inadequate resection of a malacic segment of trachea can lead to failure in surgical treatment of tracheal stenosis.[19]

Radiologic Evaluation

Radiologic evaluation of the airway is an integral part of the patient evaluation. Coronal and sagittal reconstructions of helical computed tomography (CT) images have been found to be the most useful study.[20,21] The scan is performed rapidly and results in accurate assessment of the extent of stenosis and its relation to the glottis. It also avoids the motion artifact that can occur with magnetic resonance imaging (MRI). If awake tracheoscopy is not possible, fluoroscopy may be used to estimate the amount of tracheomalacia present. Radiology of the larynx is reviewed in chapter 10.

Physiologic Testing

Pulmonary function testing can be helpful in distinguishing between pulmonary disease and laryngotracheal stenosis. The flow volume loop is also a useful measure of the extent of stenosis. A maximum inspiratory flow of less than 2 L per second denotes significant obstruction. Flattening of the inspiratory loop indicates glottic or supraglottic obstruction. Flattening of both the inspiratory and expiratory loop occurs with a fixed subglottic stenosis.

Operative Endoscopy of the Airway

The gold standard for the evaluation of airway stenosis is direct laryngoscopy and tracheoscopy. This is performed under general anesthesia. Every precaution is taken to secure the airway and avoid an airway emergency. The operative table is set up with a variety of laryngoscopes, the light sources are plugged in, and suction is ready prior to induction. A tracheotomy set is in the operating room and a moderately sized ventilating bronchoscope is also available for ventilation if airway access becomes a problem. If jet ventilation is anticipated, the circuitry and hardware are checked prior to induction as well.

Once the patient is under anesthesia, larynx and pharynx are evaluated with an operative laryngoscope, the Holinger laryngoscope (Pilling 52-2032, Research Triangle, NC) This provides the easiest access to the larynx and distorts the anatomy the least. Just as in the awake laryngoscopy, the characteristics of the posterior larynx are carefully evaluated, including the presence or absence of stenosis or joint motion impairment. The larynx is then suspended with a larger laryngoscope. The patient is usually ventilated with jet ventilation or a laser-safe endotracheal tube placed through a pre-existing tracheostoma. The full details of airway management are not presented here; the choice of spontaneous ventilation, apnea, and jet ventilation (and all of its various modes) are important and should be discussed between the surgeon and anesthesiologist prior to the entry of the patient into the operating room.

The airway is then evaluated with a long 0-degree Hopkins bronchoscopic telescope. This allows excellent visualization of the airway. At this time the length of the stenosis, its diameter and distance from the vocal folds and tracheostoma are recorded, typically in mm. Secondary stenoses are often present so care is taken to evaluate the airway down to and including mainstem bronchi. Operative intervention for the airway obstruction may take place at this first evaluation or it may be deferred to another time following further discussion with the patient.

STAGING

The purpose of staging a patient's stenoses is to help predict the outcome of surgery and compare different methods of treatment. There are a number of different staging systems used for laryngotracheal stenosis. The most often cited is that described by McCaffrey.[22] This is based on the site and length of the stenosis and the mobility of the vocal folds. This scheme may be helpful in the determining the prognosis for decannulation (see Figure 26–2). Many practitioners are also familiar with the Myer-Cotton classification[23]; this important and easy-to-use system is designed for use in the pediatric airway. Moreover, its utility is restricted to subglottic stenosis only.

McCaffrey Staging System:

Stage 1: Stenoses are confined to the subglottis or trachea and are less than 1 cm long.

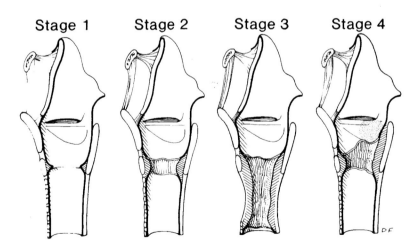

Stage 1   Stage 2   Stage 3   Stage 4

FIGURE 26–2. McCaffrey staging of laryngotracheal stenosis. **Stage 1:** Stenoses are confined to the subglottis or trachea and are less than 1 cm long. **Stage 2:** Stenoses are subglottic stenoses longer than 1 cm and do not extend to either the glottis or trachea. **Stage 3:** Stenoses where subglottic stenosis extends into the trachea but does not involve the glottis. **Stage 4:** Stenoses with glottal involvement with fixation of one or both vocal folds.[22]

Stage 2: Stenoses are subglottic stenoses longer than 1 cm and do not extend to either the glottis or trachea.

Stage 3: Stenoses where subglottic stenosis extends into the trachea but does not involve the glottis.

Stage 4: Stenoses with glottal involvement with fixation of one or both vocal folds.

In the evaluation of 75 patients, those who were stage 1 and 2 had a 90% success rate whereas those classified as stage 4 had a 40% decannulation rate. In this significant review, it should be noted that various procedures were used in the operative management of these patients. This staging system did not provide a road map for the management of these challenging cases, but rather helped to define the likelihood of success following surgical treatment. An interesting contrast to McCaffrey's experience is that of Grillo and colleagues. In one of his interval reviews of his vast experience with open airway surgery, Grillo reported on 503 patients who were treated with laryngotracheal resection only.[19] Although Grillo did not propose a staging system he noted that when a patient is treated with laryngotracheal resection the height of anastomosis had a direct correlation with success. Failure rates were 2.2% for trachea-trachea anastomosis, 6.0% for trachea-cricoid anastomosis, and 8.1% for trachea-thyroid anastomosis.

Another staging system has been widely used for the posterior glottis[24] (see Figure 26-3).

Staging System for Posterior Glottic Stenosis

(as defined by Bogdasarian and Olson[24]):

Stage 1: Interarytenoid scar band with a sinus tract posterior to the band and anormal posterior commissure.

Stage 2: Interarytenoid and posterior commissure scarring with normal arytenoid mobility.

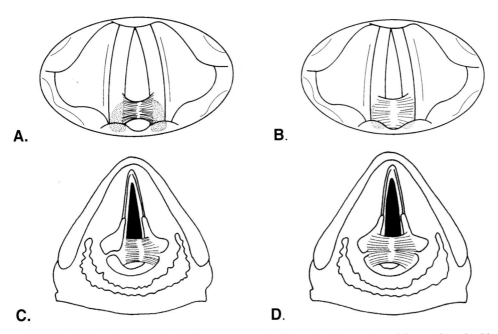

A. **B.**

C. **D.**

FIGURE 26–3. Staging of glottic stenosis. **A.** Stage 1: Interarytenoid scar band with a sinus tract posterior to the band and normal posterior commissure. **B.** Stage 2: Interarytenoid and posterior commissure scarring with normal arytenoids mobility. **C.** Stage 3: Posterior commissure scarring involving fixation of one arytenoid. **D.** Stage 4: Posterior commissure scarring involving fixation of two arytenoids.[24]

Stage 3: Posterior commissure scarring involving fixation of one arytenoid.

Stage 4: Posterior commissure scarring involving fixation of two arytenoids.

Again, this staging helps to guide treatment, predict outcome, and compare the efficacy of different surgical procedures.

Surgical Managment of Airway Stenosis

The options for the treatment of laryngotracheal stenosis are extensive. These include the placement of stents, steroid injection, microtrap door excisions, dilation alone, endoscopic CO_2 laser incision and dilation, staged reconstructive procedures, and laryngotracheal expansion or resection. This variety attests to myriad stenoses as well as to the difficulty in correcting laryngotracheal stenosis and the absence of a treatment that produces consistently reliable results in every situation. Treatment options are tailored to the extent and site of the stenosis. Outlined below are some of the more common procedures performed today. The role of tracheotomy should always be considered in every patient. With their underlying medical challenges and the recalcitrant nature of many stenoses, tracheotomy is the appropriate choice for many patients with airway stenosis.

SUBGLOTTIC AND TRACHEAL STENOSIS

CO_2 Laser Incision with Endoscopic Dilation

One of the most common endoscopic treatments for laryngotracheal stenosis is radial incision and dilation of the stenotic lesion. This was first described in 1987.[25] Prior to that time CO_2 and Nd:YAG lasers were used for complete or staged resection of laryngotracheal stenoses with variable results and high failure rates.[26-29] The rationale of the radial incision with dilation is to preserve intervening areas of mucosa to prevent scar contracture and reformation of the stenosis. A higher failure rate for this procedure has been found with stenoses that are greater then 1 cm in length, and have circumferential scarring, tracheal malacia, or cartilaginous collapse.[25,28,29] Endoscopic treatment may be attempted in such situations but the higher risk of failure and possible need for future open surgical management should be stressed to the patient. Endoscopic incision and dilation with the addition of T-tube stenting has been used even in the face of complete tracheal stenosis with a 66% success rate.[30]

Endoscopic treatment of laryngotracheal stenosis is generally performed with a CO_2 laser due to its precise cutting ability and minimal thermal spread and damage of surrounding tissue.[31] The lesion is exposed with either a laryngoscope, subglottiscope, or a CO_2 laser-coupled ventilating bronchoscope depending on the site of the lesion. The patient may be ventilated via intubation through an existing tracheotomy site, jet ventilation, or via the bronchoscope. When using a laryngoscope. or subglottiscope the laser is typically set at 4 watts with a short exposure of 0.1 seconds at 0.5 second intervals. These settings can be adjusted at the surgeon's discretion. Prior to laser treatment, many surgeons prefer to inject the area intended for treatment with a steroid preparation. The basis for this has been worked out in the animal model, although supportive evidence in human subjects has not been presented.[32]

When using a 30-cm bronchoscope, the laser may be set at 6 W, whereas it is set at 10 W for a 40-cm bronchoscope. Radial incisions are made in 3 to 5 areas of the stenosis taking care not to damage the perichondrium. After the incisions are completed, the stenosis is gently dilated with successive ventilating bronchoscopes. The goal is to pass a 7.5-mm to 8.5-mm bronchoscope. The bronchoscopes are gently inserted past the stenosis, rotated 180 degrees, and then removed. Care is taken not to damage the residual islands of mucosa (Figure 26–4).[25,28]

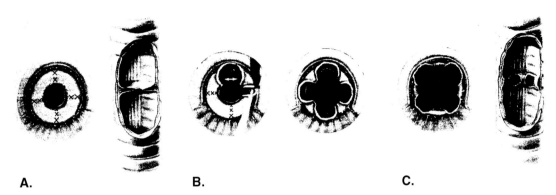

A.   **B.**   **C.**

FIGURE 26–4. Diagrammatic illustration of tracheal lumen from endoscopic view, and tracheal cross section. **A.** Fibrous concentric tracheal stenosis. x = planned radial laser incision **B.** Lumen is enlarged with radial incision and subsequent tissue retraction (*arrows*). **C.** Tracheal size after progressive dilation with a 7.5-mm and 8.5-mm rigid bronchoscopes. Island of epithelium are left intact between laser incisional areas.[35]

Recently the application of mitomycin-C has been added to the endoscopic treatment of laryngotracheal stenosis. Mitomycin-C is an antineoplastic and antiproliferative agent that preferentially inhibits fibroblast proliferation; this is believed to be the mechanism by which it reduces scar formation. Multiple reports on the use of mitomycin-C (MMC) demonstrate an improved success rate for the endoscopic treatment of laryngotracheal stenosis when compared to treatment without mitomycin-C.[12,34-36] One such study demonstrates an increase in success from 15 to 75%.[36] Most of these studies are small in scope and there are others who believe that mitomycin-C is not helpful in the treatment of a well-established stenosis.[37] A recent report by Simpson compared a historical non-MMC-treated stenosis patient group to a group managed with the adjunctive use of MMC.[38] In this comparative study, the MMC group had a significantly lower rate of recurrence and a longer interval between treatments. Although the benefit of mitomycin-C has not been proven in a large randomized controlled trial, it appears to offer significant benefit and potential cost-savings which outweigh the minimal risk encountered in the largest reported series.[39]

One technique for applying MMC to the wound is as follows. A 10-mm cottonoid pledget soaked with 0.4 mg/ml mitomycin-C is placed over the surgical site for 4 minutes. After it is removed the site is successively washed with 3 10-mm cottonoid pledgets soaked in normal saline.[36] The ideal duration and concentration of the topical MMC application has not been determined scientifically, although the outline above is typical for most centers.

Endoscopic surgery for airway stenosis can be repeated with reasonable benefit for patients, even after many procedures. The role of endoscopic surgery versus open surgery is a continuing source of debate. The impact of adjunctive treatment such as MMC may alter decision-making in this arena as more information is gathered.

Laryngotracheal Resection

Open surgical resection of laryngotracheal stenosis is undertaken when patients have failed prior endoscopic treatment or the stenosis is severe enough that successful endoscopic treatment is deemed unlikely. It is generally felt that stenoses longer than 1 cm or those that display tracheomalacia, tracheal collapse, or significant circumferential scarring are unamenable to endoscopic treatment.[25,28,29]

From the mid 1970s and into the 1990s extensive investigation of laryngotracheal resection and reconstruction (LTR) was undertaken.[40-42] Lesions isolated to the trachea were treated with a simple resection and anastomosis. Those involving the subglottis required a more extensive procedure with partial or complete anterior cricoid resection.

The technique of segmental resection removes the obstructing mucosa, scar, and cartilage from the upper airway. Tissue can be resected from any level up to the level of the inferior margin of the vocal folds. The maximum resectable length of airway is approximately 7.5 cm with the majority of resections being between 2 and 4 cm.[19] The reported success rate of LTR is between 91 and 95%.[1,2,19,41] Revision surgery for failures of laryngotracheal reconstruction comes with a higher rate of major complications, 39% compared to approximately 15% in primary procedures.[43] Ultimately these cases are as successful as primary surgery, although multiple procedures may be required. The success of revision surgery is between 91.9 and 96.5%.[43,44]

The type and extent of laryngotracheal reconstruction is dependent on the site and nature of stenosis. If the stenotic segment is confined to the trachea simple segmental resection

---

Laryngotracheal Reconstruction

In 1995 Grillo reported the results of his extensive experience with laryngotracheal reconstruction.[19] Of 503 patients who underwent either tracheal resection and/or laryngotracheal resection, 93.7% had a "satisfactory" to "good" result. The failure rate was 3.9% (2.2% for tracheal resection and 6% for laryngotracheal resection) and the mortality rate was 2.4%. In a similar study, Pearson reported on a series of 80 patients undergoing resection of subglottic airway with variable lengths of trachea.[41] Interestingly, 24 of these patients had a synchronous laryngoplasty with laryngofissure and T-tube stenting for glottic stenosis. This approach is in contrast to Dr. Grillo's practice that glottal stenosis should be treated prior to laryngotracheal reconstruction in a separate procedure. In Pearson's paper, 49 of the 56 patients who underwent sublgottic resection had no significant dyspnea with vigorous exercise; 4 had some dyspnea on exertion but required no further intervention. Two of the 56 remained with a tracheotomy in place, an overall success rate of 96%. Of the 24 patients treated simultaneously for tracheal, subglottic, and glottic pathology, 18 had no significant dyspnea with vigorous exercise, 3 had some dyspnea on exertion but require no further intervention, and, again, 2 remain trach-dependent—a 91% success rate, supporting Pearson's contention that glottal and subglottal stenosis can and should be treated simultaneously. He states that the pathology between the two sites is continuous and should be resected in one operation. Staging the operation will leave inflamed tissue of the subglottis in contact with the newly repaired glottis, decreasing the success of the glottal repair.[45] Although Pearson's results appear to confirm that a single procedure does not decrease success, systematic comparisons have not been performed so a definitive conclusion is difficult to make.

with end-to-end anastomosis can be performed as described by Wain (see Figures 26–5 and 26–6).[46] Prior to incision the patient is intubated from above whether or not a tracheotomy tube is in place. If necessary the stenosis can be dilated to assist ventilation; another option is to approach the stenosis under local anesthesia and enter the airway just at the stenosis, thus allowing for intubation of the distal trachea and general anesthesia.

The trachea is approached through a collar incision. Subplatysmal flaps are elevated from the manubrium to the hyoid. The strap muscles are divided in the midline and retracted laterally. The thyroid isthmus is then divided and also retracted laterally. The anterior aspect of the airway is exposed from the thyroid notch to several centimeters below the stenotic segment. Care is taken to minimize the disruption of the lateral blood supply of the trachea at the uninvolved segments of airway.[47] The site of stenosis is then identified by external evaluation of the trachea or intraoperative bronchoscopy with transillumination. Circumferential mobilization of the stenotic segment is then performed on the trachea to avoid injury to the recurrent laryngeal nerves. Alternatively, the airway can be entered at the stenosis and the posterior dissection can take place from the endoluminal aspect of airway. The nerves are not identified. The dissection should be confined to within 1 cm to 1.5 cm proximal or distal of the stenosis so that healthy trachea is not devascularized. The airway is then transected immediately below the stenotic lesion and the distal trachea is intubated across the field. A preoperative tracheotomy site should be resected with the stenotic segment. After resection of the stenotic segment, 2-0 Vicryl lateral traction sutures are placed proximally and distally and the head is flexed. Tension is then assessed and a suprahyoid laryngeal release is performed if necessary.[48] 4-0 Vicryl sutures are placed 3 mm apart and 3 mm from the airway margin beginning at the posterior midline. After placement, the ends of the airway are approximated by cervical flexion and the lateral stay sutures are tied. The anastomotic sutures are then tied from anterior to posterior. If the innominate artery was exposed, then interposition of

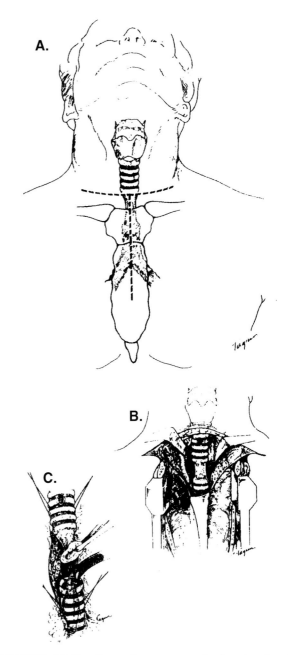

FIGURE 26–5. Operative approach for tracheal stenosis. **A.** Most cases can be approached with a low collar incision. In some cases a partial upper sternotomy is needed for access to more distal lesions. **B.** Exposure with a cervicomediastinal incision. The dissection plane is closely applied to the airway. **C.** Circumferential dissection occurs only at the level of the stenosis and at the margins of resection. Following transaction below the lesion and placement of lateral stay sutures, ventilation through the distal segment is maintained while the stenosis is excised.[49]

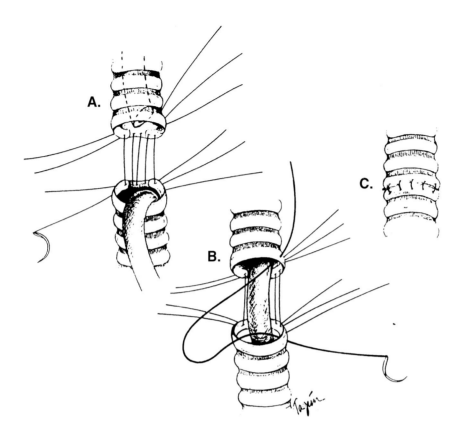

FIGURE 26–6. End-to-end tracheal anastomosis. **A.** Sutures are placed individually beginning in the midline posteriorly. **B.** The sutures are placed anterior to the mid-lateral stay sutures and the endotracheal tube is advanced into the distal tracheal segment. **C.** After cervical flexion and tying of the lateral stay sutures, the anastomotic sutures are tied from anterior to posterior.[49]

strap muscle between the artery and anastomosis is important to prevent the formation of a tracheoarterial fistula, which may be disastrous. The thyroid isthmus and strap muscles are then closed over the anastomosis. After the wound is closed a suture may be placed between the chin and presternal skin to prevent hyperextension. The patient is then awoken and extubated in the operating room. Common variations of this technique include the use of Prolene for the cartilaginous tracheal anastomosis as well as the consideration of overnight inubation to reduce air-leakage into the neck when the patient coughs.

If the stenosis involves the anterolateral subglottis, then after distal transection the stenosis dissection must proceed toward the cricoid (see Figure 26-7).[40] Circumferential dissection is performed on the airway and dissection behind the cricoid plate should not proceed more than 1 mm to 2 mm above the posterior aspect of the inferior border of the cricoid to avoid injury to the recurrent laryngeal nerves. Lateral traction sutures are placed in the lower border of the thy-

roid cartilage. The airway is divided vertically in the midline from below upward and the extent of stenosis is assessed. Once it is clear that the anterior cricoid is involved, the anterior and lateral aspects of the cricoid cartilage are then exposed via subperichondrial dissection. The stenotic area of the cricoid is then resected with rongeurs beveling laterally and inferiorly until the inferior border is reached anterior to the posterior cricoid plate. The posterior mucosa is then transected. The distal tracheal cartilage is then trimmed back in a gentle curve laterally and inferiorly mimicking the new shape of the cricoid. The head is flexed and tension is assessed. Suprahyoid laryngeal release is then performed if necessary. 4-0 Vicryl sutures are then placed as described above. Sutures pass through the full thickness of the thyroid and tracheal cartilage. Posteriorly the sutures must pass through the full thickness of the mucosa but not necessarily through the full thickness of the cricoid. The traction sutures are then tied followed by the anastomotic sutures from anterior to posterior.

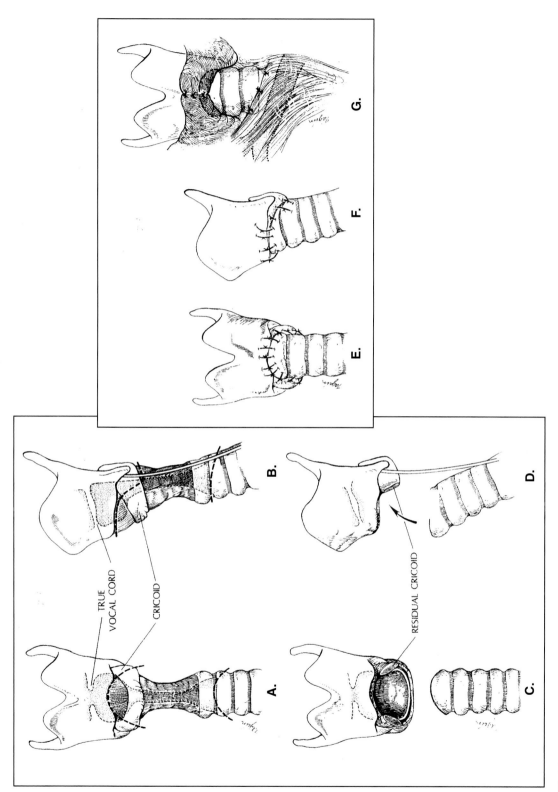

FIGURE 26–7. Operative repair of anterolateral stenosis of the subglottic larynx and trachea with crico-tracheal anastomosis. **A.** and **B.** Antero-posterior and lateral views with lines of resection. **C.** and **D.** Larynx and trachea after removal of stenotic segment. Recurrent laryngeal nerves are left intact. Mucous membrane is transected at the same level as the cartilage. **E.** and **F.** Anteroposterior and lateral views after reconstruction. **G.** Thyroid isthmus has been reapproximated to cover the anastomosis. Strap muscle shields the innominate artery from the anastomosis.

If the stenosis at the level of the cricoid is circumferential and involves the mucosa anterior to the cricoid plate further technical modification becomes necessary (see Figure 26–8). The scarred mucosa is dissected from the underlying posterior cricoid plate. The dissection may proceed to the superior aspect of the cricoid cartilage without entering and damaging the cricoarytenoid joint. The posterior mucosa of the distal trachea is then fashioned into a flap to cover the cricoid plate. Four 4-0 Vicryl sutures are placed between the laryngeal mucosa and the tracheal mucosal flap. Four more sutures are used to secure the base of the flap to the inferior margin of the cricoid. This allows the flap to lay flat and tension free.

If glottal stenosis is to be addressed at the same time as the subglottic and tracheal stenosis, a laryngofissure must be performed. This is described in detail in the following section, (isolated anterior glottic stenosis). In this case, after the posterior glottic scar is excised it is covered

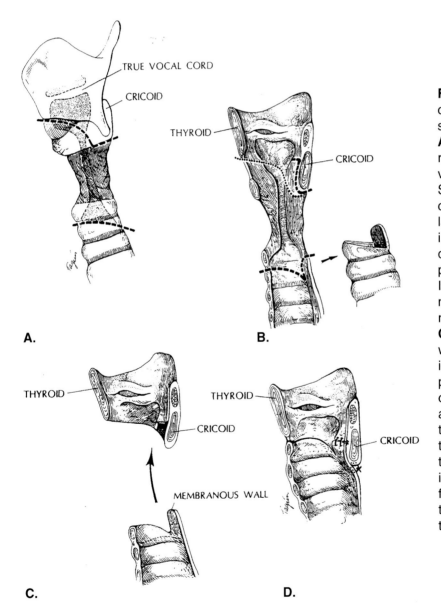

A.

B.

C.

D.

FIGURE 26–8. Operative repair of circumferential stenosis of the subglottic larynx and trachea. **A.** Lateral view with lines of resection. **B.** Lateral and interior view of lines of resection. Superior dotted line indicates cartilaginous division of the larynx. Superior dashed line indicates mucosal division after dissection of mucosa from the posterior plate of the cricoid. Inferiorly the posterior membranous wall has been retained as a broad-based flap. **C.** The flap of the membranous wall of the trachea will be fitted into the mucosal defect over the posterior cricoid. **D.** Mucosa of the larynx has been anastomosed to mucosa of the trachea. External to the lumen, the membranous wall of the trachea has been fixed to the inferior margin of the cricoid with four sutures. This will ensure that the flap will stay firmly applied to the cricoid and be tension free.[49]

with a flap from the membranous wall of the trachea. The anastomosis and glottal repair can be stented with a T-tube or Montgomery stent (Boston Medical Products, Boston, Mass) that is removed after approximately 6 weeks.

If a laryngofissure is not performed, the patient is extubated in the operating room. Reintubation is avoided unless there is clearly excessive airway obstruction from edema or the patient fails extubation. This is necessary in fewer than 5% of patients.[42,50,51] A tracheotomy or T-tube should be avoided if possible. If needed, the tracheotomy should be at least two rings below the anastomosis and strap muscle should be interposed to separate this site from the innominate artery.

Laryngotracheal Expansion

Laryngotracheal expansion (LTE) is an alternative to segmental resection. Instead of removing the diseased airway, the airway is expanded by splitting the airway and enlarging it with grafts. The indications for this surgery are the same as those for segmental resection.

McCaffrey was one of the early proponents of this technique for laryngotracheal stenosis that was within 1 cm of the vocal folds.[52] He chose this technique to prevent damage to the cricoarytenoid joint. McCaffrey was able to decannulate 40% of his patients with grade 4 stenosis. Lano et al treated patients with either laryngotracheal resection or laryngotracheal expansion. 63% of their patients were decannulated within one year. An additional 17% were decannulated after a second open procedure. Twenty percent of the patients remain cannulated.[53] Gavilan et al reported on 60 patients treated primarily with LTE. Only 70% were successfully decannulated, the average number of procedures per patient was 1.95, and the median time to decannulation was 561 days.[54] Rhee et al reviewed 15 of their patients who underwent LTE without stenting. All patients were eventually decannulated but 3 of the 15 needed an additional expansion procedure. Only 21% did not

need additional surgery. One patient required 15 endoscopic procedures prior to eventual decannulation. One patient died immediately postoperatively which the authors attributed to graft collapse.[55]

A direct comparison between LTE and segmental resection is difficult because many of the LTE series include cases that are treated with resection. When evaluating the above results, it does not appear that LTE is as successful as LTR. This may reflect the fact that the underlying stenoses are different in these reports. It is clear, however, that even in advanced cases of stenosis involving the glottis, resection may achieve a decannulation rate of 90%.[41] Most of the LTE series are less successful and require many more procedures to achieve a satisfactory result regardless of the position of the stenosis.

The technique of LTE has been described by numerous authors[53-56] (Figure 26-9). A low-collar incision is performed with subplatysmal flaps elevated to the hyoid and sternal notch. The strap muscles and thyroid isthmus are divided in the midline and lateralized. The cricoid is divided in the midline with either a knife or a saw; this incision is extended superiorly or inferiorly until normal appearing airway is encountered. If the glottis is not involved care is taken to preserve the anterior commissure orientation to minimize the impact on the patient's voice. If the cricoid is too rigid to be opened sufficiently the posterior cricoid plate is split taking care not to violate the interarytenoid muscles or esophagus. A posterior cartilage graft, if used, is then placed. This is a T-shaped graft with the flange tucked behind the posterior cricoid plate. If a stent is to be used it is then positioned at this point. If the stenosis is limited to the glottic larynx then a laryngeal stent is placed with a concomitant tracheotomy. Sutures are passed through the neck and stent ultimately tying the sutures over buttons and securing the stent in place. If the cervical trachea is involved, a T-tube is placed instead of a solid stent and tracheotomy.[54] As noted above, some authors advocate single-stage reconstruction without tracheotomy as an alternative to stenting.

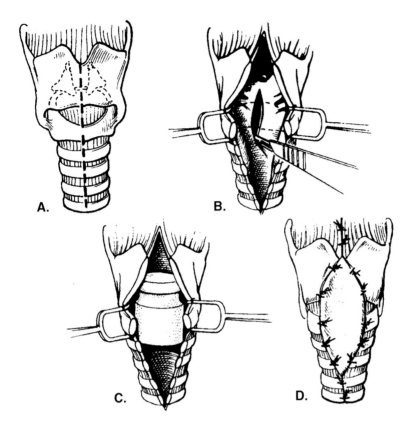

FIGURE 26–9. Laryngotracheal expansion. **A.** Vertical splitting of the area of stenosis. **B.** Splitting of posterior cricoid if necessary. **C.** Placement of stent. **D.** Graft sutured in place.[57]

The anterior cartilage graft is harvested and carved into a fusiform shape with beveled or flanged edges. It is then sutured in place with interrupted 4-0 Vicryl sutures. There are a number of different sources of graft material. A nasal septal graft can be used for stenoses up to 3 cm in length. A graft is harvested using standard septoplasty techniques. On one side of the graft the mucoperichondirum is kept intact. The mucoperichondrium will then face the lumen and be oriented so that the cilia beat superiorly.[58] Costal cartilage is harvested from the fifth or sixth rib for stenoses greater than 3 cm. The perichondrium is placed facing the lumen. After the anterior graft is secured, the thyroid and strap muscles are reapproximated and the incision is closed over drains. Stenting duration may range from 24 hours with an endotracheal tube to 4 to 6 weeks with a T-tube or a combination of laryngeal stent and tracheotomy. After this period the patient is brought back to the operating room for stent removal and CO_2 laser excision of any granulation tissue.

Complications of Surgery for Subglottic and Tracheal Stenosis

Laryngotracheal surgery can be fraught with serious complications and failed resections. In reviewing his series, Grillo identified three types of failure: incomplete diagnosis, failure in technique, and other complications not easily classified[19,59] (Table 26–2).

Incomplete diagnosis was usually due to inadequate assessment of tracheomalacia or simultaneous glottal incompetence, either incomplete abduction or adduction. A pretreatment evaluation that includes flexible tracheoscopy with the patient awake will help prevent underestimating the extent of tracheal malacia and glottic incompetence.

Idealized surgical technique has evolved over the years as clinicians have honed their techniques. The use of absorbably sutures, avoidance of intraluminal knots, the resection of all severely inflamed or damaged tissue, preservation of the lateral tracheal blood supply during dissection, and ensuring minimal tension on the anastomosis

TABLE 26–2. Complications of Laryngotracheal Reconstruction in 503 Patients[60]

	Major	Minor	Total
Granulations	11	38	49
Before 1978	10	34	44
After 1978*	1	34	5
Dehisence	28	1	29
Laryngeal Dysfunction	11	14	25
Malacia	10	0	10
Hemmorrhage	5	0	5
Edema (anastomotic)	3	1	4
Infection	12	22	34
Wound	7	8	15
Pulmonary	5	14	19
Myocardial Infarction	1	0	1
Tracheoesophageal Fistula	1	0	1
Pneumothorax	0	3	3
Line Infection	0	1	1
Atrial Fibrillation	0	1	1
Deep Venous Thrombosis	0	1	1
Totals	82	82	164

*Switched to absorbable suture

have been put forward as important techniques that may reduce the incidence of complications.

Patient factors also contribute to failure and complications. Although age, obstructive sleep apnea, congestive heart failure, recurrent pneumonia, and diabetes have been found to have a significant negative influence on outcome, only severe chronic obstructive pulmonary disease was consistently recognized as a risk factor.[2,44,53,54] Severe chronic obstructive pulmonary disease may result in prolonged intubation, need for a new tracheotomy, failure of decannulation, and even death from acute respiratory failure. In LTR the higher the anastomosis, the higher the rate of minor complications. As the anastomosis moves proximal from trachea-trachea anastomosis to trachea-cricoid and trachea-thyroid anastomosis the minor complication rate rises from 16 to 17 to 21%, respectively.

Finally, there is controversy as to whether laryngeal release is a contributing factor to postoperative morbidity. Although some maintain that the release is rarely needed others use it

routinely.[19,42,61] Grillo noted that dysphagia was significantly less with suprahyoid release as decribed by Montgomery, as compared to thyrohyoid release.[48,62] Eight of the 40 (20%) patients undergoing suprahyoid release developed complications.[19] Three experienced dysphagia, one aspiration, one malacia, and three dehiscence. This is slightly higher than the average complication rate of 15% for all patients. A confounding factor is that patients who undergo laryngeal release are already at higher risk for complications as the release is more likely to be performed in those undergoing revision operations or resections at a higher level. A recent paper provided the first otolarygology report on a series of tracheal resections in which no releasing maneuvers were performed. The success rate reported by Merati et al was 94%, comparable to the bulk of otolaryngology series in which all or nearly all patients routinely underwent these releases.[63]

GLOTTIC STENOSIS

In glottic stenosis, hoarseness or dyspnea may be the reason for surgery. Depending on the extent and position of the stenosis different procedures are applicable.

Anterior Glottic Stenosis

Anterior glottic stenosis consisting of a congenital or acquired web is treated endoscopically. After the glottis is exposed and suspended the web is lysed with either a CO_2 laser or steel instruments. A keel of 0.02-inch steel-mesh reinforced Silastic is placed in the anterior commissure preventing reformation of the scar[64] (Figure 26–10). The keel placement is achieved by threading two reusable straight needles with 2-0 Prolene. The two needles are passed transcutaneously into the larynx at the midline. One needle is placed superior to the vocal folds and the other inferior. Both needles are then pulled through the laryngoscope with an alligator forceps. One limb of the inferior suture is pulled

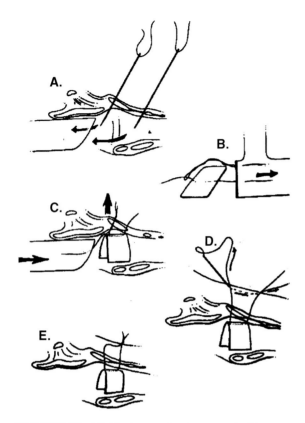

FIGURE 26–10. Endoscopic placement of laryngeal keel. **A.** Placement of superior and inferior suture. **B.** and **C.** Threading of stent and pull through of superior end of inferior suture. **D.** and **E.** Subcutaneous burying of transfixtion suture.[65]

into the larynx. This free end is then rethreaded on a needle and passed through the middle of the stent at its inferior and superior edge. The eye of the superior needle is broken and the needle is discarded. The free end of the inferior suture is passed through the loop of the superior suture. The keel is then put in place. The superior suture, acting as a pull-through device, is then pulled out of the skin of the neck pulling the free end of the lower suture with it. The superior suture is discarded and the free upper end of the remaining suture is threaded on another needle. This is passed into the subcutaneous tissues at the original entrance wound from the superior suture and passed out the entrance of the inferior suture. The lower wound is then enlarged and the suture ends are tied and buried into the subcutaneous tissue. After 2 to 3 weeks the keel is removed endoscopically as the

suture is cut after identifying it in the subcutaneous tissues. Mouney claims a nearly 100% success rate in the treatment of glottal webs with this technique.[65] Another excellent option for the endoscopic placement of laryngeal keels is the endoextralaryngeal needle carrier technique of Lichtenberger.[66,67] With this approach, the manipulations required for endoscopic suturing, keel placement, and vocal fold lateralization are made much more straightforward.

An external approach to anterior glottal stenosis is indicated when the stenosis extends to the subglottis, when there is laryngeal inlet stenosis, or after endoscopic attempts have failed. The procedure, as modified from Isshiki's description, begins with separation of the strap muscles and complete exposure of the thyroid cartilage.[68] A vertical incision is made through the midline of the thyroid cartilage using a sagittal saw. Care is taken not to damage the underlying soft tissue. A hypodermic needle is inserted at the midline. After correct positioning is confirmed with fiberoptic laryngoscopy the anterior commissure may be vertically divided, thus opening the larynx at the ideal spot; the larynx is retracted open and the scar tissue is inspected. The scar tissue is then resected and the vocal folds are shaped. The amount of scar tissue resected from the vocal folds can be determined by fiberoptic visualization with the laryngofissure temporarily closed. The areas void of mucosa are then covered with harvested buccal mucosa. The graft is sutured in place with 6-0 Dexon. Fibrin glue may be placed beneath the graft. The mucosal graft must cover the anterior commissure and must also be secured to the external perichondrium of the thyroid cartilage to prevent webbing of the anterior commissure. After this is completed, the laryngofissure is closed. The patient is decannulated once complete healing has been ensured by laryngoscopic examination.

Posterior Glottic Stenosis

Posterior glottic stenosis (PGS) is also commonly managed endoscopically. The operative procedure required is based on the staging of the stenosis as described earlier in this chapter.

For type one, the web can simply be lysed with a CO_2 laser followed by the application of mitomycin-C as described previously. It should be noted that a significant percentage of these cases also have some occult joint dysfunction.

For Bogdasarian types 2 and 3 PGS, simple lysis of the stenosis will often result in recurrence. To prevent this, a postcricoid advancement flap can be created endoscopically[69] (Figure 26–11). After exposure of the glottis and postcricoid area, the arytenoids are palpated to ensure at least one of the arytenoids is mobile. After this is confirmed, a transverse incision is made from the posterior superior aspect of one arytenoid to the other. A microscissor is then used to extend the cut from each end of the transverse incision to the base of the posterior aspect of the arytenoids, creating an inferiorly based flap. The mucosal flap is then sharply elevated from the underlying scar tissue. The scar band and interarytenoid muscle are then divided, removing tissue as needed. Care must be taken to divide all the interarytenoid muscle and avoid trauma to the cricoarytenoid joint. After this is completed, the arytenoids are separated and the mucosal flap is draped back down and sutured in place with one or two 4-0 Chromic sutures. A cuffed tracheotomy tube is kept in place with the cuff inflated for 1 week to prevent displacement of the flap secondary to coughing or phonation. Decannulation should take place 6 to 12 weeks after the procedure, after the surgical site has been allowed to heal and an adequate glottal airway is secured.

Although it represents the most advanced PGS, type 4 stenosis can also be treated endoscopically. Because these cases are defined by bilateral arytenoid fixation, the objective is to statically enlarge the fixed airway. This depends on a direct trade-off between airway and voice/ swallowing function. Ossoff et al described the CO_2 laser arytenoidectomy and partial cordectomy in 1983[70]; 24 of 26 patients with long-term follow-up were successfully managed with this procedure.[62] For this operation, the posterior larynx is exposed with a large laryngoscope. A CO_2 laser is then used to vaporize one corniculate cartilage and arytenoid cartilage and their overlying mucoperichondrium from apex to base. The posterior aspect of the vocalis muscle is also incised in anterior-medial to posterior-lateral direction beginning approximately 2 to 3 mm anterior to the vocal process. This procedure has since been modified numerous times.[72-74] Most modifications of this technique describe preservation of the medial mucosa of the arytenoid and preservation of the posterior or lateral aspect of the arytenoid. After the chosen amount of arytenoid is ablated, the preserved medial mucosal

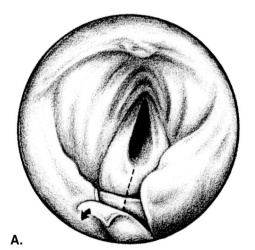
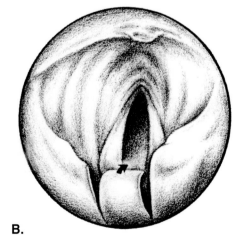

A.   **B.**

FIGURE 26–11. Isolated posterior glottic stenosis. **A.** Elevation of inferiorly based postcricoid flap. Dashed line represents incision for arytenoid separation. **B.** Inset of mucosal flap into gap created by arytenoid separation.[69]

flap is sutured laterally to cover the surgical defect. The mucosal flap aids in less tissue contraction and more predictable healing. The remnant of arytenoid decreases medial prolapse of the mucosa and is also a barrier to aspiration.

An alternative to an arytenoidectomy is a posterior transverse cordotomy which was first described in 1989 by Kashima.[75,76] After laryngoscopic exposure, a CO_2 laser posterior vestibulectomy is performed, thus exposing the floor of the ventricle and lateral true vocal fold. The laser is then used to make a horizontal cut just anterior to the vocal process. This allows the vocal fold to spring forward and enlarge the airway. Some have also advocated ablation of a small portion of the vocalis muscle without compromise of the overlying mucosa. Care is taken to minimize injury to the perichondrium of the vocal process and thyroid cartilage. If the perichondrium is damaged there is an increased risk of granuloma formation and prolonged healing that may result in a less than adequate postoperative airway. The procedure may be performed unilaterally first and then if necessary it may be performed bilaterally, although this is rarely necessary. It has been found that when compared to an arytenoidectomy, a posterior transverse cordotomy is faster and easier to perform with an equal success rate and less evidence of subclinical aspiration. Both procedures are unpredictably detrimental to the voice.[77] In younger, otherwise healthy patients, a more modest cordotomy may be performed initially; in this approach, the potential for preserving vocal function is achieved at the cost of possible revision surgery. The approach described above for PGS is also appropriate for bilateral true vocal fold paralysis, such as following thyroidectomy.

As with anterior glottic stenosis, if a patient fails endoscopic treatment a laryngofissure can be performed, as described in the previous section on isolated anterior glottic stenosis. In this case, the posterior scar is excised to enlarge the airway. An arytenoidectomy can be performed as deemed necessary. The denuded areas are covered with local mucosa flaps or free labial mucosal grafts. Care is taken not to damage the cricoarytenoid joints of mobile arytenoids. With refinement and experience of the Kashima and other endoscopic techniques, as well as with the advent of MMC, few PGS cases require open surgery.

Complete Glottal Stenosis

Complete glottic stenosis is usually the result of extralaryngeal trauma. This must be treated externally via a laryngofissure. The procedure is performed as described above for severe anterior and posterior glottic stenosis. A stent is usually sutured in place with translaryngeal sutures to support the grafts. This stent will remain in place for 4 to 6 weeks when it will be removed endoscopically. At that time any granulation tissue can be removed with CO_2 laser.

Supraglottic Stenosis

Supraglottic stenosis is uncommon. It usually results from extralaryngeal trauma or caustic injestion. In the past, supraglottic laryngectomy has been advocated as a reasonable approach to this problem; this has fallen from favor. Initial treatment of supraglottic stenosis is now performed endoscopically with a CO_2 laser.[78] If possible, areas of mucosa are left undamaged to help prevent a circumferential trauma and restenosis. Although no specific clinical studies exist to support this practice, the familiar adjunctive measures of steroid injection and MMC application may be used in the supraglottic airway as well.

Restenosis is common after an endoscopic procedure and often an external procedure is necessary. The supraglottis is approached through a laryngofissure as described previously. If the epiglottis is dislocated posteriorly, as is often seen in trauma, the base of the epiglottis is resected to enlarge the laryngeal inlet.[79] The mucosa overlying the the anterior surface of the base of the epiglottis is removed. The cartilage at the base is then dissected free from the posterior mucoperichondrium in a subperichondrial plane. The cartilaginous base is then removed. The posterior flap of mucoperichondrium is then sutured to the cut edges of the anterior mucoperichondrium, enlarging the laryngeal inlet. The remaining scar tissue in the supraglottis is resected. Areas devoid of mucosa are then covered using local flaps or free labial mucosa or skin grafts as described previously. A stent is then sutured in place with translaryngeal sutures sewn over buttons on the neck. The stent is left in place for 4 to 6 weeks as the supraglottic tissues are allowed to epithelialize and restenosis is prevented. The stent is removed endoscopically and a CO_2 laser is used to remove granulation tissue that is present.

ADDITIONAL CLINICAL CONSIDERATIONS

Wegener's Granulomatosis

The treatment paradigm for subglottic stenosis is different in cases of Wegener's granulomatosis (WG). As discussed earlier, WG is a multisystem inflammatory disease characterized by necrotizing granulomatous inflammation and vasculitis of unknown etiology. Often the disease is active and affected airway mucosa is inflamed and unhealthy. Surgical manipulation during active WG may lead to worsening of the inflammation and stenosis. A small number of patients (3–22%) with active WG may have improvement of their subglottic stenosis with medical treatment only.[9,11] This usually consists of treatment with system steroids, cyclophosphamide as indicated, and trimethoprim-sulfamethoxazole for prophylaxis. Surgical intervention should be limited to the least manipulation that will be successful. Ideally it will take place during times of quiescence when the subglottis demonstrates mature scar. Treatment may consist of intralesional injection with glucocorticoid steroids, gentle rigid dilation of the subglottis, or CO_2 laser incision with dilation. The latter two instances may be performed in conjunction with mitomycin-C application to decrease recurrent scar formation. For patients unresponsive to the above therapies, laryngotracheal expansion and tracheotomy are also options, although less desirable.

Idiopathic Subglottic Stenosis

Although it has not been proven that laryngopharyngeal reflux is the cause of ISS it may be a contributing factor.[12,16,17] 24-hour pH probe testing should be performed to determine the nature and extent of reflux. Patients with a positive 24-hour pH probe study should be treated with twice-daily proton-pump inhibitors or be considered for surgical management of reflux. Subglottic dilation with or without radial CO_2 laser incisions can be used to treat the stenosis. The procedure is the same as that described earlier. Again, stenoses that are likely to fail endoscopic treatment are those that are complex, circumferential, or greater than 1 cm in length.[12] Patients who are not cured by a few endoscopic procedures are likely to undergo repeat endoscopic treatments for progressive recurrence without cure.[12,13] In those cases, laryngotracheal resection of the stenosis is an appealing option. One can expect a long-term cure by LTR in 90% of patients.[13] LTR is contraindicated if inflammation extends to just below or involves the vocal folds. In such a case the patient should undergo repeat palliative dilations until the inflammation resolves.

Stenting

Airway stents are used to keep the airway open in benign laryngotracheal stenosis. They can be used temporarily when the patient is awaiting reconstructive surgery or permanently when either the stenosis is inoperable or the patient is a poor surgical candidate. Although the role of stenting in malignant airway compromise is fairly well established, it remains controversial in the management of benign disease.

The Montogomery T-tube is the most familiar stent used by otolaryngologists. It is a silicone tube placed via a tracheotomy. The length of the tube is fashioned so that it extends over all areas of stenosis and tracheal malacia. After placement, its position is endoscopically confirmed. If the tube must extend to the conus elasticus then the proximal end is brought through the true vocal folds to just below the false vocal folds. This helps decrease granulation tissue that often results when the top of the tube intrudes on the conus elasticus. Despite accurate placement 20% of the time the tube does not create a reliable airway. Failure is usually secondary to tube obstruction from granulation tissue.[80]

Endoluminal stents are also used. These are placed endoscopically. They are held in place by pressure exerted on the tracheal wall. The Dumon stent is a static stent made of silicone.[81] It has studs on the external surface to prevent dislodgement. The most common major complication from this stent is migration that requires repositioning under general anesthesia. Occasionally this can be an emergency due to resultant airway compromise. This migration occurs 20% of the time when used for benign stenoses.[82] As a result of this deficiency, dynamic stents that hold their position by applying radial force on the tracheal wall have been developed. Unfortunately, these stents are also fraught with the complications of granulation tissue, chronic infection, new strictures, and bronchoesophageal fistulae.[83] Due to the stent's impact on previously uninvolved airway, segmental tracheal resection may no longer be an option following stenting. As a result of the difficulties with endoluminal stents in benign airway obstruction, they are generally reserved as a secondary options or for palliation in malignant conditions.

Review Questions

1. A 66-year-old man is now 6 months status-post hospitalization following a subdural hematoma. He was "trached" during his intensive care period and was decannulated 2 months later. Cardiac and pulmonary function are fair. His vocal folds are mobile on flexible laryngoscopy. At direct laryngoscopy, you note one abnormality, as pictured below. This extends from 3.5 cm to 5.5 cm below the vocal folds. The stenosis is quite firm to palpation. You recommend:

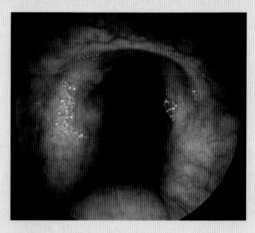

   a. Laser incision and dilation
   b. Tracheal resection and primary anastomosis
   c. Tracheal resection and hilar release for thoracic extent of stenosis
   d. Tracheotomy
   e. Stent placement

2. Mitomycin-C:
   a. Synthetic chemical that kills only fibroblasts
   b. Synthetic chemical that preferentially inhibits fibroblasts
   c. Antibiotic that kills only epithelial cells
   d. Antibiotic that kills only fibroblasts
   e. Antibiotic that preferentially inhibits fibroblasts

3. Whited, in his landmark paper,[5] estimated that _____% of patients will develop laryngotracheal stenosis following intubation for 10 days?
   a. 4
   b. 8
   c. 12
   d. 16
   e. 20

4. A patient presents with bilateral true vocal fold paralysis from thyroidectomy 2 years ago. She is 45 years old and has a family history of coronary artery disease. She undergoes the following procedure for decannulation (see picture below). This represents a:

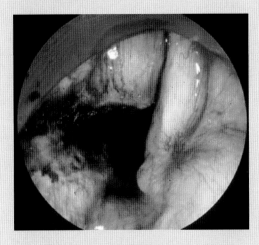

a. Left medial arytenoidectomy; her voice will be normal
b. Left medial arytenoidectomy; her voice will be impaired
c. Left posterior cordotomy; her voice will be normal
d. Left posterior cordotomy; her voice will be impaired
e. Left posterior vocal lateralization with suture; her voice will be impaired

5. All of the following except one are known risk factors for the development of endotracheal tube-related stenosis:
a. Tube size (8.0 or greater)
b. Diabetes
c. Infection
d. Duration of intubation
e. All of the above are established risk factors

REFERENCES

1. Pena J, Cicero R, Marin J, et al. Laryngotracheal reconstruction in subglottic stenosis: an ancient problem still present. *Otolaryngol Head Neck Surg.* 2001;125:397-400.
2. Rea F, Callegaro D, Loy M, et al. Benign tracheal and laryngotracheal stenosis: surgical treatment and results. *Eur J Cardiothorac Surg.* 2002;22:352-356.
3. Donnelly W. Histopathology of endotracheal intubation: an autopsy study of 99 cases. *Arch Pathol Lab Med.* 1969;88:511-520.
4. Streitz JM Jr, Shapshay SM. Airway injury after tracheotomy and endotracheal intubation. *Surg Clin North Am.* 1991;71:1211-1230.
5. Whited RE. A prospective study of laryngotracheal sequelae in long-term intubation. *Laryngoscope.* 1984;94:367-377.
6. Koitschev A, Graumueller S, Zenner HP, et al. Tracheal stenosis and obliteration above the tracheostoma after percutaneous dilational tracheostomy. *Crit Care Med.* 2003;31:1574-1576.
7. Bartels S, Mayberry JC, Goldman RK, et al. Tracheal stenosis after percutaneous dilational tracheotomy. *Otolaryngol Head Neck Surg.* 2002;126:58-62.
8. Delaere P, Feenstra L. Management of acute laryngeal trauma. *Acta Otorhinolaryngol Belg.* 1995;49:347-349.
9. Lebovics RS, Hoffman GS, Leavitt RY, et al. The management of subglottic stenosis in patients with Wegener's granulomatosis. *Laryngoscope.* 1992;102:1341-1345.
10. Langford CA, Sneller MC, Hallahan CW, et al. Clinical features and therapeutic management of subglottic stenosis in patients with Wegener's granulomatosis. *Arthritis Rheum.* 1996;39:1754-1760.
11. Gluth MB, Shinners PA, Kasperbauer JL. Subglottic stenosis associated with Wegener's granulomatosis. *Laryngoscope.* 2003;113:1304-1307.
12. Valdez TA, Shapshay SM. Idiopathic subglottic stenosis revisited. *Ann Otol Rhinol Laryngol.* 2002;111:690-695.
13. Dedo HH, Catten MD. Idiopathic progressive subglottic stenosis: findings and treatment in 52 patients. *Ann Otol Rhinol Laryngol.* 2001;110:305-311.

14. Ashiku SK, Mathisen DJ. Idiopathic laryngotracheal stenosis. *Chest Surg Clin North Am.* 2003;13:257-269.

15. Benjamin B, Jacobson I, Eckstein R. Idiopathic subglottic stenosis: diagnosis and endoscopic laser treatment. *Ann Otol Rhinol Laryngol.* 1997;106:770-774.

16. Maronian NC, Azadeh H, Waugh P, et al. Association of laryngopharyngeal reflux disease and subglottic stenosis. *Ann Otol Rhinol Laryngol.* 2001;110:606-612.

17. Koufman JA. The otolaryngologic manifestations of gastroesophageal reflux disease (GERD): a clinical investigation of 225 patients using ambulatory 24-hour pH monitoring and an experimental investigation of the role of acid and pepsin in the development of laryngeal injury. *Laryngoscope.* 1991;101(suppl 53).

18. Amin MR, Simpson CB. Office evaluation of the tracheobronchial tree. *Ear Nose Throat J.* 2004; 83:10-12.

19. Grillo HC, Donahue DM, Mathisen DJ, et al. Postintubation tracheal stenosis. Treatment and results. *J Thorac Cardiovasc Surg.* 1995;109:486-492; discussion 92-93.

20. Gluecker T, Lang F, Bessler S, et al. 2D and 3D CT imaging correlated to rigid endoscopy in complex laryngo-tracheal stenoses. *Eur Radiol.* 2001;11: 50-54.

21. Konen E, Faibel M, Hoffman C, et al. Laryngo-tracheal anastomosis: postoperative evaluation by helical CT and computerized reformations. *Clin Radiol.* 2002;57:820-825.

22. McCaffrey TV. Classification of laryngotracheal stenosis. *Laryngoscope.* 1992;102:1335-1340.

23. Myer CM, 3rd, O'Connor DM, Cotton RT. Proposed grading system for subglottic stenosis based on endotracheal tube sizes. *Ann Otol Rhinol Laryngol.* 1994;103:319-323.

24. Bogdasarian RS, Olson NR. Posterior glottic laryngeal stenosis. *Otolaryngol Head Neck Surg.* 1980; 88:765-772.

25. Shapshay SM, Beamis JF, Jr., Hybels RL, et al. Endoscopic treatment of subglottic and tracheal stenosis by radial laser incision and dilation. *Ann Otol Rhinol Laryngol.* 1987;96:661-664.

26. Strong MS, Healy GB, Vaughan CW, et al. Endoscopic management of laryngeal stenosis. *Otolaryngol Clin North Am.* 1979;12:797-805.

27. Koufman JA, Thompson JN, Kohut RI. Endoscopic management of subglottic stenosis with the CO_2 surgical laser. *Otolaryngol Head Neck Surg.* 1981;89:215-220.

28. Ossoff RH, Tucker GF, Jr., Duncavage JA, et al. Efficacy of bronchoscopic carbon dioxide laser surgery for benign strictures of the trachea. *Laryngoscope.* 1985;95:1220-1223.

29. Simpson GT, Strong MS, Healy GB, et al. Predictive factors of success or failure in the endoscopic management of laryngeal and tracheal stenosis. *Ann Otol Rhinol Laryngol.* 1982;91:384-388.

30. Shapshay SM, Beamis JF, Jr., Dumon JF. Total cervical tracheal stenosis: treatment by laser, dilation, and stenting. *Ann Otol Rhinol Laryngol.* 1989; 98:890-895.

31. Shapshay SM. Laser applications in the trachea and bronchi: a comparative study of the soft tissue effects using contact and noncontact delivery systems. *Laryngoscope.* 1987;97:1-26.

32. Campbell BH, Dennison BF, Durkin GE, et al. Early and late dilatation for acquired subglottic stenosis. *Otolaryngol Head Neck Surg.* 1986;95:566-573.

33. Shapshay SM, Beamis JF Jr, Hybels RL, et al. Endoscopic treatment of subglottic and tracheal stenosis by radial laser incision and dilation. *Ann Otol Rhinol Laryngol.* 1987;96:661-664.

34. Rahbar R, Shapshay SM, Healy GB. Mitomycin: effects on laryngeal and tracheal stenosis, benefits, and complications. *Ann Otol Rhinol Laryngol.* 2001;110:1-6.

35. Rahbar R, Jones DT, Nuss RC, et al. The role of mitomycin in the prevention and treatment of scar formation in the pediatric aerodigestive tract: friend or foe? *Arch Otolaryngol. Head Neck Surg.* 2002;128:401-406.

36. Perepelitsyn I, Shapshay SM. Endoscopic treatment of laryngeal and tracheal stenosis—has mitomycin-C improved the outcome? *Otolaryngol Head Neck Surg.* 2004;131:16-20.

37. Eliashar R, Gross M, Maly B, et al. Mitomycin does not prevent laryngotracheal repeat stenosis after endoscopic dilation surgery: an animal study. *Laryngoscope.* 2004;114:743-746.

38. James JC, Simpson CB. Efficacy of topical mitomycin-C in the Endoscopic Management of Laryngotracheal Stenosis. *Laryngoscope.* In press.

39. Ubell ML, Ettema SL, Toohill RJ, et al. Mitomycin-C application in airway stenosis surgery: analysis of safety and costs. *Otolaryngol Head Neck Surg.* 2006;134:403-406.

40. Grillo HC. Primary reconstruction of airway after resection of subglottic laryngeal and upper tracheal stenosis. *Ann Thorac Surg.* 1982;33:3-18.

41. Pearson FG, Gullane P. Subglottic resection with primary tracheal anastomosis: including synchronous laryngotracheal reconstructions. *Sem Thorac Cardiovasc Surg.* 1996;8:381-391.

42. Laccourreye O, Naudo P, Brasnu D, et al. Tracheal resection with end-to-end anastomosis for isolated postintubation cervical trachea stenosis: long-term results. *Ann Otol Rhinol Laryngol.* 1996;105:944-948.

43. Donahue DM, Grillo HC, Wain JC, et al. Reoperative tracheal resection and reconstruction for unsuccessful repair of postintubation stenosis. *J Thorac Cardiovasc Surg.* 1997;114:934-938; discussion, 938-939.

44. Wolf M, Shapira Y, Talmi YP, et al. Laryngotracheal anastomosis: primary and revised procedures. *Laryngoscope.* 2001;111:622-627.

45. Maddaus MA, Toth JL, Gullane PJ, et al. Subglottic tracheal resection and synchronous laryngeal reconstruction. *J Thorac Cardiovasc Surg.* 1992; 104:1443-1450.

46. Wain JC. Postintubation tracheal stenosis. *Chest Surg Clin North Am.* 2003;13:231-246.

47. Salassa JR PB, Payne WS. Gross and microscopical blood supply of the trachea. *Ann Thorac Surg.* 1977;24:100-107.

48. Montgomery WW. Suprahyoid release for tracheal anastomosis. *Arch Otolaryngol.* 1974;99:255-260.

49. Grillo HC. Primary reconstruction of airway after resection of subglottic laryngeal and upper tracheal stenosis. *Ann Thorac Surg.* 1982;33:3-18.

50. Grillo HC, Mathisen DJ, Wain JC. Laryngotracheal resection and reconstruction for subglottic stenosis. *Ann Thorac Surg.* 1992;53:54-63.

51. Har-El G, Krespi YP, Goldsher M. The combined use of muscle flaps and alloplasts for tracheal reconstruction. *Arch Otolaryngol. Head Neck Surg.* 1989;115:1310-1313.

52. McCaffrey TV. Management of laryngotracheal stenosis on the basis of site and severity. *Otolaryngol Head Neck Surg.* 1993;109:468-473.

53. Lano CF, Jr., Duncavage JA, Reinisch L, et al. Laryngotracheal reconstruction in the adult: a ten-year experience. *Ann Otol Rhinol Laryngol.* 1998; 107:92-97.

54. Gavilan J, Cerdeira MA, Toledano A. Surgical treatment of laryngotracheal stenosis: a review of 60 cases. *Ann Otol Rhinol Laryngol.* 1998;107: 588-592.

55. Rhee JS, Toohill RJ. Single-stage adult laryngotracheal reconstruction without stenting. *Laryngoscope.* 2001;111:765-768.

56. McCaffrey TV. Management of subglottic stenosis in the adult. *Ann Otol Rhinol Laryngol.* 1991; 100:90-94.

57. Duncavage JA, Koriwchak MJ. Open surgical techniques for laryngotracheal stenosis. *Otolaryngol Clin North Am.* 1995;28:785-795.

58. Duncavage JA, Ossoff RH, Toohill RJ. Laryngotracheal reconstruction with composite nasal septal cartilage grafts. *Ann Otol Rhinol Laryngol.* 1989; 98:581-585.

59. Grillo HC, Zannini P, Michelassi F. Complications of tracheal reconstruction. Incidence, treatment, and prevention. *J Thorac Cardiovasc Surg.* 1986; 91:322-328.

60. Grillo HC, Donahue DM, Mathiesen DJ, et al. Postintubation tracheal stenosis. Treatment and results. *J Thorac Cardiovasc Surg.* 1995;109: 486-492; discussion, 492-493.

61. Peskind SP, Stanley RB, Jr., Thangathurai D. Treatment of the compromised trachea with sleeve resection and primary repair. *Laryngoscope.* 1993;103:203-211.

62. Grillo HC. Surgical treatment of postintubation tracheal injuries. *J Thorac Cardiovasc Surg.* 1979; 78:860-875.

63. Merati AL, Rieder AA, Patel N, et al. Does successful segmental tracheal resection require releasing maneuvers? *Otolaryngol Head Neck Surg.* 2005; 133:372-376.

64. Mouney DF, Lyons GD. Fixation of laryngeal stents. *Laryngoscope.* 1985;95:905-907.

65. Mouney DF, Lyons GD. Fixation of laryngeal stents. *Laryngoscope.* 1985;95:905-907.

66. Lichtenberger G. Comparison of endoscopic glottis-dilating operations. *Eur Arch Otorhinolaryngol.* 2003;260:57-61.

67. Lichtenberger G, Toohill RJ. The endo-extralaryngeal needle carrier. *Otolaryngol Head Neck Surg.* 1991;105:755-756.

68. Isshiki N, Taira T, Nose K, et al. Surgical treatment of laryngeal web with mucosa graft. *Ann Otol Rhinol Laryngol.* 1991;100:95-100.

69. Goldberg AN. Endoscopic postcricoid advancement flap for posterior glottic stenosis. *Laryngoscope.* 2000;110:482-485.

70. Ossoff RH, Karlan MS, Sisson GA. Endoscopic laser arytenoidectomy. *Lasers Surg Med* 1983;2: 293-299.

71. Ossoff RH, Duncavage JA, Shapshay SM, et al. Endoscopic laser arytenoidectomy revisited. *Ann Otol Rhinol Laryngol.* 1990;99:764-771.

72. Rontal M, Rontal E. Endoscopic laryngeal surgery for bilateral midline vocal cord obstruction. *Ann Otol Rhinol Laryngol.* 1990;99:605-610.

73. Benninger MS, Bhattacharya N., Fried MP. Surgical management for bilateral vocal fold immobility. *Op Tech Otolaryngol Head Neck Surg.* 1998;9:1-8.

74. Remacle M, Lawson G, Mayne A, et al. Subtotal carbon dioxide laser arytenoidectomy by endoscopic approach for treatment of bilateral cord immobility in adduction. *Ann Otol Rhinol Laryngol.* 1996;105:438-445.

75. Kashima HK. Bilateral vocal fold motion impairment: pathophysiology and management by transverse cordotomy. *Ann Otol Rhinol Laryngol.* 1991;100:717-721.

76. Dennis DP, Kashima H. Carbon dioxide laser posterior cordectomy for treatment of bilateral vocal cord paralysis. *Ann Otol Rhinol Laryngol.* 1989;98:930-934.

77. Eckel HE, Thumfart M, Wassermann K, et al. Cordectomy versus arytenoidectomy in the management of bilateral vocal cord paralysis. *Ann Otol Rhinol Laryngol.* 1994;103:852-857.

78. Gregor RT. The use of carbon dioxide laser in dealing with fibrous strictures of the larynx and trachea. *J Otolaryngol.* 1988;17:16-18.

79. Montgomery WW. The surgical management of supraglottic and subglottic stenosis. *Ann Otol Rhinol Laryngol.* 1968;77:534-546.

80. Gaissert HA, Grillo HC, Mathisen DJ, et al. Temporary and permanent restoration of airway continuity with the tracheal T-tube. *J Thorac Cardiovasc Surg.* 1994;107:600-606.

81. Dumon JF. A dedicated tracheobronchial stent. *Chest.* 1990;97:328-332.

82. Noppen M, Meysman M, Claes I, et al. Screwthread vs Dumon endoprosthesis in the management of tracheal stenosis. *Chest.* 1999;115:532-535.

83. Gaissert HA, Grillo HC, Wright CD, et al. Complication of benign tracheobronchial strictures by self-expanding metal stents. *J Thorac Cardiovasc Surg.* 2003;126:744-747.

27

Surgery for Swallowing Disorders and Aspiration

Albert L. Merati, MD, FACS
Sachin Pawar, BBA

KEY POINTS

■ Relatively few patients with swallowing disorders require surgical management for these conditions.

■ Most laryngeal procedures for dysphagia and aspiration are to reduce or eliminate glottic insufficiency; most pharyngeal and esophageal procedures facilitate outflow to the esophagus.

■ Aspiration pneumonia following stroke is the leading source of morbidity and mortality related to the clinical field of laryngology.

■ There is little clinical evidence that dilation is an effective treatment for cricopharyngeal achalasia; botulinum toxin injection and cricopharyngeal myotomy are reasonable treatment options.

■ Zenker's diverticula can be managed endoscopically or transcervically; both are effective. Although the endoscopic approach appears to be quicker and have fewer complications, the long-term results are not fully described.

Swallowing disorders are responsible for the principal morbidity and mortality encountered in laryngology patients. In fact, more patients die of aspiration pneumonia complicating stroke each year than from all cases of head and neck cancer combined. Although voice is the issue most closely identified with the field of laryngology, the maintenance of safe oral intake and secretion management must be considered in all patients. The anatomy and physiology of swallowing has been discussed in previous sections of this textbook. In this chapter, operative intervention for swallowing and aspiration is reviewed.

This chapter is divided into sections by anatomic region. First, interventions directed at the oral cavity and salivary glands are outlined. The larynx and pharynx are presented next, followed by a discussion of surgical management for cricopharyngeal and esophageal disorders, particularly *cricopharyngeal achalasia* and *Zenker's diverticulum*.

THERAPEUTIC OPTIONS IN SWALLOWING DISORDERS

It is difficult to distill the management of dysphagia and aspiration into a simple decision tree. The bulk of this chapter focuses on surgical intervention although only a *minority* of patients require operative management of dysphagia. In fact, many patients with profound sensory and motor deficits may be restricted to enteral feeding via a gastrostomy tube. A significant portion of patients with dysphagia, particularly those with progressive neurodegenerative disorders, never recover from this state. Most stroke patients, however, will improve over time, with over 87% of survivors in a recent report returning to their prestroke diet.[1] Notably, more than 20% of the patients in this study developed pneumonia in the 6 months following stroke.

A complete review of nonoperative therapy for these disorders is beyond the scope of this chapter. However, important fundamentals are worth noting. Although an oral diet may be a long-term goal for an acutely or chronically dys-

phagic patient, the safety and benefit of enteral feeding must not be forgotten; even the route of feeding may matter. Norton, in a randomized, prospective study of dysphagic stroke patients in the United Kingdom, compared percutaneous enteral gastrostomy (PEG) feeding to traditional nasogastric feeding in a cohort of patients and noted significant less morbidity and *mortality* in the PEG patients.[2]

ORAL CAVITY AND SALIVARY GLANDS

It is important to distinguish the clinical management of drooling, or *ptyalism*, from aspiration related to copious oral secretions. Cerebral palsy represents the major category of patients with the primary complaint of ptyalism. Although the underlying disorders may be different, the surgical interventions for excessive saliva contributing to aspiration are similar to those for drooling.

The salivary glands produce 1.5 liters of saliva each day. Proper handling of saliva is critical for the avoidance of aspiration. Oral hygiene has been shown to be important in reducing the incidence and virulence of aspiration pneumonia.[3] Dental care and even extraction of suspect teeth may be of some benefit in patients prone to aspiration. Simple clinical inspection of dental status is quite predictive of bacterial load for patients at risk.[4]

For excessive oral secretions, therapeutic interventions include gland excision, salivary duct ligation and redirection, and chemical denervation of salivary flow using botulinum toxin.

Due to the intimate relationship of the parotid gland to the facial nerve, parotidectomy is not performed for excessive salivation or aspiration. *Salivary duct ligation*, however, has been advocated for years. The concern over secondary sialadenitis is significant, although a recent series reported on four-duct ligation (bilateral submandibular and bilateral parotid). In this study, only 1 of 21 patients developed postoperative sialadenitis, although several had prolonged salivary gland swelling.[5] In the same retrospective study, 81% of patients/families described some qualitative benefit from the procedure.

In one of the larger series published to date (again in the pediatric population), Greensmith prospectively analyzed results from 72 patients undergoing surgery for drooling.[6] All patients underwent submandibular duct transposition (to the posterolateral oral cavity); the secondary procedures were *either* sublingual gland excision or parotid duct ligation. The authors reported superior long-term results when combining sublingual gland excision with submandibular diversion.

Similar results have not been reported for surgical management of excessive salivation in adults. Botulinum toxin injection, predicated on the chemical blockade of postganglionic discharge from peripheral parasympathetic nerve supply to the salivary glands, has fostered some investigation as well as clinical usage. Botulinum toxin can be given by percutaneous injection into the submandibular (or parotid) gland with excellent efficacy and safety.[7] Electromyography is not necessary but may be useful to avoid injection into the mimetic or deglutitive musculature. A recent double-blind, placebo-controlled study has presented positive experiences with this approach in Parkinson's patients with hypersalivation.[8] It should be noted that these studies evaluate drooling alone and do not evaluate affects on aspiration. Although it is tempting to apply these principles to reduce salivary aspiration in the dysphagic patient, this has not been formally studied.

PHARYNX

Few surgical procedures of the pharynx and related structures address swallowing dysfunction. Stenosis of the pharynx, as seen following surgery or chemoradiation, may benefit from treatment by a variety of pharyngoplastic procedures, laser surgery, or dilation. Very little formal study of the outcomes for these interventions has been reported. Two areas of pharyngeal surgery are discussed in this section, velopharyngeal insufficiency and reduction pharyngoplasty for the flaccid hemipharynx following long-standing vagal paralysis.

Velopharyngeal insufficiency (VPI) is a condition in which the valve function of the soft palate, or *velum*, is impaired. It may occur as part of a cleft disorder, cranial nerve dysfunction, or following oncologic surgery of the head and neck. The principal symptom of VPI is hypernasality. VPI may also contribute to dysphagia as food and liquids pass into the nasopharynx upon pharyngeal contraction. Although palatal lift prosthetics may be beneficial to patients with a neurologically impaired but anatomically intact soft palate, augmentation of the posterior pharyngeal wall (Figure 27–1) to allow better contact to the weakened soft palate can be a useful procedure in selected cases.

Injection pharyngoplasty is an old procedure. Like injection laryngoplasty, the concept of augmenting an immobile structure to enhance closure of an incompetent or insufficient valve has been around for over a century. Remacle was one of the first modern authors to advocate injection pharyngoplasty, with the use of a cross-linked collagen[9] for augmentation. More durable materials, such as Radiesse (Bioform, Franksville, Wisc), a preparation of calcium hydroxylapatite,

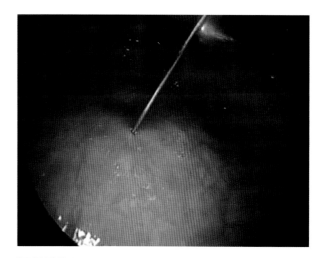

FIGURE 27–1. Transoral injection pharyngoplasty. The view is with a 70-degree endoscope looking back up into the nasopharynx. This photo was taken in the OR under general anesthesia. This procedure can also be performed transorally in the clinic setting.

can also be used (see Figure 27-1). Permanent closure of a unilateral soft palate weakness can be accomplished through the palatal adhesion procedure described by Netterville.[10,11] In this procedure, one area of the flaccid palate is closed in layers to the posterior pharynx to make a permanent contact point, or adhesion. This allows for reduction of velopharyngeal reflux without compromising the nasal airway (Figure 27-2). In his most recent report, Netterville noted that 96% of the patients had a decrease in their velopharyngeal insufficiency following the procedure.

A promising intervention for patients with flaccid paralysis affecting the pharynx is the hypopharyngeal pharyngoplasty described by Mok and Woo. The pathophysiology addressed by this procedure is the patulous hemipharynx in the dysphagia patient, typically following vagal paralysis. In these cases, the denervated pharynx becomes atonic and eventually dilates; it becomes a receptacle of the food bolus upon swallowing. It is believed that reducing the volume and capacity of the flaccid side will help direct food toward the esophageal introitus.[12] In their original series, 8 of the 9 patients reported improvement in swallowing function with no operative complications (Figure 27-3).

LARYNX

When laryngeal surgery is directed at swallowing rehabilitation, the usual aim is to improve glottic competence to some degree. Occasionally, the objective of the procedure is to close off the laryngeal airway entirely, thus sacrificing oral and nasal breathing (and necessitating *tracheotomy* or *tracheostomy*) and accepting alaryngeal communication as a trade-off.

The management of laryngeal paralysis was described in chapter 17. Again, speech and swal-

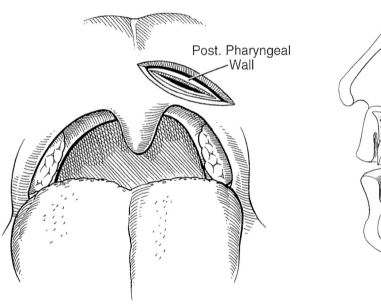

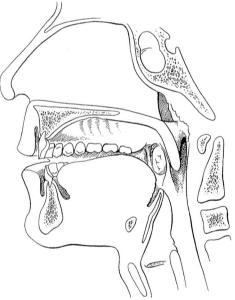

A.

B.

FIGURE 27–2. A. The palatal incision for the adhesion is created from the midline to the lateral aspect of the paralyzed side. The incision traverses all layers of the palate to allow access to the posterior pharyngeal wall for the adhesion procedure. **B.** A parasagittal view through the palate showing the healed adhesion on the weak side. The nasal airway remains patent on either side of the adhesion. (Reprinted with permission from Carrau R, Murry M. *Comprehensive Management of Swallowing Disorders.* San Diego, Calif: Plural Publishing, Inc; 1996:311.)

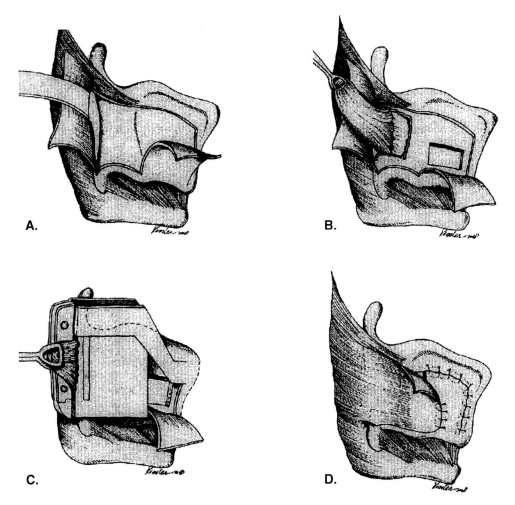

FIGURE 27–3. Hypopharyngeal pharyngoplasty after Mok and Woo. This series of diagrams shows a right-sided procedure. **A.** The posterior aspect of the thyroid lamina is exposed. **B.** The redundant mucosa is pulled through this posterior thyrotomy access. **C.** The redundant mucosa is resected with a GI stapling device. **D.** The area is then reinforced by replacing the constrictor muscle.

lowing therapy play an important role in the management of laryngeal paralysis. A recent publication focusing on the swallowing issues of laryngeal paralysis patients reported that a majority of patients benefited from swallowing evaluation and therapy.[13] Surgical treatment of laryngeal paralysis as it relates to dysphagia is worthy of review. Although *injection laryngoplasty* (Figures 27–4A and 27–4B) is a commonly performed procedure for voice and swallowing complaints related to paralysis, its benefit for the patients with dysphagia may be limited. Bhattacharyya, in an important 2002 study, reported on a large

series of patients undergoing medialization, either with injection augmentation or laryngeal framework surgery.[14] As measured by a penetration/ aspiration scale of video swallow study results, the 23 patients studied continued to demonstrate significant swallowing abnormalities following medialization. This finding was independent of the etiology of paralysis or the method of medialization. Framework surgery has been advocated in many clinical instances, such as following thoracic surgery[15]; the results for voice are excellent, the effect on swallowing function is usually positive, although this is not as well studied.

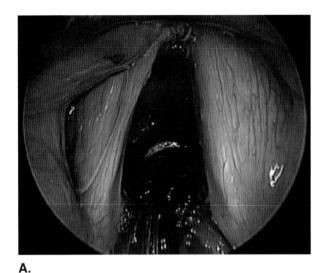

A.

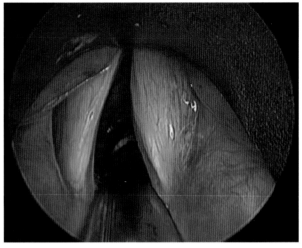

B.

FIGURE 27–4. Glottic injection laryngoplasty for the right true vocal fold paralysis shown before (**A**) and after (**B**) injection. The laryngoscope is retracting the right false fold to allow better exposure, thus making the right side appear more bulky than the left.

Laryngeal Closure Procedures

When swallowing function is not amenable to rehabilitation, or the risk of aspiration is extremely high, several more advanced options are available for the laryngeal surgeon. The key distinction among these procedures is whether or not they can be reversed. Although many of the underlying clinical conditions are unlikely to improve spontaneously, a determination of the chances of recovery must be made prior to performing one of these procedures. With all of these closure procedures, the patient must have a tracheotomy for breathing.

Perhaps the simplest procedure for obstructing the larynx to reduce aspiration is the temporary placement of an occluding stent.[16] The prototypical scenario is a neurologically impaired patient who requires tracheotomy for pulmonary toilet—in the situation where there is a reasonable chance of neurologic recovery, an occluding stent can theoretically reduce salivary soilage during this time. Although this procedure retains some hope of meaningful oral intake, only 8 of 25 patients eventually resumed an oral diet in a report by Weisberger.[16]

Another reversible procedure is the epiglottic oversew procedure[17] (Figure 27–5) in which a retroverted epiglottis is closed on the aryepiglottic folds. This allows for speech through the posterior interarytenoid area. The efficacy of this procedure has never been formally studied.

Glottic closure can also be accomplished by the Montgomery technique[18] in which the vocal folds are denuded through a laryngosfissure and closed to each other. The distinction from the above procedure, is the irreversibility of the procedure and the inability to phonate (Figures 27–6A and 27–6B).

Laryngeal Diversion and Laryngectomy

There are two versions of the *laryngotracheal separation* procedure[19,20] (Figures 27–7A and 27–7B; in both, the basic concept is to separate the mouth and pharynx from the lungs by dividing the trachea and bringing the distal trachea out as a stoma. In Lindeman's original description[19], the proximal trachea was anastomosed to the cervical esophagus. Another option was to bring the proximal trachea out to the skin

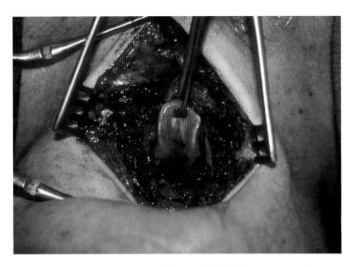

FIGURE 27–5. Epiglottic oversew. The epiglottis is exposed transcervically via a suprahyoid approach. This view is from the head of the operating table. The edges of the epiglottis are then demucosalized; it is closed to the epiglottic folds, which have been demucosalized to allow for the epiglottis to heal.

FIGURE 27–6. Montgomery closure technique. Following laryngofissure, the glottic mucosa is denuded and these sutures are placed.

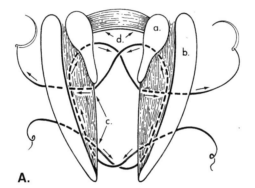

A.

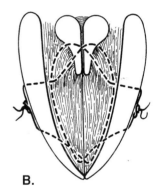

B.

(Figure 27–8). Most surgeons, however, favor closure of the proximal trachea as a blind pouch. Although leakage from the blind proximal stump or persistent retention of secretions in the tracheal remnant has been a concern with this modification, it has not been a common clinical issue.[21] The laryngotracheal separation is reversible, although the situation in which the patient needs reversal is rare. The clinical indication for this procedure involves forgoing voice for the sake of a safe and secure airway. It should be noted that many patients who are candidates for a laryngotracheal separation procedure are also dysarthric from their underlying disorder and may not speak intelligibly or communicate meaningfully. In the case where voice is desired and articulation is adequate following separation, reports have detailed successful restoration of tracheo-tracheal[22] and tracheoesophageal[23] speech by fistula creation, such as in alaryngeal speech following laryngectomy. Finally, the definitive procedure for intractable aspiration is *laryngectomy*. Of course, this procedure is irreversible but no more definitive than the separation described above. Due to the uncertainty of neurologic recovery, very few patients are willing to accept this irreversible procedure, even with life-threatening aspiration.

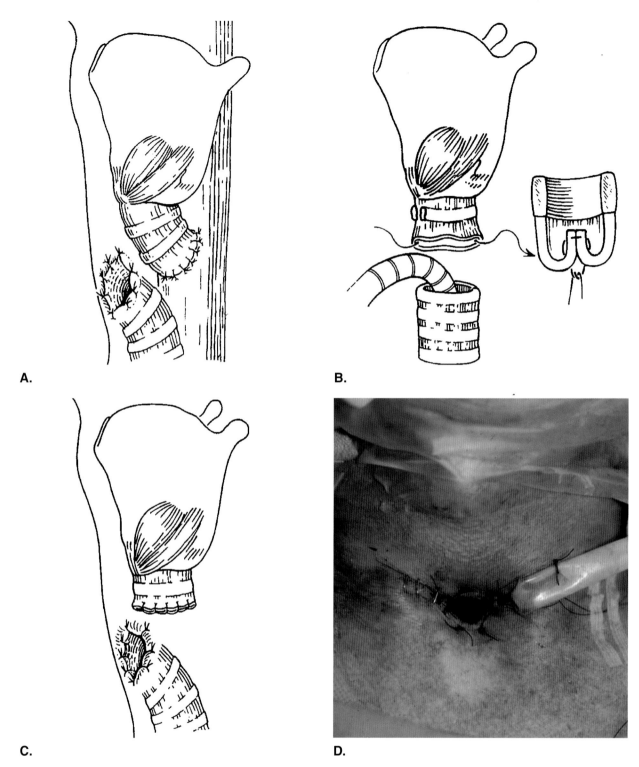

A.

B.

C.

D.

FIGURE 27–7. A. Laryngotracheal diversion (standard Lindeman procedure) involves the creation of an anastomosis between the subglottic trachea and the esophagus, and a permanent stoma from the distal trachea. **B.** and **C.** With laryngotracheal separation (modified Lindeman procedure), the proximal subglottic trachea is closed as a blind pouch and a permanent stoma is created from the distal trachea. (Reprinted from Carrau R, Murry T. *Comprehensive Management of Swallowing Disorders.* San Diego, Calif: Plural Publishing; 1996:314). **D.** The immediate postoperative appearance of the laryngotracheal separation procedure. The incision is not much more than needed for a tracheotomy. This was a 46-year-old ALS patient who was ambulatory but could not speak.

384

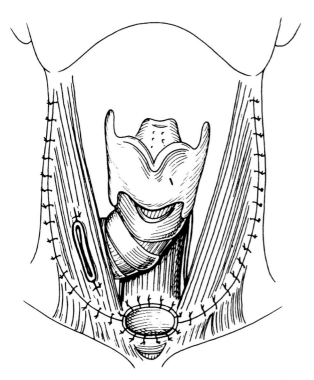

FIGURE 27–8. Laryngotrachal separation with a proximal tracheal stoma for secretions.

CERVICAL ESOPHAGUS/ UPPER ESOPHAGEAL SPHINCTER

In addition to the treatment of stenosis of the cervical esophagus by dilation, surgical procedures for dysphagia are most commonly performed for this area than any other. The two principal diagnoses reviewed in this section are *cricopharyngeal achalasia* and *Zenker's diverticulum.*

Nonsurgical therapy is a better established option for many cases of cervical dysphagia.[24] One recent important development has been the advent of the Shaker exercises, in which the patient is asked to perform repetitive head lifts from a recumbent position[25]; this is aimed at strengthening the suprahyoid muscles to elevate the larynx more effectively and enhance the passive opening of the UES. This has been shown in several excellent studies to be a promising adjunct for these patients.[26,27]

Dilation

It seems that a significant number of patients undergoing diagnostic endoscopy of the esophagus also receive therapeutic dilation directed at the upper esophageal sphincter. What is the basis for this? Diagnostic esophagoscopy is one of the most common procedures performed; the exact percentage of these patients who also undergo dilation is not known. There is very little evidence to support this common practice of dilation for nonstenotic dysphagia. In one of the few publications on this matter, 5 of 29 dysphagia patients in a Hungarian series underwent pneumatic dilation for what was described as "primary cricopharyngeal dysfunction." The diagnoses were based on radiographic imaging. Of the 5 patients dilated, 4 required no further treatment with a mean of 21 months follow-up.[28] In another series, 3 of 6 patients followed for more than 8 months had symptomatic relief dysphagia following dilation for signs of cricopharyngeal dysfunction (cricopharyngeal bar) seen on modified barium swallow.[29] Although this is promising pilot data, further investigation supporting this common procedure would be welcomed.

Botulinum Toxin Injection

For several years, botulinum toxin injection has been advocated for the management of cricopharyngeal achalasia. The basis of this approach is to interrupt the tonic contraction of the UES and allow for easier bolus transport across this segment. Though this can be performed endoscopically[30] or percutaneously in the awake patient[31] (Figures 27-9A and 27-9B); there is no clear benefit to one over the other. In Murry's review, 12 of 13 patients demonstrated improvement on the penetration/aspiration scale following injection of botulinum toxin,[31] quite similar to the results from the endoscopic approach.[30] The effects are not long lasting and may persist for 3 to 6 months. This treatment may be valuable in transient cricopharyngeal dysfunction or in patients who are apprehensive or too frail to undergo open cricopharyngeal myotomy. Patients may be

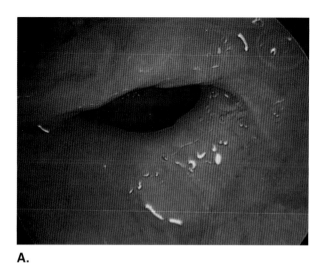
A.

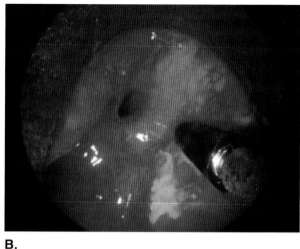
B.

FIGURE 27–9. Endoscopic view of the upper esophageal sphincter. **A.** Prior to botulinum toxin injection. **B.** During botulinum toxin injection.

"tested" for a possible response to cricopharyngeal botulinum toxin (and myotomy) by injecting the upper esophageal sphincter percutaneously with lidocaine, as described in chapter 16. The chapter authors use 2% plain lidocaine and ask the patient to try to eat different consistencies of food. The patients may report subjective changes to the physician; another option is to perform the "diagnostic" injection in the radiology suite and compare the fluoroscopic swallowing images before and after injection. This has not been studied formally.

Cricopharyngeal Myotomy

The traditional intervention for spasm or hyperfunction at the upper esophageal sphincter is the cricopharyngeal myotomy. In this procedure, a bougie or some other tubular structure (dilator, endotracheal tube) is placed in the esophagus endoscopically. Following this, the neck is opened and the viscerovertebral angle is bluntly dissected down to the muscular layer of the pharynx and esophagus. The thyroid gland often overlies the muscular layer. Once the fascia overlying the cricopharyngeus is dissected free, a myotomy or partial myectomy is performed sharply over the bougie; at least 5 cm of muscle

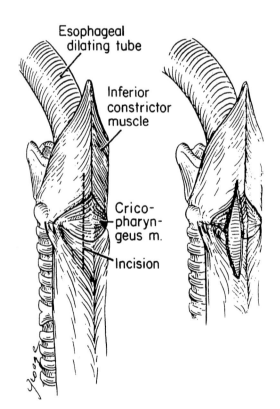

FIGURE 27–10. Posterior schematic of cricopharyngeal myotomy. With the bougie in place, the pharyngoesophageal junction is palpated; the fibers of the UES zone are sharply divided over at least 5 cm. (Reprinted from Carrau R, Murry M. *Comprehensive Management of Swallowing Disorders.* San Diego, Calif: Plural Publishing; 1996:307.)

fibers are divided (Figure 27-10). Cricopharyngeal myotomy can also be performed endoscopically, typically with a CO_2 laser[32] (Figures 27-11A and 27-11B). However it is performed, myotomy is an effective method of returning the caliber of the UES to normal dimensions as determined radiographically.[33]

One of the concerns about cricopharyngeal myotomy is the removal of a barrier against reflux from the stomach and esophagus. Although this is theoretically reasonable, a recent study has shed some light on this issue. In a series of patients undergoing cricopharyngeal myotomy, Cook and colleagues performed pre- and postoperative manometry and double pH probes. The myotomy procedures were effective, with the basal UES pressures dropping from a mean of 37 ± 5 mmHg to 19 ± 3 mmHg, a drop of 49%.[34] Even following this reduction of the UES protective barrier to reflux, the pharyngeal probe (above the cricopharyngeus) did not record a significant amount of reflux—even in the face of positive esophageal reflux events.

Surgery for Zenker's Diverticulum

Although surgical therapy continues to be the mainstay of patient management, the approach to the surgical patient has changed in the past few years. It is widely believed that the key step to any procedure for the treatment of Zenker's diverticulum is division or relief of the hyperfunctional cricopharyngeus muscle For decades, the endoscopic "Dohlman" or diathermy procedure had fallen out of favor.[35] The open diverticulectomy with or without cricopharyngeal myotomy had nearly completely replaced this approach. In recent years, the endoscopic approach has become more popular again. The endoscopic procedure depends on division of the party wall, or region between the Zenker's sac and the native esophagus (Figure 27-12). The hyperfunctional cricopharyngeus muscle represents the bulk of the tissue between the cricopharyngeus and Zenker's sac. Because the transoral approach is a midline procedure, the risk for recurrent laryngeal nerve injury is believed to be lower. This diverticulotomy (which includes a cricopharyngeal myotomy) can be accomplished with a CO_2[36] or KTP laser,[37] or with the endoscopic stapler.[37-39] In addition, advocates of the endoscopic approach point to reduced operative time and reduced morbidity for the endoscopic approach over the open technique.

Narne and colleagues, in 1999, reported on 102 patients treated with the endoscopic stapler.[38]

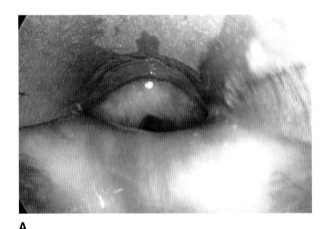

A.

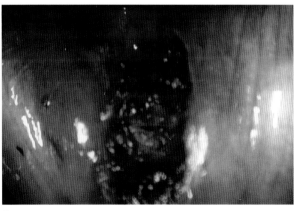

B.

FIGURE 27–11. A. Endoscopic view of cricopharyngeus prior to laser myotomy. The upper blade of the laryngoscope is placed into the esophagus and tension is created on the posterior aspect of the esophageal introitus. **B.** Using a CO_2 laser, an excision of the mucosa and muscles is undertaken to interrupt the circular fibers of the cricopharyngeal muscle.

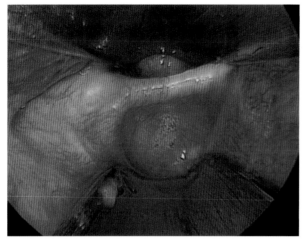

A.

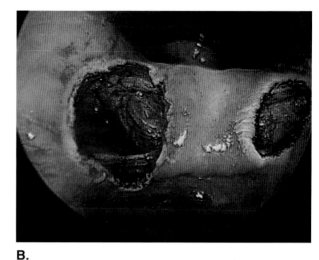

B.

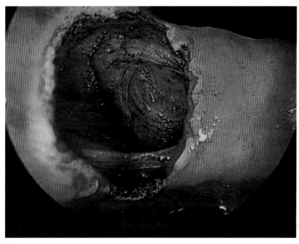

C.

FIGURE 27–12. Endoscopic Zenker's diverticulotomy with cricopharyngeal myotomy. This may be performed with an endoscopic stapler or with the laser (CO_2 or KTP). In this case, the CO_2 laser was used. **A.** Initial endoscopic view with a large sac; in this revision case, the cricopharyngeal "bar" was relatively narrow. **B.** Both sides are dissected. The central bar between the two lateral incisions is removed following distal horizontal laser cut. **C.** Closeup of the left side revealing the cricopharyngeal fibers.

They noted that the vast majority of patients required at least two cartridges to be used. Some have suggested that smaller diverticula are, paradoxically, more difficult to treat with the stapler technique as the region between the Zenker's sac and esophagus cannot be easily engaged prior to firing the stapler. The laser has been recommended by practitioners in these cases. Hoffmann and colleagues reported on a series of 103 patients, in which 90% had sustained improvement at one-year follow-up.[40]

With regard to comparative efficacy of the endoscopic and open procedures, several observations have emerged from a thorough comparative study by Chang et al.[41] In this retrospective review, it was concluded that there are benefits to the endoscopic approach, including reduced morbidity and a faster operative time. However, the authors stated that there may be a higher rate of persistence or recurrence with the endoscopic approach. Witterick and colleagues recently reported on a series of 18 patients undergoing open diverticulectomy and cricopharyngeal myotomy in which routine postoperative swallow studies were performed.[42] Eight of the 18 (44%) had persistent diverticula, although there was little association between symptomatic improvement and objective radiographic abnormalities. The authors concluded that postoperative radiography may be misleading and suggested that subjective outcomes may better reflect the success of the surgery.

Tracheotomy and Its Impact on Laryngeal Function

Tracheotomy is thought of by many physicians and speech-language pathologists as a procedure that may benefit the aspirating patient. It is true that a patient with a tracheotomy may be suctioned more easily. The point that is often lost, however, is that the very presence of a tracheotomy tube may have significant *negative* impact on laryngeal function. This occurs due to alterations of laryngeal afferent sensation, efferent activity, and the mechanics of swallowing.[43] Principally, a tracheotomy tethers the cervical skin to the trachea which interferes with the elevation of the hyolaryngeal complex required for normal swallowing.

Sasaki provided much of the basic science research along these lines, first showing that laryngeal opening is impaired following tracheotomy, believed to be a result of bypassing the upper airway and removing resistance normally sensed by thoracic receptors.[44] This vagally mediated thoracic reflex drives the posterior crico-arytenoid (PCA) muscle, the only abductor of the vocal folds, to open. When a tracheotomy is in place, the PCA muscles become dysfunctional.

More significant for swallowing dysfunction, the impact of bypassing the airway is also seen in the laryngeal closure reflex. When a tracheotomy is in place, the latency and threshold of protective laryngeal closure are increased.[45] It is not difficult to extrapolate from these animal experiments to the dysfunction seen in patients with tracheotomies.

When choosing between the open and endoscopic approaches, the surgeon must consider the ease or difficulty of endoscopic exposure. If the patient has a small mouth, jaw issues, or prominent teeth, the endoscopic view may be limited. The flexibility of the cervical spine is also an issue, of course, although this affects the feasibility of both open and endoscopic approaches.

SUMMARY

In general, surgery for swallowing disorders is limited to the prevention of aspiration and the enhancement of pharyngeal outflow. There is no commonly performed procedure to enhance sensation or motor control of the oral cavity, tongue, or pharynx. Although elegant procedures such as laryngeal reinnervation are available to rehabilitate the neurologically impaired larynx, this has been studied mostly as it relates to voice, and not swallowing. In addition, though active innervation is being restored to the larynx, it does not provide for dynamic laryngeal closure (see chapter 17, Vocal Fold Paralysis). The importance of safe oral intake cannot be overestimated; although only a minority of patients with dysphagia and aspiration undergo surgery for their laryngeal and pharyngeal dysfunction, a broad knowledge of these options is critical to manage these challenging clinical cases.

Review Questions

1. A 70-year-old male has persistent dysphagia for solids. He has a history of a left laryngeal paralysis following carotid endarterectomy 1 year ago. His voice improved following his medialization laryngoplasty 3 months ago but he is still complaining of swallowing difficulties. He is generally fit and otherwise healthy except for emphysema. A common finding on his video swallow study which would suggest the need for additional surgical management is:
   a. Shunting of the food bolus from the left to the right in the pharynx; cricopharyngeal area normal
   b. Shunting of the food bolus from the right to the left in the pharynx; cricopharyngeal area fails to open adequately
   c. Shunting of the food bolus from the right to left in the pharynx; cricopharyngeal area normal
   d. Shunting of the food bolus from the left to the right in the pharynx; cricopharyngeal area fails to open adequately
   e. Postoperative mycotic aneurysm of the carotid

2. A patient with a history of chemoradiation for a T3N0 SCCa of the larynx complains of solid food dysphagia. He has gained 30 pounds since concluding his treatment. He tolerates most liquids and some solids. He is cancer-free and has no pain. He has had no pneumonia. His larynx elevates poorly on video swallow study but he does not aspirate. His UES appears normal on the study. You recommend:
   a. Cricopharyngeal myotomy
   b. Laryngectomy
   c. Shaker exercises
   d. Botulinum toxin injection to the strap muscles
   e. PEG tube

3. A 55-year-old woman with bulbar ALS is referred from her pulmonologist for tracheotomy in anticipation of planned mechanical ventilation in the future as her neuromuscular disease progresses. She is able to phonate weakly but is profoundly dysarthric. She communicates with a board; the patient and her family are interested in supportive ventilation for the long run. You recommend:
   a. Tracheotomy
   b. Tracheostomy
   c. Laryngectomy
   d. Montgomery stent and tracheotomy
   e. Laryngotracheal separation

4. A patient is drooling following oral cavity and lip cancer surgery. After a right supraomohyoid neck dissection, he is leaking saliva due to his oral incompetence. This is exacerbated by a right marginal mandibular nerve paralysis. He has undergone 4 operative procedures in the area, including two failed procedures for the restoration of oral incompetence. As an initial treatment, you recommend:
   a. Parotidectomy
   b. Left submandibular gland removal
   c. Botulinum toxin injection to the left submandibular gland
   d. Left submandibular duct diversion
   e. Low-dose radiation therapy

5. Which of the following is responsible for the most deaths every year in the United States?
   a. Oral cavity cancer
   b. Pharyngeal cancer
   c. Laryngeal cancer
   d. a, b, and c combined
   e. Aspiration pneumonia following stroke

REFERENCES

1. Mann G, Hankey GJ, Cameron D. Swallowing function after stroke: prognosis and prognostic factors at 6 months. *Stroke.* 1999;30(4):744-748.
2. Norton B, Homer-Ward M, Donnelly MT, Long RG, Holmes GK. A randomised prospective comparison of percutaneous endoscopic gastrostomy and nasogastric tube feeding after acute dysphagic stroke. *Br Med J.* 1996;312(7022):13-16
3. Terpenning MS, Taylor GW, Lopatin DE, Kerr CK, Dominguez BL, Loesche WJ. Aspiration pneumonia: dental and oral risk factors in an older veteran population. *J Am Geriatr Soc.* 2001;49(5):557-563.
4. Abe S, Ishihara K, Adachi M, Okuda K. Oral hygiene evaluation for effective oral care in preventing pneumonia in dentate elderly. *Arch Gerontol Geriatr.* 2005. [E-pub, ahead of print]
5. Shirley WP, Hill JS, Woolley AL, Wiatrak BJ. Success and complications of four-duct ligation for sialorrhea. *Int J Pediatr Otorhinolaryngol.* 2003;67(1):1-6.
6. Greensmith AL, Johnstone BR, Reid SM, Hazard CJ, Johnson HM, Reddihough DS. Prospective analysis of the outcome of surgical management of drooling in the pediatric population: a 10-year experience. *Plast Reconstr Surg.* 2005;116(5):1233-1242.
7. Lipp A, Trottenberg T, Schink T, Kupsch A, Arnold G. A randomized trial of botulinum toxin A for treatment of drooling. *Neurology.* 2003;61(9):1279-1281.
8. Lagalla G, Millevolte M, Capecci M, Provinciali L, Ceravolo MG. Botulinum toxin type A for drooling in Parkinson's disease: a double-blind, randomized, placebo-controlled study. *Mov Disord.* 2006;21(5):704-707.
9. Remacle M, Bertrand B, Eloy P, Marbaix E. The use of injectable collagen to correct velopharyngeal insufficiency. *Laryngoscope.* 1990;100(3):269-274.
10. Netterville JL, Vrabec JT. Unilateral palatal adhesion for paralysis after high vagal injury. *Arch Otolaryngol Head Neck Surg.* 1994;120(2):218-221.
11. Netterville JL, Fortune S, Stanziale S, Billante SR. Palatal adhesion: the treatment of unilateral palatal paralysis after high vagus nerve injury. *Head Neck.* 2002;24(8):721-730.
12. Mok P, Woo P, Schaefer-Mojica J. Hypopharyngeal pharyngoplasty in the management of pharyngeal paralysis: a new procedure. *Ann Otol Rhinol Laryngol.* 2003;112(10):844-852.
13. Ollivere B, Duce K, Rowlands G, Harrison P, O'Reilly BJ. Swallowing dysfunction in patients with unilateral vocal fold paralysis: aetiology and outcomes. *J Laryngol Otol.* 2006;120(1):38-41.
14. Bhattacharyya N, Kotz T, Shapiro J. Dysphagia and aspiration with unilateral vocal cord immobility: incidence, characterization, and response to surgical treatment. *Ann Otol Rhinol Laryngol.* 2002;111(8):672-679.
15. Kraus DH, Ali MK, Ginsberg RJ, et al. Vocal cord medialization for unilateral paralysis associated with intrathoracic malignancies. *J Thorac Cardiovasc Surg.* 1996;111(2):334-339; discussion, 339-341.
16. Weisberger EC. Treatment of intractable aspiration using a laryngeal stent or obturator. *Ann Otol Rhinol Laryngol.* 1991;100(2):101-107.
17. Habal MB, Murray JE. Surgical treatment of life-endangering chronic aspiration pneumonia. Use of an epiglottic flap to the arytenoids. *Plast Reconstr Surg.* 1972;49(3):305-311.
18. Montgomery WW. Surgical laryngeal closure to eliminate chronic aspiration. *N Engl J Med.* 1975;292(26):1390-1391.
19. Lindeman RC. Diverting the paralyzed larynx: a reversible procedure for intractable aspiration. *Laryngoscope.* 1975;85(1):157-180.
20. Eibling DE, Snyderman CH, Eibling C. Laryngotracheal separation for intractable aspiration: a retrospective review of 34 patients. *Laryngoscope.* 1995;105(1):83-85.
21. Yamana T, Kitano H, Hanamitsu M, Kitajima K. Clinical outcome of laryngotracheal separation for intractable aspiration pneumonia. *J Otorhinolaryngol Relat Spec.* 2001;63(5):321-324.
22. Lombard LE, Carrau RL. Tracheo-tracheal puncture for voice rehabilitation after laryngotracheal separation. *Am J Otolaryngol.* 2001;22(3):176-178.
23. Darrow DH, Robbins KT, Goldman SN. Tracheoesophageal puncture for voice restoration following laryngotracheal separation. *Laryngoscope.* 1994;104(9):1163-1166.
24. Logemann JA. Noninvasive approaches to deglutive aspiration. *Dysphagia.* 1993;8(4):331-333.
25. Shaker R, Kern M, Bardan E, et al. Augmentation of deglutitive upper esophageal sphincter opening in the elderly by exercise. *Am J Physiol.* 1997;272(6 pt 1):G1518-G1522.
26. Shaker R, Easterling C, Kern M, et al. Rehabilitation of swallowing by exercise in tube-fed patients with pharyngeal dysphagia secondary to abnormal UES opening. *Gastroenterology.* 2002;122(5):1314-1321.

27. Easterling C, Grande B, Kern M, Sears K, Shaker R. Attaining and maintaining isometric and isokinetic goals of the Shaker exercise. *Dysphagia.* 2005; 20(2):133-138.

28. Solt J, Bajor J, Moizs M, Grexa E, Horvath PO. Primary cricopharyngeal dysfunction: treatment with balloon catheter dilatation. *Gastrointest Endosc.* 2001;54(6):767-771.

29. Wang AY, Kadkade R, Kahrilas PJ, Hirano I. Effectiveness of esophageal dilation for symptomatic cricopharyngeal bar. *Gastrointest Endosc.* 2005; 61(1):148-152.

30. Parameswaran MS, Soliman AM. Endoscopic botulinum toxin injection for cricopharyngeal dysphagia. *Ann Otol Rhinol Laryngol.* 2002;111(10): 871-874.

31. Murry T, Wasserman T, Carrau RL, Castillo B. Injection of botulinum toxin A for the treatment of dysfunction of the upper esophageal sphincter. *Am J Otolaryngol.* 2005;26(3):157-162.

32. Takes RP, van den Hoogen FJ, Marres HA. Endoscopic myotomy of the cricopharyngeal muscle with CO_2 laser surgery. *Head Neck.* 2005;27(8): 703-709.

33. Yip HT, Leonard R, Kendall KA. Cricopharyngeal myotomy normalizes the opening size of the upper esophageal sphincter in cricopharyngeal dysfunction. *Laryngoscope.* 2006;116(1):93-96.

34. Williams RB, Ali GN, Hunt DR, Wallace KL, Cook IJ. Cricopharyngeal myotomy does not increase the risk of esophagopharyngeal acid regurgitation. *Am J Gastroenterol.* 1999;94(12):3448-3454.

35. Colombo-Benkmann M, Unruh V, Krieglstein C, Senninger N. Cricopharyngeal myotomy in the treatment of Zenker's diverticulum. *J Am Coll Surg.* 2003;196(3):370-377; discussion, 377; author reply, 378.

36. Lim RY. Endoscopic CO_2 laser cricopharyngeal myotomy. *J Clin Laser Med Surg.* 1995;13(4): 241-247.

37. Kuhn FA, Bent JB 3rd. Zenker's diverticulotomy using the KTP/532 laser. *Laryngoscope.* 1992; 102(8):946-950.

38. Narne S, Cutrone C, Bonavina L, Chella B, Peracchia A. Endoscopic diverticulotomy for the treatment of Zenker's diverticulum: results in 102 patients with staple-assisted endoscopy. *Ann Otol Rhinol Laryngol.* 1999;108(8):810-815.

39. Manni JJ, Kremer B, Rinkel RN. The endoscopic stapler diverticulotomy for Zenker's diverticulum. *Eur Arch Otorhinolaryngol.* 2004;261(2):68-70.

40. Hoffmann M, Scheunemann D, Rudert HH, Maune S. Zenker's diverticulotomy with the carbon dioxide laser: perioperative management and long-term results. *Ann Otol Rhinol Laryngol.* 2003; 112(3):202-205.

41. Chang CW, Burkey BB, Netterville JL, Courey MS, Garrett CG, Bayles SW. Carbon dioxide laser endoscopic diverticulotomy versus open diverticulectomy for Zenker's diverticulum. *Laryngoscope.* 2004;114(3):519-527.

42. Witterick IJ, Gullane PJ, Yeung E. Outcome analysis of Zenker's diverticulectomy and cricopharyngeal myotomy. *Head Neck.* 1995;17(5):382-328.

43. Buckwalter JA, Sasaki CT. Effect of tracheotomy on laryngeal function. *Otolaryngol Clin North Am.* 1984;17(1):41-48.

44. Sasaki CT, Fukuda H, Kirchner JA. Laryngeal abductor activity in response to varying ventilatory resistance. *Trans Am Acad Ophthalmol Otolaryngol.* 1973;77(6):403-410.

45. Sasaki CT, Suzuki M, Horiuchi M, Kirchner JA. The effect of tracheostomy on the laryngeal closure reflex. *Laryngoscope.* 1977;87(9 pt 1):1428-1433.

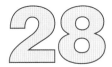

28

Pediatric Laryngology

Dana Mara Thompson, MD
Joseph E. Kerschner, MD

KEY POINTS

■ The infant larynx sits high in the neck at the level of C2 and C3. In this position, the larynx approximates with the back of the nose, velum, tongue, and epiglottis thereby functionally separating respiration from swallowing. This relationship allows infants to breathe and feed without aspirating. Anatomic anomalies or neuromuscular dysfunction that involves any of these areas can lead to airway obstruction and swallowing difficulty.

■ Airway protection is modulated through the laryngeal adductor reflex (LAR). An intact LAR is essential for normal swallow function in infants and children.

■ Laryngeal causes of dysphonia present at birth are usually congenital or neurologic.

■ Laryngeal causes of dysphonia that present after birth are more likely to be a growth, lesion, structural problem, or inflammatory cause.

■ The differential diagnosis of laryngeal causes of airway obstruction is wide. Recognizing the phase of respiration helps determine location. Inspiratory stridor is associated with supraglottic and glottic pathology, biphasic stridor is associated with subglottic pathology. Diagnosis and management requires an astute clinician, thorough endoscopic examination, and management of medical comorbidities that may contribute to disease etiology.

The field of pediatric laryngology is evolving. Traditional pediatric laryngology has included the diagnosis and management of congenital and acquired obstructing lesions of the larynx. However, as the field of adult laryngology has expanded to the management of voice and swallowing disorders, so has the field of pediatric laryngology. This chapter begins with a review of the general principles of laryngeal history and examination in children. Following this, a detailed survey of congenital and acquired obstructive lesions of the larynx as well as functional disorders and problems leading to pediatric voice and swallowing disorders is presented.

AIRWAY PATHOPHYSIOLOGY AND DIAGNOSTIC CONSIDERATIONS

The larynx is the entry point for air into the tracheobronchial tree and respiratory system. Without a functioning larynx, the remainder of the respiratory system is compromised. The phylogenetic purposes of the larynx are respiration and protection of the lower airway from aspiration. Voice is an evolutionary and secondary function of the larynx. In most organ systems, developmental biology has demonstrated that the infant and child structure and function often deviate from the mature state. This has been shown to be true, as well, in the larynx. Several investigators have demonstrated histologic variability in the lamina propria of the true vocal fold in the newborn with decreased cellular differentiation and organization compared with that of the adult.[1]

The pediatric airway also differs from the adult airway in structure and function. The infant larynx is approximately one third its adult size, measuring approximately 7 mm in the sagittal dimension and 4 mm in the coronal plane. The vocal folds are 6 to 8 mm long. The subglottic space is approximately 4.5 mm across, bounded by the cricoid cartilage, the only complete ring of cartilage in the upper airway, and is the narrowest portion of the upper airway. Therefore, only 1 mm of mucosal edema in this portion of the infant airway can obstruct the airway by 40%. As the airway space and dimensions grow with age, mucosal edema causes less compromise of the airway. The cartilaginous framework of the larynx and trachea is softer and more pliable in infancy. This can lead to a tendency to collapse under external compression or air pressure gradients, which may lead to airway obstruction as seen in laryngomalacia and tracheomalacia. As the infant grows, symptoms of these conditions often spontaneously improve and resolve without intervention.

The infant larynx sits high in the neck at the level of vertebrae C2 and C3 directly behind the nose with approximation of the velum, tongue, and epiglottis, thereby functionally separating respiration from swallowing. Because neuromuscular function for airway protection is not fully developed at this stage, this intended anatomic relationship allows the infant to safely breathe and feed at the same time without aspirating. With this anatomic relationship, however, any obstruction of the nasal cavity can cause significant obstruction of the airway, which also causes feeding difficulty. Laryngeal anomalies such as laryngomalacia may also cause feeding difficulty. In conjunction with neuromuscular maturation, the position of the larynx descends in the neck. By age two, the larynx descends to C4 thereby creating less of a functional separation between the functions of breathing and swallowing. By age six, the larynx has descended to its adult location directly behind C6. Airway and swallowing symptoms tend to be exaggerated if neuromuscular function is compromised or has not matured in conjunction with descent of the larynx.

PATIENT ASSESSMENT

History

The axiom that "pediatric patients are not just small adults" is nowhere more true in otolaryngology than in pediatric laryngology. Much of the patient history comes from a parent or caregiver;

for laryngology concerns, this can be a considerable challenge. As an example, in the child with a "hoarse voice," evaluation and intervention is often driven by someone other than the patient. Interpreting how much difficulty the patient is having associated with his or her dysphonia compared to how much the problem is "bothering" the caregiver or teacher is critical in evaluating and caring for these patients. Within the confines of these limitations, the clinician must be able to use the information provided by the caregiver as a surrogate to interpret the difficulty that a given patient is experiencing. A validated quality of life instrument, such as the Pediatric Voice Outcomes Survey, is an excellent tool that may serve to focus these discussions and quantify a patient's difficulty.[2] These questionnaires can easily be incorporated into clinical practice, serving to direct emphasis toward the social and educational impact of a patient's laryngeal dysfunction and also provide objective data to assist the clinician in quantifying these difficulties.

In the developing child, several special considerations must be made that are seldom required in the assessment of older patients. Assurance that the child has no difficulties with hearing levels, auditory input, and auditory processing should be the first consideration in a pediatric laryngology patient. The potential relationship of auditory dysfunction to laryngeal pathology is self-evident, but this can be an area that is overlooked if not carefully considered. The importance of patterning after parents, siblings, and teachers should also be recognized in that, for some patients, the nidus of their laryngeal problem is related to mimicking behaviors of those around them. Neurodevelopmental assessment also is critical in many patients as there can be an association between delays in this area to both speech and voice difficulties. Finally, the distinction and connection between *speech* quality and *voice* quality must be appreciated. In younger children, a complete laryngology evaluation requires a speech quality assessment. The clinician must consider articulation deficiencies, errors or substitutions as well as assess speech fluency, nasality, and tonsillar quality in the context of the patient's laryngeal complaints and pathology.

Examination

Examination of the pediatric laryngology patient can be quite challenging. Historically, obtaining useful information about the patient's laryngeal function has been a significant limiting factor in the assessment and intervention of pediatric patients with laryngeal pathology. Indirect mirror laryngoscopy can be accomplished in pediatric patients but often provides less than optimal visualization to make a meaningful diagnosis, especially when considering functional abnormalities. Flexible fiberoptic laryngoscopy (FFL) for evaluation of the pediatric larynx was first described in 1987[3] and has since become the standard of practice for the examination of the larynx and supraglottic airway in pediatric patients in the clinic setting. As a first-line method, FFL has been shown to be a safe and easily performed office procedure that provides invaluable information in the examination of the dynamic upper airway in neonates, infants, and children.[3-6] Reliable endoscopes that are less then 2.5 mm in diameter are widely available and provide excellent optical resolution so that virtually all pediatric patients can have a detailed evaluation in this fashion. Importantly, given the possible contribution of nasal, nasopharyngeal, palatal and oropharyngeal pathology to a patient's laryngeal difficulties, FFL allows for evaluation of each of these areas as well during the process of endoscopic laryngeal examination. The value of the FFL has been further enhanced by the ability to perform videostroboscopy with small flexible endoscopes.[7] This provides the opportunity not only to dynamically assess the pediatric patient's larynx but also, in most cases, to have that examination enhanced with videostroboscopic input. However, rigid endoscopy continues to provide the greatest optical quality in making assessments of laryngeal pathology. Advances in rigid endoscopy for children have also been made. Many children, even as young as 5 or 6 years of age, will tolerate transoral videostroboscopy with the 4.5-mm rigid 70° Storz endoscope (Figure 28–1).

In preparing the child and family for laryngeal evaluation with endoscopy, it is important to consider the patient's age and maturity. In young

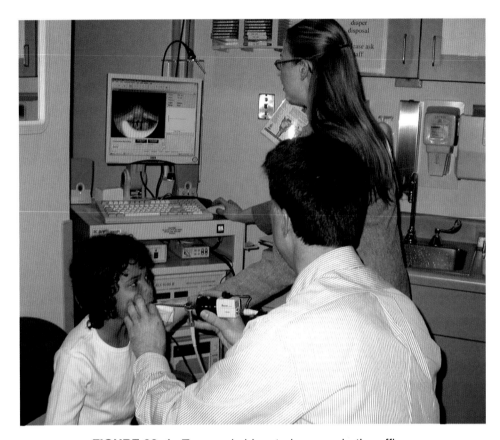

FIGURE 28–1. Transoral videostroboscopy in the office.

children, it is generally necessary to provide stabilization of the extremities to allow for an adequate examination. This can be accomplished via a papoose or with parental holding. Preschool-aged children and older children with developmental delays are often the most difficult to examine. These patients have sufficient strength to make adequate restraint difficult, but often lack the maturity to understand the procedure, its brief nature, and the need to assist with its completion. However, even for these patients, taking time to explain the procedure and reassuring the patient and family can facilitate an improved examination. Topical anesthesia is generally helpful to allow for passage of the flexible scope. Standard regimens include a decongestant as well as a topical anesthetic. The potential for cardiac stimulation with certain decongestants should be considered, especially in patients with a history of congenital cardiac disease. The impact of topical nasal anesthesia on the larynx must

also be considered in performing these procedures. Specifically, for many young children, if too large a volume is administered to the nose, there will be concomitant laryngeal anesthesia that may affect the finding obtained during the examination. This is an especially important consideration when performing FEEST on pediatric patients.

Pediatric laryngeal evaluation is often requested for neonates and infants during a hospitalization for a complex illness that required intubation or the potential for laryngeal injury from other sources such as cardiac surgery. When these evaluations are done in the nursery or in conjunction with other procedures in the operating suite, it is important that the pediatric laryngologist is aware of managing the patient's level of sedation. A mistake occasionally made by an inexperienced endoscopist is to use the increased monitoring available in these settings to allow for some degree of sedation to "facilitate" the procedure. Although this approach may

Emerging Concepts

The functional assessment of children in the outpatient setting continues to evolve. Proven technologies and techniques widely used to evaluate adult airway and swallowing function have been adapted for the pediatric population. Examples of these evolving technologies are fiberoptic endoscopic evaluation of swallowing and sensory testing (FEESST)[8] and office-based lower airway endoscopy.[9] FEESST has been successfully and safely employed in assessing children with swallowing disorders and aspiration. The advantage is the ability to evaluate laryngeal pathology as it relates to a swallowing problem or aspiration without exposing the child to radiation.[8] The details of this approach are presented later in this chapter. Evaluation of the upper airway to the level of the carina in carefully selected children can also be achieved in the office setting using a channeled flexible endoscope with the application of topical lidocaine to the larynx. Although this technique does not replace the need for direct laryngoscopy and bronchoscopy performed in the operating suite under general anesthesia, in the hands of an experienced endoscopist, it may be a valuable tool in the evaluation of laryngotracheal pathology in children and in some it may obviate the need for further diagnostic workup.

make the procedure somewhat more comfortable for the infant, it certainly alters the dynamic nature of the endoscopy and can lead to inaccurate diagnoses, especially with regard to the mobility of the vocal folds. Awake endoscopy without sedation should be accomplished at all times to avoid these difficulties.

Operative Endoscopy

Despite all the advances in outpatient endoscopy, operative assessment of the pediatric patient is certainly still required in some patients. Microsuspension laryngoscopy and bronchoscopy (MLB) allows for greater microscopic inspection of vocal fold pathology, better assessment of the distal airway, and manual palpation of laryngeal structures. There are a number of pathologic conditions where this assessment can be important. In the infant with dysphonia, mobile vocal folds, and fold irregularity an early diagnosis of respiratory papillomatosis may be greatly facilitated by MLB. Additionally, in a patient who has failed voice therapy but clearly has distinct vocal fold lesions, operative assessment of this pathology may be needed to delineate vocal fold nodules from vocal fold psuedocysts or true vocal fold cysts. Similar to adult assessment, true assessment of potential cricoarytenoid joint pathology requires manual palpation and, finally, subglottic and distal airway assessment and its relationship to laryngeal pathology can certainly be best achieved with MLB. The remainder of this chapter presents a review of laryngeal pathologies encountered in children.

CONGENITAL AND ACQUIRED OBSTRUCTIVE LESIONS OF THE LARYNX

Lesions of the larynx can present with life-threatening airway obstruction. The etiology of obstructive airway disease is often multifactorial; this includes anatomic, congenital, and inflammatory problems, many of which are managed by surgical intervention. Multiple signs and symptoms may accompany airway obstruction. The patient may demonstrate stridor, respiratory distress, apnea, cyanosis, pallor, tachypnea, use of muscles accessory to respiration and retractions, and mental status changes. *Chronic* airway obstruction presents with similar signs and symptoms; if left untreated, chronic obstruction may lead to long-term complications such as failure to thrive, poor weight gain, pulmonary hypertension, and pectus excavatum. Whether or not the airway is acutely or chronically obstructed, characterization of the stridor is the most useful noninvasive clinical examination finding for determining location of the obstruction in the airway. Stridor occurs as a result of turbulent airflow through a narrowed lumen, and is present in virtually all children with airway obstruction except those in extremis and close to complete asphyxia. The phase of respiration in which the stridor is heard will help determine the location of the lesion. *Inspiratory* stridor typically occurs in obstructive lesions above the glottis such as laryngomalacia and vocal fold paralysis. *Biphasic* stridor is heard in a fixed obstruction below the glottis in the subglottis or trachea. *Expiratory* stridor is usually represents an obstruction in the intrathoracic airway such as tracheomalacia. Obstructive lesions of the airway may be mistakenly diagnosed as asthma on the basis of a respiratory "wheeze"; therefore, a high index of suspicion and correlation with other clinical examination findings are essential as to not overlook a potentially critical or surgically correctable cause of airway obstruction.

Endoscopic evaluation of the airway has revolutionized the diagnosis and management of the obstructed airway. Endoscopic evaluations are divided into those done awake and those done under a sedation or general anesthesia. Flexible fiberoptic nasopharyngoscopy and laryngoscopy is done with the child awake. As noted in the assessment section, this technique permits for safe, rapid examination of the nose, hypopharynx, supraglottis, and glottis in virtually all children, despite age or the lack of cooperation. The awake state allows for evaluation of the dynamics of supraglottic tone, vocal fold mobility, and the impact of fixed obstructing lesions of the larynx. Examination under the influence of sedation or general anesthesia can alter the findings; therefore, a significant cause of airway obstruction particularly laryngomalacia and vocal fold paralysis could be overlooked. Direct examination of the airway under general or sedated anesthesia remains the mainstay in diagnosis and confirmation of obstructive airway pathology, particularly those below the glottis that cannot be accurately evaluated by awake fiberoptic examination, such as subglottic stenosis and tracheal stenosis.

The goal of any evaluation and management of airway obstruction caused by laryngeal disease is to establish and maintain a safe and stable airway. The number of children who require surgical intervention for airway obstruction has increased. This is due in part to the development of long-term intubation and ventilation techniques in the 1960s, which allowed increased survival rates for critically ill premature newborns. As a result of long-term intubation, these infants were able to survive, however, with an entirely new spectrum of long-term health problems including those of the airway, particularly the larynx and trachea.

LESIONS OF THE LARYNX, INCLUDING THE SUBGLOTTIS

Laryngomalacia

Laryngomalacia is the most common laryngeal anomaly and cause of stridor in infancy. The classic clinical presentation is inspiratory stridor that is worse with feeding, agitation, and supine position. The symptoms are usually present at birth or shortly thereafter. Symptoms peak at 6 to 8 months of age and usually resolve between 18 and 24 months of age.[10] Mild forms of the disease present with inspiratory stridor and usually no other constitutional symptoms. Those with moderate disease usually have feeding problems, as it can be difficult for infants to coordinate the suck-swallow breath sequence in the setting of airway obstruction. Many of these infants that fall into this category have gastroesophageal reflux (GER) and benefit from antireflux treatment and measures.[11,12] Why there is such a high incidence of GER in this patient population is poorly understood. These children may have GER because of increased intrathoracic airway pressure from the proximal airway obstruction promoting reflux. GER in this patient population, like other infant populations with airway problems and apnea, may be related to frequent relaxation events of the lower esophageal sphincter.[13] Infants with severe laryngomalacia develop life-threatening complications of airway obstruction that can lead to pectus formation, failure to thrive, chronic hypoxia, pulmonary hypertension, and cor pulmonale. These patients require surgical intervention.[14-17] The diagnosis is suspected by auscultation of the stridor but must be confirmed by flexible laryngoscopy. This examination must be done with the infant awake to demonstrate the cyclical collapse of the supraglottic tissues into the laryngeal inlet. The influence of general anesthesia can obscure these findings. Typical findings include an omega-shaped epiglottis foreshortening of the aryepiglottic folds, and forward prolapsing arytenoid cartilages and supra-arytenoid tissue obstructing airflow with poor visualization of the vocal folds (Figure 28-2). Flexible laryngoscopy is also done to ensure that no other significant supraglottic pathology is contributing to the stridor. The etiology of this condition remains elusive. Proposed theories include abnormal airway anatomy[18,19] and immature cartilage formation. Because laryngomalacia can be frequently seen in children with other neurologic diseases, some believe laryngomalacia has a neurologic etiology.

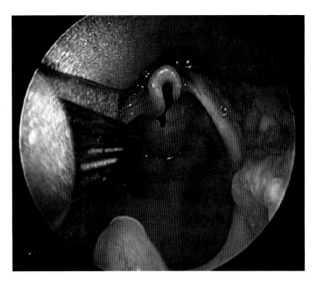

FIGURE 28–2. Tight omega-shaped epiglottis, foreshortened aryepiglottic folds, and poor visualization of the vocal folds seen in some variants of laryngomalacia

Laryngomalacia is usually a self-limiting disease that rarely requires surgical intervention. Surgical intervention is recommended in those who develop life-threatening episodes of airway obstruction or complications of hypoxia described above. Tracheotomy was the treatment of choice for this condition until the mid 1980s when techniques of supraglottoplasty were introduced.[16,20,21] Tracheotomy bypasses the site of laryngeal obstruction until the condition resolves spontaneously, usually after 18 to 24 months. Tracheotomy can be avoided by performing a supraglottoplasty. As seen in Figures 28-3A and 28-B, this is accomplished by microsurgical removal of the redundant prolapsing tissue seen in the area of the arytenoid cartilages and release of the aryepiglottic folds tethering the position of the epiglottis.[16] Long-term results with this approach have generally been excellent with a symptom reversal in 80 to 100% of cases.[14,15,17,22-25] Although, some authors report that as many as 50% of patients will require additional airway procedures, either revision supraglottoplasty or tracheotomy.[24,25] Supraglottic stenosis is the most severe complication of this operation and can occur after overzealous removal of tissue or failure to control for acid reflux disease that may enter the airway and

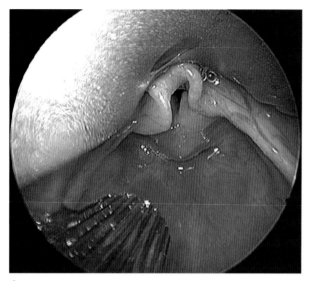

A.

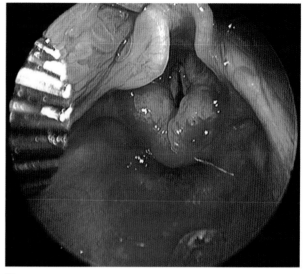

B.

FIGURE 28–3. A. Supra-arytenoid mucosa folding into the glottic inlet in an infant with laryngomalacia before supraglottoplasty. **B.** Supra-arytenoid mucosa partially removed following supraglottoplasty.

cause injury to tissue leading to haphazard scarring. Although supraglottoplasty is a superior alternative to tracheotomy, some children with multiple medical comorbidities, particularly those with severe neurologic impairment or syndromes that involve the airway, often fail supraglottoplasty and are better managed with a tracheotomy.[26]

Laryngeal Atresia and Webs

Laryngeal webs are congenital or acquired (Figure 28-4) and can sometimes be a combination of both. Congenital laryngeal webs and atresias are rare. The embryologic origin of these conditions is a failure of recannulization of the larynx during prenatal development. An atresia or a web of sufficient size will present at birth as aphonia and rapid asphyxiation if not immediately addressed. A thin web with a small residual airway may be ruptured by intubation. Often this is the only treatment needed; however, these infants should be followed closely so appropriate intervention occurs if airway obstruction develops. Thick webs and atresias make emergent intubation by standard techniques difficult if not impossible. In this setting, survival of the infant

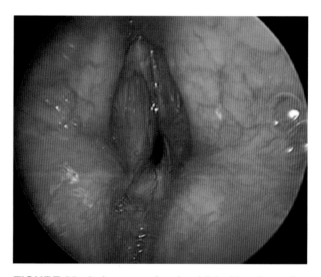

FIGURE 28–4. Laryngeal web–child with velocardiofacial syndrome, congenital anterior glottic web who developed a posterior web after prolonged intubation.

may be dependent on securing the airway with a 2.5-mm rigid bronchoscope—if that is not possible, a surgical airway must be obtained. Surgical management of thick webs and atresias may require a tracheostomy tube until the larynx is larger and more amenable for surgical intervention.[27] Surgical correction usually requires a laryngofissure with open airway division of the atretic region and placement of costal cartilage in the anterior cricoid and cervical trachea, similar to a laryngotracheal reconstruction for subglottic stenosis discussed later in this chapter. Timing or reconstruction is dependent on many factors including age of the child and surgeon experience.

Thin and moderate anterior webs are not usually diagnosed or suspected at birth and may or may not have airway obstructive symptoms. The most common presenting symptom is hoarseness. The primary goals of management are to provide a patent airway and to achieve a good voice quality. This is challenging because vocal folds have a tendency for fibrosis and granulation tissue formation after surgical interventions. Traditionally, the treatment of choice for these thin and moderate laryngeal webs is laryngofissure and placement of a stent or keel when the surgeon feels the child has grown appropriately. This is usually when the child is older than 12 months of age. Recent reports show that select laryngeal webs can be managed with endoscopic lysis and FDA off-label topical application of mitomycin-C, even in infants under one year of age.[28] This technique may allow congenital webs to be successfully managed at a younger age. However, long-term outcomes of this technique are not available, and it is unknown if infants treated by this method eventually need laryngotracheal reconstruction to maintain a patent airway. Long-term results in the management of webs depend on the severity of the original lesion. Surgically treated thin webs often heal with minimal disruption of phonation, whereas thicker plates with associated subglottic stenosis have less satisfactory results.[29]

Acquired laryngeal webs are also uncommon. Etiology is usually from direct laryngeal trauma where the medial surfaces of both vocal folds are disrupted and they heal together forming a web. This is most commonly seen in the management and treatment of laryngeal papillomas usually caused by overzealous removal of papilloma disease at the anterior glottic commissure, particularly in the setting of laryngopharyngeal reflux.[30]

Vocal Fold Immobility: Vocal Fold Paralysis and Vocal Fold Fixation

Vocal fold movement requires intact neurologic function of the vagus nerve and free rotation of the cricoarytenoid joint. The action of abduction of the vocal folds from the midline opens the glottic inlet for airflow into the tracheobronchial tree. Airflow is restricted if vocal fold abduction does not occur. Vocal fold immobility is caused by failure of the vocal folds to abduct. There are two primary etiologies of vocal fold immobility, vocal fold paralysis, and vocal fold fixation. Injury of the vagus nerve anywhere along its course from the skull-base to thoracic cavity causes neurogenic vocal fold paralysis. Paralysis can be congenital or acquired. Acquired immobility is usually caused by a stretch injury, pressure encroachment, inflammatory insult, and trauma or sectioning of the nerve itself. In this setting, the cricoarytenoid joint is mobile, but the neuromuscular function is compromised. A traumatic or inflammatory process in the cricoarytenoid joint causes vocal fold fixation. In this setting, the function of the joint that is required for mobility is fixed, but the neuromuscular function is intact. Fixation and paralysis can coexist. Regardless of the etiology of immobility, failure for one or both of the vocal folds to abduct can lead to stridor and airway obstruction.

Unilateral vocal fold immobility rarely causes stridor or airway obstruction, except occasionally in very young infants particularly in the setting of mucosal edema where the cross-sectional diameter of the airway is already small. In the setting of *bilateral* vocal fold immobility, both vocal folds lay in the midline thereby limiting airflow through the glottis. Bilateral vocal fold immobility may present with severe life-threatening symptoms and airway obstruction requiring an immediate artificial airway. Some infants and children have mild symptoms occurring only during periods of upper respiratory tract infection and may not require a tracheotomy. Most children with bilateral vocal fold immobility require tracheotomy early in the course of the disease, prior to definitive surgical therapy. Because it is bilateral immobility that most commonly leads to airway obstruction, the discussion of surgical treatment will be limited to management of bilateral immobility. Unilateral vocal fold immobility and dysphonia is discussed later in this chapter.

Management and treatment of airway symptoms of bilateral fold immobility is based on the etiology and site of involvement along the vagus nerve. In neonates and infants, bilateral vocal fold paralysis may have a central etiology and most commonly a Chiari malformation or hydrocephalus. Caudal displacement of the brainstem seen in a Chiari malformation causes pressure on the brainstem at the site of origin of the vagal nerve nuclei and nerves (Figure 28–5). Recognition and diagnosis of this is important to prevent other complications of a Chiari malformation. Vocal fold paralysis can be cured once the Chiari malformation is decompressed if done in a timely fashion. Hydrocephalus leads to increased compression of the fourth ventricle. This can also cause compression of the vagal nerve nuclei and

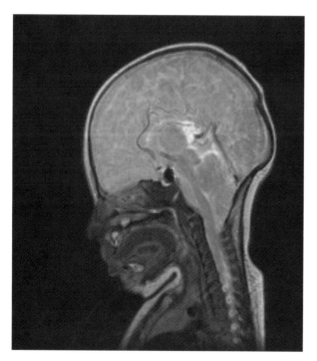

FIGURE 28–5. A 6-month-old infant with a history of hydrocephalus who presented with severe stridor and was found to have caudal displacement of the brainstem seen in a Chiari malformation as seen on this representative MRI.

nerves. Decreasing the intracranial pressure by shunt placement is often curative.[31,32] Infants with a central etiology of bilateral vocal fold paralysis who fail central decompressive procedures will require a tracheotomy for airway safety. These groups of patients also often go on to develop other lower cranial nerve problems and aspiration that keep them tracheotomy tube-dependent and not good candidates for other surgical procedures to achieve decannulation. If the vagal nerves are intact and the etiology of paralysis is a localized insult such as a stretch injury from obstetrical trauma, infection, or extrinsic compression, an observational period is often warranted if there are no acute symptoms of airway obstruction. The paralysis is often transient in these patients who are otherwise healthy. If the etiology of vocal fold paralysis is traumatic with direct nerve injury where function is not expected to return, a tracheotomy is required until another procedure can be done to expand the glottic opening. This situation may be seen in "fixed wire" neck trauma[33] with nerve injury or nerve injury as a complication of thyroid surgery.

Bilateral vocal fold immobility due to fixation occurs when the synovial joint surfaces of the cricoarytenoid joint become fixed, thereby not allowing vocal fold abduction or adduction. In this setting, the vagal nerve is usually fully functional and physically intact. The most common cause of fixation of the joint is some type of direct trauma to the joint area itself such as intubation or neck trauma dislocating the cricoarytenoid joint. Once the joint is injured, an inflammatory process occurs causing an arthritic-like process. Juvenile rheumatoid arthritis can also cause bilateral immobility.

Regardless if the cause of vocal fold immobility is paralysis or fixation, surgical approaches for treatment in children are similar. The fact that there is a wide variety of surgical approaches suggests that no one procedure is ideal. The goal is to open the posterior glottic airway enough to allow for adequate airflow without exposing the patient to increased risk of complications of aspiration. The procedures described are often done after the airway has been secured and is stable with a tracheotomy tube. More recently, many of these surgical techniques have been employed as the primary surgery with the goal of avoiding a tracheotomy. The decision to do definitive primary surgery depends on the acuity of airway obstruction, age of the child, and ability to protect the airway against aspiration.

Repositioning or removal of structures and tissue in the posterior glottis, namely the arytenoid cartilage and mucosa, are well-described techniques of opening the airway in the setting of bilateral vocal fold immobility. These include arytenoid lateralization, arytenoidopexy, partial arytenoidectomy, and cordotomy.[34-37] These procedures can be done alone or in combination with the goal of decannulation. The surgical approach can be external through a laryngofissure or endoscopic using a CO_2 laser or a combination of both. Endoscopic CO_2 laser removal of the vocal process of the arytenoid and a portion of the posterior vocal fold has been successfully employed in some series.[37] The management challenge of this technique is treatment of postoperative granulation tissue formation that may lead to airway obstruction.[38] Recent meta-analysis and retrospective studies evaluating outcomes of surgically managed bilateral vocal fold paralysis in children suggest that laryngofissure with partial arytenoidectomy combined with a vocal fold lateralization procedure results in the highest decannulation rates when compared to CO_2 arytenoidectomy and cordotomy procedures or arytenoidopexy procedures alone.[39,40] The same studies conclude that open external procedures appear to be more effective as a first-line treatment in pediatric vocal fold paralysis, with arytenoidopexy with or without partial arytenoidectomy offering an attractive first-line surgical option. They also conclude that CO_2 laser procedures, although having limited success as a primary procedure, are effective for revision. Although these procedures have been effective in achieving decannulation and maintaining airway patency, long-term outcomes on aspiration and voice are unknown.

Posterior graft laryngotracheoplasty is another effective technique to open the posterior glottis.[41-43] Through a laryngofissure with extension into the first two rings of the trachea,

the posterior cricoid lamina is incised and distracted thereby separating the arytenoid cartilages. Inserting a costal cartilage graft into the distracted posterior cricoid lamina stabilizes the position of the arytenoid cartilages,[43] Although published series of this procedure are small, the decannulation rate after posterior approaches near 100%.[39] Endoscopic posterior cricoid split and rib graft insertion has been successfully accomplished in a few children with posterior glottic and subglottic stenosis.[44]

Recurrent Respiratory Papillomatosis

Recurrent respiratory papillomatosis (RRP) is the expression of human papillomavirus (HPV) infection in the mucosa of the upper aerodigestive tract. Papillomas involving the larynx are the most common laryngeal tumor in children, and the larynx is the most common site of occurrence in the aerodigestive tract (Figure 28–6). Adult laryngeal papilloma disease is usually solitary whereas papillomas of childhood tend to occur in clusters and have an incredible propensity for recurrence. Clinical presentation of laryngeal papilloma is progressive airway obstruction, and dysphonia and may progress to aphonia. RRP

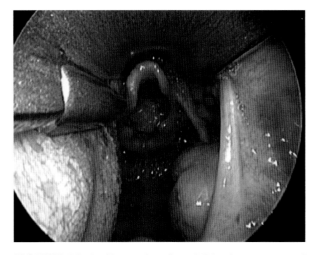

FIGURE 28–6. Example of a child who presented with progressive hoarseness and airway obstruction and laryngeal papilloma involving the false and true vocal folds.

is most commonly associated with HPV-6 and HPV-11 subtypes. Subtypes 16 and 18 are rarely associated with RRP but, if present, have a higher risk of malignant transformation. These viral particles are present in adjacent and clinically normal sites of the respiratory tract but are expressed primarily in anatomical locations of juxtaposed epithelium, hence the high predilection for the vocal fold,[45] nasal vestibule, and posterior soft palate. The other common location is at an area of mucosal injury, such as a tracheotomy site.[45] The vector of transmission is controversial. Pediatric RRP and vaginal condyloma acuminata are both caused by HPV subtypes 6 and 11, thus leading most researchers to believe that vertical transmission from mother to child is taking place in most cases. Although unusual, vertical transmission to children born by cesarean section of mothers with vaginal warts has also been documented.[46]

The natural course of RRP is extremely variable, with no obvious patient-related risk factors to aid in prognosis. The estimated mean number of procedures per child for this disease is 19.7, with an average of 4.4 procedures per year. Many cases have been seen to regress spontaneously in adolescence, but others go on to extensive disease involving the trachea and pulmonary parenchyma with a high fatality rate from untreatable airway obstruction. Even more uncommonly, the papilloma may undergo malignant degeneration to squamous cell carcinoma. For this reason, interval histologic examination of the obstruction tissue is important.

Like its adult counterpart, pediatric RRP continues to be an extremely difficult management problem for otolaryngologists. The goal of surgical treatment is to maintain a patent airway while providing a usable voice and to prevent spread of disease into the distal airway.

Although the mainstay of surgical management has traditionally been the CO_2 laser, newer surgical techniques have demonstrated efficacy in the management of pediatric RRP patients, including powered instrumentation, the laryngeal shaver[47] and the pulse-dye laser.[48] Regardless of the surgical technique employed, scarring, stenosis, and web formation in the larynx are all

the results of overly aggressive or inexpertly performed endoscopic removal of the disease. Care must be taken to avoid injury to vital structures. The papilloma should be removed down to the level of the vocal ligaments, but the folds themselves should not be incised. When working in the anterior commissure, to avoid web formation, the far anterior glottis where the vocal folds meet, bilateral resection should not be done. Even in experienced hands, the incidence of minor scarring in the anterior glottis may be as high as 25%.[49] Aggressive resection beyond that necessary to maintain a safe airway will not improve the long-term prognosis for remission, but may contribute to late morbidity.

The role of tracheotomy in the surgical management of laryngeal papilloma is controversial. Most surgeons try to avoid tracheotomy if at all possible. The mucosal injury at the tracheotomy site encourages growth of papilloma outside the larynx, thereby increasing the probability of distal spread of the disease. The rate of tracheal spread in patients requiring tracheotomy has been reported as high as 50%.[50] Given the variable degree of aggressiveness of RRP, it is possible that patients who have distal spread of disease represent a subset of the patient population with a predetermined propensity to disseminate beyond the larynx and would require a tracheotomy regardless. Patients who develop life-threatening airway obstruction from aggressive disease within or beyond the larynx that cannot be managed by endoscopic procedures should have a tracheotomy placed until the disease can be controlled with further surgical intervention and adjunctive therapy. If a tracheotomy is placed, the clinician should make every attempt possible to achieve decannulation as soon as possible, both to limit potential distal airway dissemination and to relieve the child of the burden of tracheotomy. Issues related to pediatric tracheotomy are discussed later in this chapter. The traditional adjuvant medical therapies used for pediatric RRP are interferon-[alpha]2a, retinoic acid, and indol-3-carbinol/diindolylmethane (I3C/DIM). The most recently introduced adjunctive therapy is cidofovir. Cidofovir is an acyclic nucleoside phosphonate derivative with antiviral activity used for the treatment of cytomegalovirus retinitis in patients with acquired immunodeficiency syndrome. Off-label use of cidofovir injected directly into the region after removal of laryngeal papilloma has demonstrated efficacy in selected patients. In addition, promising research efforts are being done to develop vaccination therapy for pediatric RRP. It should be noted that the long-term effects of cidofovir are not well described, such as the incidence of malignant transformation.

Laryngotracheal Stenosis and Subglottic Stenosis

Laryngotracheal stenosis may be characterized by etiology and area involved. Areas of involvement include the supraglottis, glottis, subglottis, and upper trachea. A single area or multiple areas can be involved. Stenosis of the larynx is congenital (Figure 28–7) or acquired (Figure 28–8). Congenital stenoses are believed to be the result of failure or incomplete recanalization of the laryngeal lumen that occurs by the 10th week of gestation. Congenital stenosis subglottic stenosis is histopathologically divided into a membranous stenosis and a cartilaginous stenosis (Table 28–1).

Congenital stenosis exists when the lumen of the cricoid region of the airway measures less than 4 mm in a full-term infant or 3 mm in a premature infant with no prior history of intubation. As seen in Figure 28–7, the typical appearance of a congenital cartilaginous stenosis is that of an elliptical-shaped cricoid cartilage. The definition of what may be congenital or acquired stenosis

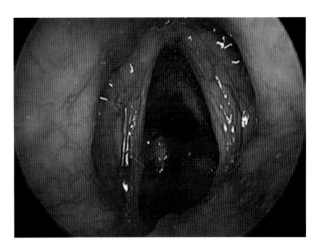

FIGURE 28–8. A 7-year-old girl with acquired subglottic stenosis who is tracheotomy tube dependent. Her medical comorbidities include multiple intubations, congenital heart disease, Down syndrome, and GERD.

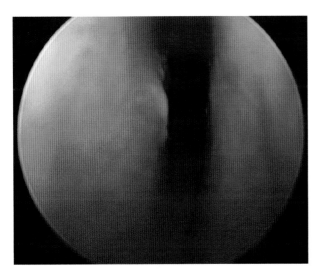

FIGURE 28–7. Elliptical-shaped cricoid cartilage seen in this 5-month-old infant who presented with biphasic stridor and congenital subglottic stenosis.

TABLE 28-1. Classification of Congenital Subglottic Stenosis

Cartilaginous Stenosis	Soft Tissue Stenosis
Cricoid cartilage deformity	Granulation tissue
Normal shape	Submucosal fibrosis
Small for infant's size	Submucosal gland hypoplasia
Abnormal shape	
Large anterior lamina	
Large posterior lamina	
Generalized thickening	
Elliptical shape	
Submucous cleft	
Other congenital cricoid stenoses	
Trapped first tracheal ring	

can be somewhat arbitrary, because children with congenital subglottic stenosis may develop secondary soft tissue stenosis and scarring from injury, thereby developing an acquired stenosis. This injury most commonly occurs from prolonged intubation, so the true incidence of congenital subglottic stenosis is difficult to determine. Of the areas involved in stenosis, the subglottis is the most common. Most subglottic stenoses that require surgical management are acquired. An example of acquired stenosis is seen in Figure 28–8. The principles of surgical management discussed are applicable to congenital and acquired disease.

Pediatric subglottic stenosis (SGS) essentially did not exist until after 1965 with the introduction of prolonged endotracheal intubation and ventilation of neonates.[51] As very low birthweight infant survival increased, so did the number of patients with secondary laryngotracheal stenosis, with the incidence of SGS in surviving neonates as high as 97%.[52] Fortunately, advances in the technique of endotracheal intubation and tube stabilization along with the implementation of softer materials for endotracheal tubes have decreased the incidence of tracheal laryngotracheal stenosis in surviving neonates to 0.9 to 8.3%.[53] With the proliferation of life-saving advancements in medicine and surgery, infants and children who are now surviving disease processes would not have survived 20 years ago. These children develop chronic diseases as a result of treatment, with subglottic stenosis being one of them. The numbers of toddlers, children, and adolescents who are now developing stenosis of the larynx have increased, but the exact percentages are unknown. The nature of the stenosis can be soft or firm and commonly a combination of both. Causes of soft tissue stenosis are submucosal mucous gland hyperplasia, ductal cysts, fibrous, granulation tissue, and laryngopharyngeal reflux of gastric acid causing mucosal edema. Firm stenoses are usually associated with an abnormally shaped or thickened cricoid cartilage or mature scar tissue. The Cotton-Myer grading system is most widely used for documentation of degree of obstruction in SGS. Endotracheal tube sizing has become the

most widely used means of grading and assessing degree of stenosis.[54]

Successful laryngotracheal reconstructive surgery requires a carefully formulated plan. This plan includes identification and management of significant medical comorbidities that have potential to contribute to poor outcomes. The plan also requires accurate identification of the type of stenosis and all areas of the larynx and upper trachea involved as the stenosis can be multilevel and require more that one type of intervention. The treatment plan is custom-tailored to the specific patient and his or her medical comorbidities and the anatomic problem. This treatment plan is best done by a multidisciplinary team approach including the pediatric otolaryngologist, pediatric surgeon, pulmonologist, gastroenterologist, anesthesiologist, intensivist, and appropriate allied health personnel.

Any laryngeal stenosis can be effectively managed by placement of a tracheotomy, thus bypassing the obstruction. Morbidity and mortality associated with tracheotomy tube placement has encouraged advancements in laryngotracheal reconstructive procedures (LTR) to either avoid tracheotomy tube placement or to achieve decannulation.

Associated medical comorbidities, particularly cardiopulmonary disease, must be addressed, stabilized, and managed prior to considering surgical intervention. Children who require significant ventilatory or medical support are not good candidates for laryngotracheal reconstruction. Evaluation of swallowing function is essential to help determine airway protection ability and aspiration risk so that preoperative and perioperative accommodations can be made to minimize the complications of aspiration. Patients with significant aspiration are usually not good candidates for LTR.

The influence of gastroesophageal reflux on laryngotracheal stenosis and wound healing cannot be overemphasized. GERD is an etiologic factor in acquired subglottic stenosis. Clinical and animal studies demonstrate that the presence of acid in the region of the larynx negatively affects healing.[55-61] Perioperative and postoperative aggressive medical and sometimes even surgical[50] antireflux therapy is recommended in the setting of LTR surgery. Prospective and retrospective studies evaluating long-term outcomes or reflux control in LTR surgery are not available.

Surgical management of laryngotracheal stenosis is individualized to the patient and no one operative approach is exactly the same. Each individual patient presents with multiple variables that must be considered, including the location and extent of the stenotic area, medical comorbidities, airway protection and swallowing function, age, and weight. Surgical options include endoscopic techniques, expansion surgery, and resection surgery. Methods employed are dependent on the degree and location of the stenosis. In general, grade I stenosis are usually managed by endoscopic techniques. Grade II stenosis may be approached with either endoscopic or open techniques depending on location and extent of the lesion. Grade III and IV lesions almost always require open surgical reconstruction.

Grade I and II stenosis can be approached with endoscopic techniques. The carbon dioxide (CO_2) and KTP lasers, because of their precise tissue characteristics, are the most widely used modalities. The laser is useful for treating early intubation injury with granulation tissue accumulation, subglottic cysts, thin circumferential webs, and crescent-shaped bands. Predisposing factors to failure of endoscopic laser treatment of SGS are previous failed endoscopic procedures; significant loss of the cartilaginous framework; thick, circumferential cicatricial scarring greater than 1 cm in vertical dimension; and posterior commissure involvement. A complication of laser treatment of SGS is exposure of perichondrium or cartilage causing perichondritis and chondritis that may lead to further scar formation.

Open surgical reconstruction is recommended when the endoscopic methods to establish a patent airway are inappropriate or have failed. Anterior cricoid split is considered one of the *expansion* surgical techniques. It is utilized predominantly in a neonate with anterior subglottic narrowing who fails multiple attempts at extubation despite adequate pulmonary reserve.

In this setting, the laryngotracheal problem due to narrowing at the level of the cricoid cartilage is relieved as the airway lumen expands and decompresses once the anterior cricoid cartilage is divided in the midline. The endotracheal tube is left in place for 5 to 10 days. Dexamethasone sodium phosphate is initiated 24 hours before extubation and continued for 5 days after extubation. This technique leads to successful extubation in 66 to 78%.[62] As seen in Table 28–2, before considering using this technique in a neonate, several clinical criteria must be met to increase the probability of successful extubation following anterior cricoid split. In the author's hands, this technique has nearly been replaced by anterior cricoid split *with* the placement of a small auricular cartilage graft followed by endotracheal intubation for 7 days. Outcomes comparing decannulation rates of cricoid split versus cricoid split with placement of the auricular cap graft have not been formally reviewed.

Multiple open procedures have been described and are used to expand the stenosed airway. These procedures and their applications have evolved over the past 30 years. Fearon and Cotton introduced laryngotracheal reconstruction (LTR) with cartilage interpositional grafting in 1972 with placement of a cartilage graft between a split anterior cricoid and upper trachea.[63] This method has become one of the most common

TABLE 28-2. Criteria for Performing an Anterior Cricoid Split

Extubation failure on at least 2 occasions secondary to subglottic laryngeal pathology

Weight greater than 1500 gm

No ventilator support for at least 10 days before repair

Supplemental O_2 requirement less than 30%

No congestive heart failure for 1 month before repair

No acute respiratory tract infection

No antihypertensive medication for 10 days before repair

techniques of expanding stenotic airway segments. Anterior grafting alone is typically used in grade II and grade III stenoses that do not involve the posterior glottis or subglottis. If there is posterior glottic or subglottic involvement in addition to the anterior stenosis, the posterior cricoid plate lamina is split with or without the placement of an interpositional graft depending on the degree of the stenosis. This problem is more commonly seen in grade III and grade IV stenosis. Partial cricotracheal resection (CTR) has evolved into another option for surgical management of selected grade III and IV stenosis.[64-69] In this operation the stenotic region of the anterior cricoid plate and any involved tracheal stenotic segment is resected, and the trachea is mobilized to allow for an end-to-end anastomosis. The posterior trachea and trachealis muscle is anastomosed with the posterior cricoid plate and its mucosa. The anterior mobilized trachea is then sewn into the removed segment of the cricoid and secured to the thyroid cartilage.[64,65,69,70]

Traditional approaches to LTR surgery involved several stages of reconstruction[71-73] at the site of expansion; a stent (Silastic or Teflon) was placed to stabilize the reconstruction. The stent is left in place above a tracheotomy stoma and tube (suprastomal stent) for 4 to 6 weeks. After removal of the stent and once the surgical site has healed with a patent subglottis the tracheotomy tube is downsized until the child tolerates and is able to breathe around a plugged trach tube. Once this is accomplished, the tracheotomy tube is removed. This process of reconstruction and decannulation can take weeks to several months. The morbidity and potential mortality of a tracheotomy tube is well recognized in children and was discussed earlier in this chapter. With staged reconstruction and stent placement, the child is left with little or no airway above the trach tube, which is life-threatening if the tube accidentally falls out or is occluded. Long-term stenting has additional morbidities of granulation tissue formation, infection, dislodgment of the stent, dysphagia, and aspiration. To address these risks and circumvent some of these problems, single stage LTR (SSLTR)

evolved. Most airway surgeons will stage procedures in children with compromised pulmonary reserve or complex, multilevel stenosis that requires prolonged stenting.

Single stage LTR (SSLTR) involves surgical correction of the stenotic airway with a short period of endotracheal intubation, thus avoiding the need for prolonged laryngotracheal stenting and tracheotomy tube dependency. The airway must have adequate cartilaginous support to consider SSLTR as a surgical option. SSLTR requires a comprehensive understanding of the principles of airway reconstruction and extensive experience on the part of the surgeon, anesthesiologist, intensivist, and nursing staff. Postoperative care of these patients can be complex.[74-76] A recent report of 200 SSLTR cases revealed that 29% were reintubated and 15% required postoperative tracheostomy. Ultimately, however, the overall decannulation rate was 96%. This study also found that the use of anterior and posterior costal cartilage grafting, age less than 4 years, sedation for more than 48 hours, a leak pressure around the endotracheal tube at greater than 20 cm H_2O, and moderate/severe tracheomalacia significantly increased the rate of reintubation. The duration of stenting did not affect outcomes. Children with anterior and posterior grafts and those with moderate or severe tracheomalacia were more likely to need a postoperative tracheostomy. SSLTR can be effectively employed in the treatment of pediatric laryngotracheal stenosis.[74] However, diligent preoperative assessment of the patient comorbidities and the patient's airway and meticulous postoperative care and surgical skill and experience are important to the success of this operation.

The ultimate goal of laryngotracheal reconstruction is tracheotomy decannulation or prevention. The rate of decannulation varies with the severity of stenosis and the method of reconstruction. Multiple operations may be required to achieve eventual extubation or decannulation; there is no specific model to predict the outcome of pediatric airway reconstruction surgery. A recent review reported that decannulation rates for double-stage laryngotracheal reconstruction in SGS patients with Myer-Cotton grades 2, 3, and 4 are 95%, 74%, and 86%, respectively. Decannulation rates for SSLTR for Myer-Cotton grades 2, 3, and 4 are 100%, 86%, and 100%, respectively. Children with Myer-Cotton grade 3 or 4 disease represent a significant challenge, and refinements of techniques are needed to address this subset of children.[77]

Surgical management of grade IV stenosis represents the most difficult group to obtain good results. Refinements in surgical technique and application of cricotracheal resection (CTR) as the primary operation for grade IV stenosis has improved the decannulation rates from 67% in the 1980s to 86% in the 1990s.[78] A recent report shows that patients who undergo CTR have higher decannulation rates than patients who have laryngotracheal reconstruction (LTR) with anterior and posterior costal cartilage grafting (92% vs 81%). CTR patients are less likely to need additional open procedures to achieve decannulation (18% vs 46%).[78] Patients with grade IV stenosis and other areas of the larynx and trachea involved often require extended CTR with the application of cartilage grafting and arytenoid procedures.[79]

HEMANGIOMA

Subglottic and tracheal hemangiomas are benign, congenital vascular malformations that are derived from mesodermal rests. The lesions are relatively uncommon, accounting for 1.5% of all congenital laryngeal anomalies, with a 2:1 female predominance.[10] Patients are usually asymptomatic at birth but present with stridor within the first few months of life; 85% present in the first 6 months,[80] and 50% have cutaneous hemangiomas present at the time of diagnosis.[81] Asymmetric subglottic narrowing is the classic finding on soft tissue neck radiographs. Endoscopic diagnosis is usually made without biopsy because of the lesion's typical appearance of a compressible, asymmetric, submucosal mass with bluish or reddish discoloration most often found in the posterolateral subglottis (Figure 28–9A).

Subglottic and tracheal hemangiomas will have a rapid growth phase that slows by 12 months, followed by slow resolution over the subsequent months to years. Most will show complete resolution by 5 years. However, subglottic hemangiomas are associated with 30 to

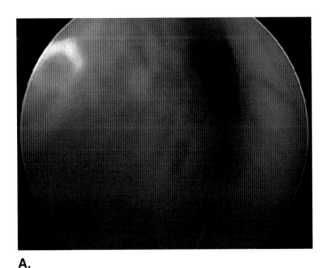
A.

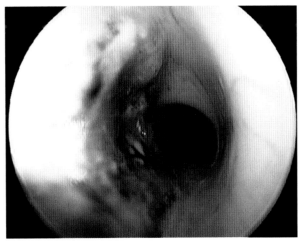
B.

FIGURE 28–9. A. A 3-month-old infant boy presents with biphasic stridor, respiratory distress, and feeding difficulty. Endoscopic examination demonstrates a prominent submucosal hemangioma in the left lateral subglottis extending to the undersurface of the left true vocal fold. **B.** Subglottic hemangioma after 2 weeks after CO_2 laser treatment and systemic steroids.

70% mortality when left untreated. Therapeutic and surgical management of this problem is directed at maintaining the airway, while minimizing potential long-term sequelae of the treatment itself. Current management options include laser partial excision, open surgical resection, systemic or intralesional steroids, systemic interferon alpha-2a, and tracheotomy.

Bypassing the obstructing lesion with a tracheotomy and waiting for the expected involution will provide for the optimal anatomic result and is considered by many to be the standard of care by which all other treatment options need to be measured. However, as previously discussed in this chapter, there are risks associated with a tracheotomy as well as the delay in speech and language that is routinely encountered when children require a tracheotomy at a young age. Early methods of treatment that are no longer used because of the associated morbidity include external beam radiation, radium and gold implants, and sclerosing agents.

Systemic corticosteroids for treatment of subglottic hemangiomas were introduced in 1969 by Cohen[82] and are used both as primary and adjuvant therapy. Steroids decrease the size of the hemangioma and accelerate involution, although the exact mechanism is not well understood. Steroids are thought to decrease hemangioma size by blocking estradiol-induced growth,[83] or by directly increasing capillary sensitivity to vasoconstrictors. Corticosteroid therapy with or without tracheotomy has been shown to be successful in 82 to 97% of cases. However, whether or not the period of tracheotomy cannulation is decreased is unknown.[84] Risks of long-term steroid use include growth retardation, Cushinoid face, and increased susceptibility to infection including life-threatening *Pneumocystis carinii* pneumonia.[85] Using an alternate-day dosing regimen in the smallest possible doses may reduce these effects. Recent reports suggest that systemic steroids followed by short-term intubation after diagnostic bronchoscopy can be used as a safe and effective alternative in the management of obstructive pediatric subglottic hemangiomas.[86] Others report successful avoidance of tracheotomy by endoscopic intralesional injection of

corticosteroids into the hemangioma, with or without short-term intubation.[87]

Endoscopic surgical management with the CO_2 laser was first reported in 1980 by Healy and colleagues.[88] Since its introduction, the CO_2 laser alone or in combination with steroids or tracheotomy has become a standard therapy. Isolated unilateral subglottic hemangiomas are usually the best type and location for CO_2 laser treatment (see Figures 28–9A and 9B). In carefully selected patients, partial resection of the hemangioma with CO_2 laser with or without systemic corticosteroids is successful.[89] Recent reports show that the KTP laser is an effective tool for management of subglottic hemangiomas with a low incidence of complications.[90,91] The KTP laser is preferentially absorbed by hemoglobin making this laser system well suited for the treatment of vascular tumors such as a hemangioma. Long-term outcomes of this technique are not available.

Interferon alpha-2a has been used recently in children with obstructing hemangioma that was unresponsive to laser and/or corticosteroid therapy, achieving a 50% or grater regression of the lesion in 73%.[92] Interferon alpha-2a requires prolonged therapy because it does not promote involution but inhibits proliferation by blocking various steps in angiogenesis. The potential side effects, which include neuromuscular impairment, skin slough, fever, and liver enzyme elevation,[92] limit its use to larger, potentially fatal lesions.

Despite the more widespread use of steroids and other treatment modalities, the requirement for tracheostomy has remained unchanged over the last 20 years. The use of laser therapy does not appear to confer any additional therapeutic benefit over and above tracheostomy alone in bringing about resolution of subglottic hemangiomas. Systemic steroids may reduce the size of the hemangioma but are associated with multiple adverse effects. The decision to use the above techniques must, therefore, be made in the light of these observations.[93] To avoid the complications and provide a more definitive treatment, the topic of open surgical excision has been revisited.[93-99] The surgical technique is similar to SSLTR. The airway is opened at the level of the cricoid cartilage, followed by a submucosal dissection with excision of the hemangioma. An anterior cartilage graft is usually placed and the patient is intubated for 5 to 7 days. A recent study concludes that surgery of severe subglottic hemangiomas is a reliable technique in selected patients and should be considered in *corticoresistant* or *corticodependent*, circular, or bilateral hemangiomas[97] and large life-threatening hemangiomas.[99] The early experience of single-stage excision suggests that this technique represents an exciting and promising surgical alternative, and its more widespread adoption may be the only way of further improving the outcome of patients with subglottic hemangiomas.[93]

LARYNGEAL AND LARYNGOTRACHEOESOPHAGEAL CLEFTS

Congenital laryngeal and laryngotracheoesophageal clefts are rare conditions that can be characterized by a posterior midline deficiency in the separation of the larynx and trachea from the hypopharynx and esophagus (Figure 28–10). The

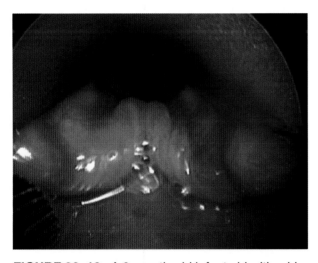

FIGURE 28–10. A 9-month-old infant girl with a history of tracheoesophageal fistula and VATER syndrome who required TEF repair at birth presents with feeding difficulty, persistent aspiration, and stridor. Microlaryngoscopy demonstrated a laryngeal cleft with partial involvement of the posterior cricoid plate.

incidence is less than 0.1% and the majority of cases are sporadic. There is a strong association with other anomalies (56%), most commonly tracheoesophageal fistula in 20 to 27%.[100] Six percent of children with tracheoesophageal fistula have a coexisting laryngeal cleft. Of the children who present with tracheoesophageal fistula (TEF), the laryngeal cleft goes undetected in three-quarters until persistent aspiration, in spite of successful tracheoesophageal fistula repair prompts further investigation.[100] Laryngeal or laryngotracheoesophageal clefting is commonly associated with a syndrome, most commonly G syndrome, VATER, VACTERL and Pallister-Hall syndrome.[101]

The degree of clefting may be relatively minor, involving only a failure of interarytenoid muscle development, or can extend to the carina and even into the mainstem bronchi. Multiple classification systems have been used to describe laryngeal clefts. Independent from the numbering system used, it is useful to differentiate to the length of the cleft as laryngeal (interarytenoid only, partial cricoid, or complete cricoid), and laryngotracheoesophageal clefts that extend into the cervical trachea, or the intrathoracic trachea.

Patients with laryngeal or laryngotracheoesophageal clefts present with congenital inspiratory stridor, cyanotic attacks associated with feeding, aspiration, and recurrent pulmonary infections. As the length of the cleft increases, so does the severity of presenting symptoms; in the most severe cleft (laryngotracheoesophageal), aspiration is present in 100% of children. Although radiographic contrast studies may suggest aspiration, the best single study for identifying a laryngeal cleft is careful endoscopic examination. The arytenoids need to be parted to obtain adequate visualization, as the larynx may be obscured by redundant esophageal mucosa prolapsing into the glottic and subglottic lumen. Most clefts that are limited to the supraglottic larynx do not require surgical intervention. The anatomic depth of these small clefts is to the interarytenoid level and stops at the vocal processes. Treatment methods include evaluation and treatment of gastroesophageal reflux and swallowing therapy.[100] When surgical intervention is required for these small clefts, endoscopic repair is successful in over 80%, with open repair reserved for endoscopic failures.[100,102]

In contrast to the interarytenoid clefts, surgical repair is required in nearly all laryngeal clefts that extend below the vocal folds. An anterior approach through a laryngofissure is most commonly used. The advantage of this approach is excellent exposure of the entire defect without risk to the laryngeal innervation. Complete laryngotracheoesophageal clefts that extend to the carina may require a posterolateral approach to allow for a two-layer closure without requiring intraoperative extracorporeal circulation. In most circumstances, a tracheotomy is present prior to or placed at the time of reconstructive surgery. However, single-stage repair utilizing endotracheal intubation as a short-term stent is being increasingly utilized and preferred by the authors.

TRACHEOTOMY

Tracheotomy is a means of managing severe airway obstruction caused by nearly all the airway lesions discussed in this chapter. The number of children who require surgical intervention for airway obstruction has increased, due in part to the development of long-term intubation and ventilation techniques in the 1960s that allowed increased survival rates for critically ill premature newborns. The three major indications for long-term tracheotomy in children are *airway obstruction*, *ventilatory support*, and *pulmonary toilet*. Most children with tracheotomy tubes in place for airway obstruction undergo the procedure as very young infants; either for acquired subglottic stenosis related to prolonged endotracheal intubation or for congenital lesions that compromise the airway. Because of morbidity and the tremendous psychosocial and developmental implications of a child with a tracheotomy, all alternative interventions before proceeding to tracheotomy should be explored and exhausted.

With increased surgical experience, improved surgical techniques, identification and management of comorbidities that affect outcomes, and improvement in postoperative care, the indica-

tions for airway expansion surgery have been extended to patients with laryngotracheal stenosis as the primary definitive operation, thus avoiding tracheotomy[74,97-99] for many of the airway lesions that may have traditionally required a tracheotomy for initial management.

FUNCTIONAL DISORDERS OF THE PEDIATRIC LARYNX

Swallowing Disorders and Airway Protection

Swallowing disorders in children not only encompass dysfunction of the process of swallowing but also include disorders of feeding. Anatomic, developmental, behavioral, and psychological factors contribute to swallowing and feeding problems in children. The etiology often is a combination of organic and nonorganic factors, differentiating the evaluation and approach of a child from an adult. The five categories of infant and pediatric feeding disorders are outlined in Table 28–3. Intact laryngeal function and airway protection is essential for safe feeding. Normal laryngeal anatomy along with normal development and maturation of laryngeal reflexes protects the lower airway from critical aspiration events.

Developmental Anatomic, Physiologic, and Behavioral Factors

An understanding of the development and maturational changes of swallowing from infancy to childhood is necessary for clinicians evaluating infant and pediatric swallowing disorders.[48,104] Feeding evolves from an infantile reflexive behavior to a mature cortically regulated behavior with concurrent development of the central nervous system, and growth, development, and maturation of the anatomy of the aerodigestive tract.[48,105] The phases of swallowing have been reviewed in chapter 5; the following discussion pertains to the growth and developmental changes in infants and children that affect the phases of swallowing.

TABLE 28–3. Five Categories of Infant and Pediatric Feeding Disorders*

Structural Abnormalities

Cleft lip/palate	Tracheoesophageal
Ankyloglossia	fistula
Macroglossia	Esophageal atresia
Pierre-Robin sequence	Esophageal mass
Laryngomalacia	Esophageal stricture
Laryngeal cleft	Vascular ring/sling

Neurologic Conditions

Cerebral palsy	Polymyositis/
Bulbar atresia	dermatomyositis
Tardive dyskinesia	Rheumatoid arthritis
Möbius syndrome	Brainstem tumors
Myasthenia gravis	Chiari malformations
Infant botulism	Myelomeningocele
Muscular dystrophy	

Cardiorespiratory Problems

Apnea/bradycardia
Recurrent pneumonia
Bronchopulmonary dysplasia
Tachypnea

Inflammatory/Metabolic Dysfunction

Adenotonsillitis	Food allergy
Deep neck space	Diabetes
infections	Crohn disease
Epiglottis	Hyperparathyroidism
Esophagitis	Cytomegalovirus
Gastroesophageal reflux	HIV
Caustic ingestion	Behçet disease
Collagen vascular disease	

Behavioral Issues/Psychological

Oral aversion	Rumination
Conditioned dysphagia	Food refusal
Depression	Poverty

*Adapted from Burklow et al.[103]

The preoral phase is also known as the oral preparatory phase. Centers for hunger and satiety in the hypothalamus receive afferent signals from a variety of sources. Appetite can also be affected by emotional state and can be negatively influenced by chronic disease allergies and food aversions. Anatomic structures involved in this stage are the lips, tongue, cheeks, buccal fat pads, palate, and dentoalveolar structures. These structures interact in receiving, formation, and transporting the bolus. Intact labial muscles are especially important in infancy to form a seal and prevent spillage. The oral phase begins with bolus formation to move food substance posteriorly toward the pharynx. Excellent tongue motion and coordination is needed for the oral phase of swallowing. In infancy, the oral phase of swallowing consists of the subcortically regulated process of suckling, characterized by primitive extension-retraction motion of the tongue.[106] The small size of the mandible, and oral cavity relative to the tongue and the presence of buccal fat pads facilitate suckling. Between 3 and 6 months of age, the anatomy of the oral cavity and pharynx begin to change, and infants begin to suppress the suckle pattern and develop voluntary suck patterns. Anatomic changes include resorption of the buccal fat pads and the inferior and forward drop of the jaw, thus increasing the intraoral space. Tongue movements mature from extension-retraction motion of suckling to up-and-down movements of sucking, facilitating bolus manipulation and thereby allowing for a more coordinated transport of food and liquid into the oral cavity. This maturation in skill allows infants to begin eating textured food from a spoon by 6 months of age. Masticatory skills begin to develop by 6 to 8 months and continue to develop as the alveolar ridges mature and deciduous teeth erupt. At 12 months, sucking patterns are minimized and children generally transition to cup drinking and no longer use the suck pattern.

The pharyngeal phase of swallowing is involuntary and is triggered by bolus contact with the tonsillar pillars and pharyngeal wall. During pharyngeal swallowing, the upper pharynx and soft palate close to seal the nasal cavity as the bolus enters the pharynx. The bolus is propelled to the esophagus by contraction of the pharyngeal muscles. During pharyngeal contraction, the larynx elevates, the glottis closes, and respiration ceases to protect the lower airway from aspiration. Because the pharynx is the common chamber for the respiration and digestive pathways, important developmental changes occur to allow for safe swallowing. In the infant, the larynx sits high in the neck at the level of vertebrae C1 to C3 allowing for the velum, tongue, and epiglottis to approximate, thereby functionally separating the respiratory and digestive tracts. This allows the infant to safely breathe and feed. By age 2 to 3 years the larynx descends decreasing the separation of the swallowing and digestive tracts. Intact oral motor skills and laryngeal function are essential to prevent complications of aspiration as this occurs.

The esophageal phase begins as the bolus enters the esophagus after cricopharyngeal muscle relaxation. This phase is involuntary and does not seem to have developmental differences with age and maturation.

Evaluation of Infant and Pediatric Swallowing Disorders

Standard evaluative test of the feeding and swallowing process used in the assessment of adult dysphagia are translational to infants and children; however, modifications and accommodations in technique and interpretation are essential. As feeding and swallowing disorders can be serious and even life-threatening, prompt and thorough evaluation is critical to avoid complications.

Airway protection against aspiration is modulated through the laryngeal adductor reflex (LAR). The laryngeal adductor reflex is induced by stimulation of mechanoreceptors located in the aryepiglottic folds which are innervated by the superior laryngeal nerve (see chapter 4, Physiology of Airway Regulation). Stimulation of these receptors sends sensory afferent information along the superior laryngeal nerve to the brainstem for integration via the nucleus tractus solitarius and the nucleus ambiguus. Involuntary efferent impulses travel along the vagus nerve and reach the larynx through the recurrent laryngeal nerve to adduct the vocal folds and initiate a swallow response. This reflex arc is important for the protection of the upper airway from aspiration of saliva and food materials. Anything that alters the integrity of the LAR will alter the function of the larynx to protect against aspiration. This predisposes the infant or child to aspiration and feed-

ing difficulty. The LAR can be altered at the peripheral level from acid exposure, leading to a functional denervation and altered laryngeal sensation that leads to poor airway protection and swallowing dysfunction. Alteration of the LAR from central causes such as a Chiari malformation or hydrocephalus can present with vocal fold dysfunction[107] and swallowing difficulty from poor airway protection and altered laryngeal sensation.

Airway protection in relation to swallowing function can be easily evaluated by an endoscopic swallowing study. Flexible endoscopic evaluation of swallowing (FEES), initially introduced as an adjunct to the adult feeding evaluation, has been successfully used in infants and children of all ages. This test combines flexible endoscopy of the nose, pharynx, and larynx with a feeding assessment. This examination is performed conjointly by a feeding therapist and an otolaryngologist.[108-111] A flexible fiberoptic laryngoscope is passed through the nose to visualize the larynx and pharynx. An assessment of the anatomy of the nose, velopharynx, pharynx, and larynx is done prior to the feeding assessment. An assessment of laryngeal function and structure is performed to rule out concomitant laryngeal pathology and to evaluate vocal fold closure and airway protection. With simultaneous endoscopic visualization and feeding, FEES allows for assessment of velopharyngeal closure and its impact on swallowing, pharyngeal contractility and proficiency, secretion management, vocal fold closure, laryngeal penetration, and aspiration. Patients who are unable or unwilling to feed can be assessed for aspiration risk by placing green food coloring into the oral cavity to mix with the patient's own secretions. Visualization of the path of secretions and how the child handles them by spontaneous or voluntary swallows can help determine aspiration risk. Swallowing safety by modifications in food consistencies and volumes and compensatory postural changes can be assessed by the FEES examination without exposing the patient to radiation. FEES not only provides an assessment of feeding but also provides an assessment of potential pharyngeal and laryngeal anomalies that affect the feeding process and ability to protect the lower airway from aspiration.

Sensory testing can be added to the FEES examination and is know as flexible endoscopic evaluation of swallowing with sensory testing (FEESST). Laryngopharyngeal sensory testing (LPST) allows for objective, quantifiable evaluation of the sensorimotor integrative function of airway protection by testing the integrity of the LAR. A duration (50 msec) and intensity (2.5-10 mmHg) controlled air pulse is applied to the aryepiglottic fold while observing a response of glottic closure and swallow. Normal adult LPST thresholds range from 2 to 4 mmHg and average at 2.3 mmHg.[112,113] Normative data are not available for infants and children; however, average thresholds in infants without neurologic disease or developmental delay who were evaluated for airway obstruction are 4.3 mm Hg.[114] LPST thresholds of greater than 5 mm Hg correlate with an abnormality or pathology somewhere along the afferent, brainstem, or efferent limb of the reflex arc and are most often implicated in sensory abnormalities of the larynx.[110] Thresholds of greater than 5 mmHg also correlate with poor airway protection and swallowing difficulty. Thresholds greater than 6 mmHg are seen in children with neurologic disease that includes CNS and brainstem pathology.[110,113,115-117] Elevated LPST thresholds of 6.3 mmHg in infants and children[118] and 5.8 mmHg in adults are seen in the setting of chronic laryngopharyngeal reflux (LPR).[110,119-121] Decreased LPST thresholds of 3.5 mmHg and 3.8 mmHg, respectively, in infants and children and adults are seen after antireflux treatment for LPR.[118,119] This finding shows that there is a greater response of the sensorimotor reflex and that sensation is improved after receiving reflux treatment.[118,119] This information shows that control of acid disease likely has an important role in laryngeal function in swallowing disorders in children.

A videofluoroscopic swallow study (VSS) should be considered in all infants and children with a feeding or swallowing disorder. If the esophagus and upper gastrointestinal tract have not been evaluated, an upper gastrointestinal (UGI) exam should also be considered. A speech pathologist or occupational therapist in conjunction with a radiologist perform this examination. The advantage of this evaluation is that it provides a dynamic assessment of all phases of swallowing simultaneously, thereby providing an assessment of velopharyngeal closure, pharyngeal contraction, and laryngeal penetration or aspiration and esophageal propagation. This study, however, is limited in its ability to evaluate specific laryngeal pathology in relation to a swallowing problem. Additionally, this evaluation can outline any obstructive or congenital pathology of the esophagus that can interfere with swallowing. An assessment of gastroesophageal reflux can be made by this study but it is unable to specifically determine if reflux is pathologic. Food substances given during this examination typically mirror what was determined tolerable during the oral motor evaluation. Infants are fed barium through a nipple or given a thin barium-coated puree. Children older than 12 months of age are assessed by three textures, a liquid, puree, and solid. The primary limitation of the use of VSS in children is that repeated exposure to radiation limits its use for extensive teaching of compensatory maneuvers and repeat assessment of swallowing over time to evaluate progress. Additionally, infants and children with oral aversion and feeding disorder may not ingest an adequate amount of barium to provide a meaningful study. Airway protection in orally averted infants may be better evaluated by the FEES technique.

PEDIATRIC VOICE DISORDERS

The area of pediatric laryngology has expanded to the evaluation and management of voice disorders. The larynx is often involved and may include inflammatory disorders, neoplastic lesions, and neurologic and iatrogenic causes of laryngeal dysphonia.

Laryngeal causes of dysphonia that present at birth are usually congenital or neurologic. Congenital causes that present in infancy are usually associated with airway obstruction or difficulty in swallowing. Examples include laryngeal webs and laryngeal clefts. Neurologic causes are usually related to unilateral paralysis of the vocal fold, leading to a weak cry. Central causes including Chiari malformation and hydrocephalus must be excluded as to not overlook a serious condition,[107] In infants, vocal fold function often returns once the central cause is corrected.

It is important to take a careful history to help differentiate causes. Dysphonia that presents after birth is more likely related to a growth or lesion, structural problem, or inflammatory cause. Dysphonia that is progressive is usually due to a growth or lesion on the vocal fold. For a child who presents with intermittent dysphonia, it is important to distinguish intermittent or recurrent dysphonia from persistent or progressive dysphonia. Intermittent dysphonia may be worse in the morning, which suggests laryngopharyngeal reflux as a cause; if worse in the evening after voice use, it suggests an anatomic problem such as vocal nodules. Persistent, progressive dysphonia suggests the presence of an enlarging neoplasm, most commonly laryngeal papilloma. Progressive dysphonia may also be fluctuant. The key differentiation between intermittent and fluctuating progressive hoarseness, however, is that the general baseline of the voice disorder also slowly worsens, which may indicate a more serious and potentially life-threatening problem such as a growing neoplasm or papilloma.[122]

Extraesophageal reflux disease, also referred to as laryngopharyngeal reflux (LPR), can lead to dysphonia in children as it does in adults (Figure 28-11). LPR causes direct inflammation to the vocal folds leading to changes in vibratory motion. However, determining the presence of reflux in children and infants based on history can be difficult. Common presentations of GERD and LPR in children include frequent emesis events, wet burps, and recurrent cough, especially in the morning. Reflux also is thought to be associated with chronic hoarseness and formation of vocal nodules in children.[122] No criterion for diagnosis exists for significant gastroesophageal reflux inducing laryngeal pathology in children; however, the criteria for adults may be applicable.[123,124] Once the other causes for dysphonia have been ruled out, an empiric trial of reflux management may be a useful diagnostic tool.

Vocal fold nodules (Figure 28-12) and cyst (Figure 28-11) are the most common finding in children who present with dysphonia. The etiology is unknown, but thought to be strongly associated with LPR. Treatment is evolving and includes voice use modification and therapy along with reflux management. The role and timing of surgical removal is controversial.

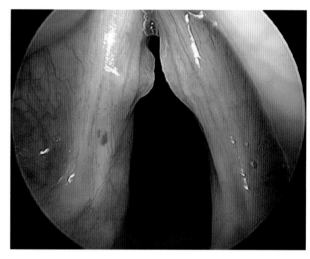

FIGURE 28–11. A 4-year-old child with laryngopharyngeal reflux documented on dual 24-hour pH metry who presented with chronic dysphonia.

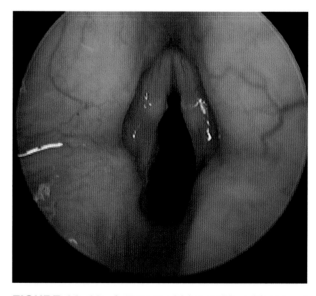

FIGURE 28–12. A 7-year-old boy with a history of voice abuse and intermittent hoarseness diagnosed with vocal fold nodules.

Iatrogenic causes of laryngeal dysphonia are usually related to direct trauma to the larynx. Blunt neck trauma may lead to arytenoid dislocation and subsequent dysphonia. Endotracheal tube intubation may lead to formation of contact granulomas, especially if the endotracheal tube is inappropriately large. Prolonged intubations with cuffed endotracheal tubes in children also lead to glottic and subglottic pathology that can cause dysphonia. Subglottic pathology leads to turbulent airflow through the glottis that can alter voice quality.

Unilateral vocal fold paralysis can lead to a weak cry in infants or hoarseness in children. Causes of unilateral paralysis in children are central or peripheral. Central causes are either due to hydrocephalus or brainstem pathology (Chiari malformation, atlanto-axial subluxation, or tumor). Peripheral causes can occur anywhere along the course of the vagal nerve and include compressive effect from neck or mediastinal tumors; direct injury during neck, spinal, or intrathoracic surgery; or injury from blunt or fix-wire neck trauma. An additional but rare cause of vocal fold paralysis in children is postviral vagal neuropathy. Most children with unilateral vocal fold paralysis, however, compensate and the degree of dysphonia is negligible and intervention is rarely indicated. Vocal fold medialization techniques including vocal fold injection[125] and type I thyroplasty used in adults are applicable in select children.[126,127]

Essential to the diagnosis of a pediatric voice disorder is direct visualization of the larynx. A dynamic examination by flexible laryngoscopy in an awake child or infant allows for evaluation of function in addition to assessing for lesions, structural abnormalities, or inflammatory processes. The role of stroboscopic evaluation of the larynx in children is evolving. Normative data are not widely available.[128] An examination under general anesthesia may be required to confirm neoplastic disorders and other lesions of the larynx. Laryngeal electromyography (EMG) has been used on occasion in the assessment of children with vocal and motion abnormalities, but technical difficulties have made this procedure problematic. EMG may be helpful, however, in distinguishing fixation of the vocal fold from vocal fold paralysis, as well as to follow reinnervation after recurrent laryngeal nerve injury. This procedure remains investigational in children, however, because of its technical difficulties.[122]

Review Questions

1. A 3-month-old infant boy presents with inspiratory stridor since birth that is worse with feeding and sleeping supine. He has frequent episodes of emesis. He is at the 5th percentile for weight. Clinical examination shows a transcutaneous oxygen saturation level of 85% and inspiratory stridor with pectus excavatum. The next best step in management is:
   a. Antireflux treatment with proton pump inhibitor
   b. Antireflux treatment with Nissen fundoplication
   c. Tracheotomy and feeding tube
   d. Supraglottoplasty and proton pump inhibitor
   e. Supraglottoplasty and feeding tube

2. Grade III subglottic stenosis is best treated by:
   a. CO_2 laser
   b. KTP Laser
   c. CO_2 laser and tracheotomy
   d. KTP laser and tracheotomy
   e. Open surgical reconstruction

3. A 10-month-old infant girl presents with a history of inspiratory stridor, recurrent cyanosis with feeding, and recurrent pneumonia. Her past medical history includes a PDA, right choanal atresia, and hydronephrosis. The most likely laryngeal anomaly is:
   a. Right vocal cord paralysis
   b. Laryngomalacia
   c. Laryngeal cleft
   d. Laryngeal web
   e. Subglottic stenosis

4. A 4-year-old otherwise healthy boy with a 5-month history of intermittent dysphonia and hoarseness presents with progressive respiratory distress. The most common cause is:
   a. Severe gastroesophageal reflux disease with laryngopharyngeal reflux
   b. Laryngeal papilloma
   c. Laryngeal web
   d. Hydrocephalus
   e. Subglottic stenosis

5. A 3-year-old is brought in by her parents with multiple concerns. She is described as a picky eater, who has coughing and choking episodes during feeding. She is at the 10th percentile for weight. The parents also express concern about the quality of her voice, and describe it as raspy, and worse at the end of the day. She is a former 33-week preemie, who required intubation for the first 3 weeks of life. She has a history of recurrent emesis and colic during the first year of life. The best next step in the evaluation and management of this child is:
   a. Trial of empiric reflux management with PPI therapy
   b. MRI to rule out Chiari malformation
   c. Direct laryngoscopy and esophagoscopy under general anesthesia
   d. Videofluoroscopic swallow study
   e. FEES examination

6. The child described in question 5 is found to have bilateral vocal fold cyst and laryngeal penetration with cough during a feeding assessment and pooling of secretions in the hypopharynx. The next best step in her management is
   a. Direct laryngoscopy and esophagoscopy under general anesthesia

   b. Trial of empiric reflux management with PPI therapy
   c. MRI to rule out Chiari malformation
   d. Videofluoroscopic swallow study
   e. Secretion management with glycopyrrolate

REFERENCES

1. Hartnick CJ. Rehbar R. Prasad V. Development and maturation of the pediatric human vocal fold lamina propria. *Laryngoscope.* 2005;115(1): 4-15.
2. Boseley ME, Hartnick CJ. Assessing the outcome of surgery to correct velopharyngeal insufficiency with the pediatric voice outcomes survey. *Intl J Pediatr Otorhinolaryngol.* 2004; 68(11):1429-1433.
3. Hawkins DB, Clark RW. Flexible laryngoscopy in neonates, infants, and young children. *Ann Otol Rhinol Laryngol.* 1987;96:81-85.
4. Chait DH, Lotz WK. Successful pediatric examinations using nasoendoscopy. *Laryngoscope.* 1991;101:1016-1018.
5. Schechtman FG. Office evaluation of pediatric upper airway obstruction. *Otolaryngol Clin North Am.* 1992;25:857-865.
6. Berkowitz RG. Neonatal upper airway assessment by awake flexible laryngoscopy. *Ann Otol Rhinol Laryngol.* 1998;107:75-80.
7. Hartnick CJ. Zeitels SM. Pediatric video laryngostroboscopy. *Intl J Pediatr Otorhinolaryngol.* 2005;69:215-219.
8. Link DT, Willging JP, Miller CK, Cotton RT, Rudolph CD. Pediatric laryngopharyngeal sensory testing during flexible endoscopic evaluation of swallowing: feasible and correlative. *Ann Otol Rhinol Laryngol.* 2000;109:899-905.
9. Lindstrom DR, Book DT, Conley SF, Flanary VA, Kerschner JE. Office-based lower airway endoscopy in pediatric patients. *Arch Otolaryngol Head Neck Surg.* 2003;129(8):847-853.
10. Holinger PH, Brown W. Congenital webs, cyst, laryngoceles and other anomalies of the larynx. *Ann Otol Rhinol Laryngol.* 1967;76:744-752.

11. Giannoni C, Sulek M, Friedman EM, Duncan NO, 3rd. Gastroesophageal reflux association with laryngomalacia: a prospective study. *Intl J Pediatr Otorhinolaryngol.* 1998;43(1):11-20.

12. Remacle M, Bodart E, Lawson G, Minet M, Mayne A. Use of the CO_2-laser micropoint micromanipulator for the treatment of laryngomalacia. *Eur Arch Oto-Rhino-Laryngol.* 1996;253(7):401-404.

13. Rudolph CD, Mazur LJ, Liptak GS, et al. Guidelines for evaluation and treatment of gastroesophageal reflux in infants and children: recommendations of the North American Society for Pediatric Gastroenterology and Nutrition. [see comment]. *J Pediatr Gastroenterol Nutr.* 2001;32(2):S1-S31.

14. Holinger LD, Konior RJ. Surgical management of severe laryngomalacia. *Laryngoscope.* 1989;99(2):136-142.

15. Polonovski JM, Contencin P, Francois M, Viala P, Narcy P. Aryepiglottic fold excision for the treatment of severe laryngomalacia. *Ann Otol Rhinol Laryngol.* 1990;99(8):625-627.

16. Zalzal GH, Anon JB, Cotton RT. Epiglottoplasty for the treatment of laryngomalacia. *Ann Otol Rhinol Laryngol.* 1987;96(1 pt 1):72-76.

17. Roger G, Denoyelle F, Triglia JM, Garabedian EN. Severe laryngomalacia: surgical indications and results in 115 patients. *Laryngoscope.* 1995;105(10):1111-1117.

18. Baxter MR. Congenital laryngomalacia. *Can J Anaesthes.* 1994;41(4):332-339.

19. McSwiney PF, Cavanagh NP, Languth P. Outcome in congenital stridor (laryngomalacia). *Arch Dis Childhood.* 1977;52(3):215-218.

20. Seid AB, Park SM, Kearns MJ, Gugenheim S. Laser division of the aryepiglottic folds for severe laryngomalacia. *Intl J Pediatric Otorhinolaryngol.* 1985;10(2):153-158.

21. Lane RW, Weider DJ, Steinem C, Marin-Padilla M. Laryngomalacia. A review and case report of surgical treatment with resolution of pectus excavatum. *Arch Otolaryngol.* 1984;110(8):546-551.

22. Jani P, Koltai P, Ochi JW, Bailey CM. Surgical treatment of laryngomalacia. *J Laryngol Otol.* 1991;105(12):1040-1045.

23. Marcus CL, Crockett DM, Davidson Ward SL. Evaluation of epiglottoplasty as a treatment for severe laryngomalacia. *J Peds.* 1990;117(5):706-710.

24. McClurg FL, Evans DA. Laser laryngoplasty for laryngomalacia. *Laryngoscope.* 1994;104(3 pt 1):247-252.

25. Toynton SC, Saunders MW, Bailey CM. Aryepiglottoplasty for laryngomalacia: 100 consecutive cases. *J Laryngol Otol.* 2001;115(1):35-38.

26. Denoyelle F, Mondain M, Gresillon N, Roger G, Chaudre F, Garabedian EN. Failures and complications of supraglottoplasty in children. *Arch Otolaryngol Head Neck Surg.* 2003;129(10):1077-1080; discussion 1080.

27. Milczuk HA, Smith JD, Everts EC. Congenital laryngeal webs: surgical management and clinical embryology. *Intl J Pediatr Otorhinolaryngol.* 2000;52(1):1-9.

28. Unal M. The successful management of congenital laryngeal web with endoscopic lysis and topical mitomycin-C. *Intl J Pediatr Otorhinolaryngol.* 2004;68(2):231-235.

29. Benjamin BN. Congenital laryngeal webs. *Ann Otol Rhinol Laryngol.* 1983;92:317-326.

30. Holland BW, Koufman JA, Postma GN, McGuirt WF, Jr. Laryngopharyngeal reflux and laryngeal web formation in patients with pediatric recurrent respiratory papillomas. *Laryngoscope.* 2002;112(11):1926-1929.

31. Pollack IF, Kinnunen D, Albright AL. The effect of early craniocervical decompression on functional outcome in neonates and young infants with myelodysplasia and symptomatic Chiari II malformations: results from a prospective series. *Neurosurgery.* 1996;38(4):703-710.

32. Yamada H, Tanaka Y, Nakamura S. Laryngeal stridor associated with the Chiari II malformation. *Childs Nerv Syst.* 1985;1(6):312-318.

33. Link DT, Cotton RT. The laryngotracheal complex in pediatric head and neck trauma: securing the airway and management of external laryngeal injury. *Fac Plast Surg Clin North Am.* 1999;7(2):133-144.

34. Bower CM, Choi SS, Cotton RT. Arytenoidectomy in children. *Ann Otol Rhinol Laryngol.* 1994;103(4 pt 1):271-278.

35. Triglia JM, Belus JF, Nicollas R. Arytenoidopexy for bilateral vocal fold paralysis in young children. *J Laryngol Otol.* 1996;110(11):1027-1030.

36. Narcy P, Contencin P, Viala P. Surgical treatment for laryngeal paralysis in infants and children. Ann Otol Rhinol Laryngol. 1990;99(2 pt 1):124-128.

37. Friedman EM, de Jong AL, Sulek M. Pediatric bilateral vocal fold immobility: the role of carbon dioxide laser posterior transverse partial cordectomy. *Ann Otol, Rhinol Laryngol.* 2001;110(8):723-728.

38. Rimell FL, Dohar JE. Endoscopic management of pediatric posterior glottic stenosis. *Ann Otol Rhinol Laryngol.* 1998;107(4):285-290.

39. Hartnick CJ, Brigger MT, Willging JP, Cotton RT, Myer CM, 3rd. Surgery for pediatric vocal cord paralysis: a retrospective review. *Ann Otol Rhinol Laryngol.* 2003;112(1):1-6.

40. Brigger MT, Hartnick CJ. Surgery for pediatric vocal cord paralysis: a meta-analysis. *Otolaryngol Head Neck Surg.* 2002;126(4):349-355.

41. Gray SD, Kelly SM, Dove H. Arytenoid separation for impaired pediatric vocal fold mobility. *Ann Otol Rhinol Laryngol.* 1994;103(7):510-515.

42. Younis RT, Lazar RH, Astor F. Posterior cartilage graft in single-stage laryngotracheal reconstruction. *Otolaryngol Head Neck Surg.* 2003;129(3):168-175.

43. Rutter MJ, Cotton RT. The use of posterior cricoid grafting in managing isolated posterior glottic stenosis in children. *Arch Otolaryngol Head Neck Surg.* 2004;130(6):737-739.

44. Inglis AF, Jr., Perkins JA, Manning SC, Mouzakes J. Endoscopic posterior cricoid split and rib grafting in 10 children. *Laryngoscope.* 2003;113(11):2004-2009.

45. Kashima H, Leventhal B, Clark K, et al. Interferon alfa-n1 (Wellferon) in juvenile onset recurrent respiratory papillomatosis: results of a randomized study in twelve collaborative institutions. *Laryngoscope.* 1988;98(3):334-340.

46. Shah K, Kashima H, Polk BF, Shah F, Abbey H, Abramson A. Rarity of cesarean delivery in cases of juvenile-onset respiratory papillomatosis. *Obstet Gynecol.* 1986;68(6):795-799.

47. Parsons DS, Bothwell MR. Powered instrument papilloma excision: an alternative to laser therapy for recurrent respiratory papilloma. *Laryngoscope.* 2001;111(8):1494-1496.

48. Derkay CS, Schechter GL. Anatomy and physiology of pediatric swallowing disorders. *Otolaryngol Clin North Am.* 1998;31(3):397-404.

49. Wetmore S, Key J, Suen J. Complications of laser surgery for laryngeal papillomatosis. *Laryngoscope.* 1985;95:798-801.

50. Cole RR, Myer CM, 3rd, Cotton RT. Tracheotomy in children with recurrent respiratory papillomatosis. *Head Neck.* 1989;11(3):226-230.

51. McDonald I, Stock J. Prolonged nasotracheal intubation. *Br J Anesthesia.* 1965;37:161-173.

52. Holinger PH, Kutnick SL, Schild JA, Holinger LD. Subglottic stenosis in infants and children. *Ann Otol Rhinol Laryngol.* 1976;85:591-599.

53. Ratner I, Whitfield J. Acquired subglottic stenosis in the very-low-birth-weight infant. *Am J Dis Child.* 1983;137(1):40-43.

54. Myer CM, 3rd, O'Connor DM, Cotton RT. Proposed grading system for subglottic stenosis based on endotracheal tube sizes. *Ann Otol Rhinol Laryngol.* 1994;103(4 pt 1):319-323.

55. Little FB, Koufman JA, Kohut RI, Marshall RB. Effect of gastric acid on the pathogenesis of subglottic stenosis. *Ann Otol Rhinol Laryngol.* 1985;94:516-519.

56. Gilger MA. Pediatric otolaryngologic manifestations of gastroesophageal reflux disease. *Curr Gastroenterol Rep.* 2003;5(3):247-252.

57. Yellon RF, Goldberg H. Update on gastroesophageal reflux disease in pediatric airway disorders. *Am J Med.* 2001;111(suppl 8A):78S-84S.

58. Maronian NC, Azadeh H, Waugh P, Hillel A. Association of laryngopharyngeal reflux disease and subglottic stenosis. *Ann Otol Rhinol Laryngol.* 2001;110(7 pt 1):606-612.

59. Suskind DL, Zeringue GP, 3rd, Kluka EA, Udall J, Liu DC. Gastroesophageal reflux and pediatric otolaryngologic disease: the role of antireflux surgery. *Arch Otolaryngol Head Neck Surg.* 2001;127(5):511-514.

60. Walner DL, Stern Y, Gerber ME, Rudolph C, Baldwin CY, Cotton RT. Gastroesophageal reflux in patients with subglottic stenosis. *Arch Otolaryngol Head Neck Surg.* 1998;124(5):551-555.

61. Halstead LA. Gastroesophageal reflux: a critical factor in pediatric subglottic stenosis. *Otolaryngol Head Neck Surg.* 1999;120(5):683-638.

62. Cotton RT, Myer CM, 3rd, Bratcher GO, Fitton CM. Anterior cricoid split, 1977-1987. Evolution of a technique. *Arch Otolaryngol Head Neck Surg.* 1988;114(11):1300-1302.

63. Fearon B, Cotton R. Surgical correction of subglottic stenosis of the larynx. Preliminary report of an experimental surgical technique. *Ann Otol Rhinol Laryngol.* 1972;81(4):508-513.

64. Rutter MJ, Hartley BE, Cotton RT. Cricotracheal resection in children. *Arch Otolaryngol Head Neck Surg.* 2001;127(3):289-292.

65. Stern Y, Gerber ME, Walner DL, Cotton RT. Partial cricotracheal resection with primary anastomosis in the pediatric age group. *Ann Otol Rhinol Laryngol.* 1997;106(11):891-896.

66. Hartley BE, Cotton RT. Paediatric airway stenosis: laryngotracheal reconstruction or cricotracheal resection? *Clin Otolaryngol Allied Sci.* 2000;25(5):342-349.

67. Walner DL, Stern Y, Cotton RT. Margins of partial cricotracheal resection in children. *Laryngoscope.* 1999;109(10):1607-1610.

68. Monnier P, Lang F, Savary M. Partial cricotracheal resection for pediatric subglottic stenosis: a single institution's experience in 60 cases. *Eur Arch Oto-Rhino-Laryngol.* 2003;260(6):295-297.

69. Triglia JM, Nicollas R, Roman S. Primary cricotracheal resection in children: indications, technique and outcome. *Intl J Pediatr Otorhinolaryngol.* 2001;58(1):17-25.

70. Hartley BE, Rutter MJ, Cotton RT. Cricotracheal resection as a primary procedure for laryngotracheal stenosis in children. *Intl J Pediatr Otorhinolaryngol.* 2000;54(2-3):133-136.

71. Cotton RT, Myer CM, 3rd. Contemporary surgical management of laryngeal stenosis in children. *Am J Otolaryngol.* 1984;5(5):360-368.

72. Cotton RT, Gray SD, Miller RP. Update of the Cincinnati experience in pediatric laryngotracheal reconstruction. *Laryngoscope.* 1989;99(11):1111-1116.

73. Zalzal GH, Cotton RT, McAdams AJ. Cartilage grafts—present status. *Head Neck Surg.* 1986;8(5):363-374.

74. Gustafson LM, Hartley BE, Liu JH, et al. Single-stage laryngotracheal reconstruction in children: a review of 200 cases. *Otolaryngol Head Neck Surg.* 2000;123(4):430-434.

75. Jacobs BR, Salman BA, Cotton RT, Lyons K, Brilli RJ. Postoperative management of children after single-stage laryngotracheal reconstruction. *Crit Care Med.* 2001;29(1):164-168.

76. Hartley BE, Gustafson LM, Liu JH, Hartnick CJ, Cotton RT. Duration of stenting in single-stage laryngotracheal reconstruction with anterior costal cartilage grafts. *Ann Otol Rhinol Laryngol.* 2001;110(5 pt 1):413-416.

77. Hartnick CJ, Hartley BE, Lacy PD, et al. Surgery for pediatric subglottic stenosis: disease-specific outcomes. *Ann Otol Rhinol Laryngol.* 2001;110(12):1109-1113.

78. Gustafson LM, Hartley BE, Cotton RT. Acquired total (grade 4) subglottic stenosis in children. *Ann Otol Rhinol Laryngol.* 2001;110(1):16-19.

79. White DR, Cotton RT, Bean JA, Rutter MJ. Pediatric cricotracheal resection: surgical outcomes and risk factor analysis. *Arch Otolaryngol Head Neck Surg.* 2005;131(10):896-899.

80. Choa DI, Smith MC, Evans JN, Bailey CM. Subglottic hemangioma in children. *J Laryngol Otol.* 1986;100:447.

81. Leikensohn B, Cotton. Subglottic hemangioma. *J Otolaryngol.* 1976;5:487-492.

82. Cohen SR. Unusual lesions of the larynx, trachea, and bronchial tree. *Ann Otol Rhinol Laryngol.* 1969;78:476-489.

83. Hawkins DB. Corticosteroid managment of airway hemangiomas: Long term follow-up. *Laryngoscope.* 1984;94:633-637.

84. Shikhani AH. Infantile subglottic hemangiomas. *Ann Otol Rhinol Laryngol.* 1986;95:336-347.

85. Aviles R, Boyce TG, Thompson DM. *Pneumocystis carinii* pneumonia in a 3-month-old infant receiving high-dose corticosteroid therapy for airway hemangiomas. *Mayo Clin Proc.* 2004; 79(2):243-245.

86. Al-Sebeih K, Manoukian J. Systemic steroids for the management of obstructive subglottic hemangioma. *J Otolaryngol.* 2000;29(6):361-366.

87. Meeuwis J, Bos C, Hoeve L, van der Voort E. Subglottic hemangiomas in infants: treatment with intralesional corticosteroid injection and intubation. *Intl J Pediatr Otorhinolaryngol.* 1990;19:145-150.

88. Healy GB. Treatment of subglottic hemangioma with the carbon dioxide laser. *Laryngoscope.* 1980;90:809-813.

89. Sie KC, McGill T, Healy GB. Subglottic hemangioma: ten year's experience with the carbon dioxide laser. *Ann Otol Rhinol Laryngol.* 1994; 103:167-172.

90. Kacker A, April M, Ward RF. Use of potassium titanyl phosphate (KTP) laser in management of subglottic hemangiomas. *Intl J Pediatr Otorhinolaryngol.* 2001;59(1):15-21.

91. Madgy D, Ahsan SF, Kest D, Stein I. The application of the potassium-titanyl-phosphate (KTP) laser in the management of subglottic hemangioma. *Arch Otolaryngol Head Neck Surg.* 2001;127(1):47-50.

92. Ohlms LA, Jones DT, McGill T, Healy GB. Interferon alpha-2A therapy for airway hemangiomas. *Ann Otol Rhinol Laryngol.* 1994;103:1-8.

93. Chatrath P, Black M, Jani P, Albert DM, Bailey CM. A review of the current management of infantile subglottic haemangioma, including a comparison of CO_2 laser therapy versus tracheostomy. *Intl J Pediatr Otorhinolaryngol.* 2002;64(2):143-157.

94. Seid AB, Pransky SM, Kearns DB. The open surgical approach to subglottic hemangioma [comment]. *Intl J Pediatr Otorhinolaryngol.* 1993;26(1):95-96.

95. Seid AB, Pransky SM, Kearns DB. The open surgical approach to subglottic hemangioma [see comment]. *Intl J Pediatr Otorhinolaryngol.* 1991;22(1):85–90.

96. Naiman AN, Ayari S, Froehlich P. Controlled risk of stenosis after surgical excision of laryngeal hemangioma. *Arch Otolaryngol Head Neck Surg.* 2003;129(12):1291–1295.

97. Van Den Abbeele T, Triglia JM, Lescanne E, et al. Surgical removal of subglottic hemangiomas in children. *Laryngoscope.* 1999;109(8):1281–1286.

98. Wiatrak BJ, Reilly JS, Seid AB, Pransky SM, Castillo JV. Open surgical excision of subglottic hemangioma in children. *Intl J Pediatr Otorhinolaryngol.* 1996;34(1–2):191–206.

99. Froehlich P, Seid AB, Morgon A. Contrasting strategic approaches to the management of subglottic hemangiomas. *Intl J Pediatr Otorhinolaryngol.* 1996;36(2):137–146.

100. Evans KL, Courteney-Harris R, Bailey CM, Evans JN, Parsons DS. Management of posterior laryngeal and laryngotracheoesophageal clefts. *Arch Otolaryngol.* 1995;121:1380–1385.

101. Eriksen C, Zwillenberg D, Robinson N. Diagnosis and management of cleft larynx: literature review and case report. *Ann Otol Rhinol Laryngol.* 1990;99(9 pt 1):703–708.

102. Bent JP. Endoloscope repair of tpe IA laryngeal clefts. *Laryngoscope.* 1997;107:282–286.

103. Burklow KA, Phelps AN, Schultz JR, McConnell K, Rudolph C. Classifying complex pediatric feeding disorders. *J Pediatr Gastroenterol Nutr.* 1998;27(2):143–147.

104. Darrow DH, Harley CM. Evaluation of swallowing disorders in children. *Otolaryngol Clin North Am.* 1998;31(3):405–418.

105. Donner MW, Bosma JF, Robertson DL. Anatomy and physiology of the pharynx. *Gastrointest Radiol.* 1985;10(3):196–212.

106. Morris SE, Klein MD. *Prefeeding Skills: A Comprehensive Resource for Feeding Development.* Tucon, Ariz: Therapy Skill Builders; 1987.

107. Bluestone CD, Delerme AN, Samuelson GH. Airway obstruction due to vocal cord paralysis in infants with hydrocephalus and meningomyelocele. *Ann Otol Rhinol Laryngol.* 1972;81(6):778–783.

108. Willging JP. Swallowing disorders in children. *Curr Opin Otolaryngol Head Neck Surg.* 1994;2:504–507.

109. Willging JP, Miller CK, Rudloph CD. Feeding disorders in children. In: Cotton RT, Myer CM, eds. *Practical Pediatric Otolaryngology.* 1st ed. Philadelphia, Pa: Lippincott-Raven; 1999:603–312.

110. Link DT, Willging JP, Miller CK, Cotton RT, Rudolph CD. Pediatric laryngopharyngeal sensory testing during flexible endoscopic evaluation of swallowing (FEES): feasible and correlative. *Ann Otol Rhinol Laryngol.* 2000;109(10):899–905.

111. Hartnick CJ, Hartley BE, Miller C, Willging JP. Pediatric fiberoptic endoscopic evaluation of swallowing. *Ann Otol Rhinol Laryngol.* 2000;109(11):996–999.

112. Aviv JE. Sensory discrimination in the larynx and hypopharynx. *Otolaryngol Head Neck Surg.* 1997;116(3):331–334.

113. Aviv JE, Martin JH, Jones ME, et al. Age-related changes in pharyngeal and supraglottic sensation. *Ann Otol Rhinol Laryngol.* 1994;103(10):749–752.

114. Thompson DM, Rutter M, Willging JP, Rudolph C, Cotton RT. Altered laryngeal sensation: a potential etiology of apnea of infancy. *Ann Otol Rhinol Laryngol.* 2005;114(4):258–263.

115. Aviv JE, Martin JH, Sacco RL, et al. Supraglottic and pharyngeal sensory abnormalities in stroke patients with dysphagia. *Ann Otol Rhinol Laryngol.* 1996;105(2):92–97.

116. Aviv JE. Effects of aging on sensitivity of the pharyngeal and supraglottic areas. *Am J Med.* 1997;103(5A):74S–6S.

117. Aviv JE, Sacco RL, Thomson J, et al. Silent laryngopharyngeal sensory deficits after stroke. *Ann Otol Rhinol Laryngol.* 1997;106(2):87–93.

118. Suskind DL, Thompson DM, Gulati M, Hudleston P, Liu DC, Baroody F. Improved infant swallowing after GER treatment: a function of improved laryngeal sensation? *Laryngoscope.* 2006: In press.

119. Aviv JE, Liu H, Parides M, Kaplan ST, Close LG. Laryngopharyngeal sensory deficits in patients with laryngopharyngeal reflux and dysphagia. *Ann Otol Rhinol Laryngol.* 2000;109(11):1000–1006.

120. Aviv JE, Martin JH, Kim T, et al. Laryngopharyngeal sensory discrimination testing and the laryngeal adductor reflex. *Ann Otol Rhinol Laryngol.* 1999;108(8):725–730.

121. Close LG. Laryngopharyngeal manifestations of reflux: diagnosis and therapy. *Eur J Gastroenterol Hepatol.* 2002;14(suppl 1):S23–S27.

122. McMurray JS. Disorders of phonation in children. *Pediatr Clin North Am.* 2003;50(2):363–380.

123. Koufman JA. Laryngopharyngeal reflux is different from classic gastroesophageal reflux disease. *Ear Nose Throat J.* 2002;81(9 suppl 2):7-9.

124. Koufman JA, Belafsky PC. Unilateral or localized Reinke's edema (pseudocyst) as a manifestation of vocal fold paresis: the paresis podule. *Laryngoscope.* 2001;111(4 pt 1):576-580.

125. Patel NJ, Kershner JE, Merati AL. The use of injectable collagen in the management of pediatric unilateral vocal fold paralysis. Int *J Pediatr Otolaryngol.* 2003;67(12):1355-1360.

126. Gardner GM, Altman JS, Balakrishnan G. Pediatric vocal fold medialization with Silastic implant: intraoperative airway management. *Intl J Pediatr Otorhinolaryngol.* 2000;52(1):37-44.

127. Link DT, Rutter MJ, Liu JH, Willging JP, Myer CM, Cotton RT. Pediatric type I thyroplasty: an evolving procedure. *Ann Otol Rhinol Laryngol.* 1999;108(12):1105-1110.

128. Hartnick CJ, Zeitels SM. Pediatric video laryngostroboscopy. *Intl J Pediatr Otorhinolaryngol.* 2005;69(2):215-219.

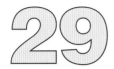

Postlaryngectomy Speech Rehabilitation

Bruce H. Campbell, MD, FACS
Mary Brawley, MA, CCC-SLP

KEY POINTS

■ Postlaryngectomy speech rehabilitation options include electrolarynx, esophageal, and tracheoesophageal puncture (TEP) speech.

■ Esophageal speech is difficult or impossible for the majority of laryngectomy patients to master.

■ TEP fistula speech requires a significant commitment by both patient and health care provider aimed at stoma and prosthesis care.

■ Both primary and secondary TEP fistula speech are options for the properly motivated patient.

Since the procedure was first successfully performed in 1874, laryngectomy has cured cancer at the cost of oral speech communication. However, a consistent secondary goal has been the restoration of speech after laryngectomy. Even the earliest laryngeal cancer surgeries included the use of mucosally lined shunts and partial laryngeal resection procedures. Until the 1980s, postlaryngectomy speech rehabilitation relied on esophageal speech, electrolarynx speech, or the creation of mucosa-lined shunts and partial laryngectomy procedures. In general, the nonsurgical approaches were either difficult for the patient to master or sounded artificial. The surgical approaches were technically challenging for the surgeon and were often associated with intractable aspiration, functional failure, and dysphagia. In the 1980s, tracheoesophageal puncture (TEP) speech became widely available, simplifying voice restoration for the surgeon and speech-language pathologist (SLP) while reducing risk and increasing success rates for the patient. Despite challenges including leakage, lack of fluency, prosthesis failure, and discomfort of stoma manipulation, the use of TEP speech has become the centerpiece of postlaryngectomy speech rehabilitation.

As the approaches to successful speech rehabilitation evolved, so have the indications for laryngectomy. Prior to the 1980s, total laryngectomy was routinely offered as the primary treatment option for all but the earliest stage laryngeal and hypopharyngeal cancers. With the publication of organ preservation protocols including the VA Cooperative Study 268,[1] the treatment of advanced laryngeal cancers shifted from total laryngectomy to a combination of chemotherapy with radiation therapy (CTX/RT). [2,3] Subsequent organ preservation studies including RTOG 91-11[4] further refined CTX/RT approaches by demonstrating that destructive laryngeal cancers (primarily T4 lesions) still had better outcomes with a primary laryngectomy while confirming that T3 cancers could be successfully managed nonoperatively in many patients. This evidence supported total laryngectomy as the best treatment for only the most advanced laryngeal and hypopharynx cancers. These studies also support the use of total laryngectomy for patients who failed initial control with a nonsurgical treatment.

In addition, laryngectomy speech rehabilitation shifted away from an emphasis on esophageal speech toward TEP speech, and, as surgeons and SLPs became more comfortable with the techniques, more patients underwent primary TE fistula creation at the time of laryngectomy. TEP speech was an attractive alternative because it did not compromise oncologic principles, did not require complicated reconstructive procedures, carried little risk of aspiration, and simplified speech training.[5] In this chapter, current considerations for speech rehabilitation after laryngectomy are reviewed from the perspective of the surgeon and the SLP.

PREOPERATIVE CONSIDERATIONS

A team approach to preoperative counseling is crucial to successful postlaryngectomy outcome. The SLP is instrumental in reinforcing preoperative teaching about the surgical procedure and the expected postoperative physical and psychological changes. An overwhelming amount of information is provided in a very short period of time and the experienced SLP is faced with the challenge of teaching an unfamiliar subject to a dazed and confused patient and his or her family. Much of the information is repeated and provided whenever possible in written form. Many centers recruit survivors who have undergone laryngectomy to serve as role models for newly diagnosed patients.

The selection of a speech rehabilitation approach depends on a number of factors including the patient's anticipated social support, self-care potential, pulmonary function, and hand-eye coordination. Patients who would be expected to have significant problems caring for a stoma because of limited visual acuity, poor hand-eye coordination, and/or aversion to dealing with secretions are generally poor candidates for primary TEP speech. If they elect TEP speech, these individuals might have more success with an indwelling prosthesis rather than one version that requires regular removal and replacement. Some individuals are uncertain which type of speech rehabilitation they will pursue. In this case, the surgeon may elect to create a TE fistula at the time of the laryngectomy and allow it to heal if the patient later decides against TEP speech.[6]

From the surgeon's perspective, the site of the primary tumor or the expected reconstruction can also affect the selection of speech rehabilitation. The best candidates for a primary TEP fistula speech are those where little pharyngeal mucosa will be sacrificed and the remainder of the cervical anatomy is normal. Relative contraindications to the primary creation of a TE fistula include an unusually tight pharyngeal closure or the need for microvascular pharyngeal reconstruction in the planned TE fistula site. Relative contraindications for secondary TE fistula creation include poor pulmonary function, a small tracheal stoma, tight cricopharyngeus muscle anatomy, and the inability to pass an air insufflation test. The air insufflation test is a technique in which a device is used to temporarily introduce air into the esophagus. A valve is placed over the stoma and this valve is connected to tubing that is introduced into the esophagus by a transnasal route.

In addition, because most secondary TE fistula creation techniques require passage of a cervical esophagoscope to the level of the stoma, anatomic relative contraindications to secondary TE fistula creation include significant cervical kyphosis, tight pharyngeal stenosis, and severe trismus.

ELECTROLARYNX

The electrolarynx remains the only type of speech rehabilitation for many postlaryngectomy cancer survivors. The electrolarynx can either serve as the main or an alternative speech technique throughout the individual's life. The neck-placed device produces sound vibrations that are transmitted through the neck tissues. Neck placement depends on identification of a "sweet spot." Finding the "sweet spot" is a matter of trial and error and can be particularly difficult for hearing-impaired individuals. The communication partner often provides valuable feedback. Alternatively, an intraoral vibrating plastic tube can be held in the side of the mouth between the tongue and molar teeth. Intraoral devices can serve as a bridge to the use of neck placement in the early postoperative period when neck swelling is still present. Vibrating devices can be permanently implanted in a denture although this is less widely available. The SLP teaches the patient how to operate the device and optimize placement. Once the patient has mastered the basics of electrolarynx use, little additional training is needed. The devices are an excellent choice for cancer survivors who cannot master esophageal speech and who are not able to travel to a medical center regularly.

ESOPHAGEAL SPEECH

Esophageal speech was, for several decades, the primary goal of postlaryngectomy speech rehabilitation. Esophageal sound is produced by first trapping air in the cervical esophagus and/or neopharynx and then voluntarily releasing it back through the mouth. As the air passes, the tissue pulsates and produces a sound. Esophageal speech has always been difficult to teach and learn; reported mastery rates in the era prior to the availability of TE fistula speech were generally around 25%.[7] When effective, it can be consistently understandable, dynamic, and relatively fluent. Esophageal speech provides a level of independence not available to TE fistula speakers; it is a hands-free technique that requires no equipment or devices. Despite an initial steep learning curve, once the technique is mastered, there are few visits to the hospital or clinic for speech intervention. Esophageal speech training has not been employed by most clinicians since the introduction of the TEP speech.

Nevertheless, esophageal speech remains a viable alternative, and it is possible that higher than historical success rates could be achieved by combining neopharynx construction that decreases pharyngeal tightness, improved radiation therapy techniques, and the judicious use of botulinum toxin.

TRACHEOESOPHAGEAL PROSTHESIS

TEP speech is produced by directing pulmonary air directly from the lungs into the pharynx via a prosthesis. Because the pulmonary air column powers speech, spoken phrases can be longer, louder, more fluent, and more flexible than with esophageal speech. The fistula can be created either primarily (at the time of the laryngectomy) or secondarily (at a subsequent procedure). Although secondary TE fistulas can be created in the awake patient,[8] most procedures are performed in the operating room under general anesthesia.

Although 90% of patients can achieve TEP fistula speech on the first day of treatment,[9] long-term successful use of the devices is 75 to 85%.[10-12] Prostheses have variable durability depending on the model and local tissue conditions. The TEP speech patient's long-term care requires significantly more ongoing interaction with the SLP than for electrolarynx or esophageal speakers because of the need for prosthesis replacement and troubleshooting. Complications and the need for troubleshooting are fairly common with TE fistulas and include *Candida* infestations, hypertrophy of the fistula tract, leakage around or through the prosthesis, unexpected displacement of the prosthesis, migration or closure of the fistula tract, and loss of fluency.[6] Therefore, the patient must understand that the improved speech quality and ease of mastery will require a significant commitment to participate in the management of the tract and prosthesis. Despite this, successful TEP speech is associated with higher quality of life scores than other types of speech rehabilitation.[13]

Improving Speech Success Rates for Primary TEP Fistula Formation

Several modifications of the standard laryngectomy technique have been described to ensure successful speech rehabilitation. The goal of these techniques is to maintain a solid pharyngeal closure and adequate airway yet allow for relaxed pharyngeal tone and a stoma opening that is flush to the anterior cervical skin.

The surgical optimization of speech rehabilitation begins during the laryngeal resection. By intentionally dissecting the mucosa away from the constrictors and the thyroid cartilage prior to making the mucosal cuts, the final pharyngeal size will be as large as possible. For cancers confined to the endolarynx, the pharyngeal mucosal cuts hug the aryepiglottic folds as closely as possible, and are joined high across the postcricoid mucosa.

To decrease pharyngeal tone and improve fluency, Singer described a selective pharyngeal constrictor myotomy and division of the pharyngeal plexus nerves.[14,15] Either approach relaxes the tonicity of the pharynx and improves the efficient passage of air from the level of the fistula to the oral cavity. The cricopharyngeus and proximal esophageal muscles are usually sectioned at the time of laryngectomy to optimize a relaxed neopharynx.

The TE fistula can be created 10 to 15 mm below the mucosal margin of the cut trachea by passing a right-angle hemostat from the open pharynx into the cervical esophagus and then tenting up the posterior tracheal wall (Figure 29-1). A feeding tube or catheter is passed via the tract to the stomach.

To decrease potential scar formation, muscle spasm, and constriction of the pharyngeal

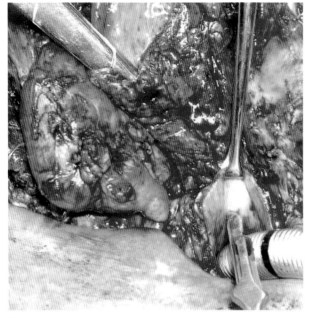 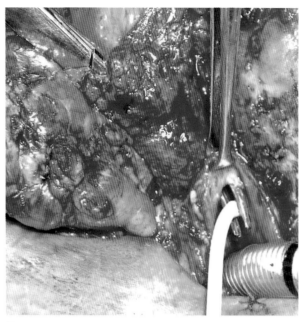

A. **B.**

FIGURE 29–1. A. The proposed primary TE fistula site is tented up over a right angle hemostat that is passed to the level of the upper trachea via the pharynx at the time of laryngectomy. A 15 blade is about to make the incision. **B.** The right-angle clamp grasps the feeding tube which is passed via the fistula into the stomach.

lumen, the pharyngeal closure can be left unreinforced by omitting the reapproximation of the pharyngeal constrictors. Alternatively, the pharynx can be oversewn with a "half-closure" where the muscle on one side is mobilized and approximated to the deep submucosa beyond the pharyngeal closure itself.[16] Because a single layer or half-closure technique can potentially be less secure than a standard multilayer closure, the integrity of the closure is tested by insufflating the oral cavity and pharynx with saline under pressure while occluding the nostrils and distal pharynx.

Having a "flat," or vertical stoma to the surrounding plane of skin improves the eventual use of a hands-free voicing system (Figure 29–2). To improve the position of the stoma and flatten the airway to the skin, the sternal heads of both sternocleidomastoid muscles are divided (Figure 29-3). This avoids a "deep" stoma in many individuals and allows better access and visibility for the patient and SLP. A silicone laryngectomy tube or tracheotomy tube is used postoperatively to maintain airway size.

Improving Speech Success Rates for Secondary TE Fistula Formation

Secondary tracheoesophageal puncture techniques vary between institutions; however, the goal is to create a small opening in the midline of the posterior tracheal wall approximately 10 mm below the tracheocutaneous junction. A large opening can lead to leakage; an off-center opening can complicate subsequent prosthesis placement. Some techniques place the prosthesis at the time of the TE fistula creation[17]; others place a

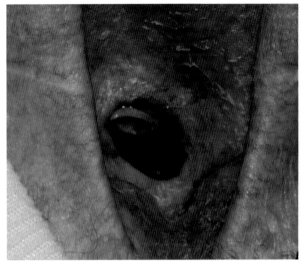

A.

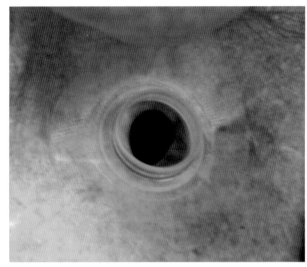

B.

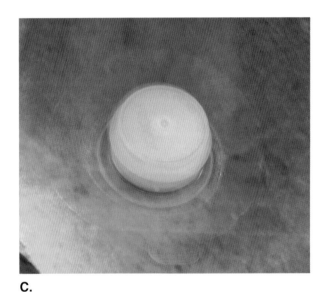

C.

FIGURE 29–2. A. Deep stoma in patient whose sternal heads were not divided. This stoma presentation makes fitting of a hands-free device difficult. **B.** Flat stoma presentation in a patient who underwent sternal head divisions. Hands-free housing in place. **C.** Housing with humidification cassette in place.

catheter in the tract for a few days prior to final placement of the prosthesis.

One technique for secondary TEP creation is shown here (Figures 29-4 through 29-11). A 16 Fr 24-inch (61-cm) central line catheter is modified for use by creating a gentle curve in the 14 Fr introducing needle. The needle is then inserted from the stoma into the tip of an inverted cervical esophagoscope under direct vision using the light from the esophagoscope as a target. The plastic connector tip of the guide wire is removed

and the wire is passed through the needle until it emerges from the esophagoscope. The needle is then removed from the tract. The fistula tract is dilated around the wire with either a hemostat or a dilator. The tip of an appropriately sized red rubber catheter (usually 14 or 16 Fr) is trimmed off and the wire is passed through the new opening in the catheter and out one of the eyeholes and twisted on itself, thus securing the catheter to the wire. The wire and catheter are then advanced into the esophagoscope while main-

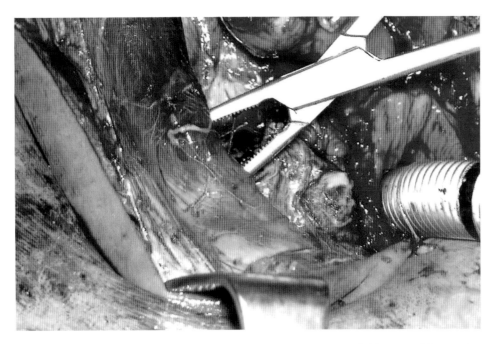

FIGURE 29–3. The inferior sternal head of the right sternocleidomastoid muscle is being divided to improve stoma presentation.

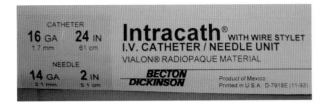

FIGURE 29–4. Packaging from needle and wire used to create a secondary TEP.

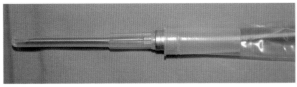

A.

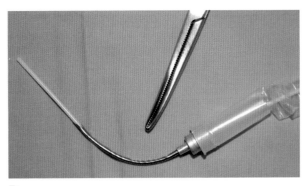

B.

FIGURE 29–5. A. The needle prior to modification. **B.** Using a heavy hemostat, the needle is gently curved to simplify eventual insertion into the pharynx. The bend is created with the plastic catheter in place to prevent kinking of the needle shaft, which would prevent passage of the wire.

taining traction on the wire. Once the catheter has been fully advanced through the fistula site and through the esophagoscope, the wire is removed. The tip of the catheter is grasped with a long cup forceps, and the catheter is returned back through the esophagoscope and gently guided down the esophagus. Correct placement is visually confirmed and the esophagoscope removed. The catheter is secured. Once initial healing has taken place (usually 3–5 days) the catheter is removed and the speech prosthesis is placed.

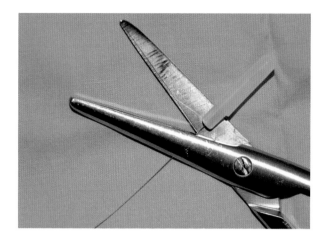

FIGURE 29–6. The plastic connector is removed from the guide wire. This is the end that will be eventually attached to the catheter.

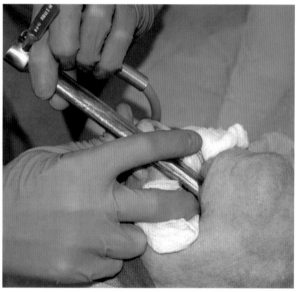

A.

FIGURE 29–7. A. and **B.** The cervical esophagoscope is inserted to the level of the stoma and then flipped over to allow the bevel of the scope to face the stoma from the pharynx.

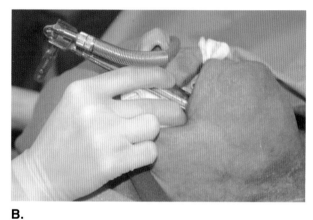

B.

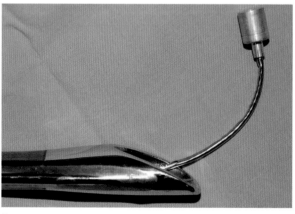

A.

B.

FIGURE 29–8. A. With an assistant watching through the esophagoscope, the surgeon passes the needle into the tip of the scope 10 mm below the tracheocutaneous junction. **B.** The guide wire is passed through the needle until it reaches the opposite end of the esophagoscope. The needle is removed and set aside.

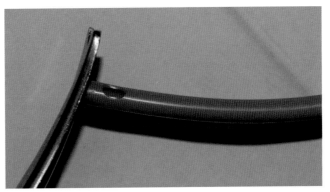

A.

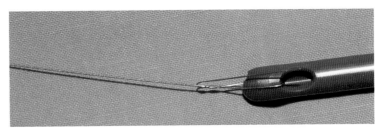

B.

FIGURE 29–9. **A.** The very tip of a red rubber catheter is trimmed off to allow the wire to pass first along the axis of the catheter. **B.** The wire passes through the new cut, out an eyehole, and then is twisted on itself. **C.** and **D.** After dilating the tract around the wire, the catheter is passed through the tract and into the esophagoscope with the wire under tension from the assistant.

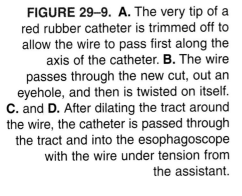

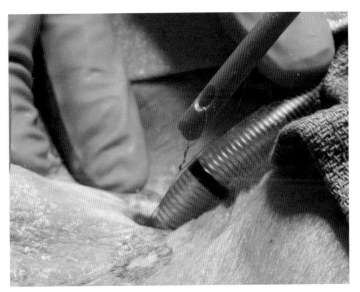

C.

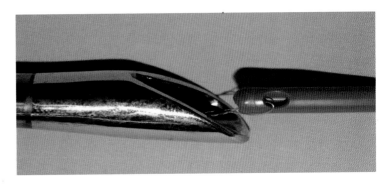

D.

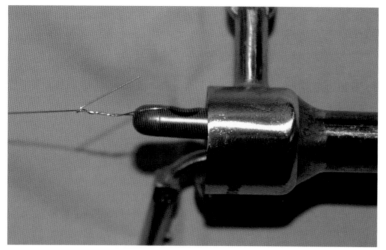

A.

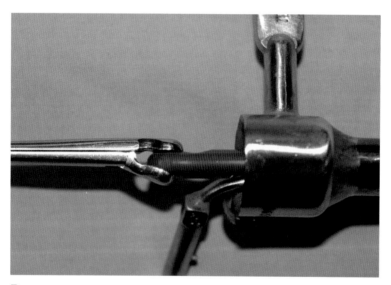

B.

FIGURE 29–10. A. The wire is removed. **B.** The catheter is grasped with a long cup forcep and passed back down the esophagoscope. **C.** After the catheter reaches the level of the fistula tract, it is advanced down the esophagus.

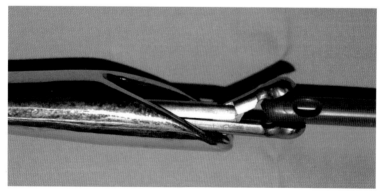

C.

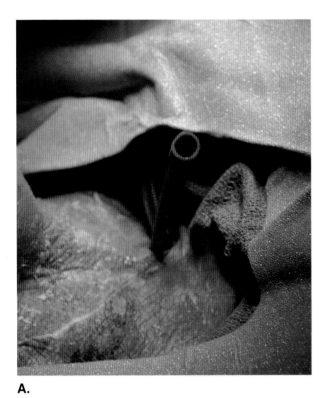

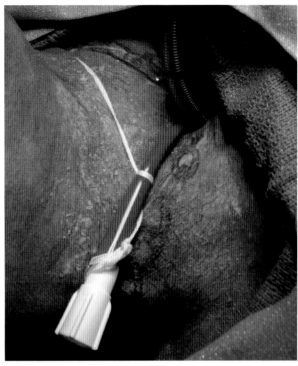

A.   B.

FIGURE 29–11. A. The catheter in place. **B.** The catheter secured with a catheter plug and twill tape.

Long-Term Issues

Postlaryngectomy speech rehabilitation is an ongoing concern for patients, surgeons, SLPs, and caregivers and requires preoperative planning (Figure 29-12). Despite early voicing success, the late effects of radiation, progressive postoperative scar formation, and the effects of aging can lead to deteriorating speech for each of the techniques. Survivors and caregivers must understand and be open to the option of alternative speech approaches at some point. On occasion, the TE fistula can migrate out of the stoma or become nonfunctional. For these patients, surgical closure or use of a dummy prosthesis might be necessary. The stoma can become unexpectedly smaller or larger and the use of laryngectomy tubes or stoma revision becomes necessary.

Pharyngeal hypertonicity can prevent speech fluency for both TE fistula and esophageal speakers. Tightness can be noted immediately or can develop months after the initial procedure. After an initial test injection with a local anesthetic, some patients can benefit from the use of botulinim toxin injections into the pharyngeal constrictors.[18]

Interestingly, even with excellent speech skills, laryngectomy survivors are sometimes reluctant to use their postlaryngectomy voice in public situations. The care providers need to be supportive and understanding when patients refuse to talk even when they are fully capable. In addition, many survivors who might be good candidates for secondary TEP fistula will decline additional procedures.

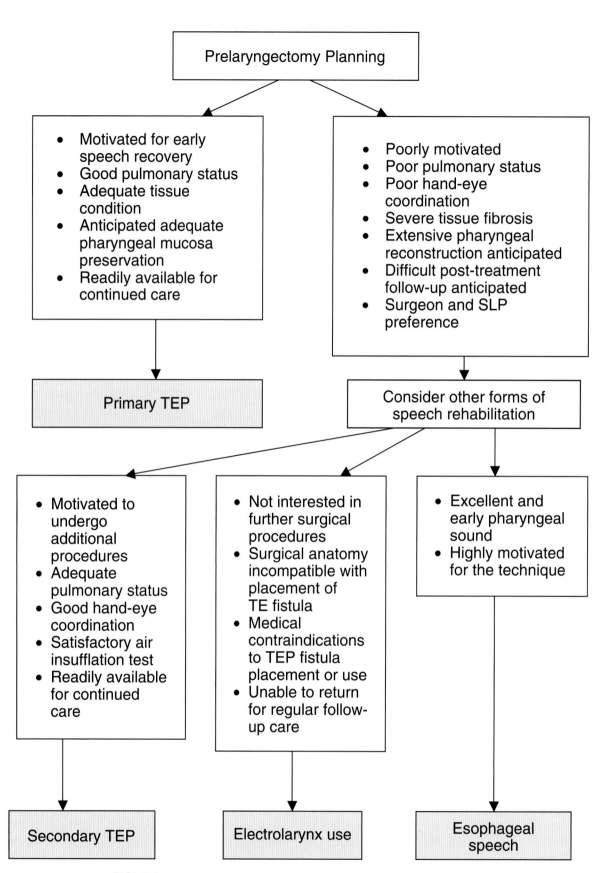

FIGURE 29–12. Management tree for postlaryngectomy speech.

Controversy: Primary Versus Secondary Tracheoesophageal Puncture (TEP) Speech

Placement of a Primary TE Speech Fistula

Advantages:

■ Shortens rehabilitation time from surgery to final speech result
■ Requires fewer surgical procedures and visits

Disadvantages:

■ Speech outcome is more difficult to predict preoperatively because an air insufflation test is not possible
■ The prosthesis must be successively resized as postoperative swelling diminishes. It becomes an additional potential problem in the early postoperative care of an already stressed patient.

Placement of a Secondary TE Speech Fistula

Advantages:

■ Permits simplified stoma care in the immediate postoperative period
■ Requires fewer issues to be addressed simultaneously
■ Allows patient to attempt esophageal speech prior to placement of the TE speech fistula

Disadvantages:

■ Patients may be very reluctant to undergo any additional surgical procedures
■ Increased costs of additional surgery
■ Prolongs rehabilitation until final speech outcome
■ Possibly has a lower success rate than primary TEP[19]

In summary, postlaryngectomy speech rehabilitation can be performed with a variety of techniques either primarily or secondarily. A significant majority of postlaryngectomy cancer survivors will develop effective techniques that allow them to communicate successfully with others in social and emergency situations.

Review Questions

1. In the era prior to the introduction of tracheoesophageal puncture (TEP) speech, the success rates of patients learning esophageal speech was approximately:
   a. 10%
   b. 25%
   c. 50%
   d. 60%
   e. 85%

2. An absolute contraindication to the most common technique for secondary TE fistula creation includes:
   a. Severe trismus
   b. Flap reconstruction of the pharynx
   c. Radiation therapy
   d. Decreased pulmonary function
   e. Failed electrolarynx use

3. Which of the following techniques of speech rehabilitation after laryngectomy requires the most long-term follow-up visits?
   a. Esophageal speech
   b. Electrolarynx speech
   c. TE fistula speech

4. Techniques that can improve post-laryngectomy speech efficiency include all of the following EXCEPT:
   a. Pharyngeal plexus neurectomy
   b. Cricopharyngeal muscle myotomy
   c. Pharyngeal constrictor muscle myotomy
   d. Botox injections
   e. Adequate muscle reinforcement of the mucosal closure

5. Which of the following represents an advantage of secondary placement of a TE speech fistula over primary placement?

a. Earlier overall speech rehabilitation
b. Higher ultimate success rate
c. Lower cost
d. Fewer initial post-operative issues
e. Air insufflation test is less predictable

REFERENCES

1. The Department of Veterans Affairs Laryngeal Cancer Study Group. Induction chemotherapy plus radiation compared with surgery plus radiation in patients with advanced laryngeal cancer. *N Engl J Med.* 1991;324:1685–1690.
2. Hoffman HT, Karnell LH, Funk GF, Robinson RA, Menck HR. The National Cancer Data Base report on cancer of the head and neck. *Arch Otolaryngol Head Neck Surg.* 1998;124:951–962.
3. Forastiere A, Koch W, Trotti A, Sidransky D. Head and neck cancer. *N Engl J Med.* 2001;345:1890–1900.
4. Forastiere A, Goepfert H, Maor M, et al. Concurrent chemotherapy and radiotherapy for organ preservation in advanced laryngeal cancer. *N Engl J Med.* 2003;349:2091–2098.
5. Singer MI. The development of successful tracheoesophageal voice restoration. *Otolaryngol Clin North Am.* 2004;37:507–517.
6. Pou AM. Tracheoesophageal voice restoration with total laryngectomy. *Otolaryngol Clin North Am.* 2004;37:531–545.
7. Gates GA, Ryan W, Cooper JC, Lawlis GF, Cantu E, Hayaski T, et al. Current status of laryngectomy rehabilitation: results of therapy. *Am J Otolaryngol.* 1982;3:1–7.
8. Desyatnikova S, Caro JJ, Andersen PE, Cohen JI, Wax MK. Tracheoesophageal puncture in the office setting with local anesthesia. *Ann Otol, Rhinol Laryngol.* 2001;110:613–616.
9. Lavertu P, Guay ME, Meeker SS, et al. Secondary tracheoesophageal puncture: factors predictive of voice quality and prothesis use. *Head Neck.* 1996;18:393–398.
10. Jacobson MC, Franssen E, Birt BD, Davisdon MJ, Gilbert RW. Predicting postlaryngectomy voice

outcome in an era of primary tracheoesophageal fistulization: a retrospective evaluation. *J Otolaryngol.* 1997;26:171–179.

11. Makitie AA, Niemensivu R, Juvas A, Aaltonen LM, Back L, Lehtonen H, Postlaryngectomy voice restoration using a voice prosthesis: a single institution's ten-year experience. *Ann Otol, Rhinol Laryngol.* 2003;112:1007–1010.

12. Stafford FW. Current indications and complications of tracheoesophageal puncture for voice restoration after laryngectomy. *Curr Opin Otolaryngol Head Neck Surg.* 2003;11:89–95.

13. Finizia C, Bergman B. Health-related quality of life in patients with laryngeal cancer: a post-treatment comparison of different modes of communication. *Laryngoscope.* 2001;111:918–923.

14. Singer MI, Blom ED. Selective myotomy for voice restoration after total laryngectomy. *Arch Otolaryngol Head Neck Surg.* 1981;107:670–673.

15. Singer MI, Blom ED, Hamaker RC. Pharyngeal plexus neurectomy for alaryngeal speech rehabilitation. *Laryngoscope.* 1986;96:50–53.

16. Deschler DG, Doherty ET, Reed CG, et al. Prevention of pharyngoesophageal spasm after laryngectomy with a half-muscle closure technique. *Ann Otol Rhinol Laryngol.* 2000;109:514–518.

17. Lichtenberger G. Simple and safe puncture technique for voice prosthesis implantation. *Otolaryngol Head Neck Surg.* 2003;128:835–840.

18. Lewin JS, Bishop-Leone JK, Forman AD, Diaz EM. Further experience with Botox injection for tracheoesophageal speech failure. *Head Neck.* 2001; 23:256–260.

19. Chone CT, Gripp FM, Spina AL, Crespo AN. Primary versus secondary tracheoesophageal puncture for speech rehabilitation in total laryngectomy: long-term results with indwelling voice prosthesis, *Otolaryngol Head Neck Surg.* 2005;133:89–93.

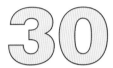

Endocrine Disorders of the Larynx

Mai Thy Truong, MD
Edward J. Damrose, MD

KEY POINTS

■ Changes in the male larynx during puberty are a result of androgen stimulation, leading to lengthening and thickening of the vocal folds, causing lowering of the voice by an octave; puberty in the female is characterized by less dramatic changes in the larynx with gradual, age-dependent changes resulting in a voice lowered by one third of an octave.

■ Androgen stimulation of the larynx causes irreversible changes, including hypertrophy and hyperplasia of muscle, thickening of the epithelium, growth of the cartilaginous framework, lengthening of the vocal folds, and lowering of the fundamental frequency. Estrogens have a hypertrophic effect on laryngeal mucosa and cause an increase in secretion of glandular cells. Progesterone has an antiproliferative effect, decreasing glandular secretion while increasing acidity and viscosity, leading to desquamation and dryness.

■ A premenstrual vocal syndrome has been described in professional singers, with vocal symptoms that result from the surge in estrogen and progesterone prior to menses. Menopause has been implicated in vocal symptoms due to the decrease in estrogen and progesterone, and an increase in androgens, which may be alleviated by hormone replacement therapy.

■ Modern formulation oral contraceptives likely contribute to hormone stability that results in improved vocal quality and stability. Another example of hormone-related dysphonia is seen in thyroid disease.

HORMONES AND THE LARYNX: AN OVERVIEW

The larynx is a target organ of the hormonal environment. This is obvious when the exquisite differences between male and female voices are considered. Dysphonia and vocal alterations may also occur in states of hormonal imbalance and may be the presenting symptom in systemic disease. As early as 400 BC, Aristotle described the effect of castration on the songbird.[1] In the 16th century, women's voices were precluded from the Roman church, and to preserve the feminine voice in the Sistine Chapel choir, the practice of castration was begun.[2] One approach to thinking about the impact of hormones on the larynx is by examining the effects they may have on anatomic components of the organ itself.

1. **Extravascular spaces**—Fluid shifts within these spaces can result in laryngeal edema or dry states in response to hormonal fluctuations, which can affect voice quality and function. These can be demonstrated in states of hypothyroidism, acromegaly, and menopause.
2. **Epithelium and glandular cells**—Dysfunction and changes in glandular secretion in response to hormonal states can lead to dehydration and dysphonia.[3]
3. **Muscles**—Androgens cause hypertrophy of laryngeal striated muscle.[4] Studies in the African clawed frog, *Xenopus laevus,* also demonstrate alterations in muscle fiber type after exposure to androgens. Muscle atrophy may be seen with other endocrine disorders.[5]
4. **Laryngeal framework**—Androgens and growth hormone, particularly as seen in puberty, promote growth and calcification of cartilaginous structures of the larynx.
5. **Neurovascular structures**—Laryngeal neuropathy may be secondary diabetic states.

Numerous studies have described the larynx as an active target for hormone action. Newman et al[6] demonstrated the presence of hormone receptors in the nucleus and cytoplasm of cells of cadaveric vocal folds, with receptor differences depending on age and gender. Androgen receptors were found in glandular cell cytoplasm, estrogen receptors in epithelial cell cytoplasm, and progesterone receptors were found in glandular cell nuclei. Androgen and progesterone receptors were found more commonly in male subjects.[6] Thyroid hormone receptors have been found in the lamina propria, the cartilage, and the glandular elements of the larynx.[7] Although hormonal influence on the larynx has long been acknowledged, further studies will elucidate the anatomic changes, cellular processes, and characteristic histologic changes involved.

Following a review of puberty and development as it relates to the larynx, this chapter details the specific hormonal effects related to the sex hormones and to systemic endocrinologic disorders, such as diabetes and thyroid dysfunction.

DEVELOPMENT AND PUBERTY

Puberty and the Male Larynx

Testosterone is produced in small amounts by the cortex of the adrenal gland with other androgenic steroids. Early stages of development happen similarly in females, moderated by the androgens secreted by the adrenal cortex, which stimulate sebaceous gland development and growth of pubic hair. Later, the majority of testosterone in the male is produced by the Leydig cells of the testes, controlled by the hypothalamic-pituitary-gonadal axis. The hypothalamus produces releasing factors that stimulate the pituitary to release luteinizing hormone (LH), which in turn stimulates the Leydig cells to produce testosterone, which then feeds back to the hypothalamus. The factors that determine the onset of puberty are poorly understood. Testosterone affects the maturation of secondary sex characteristics and genitalia, promotes growth and strength of muscle, and leads to the closure of growth plates. In males, pubertal changes take place between ages 9 and 17.[8,9]

Androgens are responsible for the irreversible changes that occur in the male larynx at puberty, resulting in an adult voice that is approximately one octave lower than that of a child (Table 30-1). Anatomically, there is an increase in the anteroposterior length of the thyroid cartilage and the thyroid ala enlarges to produce a more prominent notch, resulting in an "Adam's apple." The vocal cords lengthen and become more rounded, the epithelium thickens and forms three distinct layers, laryngeal mucus becomes more viscous, the arytenoids grow, the thyroarytenoid ligaments become thicker, and the cricothyroid muscle broadens.[3,10]

Vocal tract morphology was investigated in a study by Fitch et al analyzing magnetic resonance imaging of 129 normal humans, ages 2 to 25.[10] The authors found that, prior to puberty, there were few sex differences in laryngeal morphology. Following puberty, however, males had a significant increase in vocal tract length, a measurement that was taken from a line drawn from the lips to the glottis. The authors attributed this difference to a descent of the male larynx occurring at puberty. This descent likely changes the resonance of the voice, ultimately changing the timbre, or overall quality. This descent happens in conjunction with a near doubling of the anteroposterior length of the glottis. The lengthening of the vocal fold contributes to the change in fundamental frequency of the male voice, resulting in a deeper voice. Previous studies that show baritones and bases have longer vocal folds than tenors support this.[11-13] Measurements taken from 30 cadavers comparing prepubertal and pubertal larynges in males and females showed male vocal cords had an increase in length by 67% in adult men compared with prepubertal boys, whereas in the female the increase is only 24%.[14]

The drop in fundamental frequency of the male voice occurs later in puberty, between Tanner stages III and IV.[15] As these dramatic changes progress, the adolescent male voice cracks often. This has been speculated to be due to imbalance between the childlike glottis and the wind power of the adult thoraco-abdominal structure, with fluctuations in power resulting in a yodeling voice.[3] Alternatively, the breaking voice has been attributed to the substitution of the chest voice (or heavy mechanism) for the head voice (or light mechanism) in an adolescent who is still speaking

TABLE 30-1. Changes in the Male Larynx in Puberty[3,10]

1. Growth of the cartilaginous framework; development of the thyroid prominence, or "Adam's apple."

2. Descent of the larynx.

3. Lengthening and thickening of vocal folds.

4. Thickening of the epithelium of the vocal fold, forming three distinct layers.

5. Growth of the arytenoids.

6. Thickening of the thyroarytenoid ligaments.

7. Broadening of the cricothyroid muscle.

in a childlike voice.[16] Finally, King et al proposed that the breaking voice results from the maturing male learning to adapt to the developing laryngeal muscle and its increase in strength and size that arises from androgenic stimulation.[8]

These anatomic and physiologic changes in the male larynx that occur with puberty are the result of the secretion of testosterone and other androgens such as dihydrotestosterone. A historical example of hormonal "manipulation" of laryngeal development is seen in the *castrati*. Beginning in the late 16th century for the Church of Rome, males were castrated at ages 7 to 9 to preserve the unbroken voice. The small larynx of a child paired with fully grown thoracoabdominal cavities and adult resonating chambers of the pharynx, oral cavities, and sinuses resulted in powerful voices that were reported to range up to three or four octaves. The castrati had a strong presence in Italian opera, as well as a place in the Sistine Chapel for three centuries.[2]

Puberty and the Female Larynx

Puberty in females occurs 1 to 3 years before males. Similarly to males, early development is dominated by androgens secreted by the adrenal cortex during adrenarche. Menarche marks the completion of the maturation of the reproductive system controlled by the hypothalamic-pituitary-gonadal axis. Cyclical secretion involves a positive feedback mechanism by which an increased estrogen level above a certain point triggers the simultaneous release of luteinizing hormone (LH) and follicle-stimulating hormone (FSH), involved in ovulation and menses. The ovaries are the primary source of estradiol and also produce a small amount of testosterone. The average age of onset of menses is 12.6 years (9.1–16.2 year range).[17]

A woman's voice is one third of an octave lower than a child's voice. The female larynx is thought to mature gradually as a child gets older, without the dramatic changes that are seen in a male larynx at puberty. Fitch et al found that female vocal tract growth was steady throughout

puberty and adulthood.[10] The thyroid cartilage has little development during puberty compared to what is seen in a male. It is reported that the thyroid cartilage reaches adult size by the onset of puberty. The vocal muscle remains narrow though may thicken slightly.[3]

In a study by Pedersen et al, voice frequency was studied as a secondary sex characteristic during puberty in females. The authors found that tone range and lowest tone were significantly different in females in three progressive age groups. Fundamental frequency in continuous speech dropped progressively by 15 Hz in the three age groups, aged 8 to 19. This study showed a continued age dependence in vocal changes, demonstrating that gradual vocal changes occur in females during puberty in contrast to males.[18]

SPECIFIC HORMONE CLASSES AND THEIR EFFECTS ON THE LARYNX

Androgens

The changes marked in male puberty can be attributed to testosterone. Testosterone itself is known to result in an increase in muscle mass in castrated animals, as well as in normal men as demonstrated in triceps and quadriceps.[19,20] Androgen therapy and supplementation have been investigated in various populations. Akcam et al studied the effects of androgen therapy on males with idiopathic hypogonadotropic hypogonadism (IHH). Prior to treatment, the IHH males were found to have a mean fundamental frequency that was in between normal male controls and normal female controls. After 3 months of androgen therapy, the fundamental frequency approached that of normal males. These changes were attributed to permanent changes in laryngeal muscle mass.[21]

Androgen exposure to the female larynx had broad effects as shown in histologic studies of the mouse model. When exposed to anabolic steroids, the thyroarytenoid muscle demonstrated hypertrophy and hyperplasia. Histologic changes

Comparative Laryngology and Sexual Development

The developing larynx of the African clawed frog, *Xenopus laevis,* is greatly affected by androgens and serves as a unique model of laryngeal development. The male larynx is larger as a result of greater cell numbers in both cartilage and muscle. Prior to metamorphosis, the male and female larynges are monomorphic. After metamorphosis, the dilator laryngis muscle of the male gains 6 to 7 times more muscle fibers than that of the female. If androgen exposure is prevented, the larynx fails to masculinize, with a femalelike pattern and cell number.[24] Androgens given prior to metamorphosis stimulate laryngeal development prematurely and stimulate cell proliferation, especially of laryngeal muscle and within elastic precartilage zones. This is in parallel with an increase in androgen receptor mRNA production.[25] Androgens were also shown to convert laryngeal muscle of *Xenopus laevis* from mixed slow and fast twitch muscle, to all fast twitch muscle, a change that was independent from innervated versus dennervated muscle.[5]

The *Xenopus laevis* model has also provided compelling information regarding estrogen and its effect on the larynx, particularly at the neuromuscular junction. Investigators have demonstrated that estrogen plays a key role in the sexual dimorphism of song production. The laryngeal synapse is estrogen sensitive; females have stronger synapses than males and synaptic strength relies on estrogen exposure during development. Females produce distinct types of calls depending on sexual state. Sexually unreceptive females usually tick, while sexually receptive females usually rap. Rapping is faster and louder than ticking. Wu et al found that chronic estrogen exposure induced sexual receptivity by increasing laryngeal synaptic strength. The authors suggested that stronger synaptic strength is associated with the rapping call type. This is supported in studies that show exogenous estrogen treatment strengthens juvenile laryngeal synapses in both sexes whereas ovariectomy in immature females prevents synaptic strengthening as adults.[28,29] The differences between male and female voices is complex; these studies show that hormones may play a role in modulating sound at a level not previously studied, the neuromuscular junction.

---

of the epithelium also include basal cell hyperplasia, parakeratosis of the vocal cord epithelium, and squamous metaplasia of the laryngeal mucosa. Hyperplasia of seromucinous glands and increased vascularity, vascular congestion, and slight edema were noted in the connective tissue stroma. Ballooning and signet ring appearance of the cartilage cells was noted in laryngeal cartilage.[4] In humans, females with congenital adrenal hyperplasia have an elevated state of androgens and their voices are classically masculine, changes that are irreversible.[22]

Androgen stimulation of the sheep larynx causes changes in the thyroid cartilage framework ultimately resulting in a lengthening of the vocal tract. Distances between the vocal process and the base of the arytenoid increases, as with the distance between the vocal process to the muscular process.[23]

Estrogen and Progesterone

Estrogens are reported to have a hypertrophic effect on the laryngeal mucosa, as well as cause an increase in secretion from the laryngeal glandular cells. Estrogens cause a differentiation and maturation of fat cells. In periods of elevated estrogen, such as during pregnancy, the larynx has been described as hyperemic with congested mucosa.[26] Estrogens act in a cyclical fashion with progesterone. Progesterone has been reported to have an antiproliferative effect on mucosa, accelerating desquamation and decreasing glandular cell secretion while increasing viscosity and acidity, leading to dryness. Also, progesterone has been implicated in inhibiting capillary permeability, trapping extracellular fluid and causing edema. Some synthetic progesterones have been shown to have androgenic effects.[27] However, true animal or human experiments need to be done to confirm these histologic findings in the larynx.

The Menstrual Cycle

During the follicular phase of the menstrual cycle, release of FSH from the pituitary results in the maturation of the primary ovarian follicle which produces estrogen. Estrogen secretion steadily increases until it reaches a peak which results in an LH surge on day 14, stimulating ovulation. The release of the ovum from the follicle marks the luteal phase, during which the corpus luteum begins secreting significant quantities of progesterone and estrogen. If fertilization does not occur, the corpus luteum degenerates, and progesterone levels fall. Without progesterone, the endometrial lining is sloughed off, resulting in menstruation.

The Premenstrual Vocal Syndrome

Vocal symptoms have been described during the premenstrual phase, mostly in trained vocal professionals, in a condition also known as *laryngopathia premenstrualis* (Table 30-2). It has been reported that 33% of nonprofessional voice users, and a higher percentage of professionals, experience these voice symptoms.[27,30] In some opera performer contracts, "grace days" are allotted for voice rest for this reason. It has been reported that the elevations in estrogen and progesterone cause structural changes in laryngeal mucosa resulting in changes in vocal tone. Prior to menstruation, estrogen elevation causes a thickening of mucus as rising progesterone levels cause the viscosity and acidity of glandular secretions to increase, ultimately leading in dryness.

Abitbol et al demonstrated a correlation between cervical and vocal cytological smears during the premenstrual period.[27] This study showed the larynx to be hormonally receptive in a fashion similar to the cervix. Videostroboscopy may show reduced tonicity of the laryngeal muscle, less supple epithelium, reduced vibratory amplitude, vibratory asymmetry, edema of the vocal cords, and venous dilation. Chernobeisky et al found that these premenstrual symptoms were aggravated and more prevalent in vocal abusers, showing that the vocal folds may be even more susceptible and vulnerable to stressors during this premenstrual period.[31]

This clinical entity still requires further investigation as these symptoms have been described mostly by the professional singer through questionnaire or survey techniques. Chae et al com-

TABLE 30–2. Premenstrual Vocal Syndrome Symptoms[27,30]

1. Vocal fatigue.

2. Decreased range, with higher tones more susceptible for loss.

3. Loss of vocal power.

4. Decline in high harmonics.

pared acoustic measurements made during the follicular phase and the premenstrual phase in 28 women. Each participant was asked to produce an "a" sound for 5 seconds at the midfollicular phase of the menstrual cycle and then 2 to 3 days before menstruation. Analysis of each voice found that jitter was significantly increased in the premenstrual phase.[32] This syndrome may simply be a clinical entity that is more apparent to vocal professionals who have more demands on their voice and who are more sensitive to any vocal perturbations.

Pregnancy

Voice changes associated with pregnancy are termed *laryngopathia gravidarum*. It is generally associated with vocal symptoms similar to those seen premenstrually as a result of elevated levels of estrogen and progesterone. These voice changed have been reported in 15 to 20% of pregnant women in the last 5 months of pregnancy.[3] Vocal changes during pregnancy have also been attributed to abdominal distention, which interferes with abdominal muscle function and the severity of reflux.[33]

Laryngopathia gravidarum has also been described as a rare complication during pregnancy that is associated with pre-eclampsia, with different degrees of severity ranging from simple hoarseness to dangerous states of airway obstruction. Generalized edema is seen commonly in women with severe pre-eclampsia. Edema of the larynx and upper airway may cause dysphonia, or even airway obstruction, and may be the presenting symptom of severe pre-eclampsia.[34] Pre-eclamptic women who will be undergoing general anaesthesia may need a preoperative assessment of the airway. If the airway is compromised, awake fiberoptic intubation may be required.[35-38] In severe cases, planned prolonged intubation and ICU monitoring should be considered until the airway resolves.[39] Planned prolonged intubation and ICU monitoring should also be considered until resolution of edema.[39] Reports in the literature describe that morpho-

logic and functional findings disappear after the end of pregnancy.[40]

Menopause

Menopause is defined as the cessation of menstruation, when ovarian follicles become atretic. It occurs at a mean age of 51 years in normal women in the United States. During menopause, there is a loss of ovarian sensitivity to gonadotropin stimulation, and estrogen production declines with the cessation of ovarian follicular activity. Serum gonadotropin concentrations increase in response, FSH rises more than LH. The ovary continues to secrete androgens because of the high serum LH concentrations. A major contribution to estrogen in the circulation then comes from the peripheral aromatization of androstenedione of both ovarian and adrenal origin. The drop in estrogen results in the classic symptoms of menopause, including "hot flashes," sweats, mood instability, and depression, as well as findings of vaginal, urethral, and cervical atrophy.[41]

The drop in estrogen and progesterone with the increase in androgens has been reported to result in a menopausal vocal syndrome (Table 30-3). Vocal changes during menopause have long been reported, but few studies have been done to fully investigate these changes. It has been reported that fewer glandular cells in laryngeal mucosa result in more dry conditions during

TABLE 30–3. Menopausal Vocal Syndrome Symptoms[27,43]

1. Lowering of vocal intensity.
2. Vocal fatigue.
3. Decreased range with loss in high notes.
4. Change in timbre in spoken and singing voices.
5. Loss of power.
6. Loss of "brilliance."
7. Loss of stability.
8. Huskiness.

phonation which contribute to more dysphonia and vocal fatigue.[42]

In a survey of 48 female and 24 male professional singers, Boulet et al examined voice changes during the 5th decade in life, comparing male and female voice changes to reveal the impact of menopause. The authors found that 77% of women and 71% of men reported vocal changes. Compared to men, women reported more problems with huskiness, loss of range in high registers, and impaired steadiness of voice. Both sexes reported change in timbre. In the survey, of those women who experience negative voice changes, the majority attributed vocal changes to menopause.[43]

Abitbol et al studied 100 menopausal women, 17 of whom were identified to have menopausal vocal syndrome. Laryngeal assessment and cytologic studies were performed on these women to further characterize the syndrome. The authors found that cervical smears matched laryngeal smears, revealing mucosal subatrophy with basophils and significant reduction in glandular cells, further supporting the parallel in hormonal response between the larynx and the cervix. Muscular atrophy, thinning of vocal fold mucosa, reduction of amplitude during phonation, asymmetry between right and left vocal folds, and a decreased vocal range were reported. The authors went on to supplement the 17 women with hormone replacement therapy and reported 14 of the women maintained normal muscular contour, amplitude of vibrations returned to normal, and improvement in vocal timbre was reported.[27]

The effect of estrogen replacement therapy (ERT) on the postmenopausal larynx was further investigated by Caruso et al, who looked at 77 women, comparing laryngeal and cervical smears in 38 women on ERT and 31 controls. They found that the laryngeal and cervical smears showed indistinguishable cytologic aspects, supporting findings from Abitbol et al. Control subjects demonstrated more atrophy-dystrophy in the smears compared to smears from subjects treated with ERT. Those on ERT were found to have decreased voice complaints, including decreased reports of hoarseness, change in timbre, instability, voice fatigue, and voice lowering.[44]

Lindholm et al compared changes in measured vocal values and subjective symptoms in postmenopausal women receiving estrogen alone or combined estrogen-progestin therapy to those not receiving hormonal therapy. Looking at 42 nonprofessional voice users, the authors compared fundamental frequency (F_0) and sound pressure levels (SPLs), which correlate to loudness, over a 1-year span. In the group without hormone therapy, the authors found a significant drop in F_0 and SPL, and reported less of a drop in both groups receiving hormone therapy, with the fewest subjective symptoms in those on estrogen therapy alone. This study supports hormone therapy to preserve vocal quality in postmenopausal women. However, further studies are needed to define more fully the postmenopausal syndrome, its vocal characteristics, and the possible therapeutic effects of hormone therapy.[45]

Oral Contraceptives

Oral contraceptives vary in hormone content, from progestin only to estrogen-progestin combinations, with variable doses of hormone from monophasic to triphasic formulations. There is a traditional view that oral contraceptives propose a risk to vocal quality.[33] However, old formulations of oral contraceptives contained much higher doses of hormones, with high levels of certain progestins, which resulted in more potential androgenic virilizing effects on the larynx.[46] In contrast, modern oral contraceptives have significantly reduced levels of estrogens and progestins, and current research suggests that these low-dose formulations may provide more stable hormone levels resulting in more vocal stability.

Several studies regarding oral contraceptives and the voice are presented here. Wendler et al found no differences in mean speaking frequency, pitch range, dynamic range, or voice sound quality in subjects before and after oral contraceptive consumption in a 1-year study.[46] Amir et al analyzed multiple voice parameters, comparing seven women taking low-dose, monophasic combination estrogen-progestin oral contraceptives, to seven controls. The authors found lower frequency perturbations, amplitude perturbations, and noise parameters in women taking oral contraceptives, showing improvement in quality and stability.[47] Follow-up studies with more subjects and variations of oral contraceptives, all combination low-dose estrogen-progestin pills, found similar results.[47,48] Gorham-Rowan et al analyzed the effect of oral contraceptives on vocal characteristics during normal speech, finding no significant difference between the two groups.[49] In a follow-up study, the authors found that women taking oral contraceptives demonstrated higher pitch levels and greater stability during phonation than women not taking oral contraceptives, further supporting the safety and potential benefits of oral contraceptives on vocal control.[50]

THYROID FUNCTION AND THE LARYNX

The thyroid gland has multiple effects on development, growth, and metabolism. The larynx has been shown to be a thyroid hormone target. Altman et al identified thyroid hormone receptors in the larynx of a human male and a human female cadaver.[7] Studies of *Xenopus laevis* have also revealed the key role thyroid hormone plays in androgen competency in the developing larynx. If thyroid hormone secretion is blocked, androgens cannot stimulate normal laryngeal growth. Developing *Xenopus laevis* laryngeal cartilage and muscle have been found to express thyroid receptor mRNA, and because these receptors are nuclear transcription factors, thyroid hormone has been implicated in playing a role in the development cascade in masculinization.[51] This section focuses on the known effects of thyroid function and dysfunction on the larynx; the treatment of thyroid disorders is reviewed here.

Hypothyroidism

Hypothyroidism is a state of low production of thyroid hormone. Signs and symptoms of the disease vary in relation to the amount of hormone

deficiency, and the acuteness with which the deficiency developed. If congenital and untreated, the state of cretinism has been associated with a small larynx. Hypothyroid states have been associated with hoarseness, vocal fatigue, muffling of the voice, loss of range, and a feeling of a lump in the throat.[33] The dysphonia of hypothyroidism has been described as coarse or gravelly and low-pitched. Ataxic dysarthria and lingual articulatory imprecision due to tongue swelling and macroglossia are also described, aggravating laryngeal symptoms.[52] On clinical exam, Ferlito describes "cramps" of the vocal folds, muscle stiffness, dry epithelium with narrow vibratory amplitude, mucinous edema, cricoarytenoid joint stiffness, and pale vocal folds with edema of Reinke's space.[3]

Hypothyroidism has been reported to cause myxedema of the laryngeal muscle and vocal folds, grossly similar to Reinke's edema, with a resultant lowering of pitch. Biopsy shows mild exudation of fibrin and basophilic material with some proliferation of fibroblasts in Reinke's space.[53] An increased level of acid mucopolysaccharides has also been described submucosally in the vocal folds, resulting in an osmotic increase in fluid content, leading to edema and decreased vibration.[54] Severe hypothyroidism and myxedema have been reported to be associated with decreased vocal muscle strength and even vocal fold paralysis.[33]

Hyperthyroidism

Hyperthyroidism is due to thyroid hormone overproduction. Mild hyperthyroidism is not likely associated with laryngeal pathology; however, severe thyrotoxicosis may reveal submucosal vocal fold changes and muscle weakness, as well as symptoms similar to those seen in hypothyroid states.[33] Dysphonia has not been carefully described, but breathy voice quality and reduced loudness have been reported, presumably due to weakness of the laryngeal musculature.[52] Tremulousness of the voice and hoarseness has been associated with anxiety, whereas gastroesophageal reflux in the hyperthyroid state may worsen laryngeal symptoms. Ferlito described the clinical appearance of the larynx as featuring weakened vocal fold muscles and the presence of a glottic chink during phonation resulting in a breathy, hoarse voice.[3]

DIABETES AND THE LARYNX

Laryngeal manifestations of diabetes have not been extensively characterized. Authors have suggested a general neuropathy that, in a professional voice user, may result in impaired tactile and sensory information needed for vocal control. Advanced neuropathy has been reported to result in vocal cord paralysis.[3,33] Bilateral and unilateral vocal cord paralysis have been attributed to diabetic neuropathy in various case reports, with some reports documenting return of function with hyperglycemic control.[55-58]

In general, diabetes is associated with an increased risk of infection. Serious infections of the larynx have been described in diabetics, including severe bacterial and fungal infections. Chronic granulomatous infections from fungal sources such as histoplasmosis or cryptococcus can mimic carcinoma on presentation, leading to improper treatment and surgical excision.[59,60] In the diabetic host, infection can be severe and may even lead to airway obstruction, as has been reported with murcomycosis.[61]

Diabetes may have a greater *indirect* impact on laryngeal disease beyond that described above. Patients with diabetes have a significant risk for cardiovascular disease and critical illness; a recent study has suggested that diabetics may be at increased risk of airway stenosis, perhaps related to a higher likelihood of cricitcal illness with prolonged intubation.[62] This may be compounded by the association between diabetes and reflux.[63,64] Lower esophageal sphincter function, a key physiologic barrier against the refluxate of gastric contents, is impaired in diabetes.[65] Along with neural impairment of motility, such as in gastric atony, these changes make laryngeal and pharyngeal damage from reflux more likely in diabetics.

HYPOPHYSEAL DISORDERS

Acromegaly

Acromegaly is the clinical syndrome that results from excessive secretion of growth hormone (GH). Its annual incidence is three to four cases per million persons. The mean age at diagnosis is 40 to 45 years; the characteristic findings are macrognathia and enlarged, swollen hands and feet, which result in increasing shoe and glove size and the need to enlarge rings. The facial features become coarse, with enlargement of the nose and frontal bones as well as the jaw, and the teeth become spread apart. The most common cause of acromegaly is a GH-secreting adenoma of the anterior pituitary.[66]

Vocal changes have been described as a deepening of the voice with narrow register and intensity. Tissue from the oral cavity down to the pharynx thickens, both of which lead to a change in vocal resonance. Ferlito describes clinically that the epiglottis and thyroid cartilage enlarge, the cricoarytenoid joint has decreased mobility, and the vocal folds develop thickened epithelium.[3] True and false vocal cords thicken as well, and a widening of the larynx is associated with pitch changes.[67] In a study by Williams et al, the mean fundamental frequency in acromegalic patients was found to be significantly lower in comparison to normal controls. Interestingly, the authors reported a rapid increase in fundamental frequency after hypophysectomy, demonstrating these vocal changes to be reversible.[68]

Review Questions

1. All of these are known effects of androgens, *except:*
   a. Decrease in fundamental frequency, a reversible change.

b. Hypertrophy and hyperplasia of laryngeal muscle

c. Increase in the anteroposterior length of the thyroid cartilage in pubescent males

d. Thickening of the epithelium of the vocal fold

e. All of the above are known effects of androgens

2. All are changes of the human larynx during puberty, *except:*

a. A lengthening of the vocal folds by 67% in males and 24% in females

b. A gradually progressive decrease in fundamental frequency in females

c. A decrease in the adult male voice by one octave, changes which occur in early stages of puberty

d. A descent of the larynx

e. All the above are changes of the human larynx during puberty

3. Premenstrual vocal syndrome:

a. Is likely due to the sudden drop in estrogen and progesterone levels during menstruation

b. Is mostly reported in professional voice users, and is characterized by vocal fatigue, loss in vocal power, and decreased range

c. Is not a true clinical entity as the larynx is not affected by circulating estrogen or progesterone levels

d. Is not aggrevated by vocal abusers

4. Diabetes may be linked to:

a. Infections of the larynx mimicking surgical lesions

b. Hypertrophy and hyperplasia of laryngeal muscle

c. Thickening of laryngeal secretions

d. Diabetes is not associated with laryngeal pathology

e. Failure of ossification affecting the cricoid

REFERENCES

1. Aristotle. *Historia animalia.* 1853.

2. Jenkins JS. The lost voice, a history of the castrato. *J Pediatr Endocrinol Metab.* 2000;13(suppl 6): 1503-1508.

3. Ferlito A, ed. *Diseases of the Larynx.* New York, NY: Oxford University Press; 2000:xvii.

4. Talaat M, Talaat AM, Kelada I, et al. Histologic and histochemical study of effects of anabolic steroids on the female larynx. *Ann Otol Rhinol Laryngol.* 1987;96:468.

5. Tobias ML, Marin ML, Kelley DB. The roles of sex, innervation, and androgen in laryngeal muscle of *Xenopus laevis. J Neurosci.* 1993;13:324.

6. Newman SR, Butler J, Hammond EH, et al. Preliminary report on hormone receptors in the human vocal fold. *J Voice.* 2000;14:72.

7. Altman KW, Haines GK, Vakkalanka SK, et al. Identification of thyroid hormone receptors in the human larynx. *Laryngoscope.* 2003;113:1931.

8. King A, Ashby J, Nelson C. Effects of testosterone replacement on a male professional singer. *J Voice.* 2001;15:553.

9. Larsen PR KH, Melmed S, Polonsky KS. *Williams Textbook of Endocrinology.* 10th ed. Amsterdam:Elsevier; 2003.

10. Fitch W, Giedd J. Morphology and development of the human vocal tract: a study using magnetic resonance imaging. *J Acoust Soc Am.* 1999;106: 1511-1522.

11. Dmitriev L, Kiselev A. Relationship between the formant structure of different types of singing voices and the dimensions of supraglottic cavities. *Folia Phoniatr.* 1979;31:238.

12. Cleveland TF. Acoustic properties of voice timbre types and their influence on voice classification. *J Acoust Soc Am.* 1977;61:1622.

13. Hollien H, Green R, Massey K. Longitudinal research on adolescent voice change in males. *J Acoust Soc Am.* 1994;96:2646.

14. Kahane JC. Growth of the human prepubertal and pubertal larynx. *J Speech Hear Res.* 1982;25: 446-455.

15. Harries M, Hawkins S, Hacking J, Hughes I. Changes in the male voice at puberty: vocal fold length and its relationship to the fundamental frequency of the voice. *J Laryngol Otol.* 1998;112: 451-454.

16. Amy de la Breteque B. Rehabilitation of disorders of the breaking of voice [in French]. *Rev Laryngol Otol Rhinol.* 1995;116:271.

17. Wein A, et al. *Campbell-Walsh Urology.* 8th ed. Philadelphia, PA: WB Saunders; 2007.

18. Pedersen M, Muller S, Krabbe S, Bennett P, Svenstrup B. Fundamental voice frequency in female puberty measured with electroglottography during continuous speech as a secondary sex characteristic. A comparison between voice, pubertal stages, oestrogens and androgens. *Int J Pediatr Otorhinolaryngol.* 1990;20:17–24.

19. Griggs RC, Kingston W, Jozefowicz RF, et al. Effect of testosterone on muscle mass and muscle protein synthesis. *J Appl Physiol.* 1989;66:498.

20. Bhasin S, Storer TW, Berman N, et al. The effects of supraphysiologic doses of testosterone on muscle size and strength in normal men. *New Engl J Med.* 1996;335:1.

21. Akcam T, Bolu E, Merati AL, et al. Voice changes after androgen therapy for hypogonadotrophic hypogonadism. *Laryngoscope.* 2004;114:1587.

22. Furst-Recktenwald S, Dorr HG, Rosanowski F. Androglottia in a young female adolescent with congenital adrenal hyperplasia and 21-hydroxylase deficiency. *J Pediatr Endocrinol.* 2000;13:959.

23. Beckford NS, Rood SR, Schaid D, et al. Androgen stimulation and laryngeal development. *Ann Otol Rhinol Laryngol.* 1985;94:634.

24. Sassoon D, Kelley DB. The sexually dimorphic larynx of *Xenopus laevis*: development and androgen regulation. *Am J Anat.* 1986;177:457.

25. Fischer LM, Catz D, Kelley DB. Androgen-directed development of the *Xenopus laevis* larynx: control of androgen receptor expression and tissue differentiation. *Dev Biol.* 1995;170:115.

26. Maceri DR. Head and neck manifestations of endocrine disease. *Otolaryngol Clin North Am.* 1986;19:171.

27. Abitbol J, Abitbol P, Abitbol B. Sex hormones and the female voice. *J Voice.* 1999;13:424–446.

28. Wu KH, Tobias ML, Kelley DB. Estrogen receptor expression in laryngeal muscle in relation to estrogen-dependent increases in synapse strength. *Neuroendocrinology.* 2003;78:72.

29. Wu KH, Tobias ML, Kelley DB. Estrogen and laryngeal synaptic strength in *Xenopus laevis*: opposite effects of acute and chronic exposure. *Neuroendocrinology.* 2001;74:22.

30. Davis C, Davis ML. The effects of premenstrual syndrome (PMS) on the female singer. *J Voice.* 1993;7:337–353.

31. Chernobelsky SI. A study of menses-related changes to the larynx in singers with voice abuse. *Folia Phoniatr Logop.* 2002;54:2.

32. Chae SW, Choi G, Kang HJ, et al. Clinical analysis of voice change as a parameter of premenstrual syndrome. *J Voice.* 2001;15:278.

33. Sataloff RT. *Professional Voice: The Scince and Art of Clinical Care.* 2nd ed. San Diego, Calif: Singular Publishing Group; 1997:1069.

34. Perlow JH, Kirz DS. Severe preeclampsia presenting as dysphonia secondary to uvular edema. A case report. *J Reproduct Med.* 1990;35:1059.

35. Heller PJ, Scheider EP, Marx GF. Pharyngolaryngeal edema as a presenting symptom in preeclampsia. *Obstet Gynecol.* 1983;62:523.

36. Seager SJ, Macdonald R. Laryngeal oedema and pre-eclampsia. *Anaesthesia.* 1980;35:360.

37. Brock-Utne JJG, Downing JJW, Seedat FF. Laryngeal oedema associated with pre-eclamptic toxaemia. *Anaesthesia.* 1977;32:556.

38. Brimacombe J. Acute pharyngolaryngeal oedema and pre-eclamptic toxaemia. *Anaesthesia Intens Care.* 1992;20:97.

39. Rocke DA, Scoones GP. Rapidly progressive laryngeal oedema associated with pregnancy-aggravated hypertension. *Anaesthesia,* 1992;47:141.

40. Hoing R, Seitzer D. Clinical aspects of laryngopathia gravidarum [in French]. *Laryngol Rhinol Otol.* 1988;67:564.

41. Mattingly RF, Huang WY. Steroidogenesis of the menopausal and postmenopausal ovary. *Am J Obstet Gynecol.* 1969;103:679.

42. Buchsbaum HJ. *The Menopause.* New York, NY: Springer Verlag; 1983.

43. Boulet M, Oddens B J. Female voice changes around and after the menopause—an initial investigation. *Maturitas.* 1996;23:15–21.

44. Caruso S, Roccasalva L, Sapienza G, et al. Laryngeal cytological aspects in women with surgically induced menopause who were treated with transdermal estrogen replacement therapy. *Fertil Steril.* 2000;74:1073.

45. Lindholm P, Vilkman,E, Raudaskoski T, Suvanto-Luukkonen E, Kauppila A. The effect of postmenopause and postmenopausal HRT on measured voice values and vocal symptoms. *Maturitas.* 1997;28:47–53.

46. Wendler J, Siegert C, Schelhorn P, et al. The influence of Microgynon and Diane-35, two sub-fifty ovulation inhibitors, on voice function in women. *Contraception.* 1995;52:343.

47. Amir O, Kishon-Rabin L. Association between birth control pills and voice quality. *Laryngoscope.* 2004;114:1021.

48. Amir O, Biron-Shental T, Tzenker O, et al. Different oral contraceptives and voice quality—an observational study. *Contraception.* 2005;71:348.

49. Gorham-Rowan M, Langford A, Corrigan K, et al. Vocal pitch levels during connected speech associated with oral contraceptive use. *J Obstet Gynecol.* 2004;24:284.

50. Gorham-Rowan M. Acoustic measures of vocal stability during different speech tasks in young women using oral contraceptives: a retrospective study. *Eur J Contracep Reprod Health Care.* 2004;9:166.

51. Cohen MA, Kelley DB. Androgen-induced proliferation in the developing larynx of *Xenopus laevis* is regulated by thyroid hormone. *Dev Biol.* 1996; 178:113.

52. Aronson A. *Clinical Voice Disorders.* New York, NY: Brian C. Decker; 1980:261.

53. Michaels L. *Pathology of the Larynx.* New York, NY: Springer-Verlag; 1984:353.

54. Ritter F. *Otolaryngology.* Philadelphia, Pa: WB Saunders; 1973:727-734.

55. Sommer D, Freeman JL. Bilateral vocal cord paralysis associated with diabetes mellitus: case reports. *J Otolaryngol.* 1994;23:169.

56. Semiz S, Fisenk F, Akcurin S, et al. Temporary multiple cranial nerve palsies in a patient with type 1 diabetes mellitus. *Diabetes Metab.* 2002; 28:413.

57. Kabadi UM. Unilateral vocal cord palsy in a diabetic patient. *Postgrad Med.* 1988;84:53, 55.

58. Shuman CR Weissman B. Recurrent laryngeal nerve involvement as a manifestation of diabetic neuropathy. *Diabetes Metab.* 1968;17:302.

59. Klein AM, Tiu C, Lafreniere D. Malignant mimickers: chronic bacterial and fungal infections of the larynx. *J Voice.* 2005;19:151.

60. Sulica L. Laryngeal thrush. *Ann Otol Rhinol Laryngol.* 2005;114:369.

61. Schwartz JR, Nagle MG, Elkins RC, et al. Mucormycosis of the trachea: an unusual cause of acute upper airway obstruction. *Chest.* 1982;81:653.

62. Ettema SL LT, Toohill RJ, Merati AL. Prevalence of diabetes in patients with subglottic stenosis. *Ear Nose Throat J.* In press.

63. Nishida T, Tsuji S, Tsujii M, et al. Gastroesophageal reflux disease related to diabetes: Analysis of 241 cases with type 2 diabetes mellitus. *J Gastroenterol Hepatol.* 2004;19:258.

64. Lluch I, Ascaso JF, Mora F, et al. Gastroesophageal reflux in diabetes mellitus. *Am J Gastroenterol.* 1999;94:919.

65. Zhang Q, Horowitz M, Rigda R, et al. Effect of hyperglycemia on triggering of transient lower esophageal sphincter relaxations. *Am J Physiol Gastrointest Liver Physiol.* 2004;286:G797.

66. Bengtsson BA ES, Ernest I, Oden A, Sjogren B. Epidemiology and long-term survival in acromegaly. A study of 166 cases diagnosed between 1955 and 1984. *Acta Med Scand.* 1988:327-335.

67. Morewood DJ BP, Evans CC, Whitehouse GH. The extrathoracic airway in acromegaly. *Clin Radiol.* 1986:243-246.

68. Williams RS, Mills RG, Eccles R. Voice changes in acromegaly. *Laryngoscope.* 1994;104:484-487.

31

Rhinologic Disease and Its Impact on the Larynx

Kenneth W. Altman, MD, PhD

KEY POINTS

- Rhinologic disease is often overlooked in the evaluation of laryngologic problems.

- The underlying principle of rhinolaryngeal disease is that the upper and lower airways form a common respiratory tract that is lubricated in mucus.

- The larynx is at the epicenter of this airway, and sensitive to perturbations from respiratory tract disease.

- In the absence of a lesion, hoarseness may be modeled by chronic cough which is often multifactorial in etiology.

- Reasonable suspicion and a comprehensive approach to management is warranted.

Rhinologic disease is significantly underestimated and often overlooked in the workup and diagnosis of laryngological problems.[1] The underlying principle of rhinolaryngeal disease is that the upper and lower respiratory tracts form a common airway with the larynx at the epicenter. There are a number of reasons why it is often overlooked, and failure to treat associated rhinologic disease often results in suboptimal resolution of symptoms and signs of laryngeal irritation.

Sinonasal disease including allergic rhinitis and sinusitis is often *asymptomatic*, so patients may present with complaints of other symptoms, such as laryngeal irritation in response to the infected mucus draining from the nasopharynx. Because this drainage is often intermittent, it may not be routinely seen on physical examination of the posterior oropharynx. When a patient presents with laryngeal or voice-related complaints, the otolaryngologist often targets the larynx during the examination, which is often evaluated with a mirror or 70-degree Hopkins rod telescope. Flexible fiberoptic nasopharyngeal laryngoscopy would certainly afford visualization of the nasal mucosa, sinonasal outflow tracks, and the presence of inflammation or polyps; however, these findings are also sometimes overlooked when the larynx is "targeted" during the physical examination.

There has also been significantly increasing awareness of the *prominent role of laryngopharyngeal reflux* (LPR) in laryngeal disease.[2-4] (See Chapter 23, Reflux and Its Impact on Laryngology.) This results in a pattern of findings in the larynx including posterior hyperplasia with pachydermia,[5] pseudosulcus vocalis,[6] ventricular effacement, and arytenoid edema and erythema. Although many of these findings are common to LPR, they may not be highly specific to LPR.[7,8] Consequently, LPR may be overrecognized at times and relatively occult rhinologic disease may be an underrecognized contributor to voice and laryngeal problems.

PATHOPHYSIOLOGY OF RHINOLARYNGEAL DISEASE

The sinonasal cavity is responsible for the production of almost one liter of mucus each day to augment the function of the paranasal sinuses,[9] which includes warming and humidifying inspired air through the nares, lubricating and protecting the surface of the nasal cavity from irritants and allergens, as well as providing mucus and sol layers to facilitate ciliary clearance of these secretions.[10,11] The course of the mucus produced in the sinonasal cavities is generally toward naturally occurring sinus ostia, posteriorly toward the nasopharynx, with gravity-dependent drainage to the inferior oropharynx; at that point it is swallowed along with saliva produced in the oral cavity.[10] This pathway of mucus produced in the sinonasal cavity toward the posterior glottis explains many laryngeal symptoms and inflammation in response to rhinologic disease. The tracheobronchial tree also produces mucus, whose clearance pathway is superiorly toward the larynx, similarly explaining voice problems in response to aberrant mucus produced in response to pulmonary disease such as bronchitis (Figure 31–1).

Inhalant allergy has a common effect on the entire respiratory tract, resulting in nasal symptoms such as congestion, rhinorrhea, and itchy eyes and nose. Because the respiratory tract acts as a physiologic unit in response to allergy, there is consequently a high association between

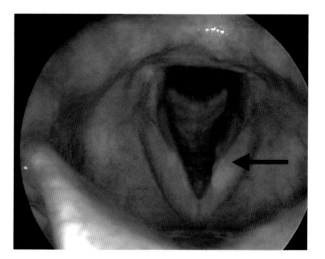

FIGURE 31–1. Tracheobronchitis in a professional opera singer. Note the white mucus emerging from the subglottis (*arrow*), with baseline inflammation on the posterior and infraglottic vocal folds associated with laryngopharyngeal reflux.

allergic rhinitis and *asthma*, with multiple studies documenting improvement in asthma scores with additional treatment for allergic rhinitis.[12]

The larynx is at the epicenter of the upper and lower respiratory tract and it is highly sensitive to perturbations, such as the presence of aberrant inflamed mucus produced in this reactive airway disease. The larynx mucosa may manifest *direct effects* of the allergy associated with the generalized respiratory inflammation,[13] as well as *indirect effects* of the inflammatory mediators in the allergic mucin (Figure 31-2).[14] Inhaled medications to treat asthma also have to pass through the laryngeal inlet, predisposing the larynx to secondary effects. These include the effects of steroids (which may result in candidiasis, Figure 31-3), as well as the desiccating effects and particulate deposition associated with some pulmonary inhalers.[15]

Bacterial sinusitis has been studied extensively and is a common complication associated with approximately 15% of upper respiratory infections. The paranasal sinuses drain through narrow bony channels, such as the osteomeatal complex (Figure 31-4) for the downstream

drainage pathway from the frontal recess, ethmoid complex, and maxillary sinuses. This can become obstructed from nasal mucosal edema associated with allergic and nonallergic rhinitis as well. Anatomic conditions such as a deviated nasal septum, concha bullosa formation of the middle turbinates, and the presence of infraorbital

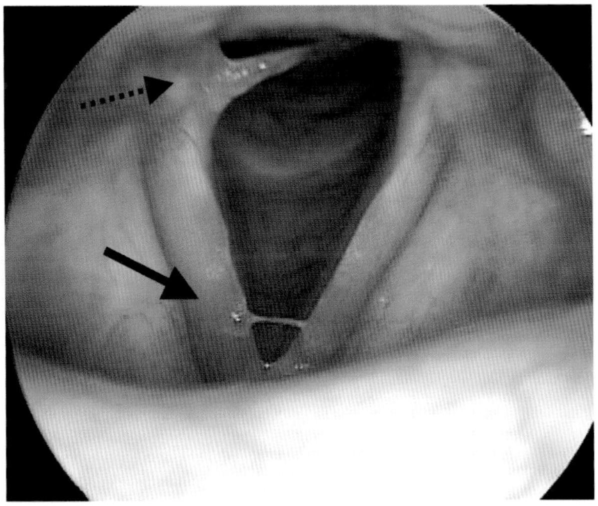

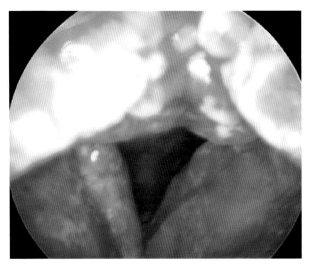

FIGURE 31–3. Laryngeal candidiasis in this diabetic patient with steroid-inhaler dependent asthma. Note the diffuse white patches over the posterior glottis, and boggy edema of the true vocal folds.

FIGURE 31–2. Allergic rhinitis in a patient with asthma. The classic "string sign" of sticky clear mucus bridging between the vocal folds anteriorly (*arrow*) is present, associated with thick tenacious mucus posteriorly (*dashed arrow*) produced in the tracheobronchial tree. The vocal folds also manifest mild edema.

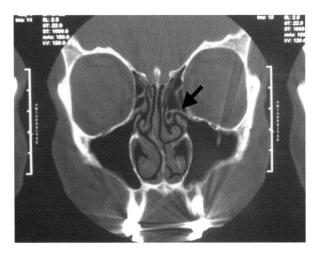

FIGURE 31–4. Computed tomography of the paranasal sinuses (*coronal section through the osteomeatal complex, arrow*). Note the complex deviated septum and paradoxic curvature of the middle turbinates.

ethmoidal cells predispose to obstruction of the sinonasal mucus outflow tracts. Sinusitis certainly alters the quality and character of sinonasal mucus that drains posteriorly to the glottis (Figure 31–5). Sinusitis has also been implicated in bronchitis as well as asthma, complicating the cycle of inflammation in the upper and lower respiratory tracts.[16-18]

Chronic cough is a good model for studying the effects of rhinologic and respiratory tract disease on the larynx, because most cough is produced from a direct adverse effect at the level of the larynx.[19] Postnasal drainage from allergy, nonallergic rhinitis, and sinusitis is among the most common causes of adult and pediatric chronic cough. Asthma, chronic bronchitis, and other pulmonary diseases are also highly associated with chronic cough. Not surprisingly, chronic cough has multifactorial etiologies in two-thirds of patients.[19]

The effects of chronic laryngeal irritation compounded by maladaptive behaviors such as cough and throat-clearing also predispose to the *development of laryngeal lesions.*[20] For exam-

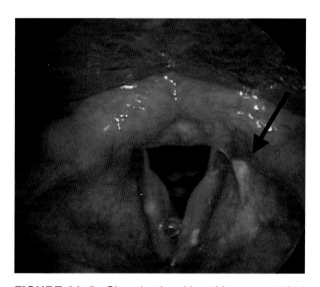

FIGURE 31–5. Chronic sinusitis, with pus noted at the posterior aspect of the aryepiglottic fold (*arrow*) draining anteromedially to the glottic inlet. Also note this patient to has a right vocal fold hemorrhagic polyp with edema and resolving right vocal fold hemorrhage.

ple, inflammation increases vascularity and the combined effects of the laryngeal trauma from coughing predispose to microhemorrhage and, ultimately, clot organization and the development of a vocal fold polyp. Also, chronic laryngeal inflammation actually reduces sensation in the glottis, which may result in muscle tension patterns of phonation and ultimately in the development of other vocal lesions such as nodules.

Laryngopharyngeal reflux (LPR) should not be dismissed in the presence of rhinologic disease, as there is often more than one contributing factor to laryngeal problems, and LPR may also be relatively asymptomatic. Furthermore, a number of studies support a causal relationship between LPR and sinusitis with documented pharyngeal pH changes in patients with chronic sinusitis.[21-23] Although the emerging diagnosis of eosinophilic esophagitis (see Controversy box for this chapter: Emerging Concepts) supports a possible link with allergy, it appears that gastroesophageal reflux (GER) is more of a concomitant disease rather than there being a true allergy-GER association.[24-26] The possible link between postnasal drip (PND) and reflux was recently investigated in a double-blind, randomized, prospective study.[27] Fifty subjects with the *primary* complaint of postnasal drip underwent pH probe examinations[28] and subsequently were randomized to a twice-daily proton pump inhibitor or a placebo. These patients had no clinical or endoscopic evidence of rhinologic disease. The subjects with PND had a higher acid exposure time than controls, indicating a possible association between PND and reflux; although the therapeutic arm did not reach statistical significance, there was a stronger trend toward symptomatic improvement of PND in the PPI group than in the placebo group.

It is common for patients with chronic and recurring problems related to rhinolaryngeal disease to fall into a cycle that reflects this interrelated pathophysiology, with each component contributing to laryngeal symptoms and hoarseness. This cycle of inflammation with multifactorial contributions is described in Figure 31–6. In its more extreme presentation, this may also be

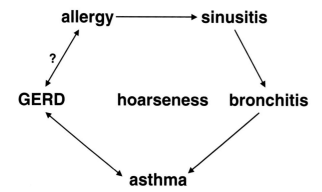

FIGURE 31–6. One common cycle of upper and lower respiratory inflammation, each component having the potential to affect the larynx and cause voice disturbance. The possible connection between allergy and gastroesophageal reflux may be explained by overlapping diagnoses in eosinophilic esophagitis.

associated with hypersensitive conditions such as an "irritable larynx," which occurs as a result of chronic adverse stimuli and may have an association with paradoxic vocal fold motion.[19, 29]

HISTORY AND PHYSICAL EXAMINATION

It is important to obtain an appropriate history when a patient presents with laryngeal complaints. An important clue is a prior history of sinusitis, allergy, nonallergic rhinitis, bronchitis, asthma, or other pulmonary disease. There should be particular suspicion for a causal relationship between rhinologic disease and laryngeal symptoms when the timing of the hoarseness is associated with nasal or upper respiratory symptoms. Even though there may not be a specific rhinologic symptom, it is important to ask the patient about the nature of mucus and where they sense it. For example, a complaint of "postnasal drip" is more likely to be associated with LPR if the patient only feels it at the level of the larynx or cricoid cartilage. However, rhinologic disease and true inflamed or infected posterior nasopharyngeal drainage should be suspected when a patient states that he or she is aware of the pathway

Emerging Concepts and Controversy— Eosinophilic Esophagitis

Is there a link between allergy and gastroesophageal reflux?

Eosinophilic esophagitis is an intriguing concept that describes the presence of eosinophils in esophageal biopsies from patients with symptomatic esophagitis.[25] Initially found more commonly in children, there is increasing recognition of this seemingly distinct clinicopathologic entity in the adult population as well.[30] Eosinophils are generally present in allergic-related inflammation, and their presence in esophageal biopsies suggested a potential link between allergy and gastroesophageal reflux (GERD). This relationship between eosinophils and possible gastroesophageal reflux was recognized by Winter et al,[31] who correlated the presence of esophageal eosinophils with prolonged esophageal acid clearance in children.

    More recent studies included the recognition of a likely allergic component in a subpopulation of pediatric patients with esophagitis. Walsh et al[24] studied 28 patients with intraepithelial esophageal eosinophils after antireflux therapy. Patients with an incomplete response to antireflux medication were noted to have a significantly greater concentration of eosinophils (28–31 per high-powered field [HPF] compared to 5 per HPF). These patients also had abnormal allergy skin testing results and tended to have clinical improvement on concomitant antiallergy treatment.

Mishra et al[32] studied experimental esophagitis in the murine model. They challenged mice to respiratory allergens, which subsequently resulted in development of esophageal eosinophils. Exposure to oral or intragastric allergen did not promote eosinophilic esophagitis. In the absence of interleukin-5 (IL-5), eosinophilic accumulation and epithelial hyperplasia were abated. This link between eosinophilic accumulation, eotaxin, and IL-5 is well-recognized and has been shown on subsequent studies.[33,34] It is now generally accepted that, although the presence of eosinophils is expected in pediatric esophagitis, it is the concentration of eosinophils that determines whether its response is primarily allergy (greater that 24 per HPF) or traditional gastroesophageal reflux (less than 7 per HPF).[35] Controversy remains in a number of different areas, including the "transitional zone" of 7 to 24 eosinophils per HPF that is believed to be a multifactorial esophagitis induced by GERD and allergy.

Controversy also remains in the adult population with eosinophilic esophagitis. This group tends to present with dysphagia due to esophageal stricture with no history of allergy or childhood symptoms of esophagitis,[36–38] It is not surprising that this adult population requires ongoing treatment of GERD despite a presumed "allergy" as the incipient cause. A simple explanation for this controversy is that multifactorial disease processes, each of which is relatively asymptomatic, result in a synergisitic pathophysiology inducing the esophageal stricture. However, it is likely more of a complex disease process that is still not fully understood.

One possibility that has not been discussed in the literature is that there is a common mediator to both disease processes (allergy and GERD) that results in a synergistic exacerbation of each disease. As discussed, IL-5 is a promoter of the eosinophilic and allergic response.[32,33] Interleukin-8 (IL-8) has been implicated in pre-esophagitis GERD.[39,40] Not surprisingly, IL-5 and IL-8 have commonly been identified in patients with bronchial hyperreactivity,[41,42] and allergy.[43,44] In fact, IL-5 has been shown to modulate IL-8 secretion in eosinophilic inflammation.[45] One may speculate as to the role of interleukins in this "link." Nevertheless, eosinophilic esophagitis is an entity that likely emphasizes the multifactorial and interrelated nature of diseases that may affect the larynx.

of mucus from the back of the nose to the throat to the larynx. It is important to remember that a significant portion of patients with evidence of rhinologic disease do not have predominant rhinologic symptoms.

Professional voice users such as singers are particularly sensitive to changes that can affect their voices. Because the nasal cavity is critical to the pathway for some air egress during phonation, there may only be a complaint of hyponasality or a subtle decreased nasal resonance. Voice breaks are another common complaint among singers, where there is a phonatory "break" while holding a note or during a vocal glide. Singers are more sensitive to these voice breaks around the passaggio (transition) between the "chest" voice and the "head" voice (falsetto). Although these voice breaks may be associated with subtle superior laryngeal nerve paresis, they may also occur with aberrant mucus on the vocal folds, which would be evident on strobolaryngoscopy.

On physical examination, it is important to recognize the character of mucus or pus in the posterior oropharynx. As the paranasal sinuses are lateral to the midline, inflamed or infected mucus tends to drain along the lateral aspects of the posterior oropharynx. Rather than discrete mucus or pus, one may only note a streak of erythema or hyperemia along these lateral pathways. There is also considerable evidence to support the observation that inflamed mucus and mucosa may remain long after resolution of an acute infection. One example is the lingering cough that may last up to 2 weeks after resolution of a viral upper respiratory infection.

Nasal endoscopy after the use of nasal decongestion is considered to be standard workup when one suspects contributions of rhinologic disease associated with laryngeal problems. This may be performed in association with flexible fiberoptic laryngoscopy, provided the examining physician takes note of pertinent findings. Although the technique and spectrum of findings goes beyond the scope of this chapter, findings include patency of the nasal airway, edematous appearance of nasal mucosa (particularly after attempts

at decongestion), symmetry of the nasal vestibule and septum, the presence of polyps or obstructing lesions, the presence of middle turbinate erythema, and patency and presence of pus in the middle meatus, sphenoethmoidal recess, and eustachian tube orifices.

Computed tomography (CT) of the paranasal sinuses is an important step in the workup of patients with suspected rhinologic disease. This study is often used as an adjunct to nasal endoscopy to characterize disease persistence after treatment, and also serves as a "road-map" if surgical intervention is warranted. Formal allergy evaluation is also imperative to maximize management of rhinologic disease, particularly as it relates to chronic sinusitis. Asthma is also underdiagnosed in this population and should be considered if the patient has lower respiratory symptoms or allergy is present.

MULTIFACTORIAL TREATMENT STRATEGY

Although the spectrum of treatment options for each of the rhinologic and respiratory tract diseases goes well beyond the scope of this chapter, certain fundamental principles remain: (1) it is imperative to treat acute disease that is evident on physical examination, (2) maximizing the treatment of preexisting respiratory tract disease, and (3) having a reasonable suspicion to extend the formal diagnostic evaluation (ie, with CT of the sinuses and formal allergy evaluation) when patients fail to respond as expected (see the management tree in Figure 31–7). There is ongoing debate whether "step-up" therapy or "step-down" therapy is most effective for different conditions. Because rhinologic and respiratory diseases are often not the only issues affecting laryngeal problems, polypharmacy (using more than one medication) is employed which requires a careful approach in management.

Medication options for allergic disease generally include antihistamines (traditional and

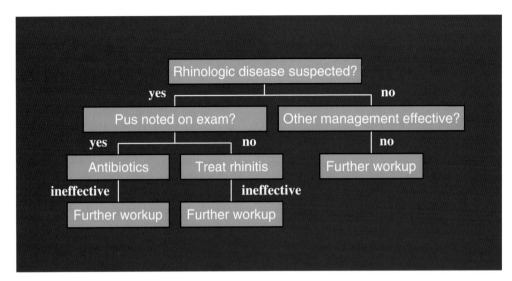

FIGURE 31–7. Management algorithm for suspected rhinologic disease.

nonsedating), antileukotrienes, oral and inhaled decongestants, oral and intranasal corticosteroids, and intranasal mast cell stabilizers. When reactive airway disease is associated with allergy, this regimen is usually supplemented with orally inhaled corticosteroids, bronchodilators, and (historically) theophyllines. Sinusitis (and bronchitis) are additionally treated with oral and intranasal antibiotics (bacterial and fungal), as well as a plethora of options regarding intranasal irrigation and humidification. Generally, decongestants are used with caution in the professional voice user as they tend to dry secretions that are otherwise important in lubricating the vocal folds. Hydration is also imperative to lubricate mucous secretions.

Rhinolaryngeal disease is an often overlooked component of laryngeal problems. A comprehensive approach to evaluation and treatment is necessary due to the complex nature of its pathophysiology. Hygiene, including maintenance of hydration and avoidance of irritants, is particularly important when excessive or problematic mucus is affecting laryngeal function. Future research will better characterize the interaction between the organs of the upper aerodigestive tract, including allergic and neurologic interconnections.

Review Questions

1. A 40-year-old male has some dysphagia and reflux symptoms. He is found to have a mild esophageal stricture; his biopsy is shown below. He has no prior allergic history. He has been on twice-daily PPIs with modest benefit. You recommend:

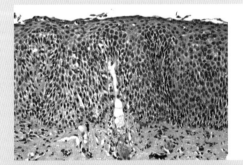

From: http://dave1.mgh.harvard.edu/movies/thumbs/Path_And_Rad/jpeg.e.inf.eos.ooo.bio.0p1.lu040622.jpg

a. addition of a nighttime H2 blocker
b. Nissen fundoplication
c. anti-trypanosomal therapy
d. steroids
e. esophagectomy

2. Bacterial sinusitis complicates approximately what percentage of URIs?
   a. 5
   b. 15
   c. 25
   d. 35
   e. 45

3. Chronic cough in a nonsmoker with a negative methacholine challenge test is most likely to represent:
   a. asthma
   b. COPD
   c. sinusitis
   d. laryngopharyngeal reflux
   e. laryngeal tic

4. Inhaled steroids for the treatment of asthma and rhinitis:
   a. have a uniformly negative effect on the voice
   b. result in laryngeal candidiasis in immunoincompetent individuals only
   c. are no longer indicated
   d. may enhance breath support and improve the voice in patients with obstructive disease
   e. should be substituted with oral steroids whenever possible in the performing artist

REFERENCES

1. Chadwick SJ. Allergy and the contemporary laryngologist. *Otolaryngol Clin North Am.* 2003;36: 957-988.
2. Koufman JA, Aviv JE, Casiano RR, Shaw GY. Laryngopharyngeal reflux: position statement of the committee on speech, voice, and swallowing disorders of the American Academy of Otolaryngology-Head and Neck Surgery. *Otolaryngol Head Neck Surg.* 2002;127:32-35.
3. Shaker R, Milbrath M, Ren J, Toohill R, Hogan WJ, Li Q, Hoffman CL. "Esophagopharyngeal distribution of refluxed gastric acid in patients with reflux laryngitis. *Gastroenterology.* 1995;109:1575-1582.
4. Weiner GJ, Koufman JA, Wu W, Cooper JB, Richter JE, Castell DO. Chronic hoarseness secondary to gastroesophageal reflux disease: documentation with 24-h ambulatory pH monitoring," *Am J Gastroenterol.* 1989;84:1503-1508.
5. Kambic V, Radsel Z. Acid posterior laryngitis. Aetiology, histology, diagnosis and treatment. *J Laryngol Otol.* 1984;98:1237-1240.
6. Belafsky PC, Postma GN, Koufman JA. The association between laryngeal pseudosulcus and laryngopharyngeal reflux. *Otolaryngol Head Neck Surg.* 2002;126:649-652.
7. Noordzij JP, Khidr A, Desper E, Meek RB, Reibel JF, Levine PA. Correlation of pH probe-measured laryngopharyngeal reflux with symptoms and signs of reflux laryngitis. *Laryngoscope.* 2002; 112:2192-2195.
8. Hill RK, Simpson CB, Velazquez R, Larson N. Pachydermia is not diagnostic of active laryngopharyngeal reflux disease. *Laryngoscope.* 2004; 114:1557-1561.
9. Tos M. Mucous elements in the nose. *Rhinology.* 1976;14:155-162.
10. Rice DH, Gluckman JL. Physiology. In: Donald PJ, Gluckman JL, Rice DH, eds, *The Sinuses.* New York, NY: Raven Press; 1995:49-56.
11. Widdicombe JG. Airway surface liquid: concepts and measurements. In: Rogers DF, Lethem MI, eds. *Airway Mucus: Basic Mechanisms and Clinical Perspectives.* Boston: Birkhauser Verlag; 1997:1-18.
12. Hurwitz B. Nasal pathophysiology impacts bronchial reactivity in asthmatic patients with allergic rhinitis. *J Asthma.* 1997;34:427-431.
13. Jackson-Menaldi CA, Dzul AI, Holland RW. Allergies and vocal fold edema: a preliminary report. *J Voice.* 1999;13:113-122.
14. Corey JP, Gungor A, Karnell M. Allergy for the laryngologist. *Otolaryngol Clin North Am.* 1998; 31(1):189-205.
15. Mirza N, Kasper Schwartz S, Antin-Ozerkis D. Laryngeal findings in users of combination corticosteroid and bronchodilator therapy. *Laryngoscope.* 2004;114:1566-1569.
16. Meltzer EO, Szwarcberg J, Pill MW. Allergic rhinitis, asthma, and rhinosinusitis: diseases of the integrated airway. *J Man Care Pharm.* 2004;10: 310-317.
17. Braunstahl GJ, Fokkens W, "Nasal involvement in allergic asthma. *Allergy.* 2003;58:1235-1243.
18. Batra PS, Kern RC, Tripathi A, et al. Outcome analysis of endoscopic sinus surgery in patients

with nasal polyps and asthma. *Laryngoscope.* 2003;113:1703–1706.

19. Altman KW, Simpson CB, Amin MR, Abaza M, Balkisson R, Casiano RR. Cough and paradoxical vocal fold motion. *Otolaryngol Head Neck Surg.* 2002;127:501–511.

20. Kuhn J, Toohill RJ, Ulualp SO, et al. Pharyngeal acid reflux events in patients with vocal cord nodules. *Laryngoscope.* 1998;108:1146–1149.

21. Ulualp SO, Toohill RJ, Hoffmann R, Shaker R. Possible relationship of gastroesophagopharyngeal acid reflux with pathogenesis of chronic sinusitis. *Am J Rhinol.* 1999;13:197–202.

22. Cotencin P, Narcy P. Nasopharyngeal pH monitoring in infants and children with chronic rhinopharyngitis. *Int J Ped Otorhinolaryngol.* 1991;22:249–256.

23. Bothwell MR, Parsons DS, Talbot A, Barbero GJ, Wilder B. Outcome of reflux therapy on pediatric chronic sinusitis. *Otolaryngol Head Neck Surg.* 1999;121:255–262.

24. Walsh SV, Antonioli DA, Goldman H, et al. Allergic esophagitis in children: a clinicopathologic entity. *Am J Surg Pathol.* 1999;23:390–396.

25. Markowitz JE, Liacouras CA. Eosinophilic esophagitis. *Gastroenterol Clin North Am.* 2003;32: 949–966.

26. Liacouras CA, Ruchelli E. Eosinophilic esophagitis. *Curr Opin Pediatr.* 2004;16:560–566.

27. Gill MT, Merati AL, Toohill RJ, Smith TL, Loehrl TA. The effect of PPI treatment on patients presenting with post-nasal drip: a double-blind, randomized, placebo-controlled trial. Paper presented at: Middle Section, Triological Society Meeting; February 3, 2006; San Diego, Calif. *Laryngoscope.* In press .

28. Loehrl TA, Smith TL, Toohill RJ, Hoffmann R, Merati AL. Pharyngeal pH probe findings in patients with post-nasal drip. *Am J Rhinol.* 2005; 19(4):340–343.

29. Perkner JJ, Fenelly KP, Balkissoon R, et al. Irritant-associated vocal cord dysfunction. *J Occup Environ Med.* 1998;40:136–143.

30. Furuta GT. Clinicopathologic features of esophagitis in children. *Gastrointest Endosc Clin North Am.* 2001;11:683–715.

31. Winter HS, et al. Intraepithelial eosinophils: a new diagnostic criterion for reflux esophagitis. *Gastroenterology.* 1982;83:818–823.

32. Mishra A, Hogan SP, Brandt EB, Rothenberg ME. An etiological role for aeroallergens and eosinophils in experimental esophagitis. *J Clin Invest.* 2001;107:83–90.

33. Mishra A, Hogan SP, Brandt EB, Rothenberg ME.

IL-5 promotes eosinophil trafficking to the esophagus. *J Immunol.* 2002;168: 2464–2469.

34. Fujiwara H, Morita A, Kobayashi H, et al. Infiltrating eosinophils and eotaxin: their association with idiopathic eosinophilic esophagitis. *Ann Allergy Asthma Immunol.* 2002;89:429–432.

35. Rothenberg ME, Mishra A, Collins MH, Putnam PE. Pathogenesis and clinical features of eosinophilic esophagitis. *J Allergy Clin Immunol.* 2001;108: 891–894.

36. Landres RT, Kuster GG, Strum WB. Eosinophilic esophagitis in a patient with vigorous achalasia. *Gastroenterology.* 1978;74:298–1301.

37. Arora AS, Perrault J, Smyrk TC. Topical corticosteroid treatment of dysphagia due to eosinophilic esophagitis in adults. *Mayo Clin Proc.* 2003;78: 830–835.

38. Khan S, Orenstein SR, Di Lorenzo C, et al. Eosinophilic esophagitis: strictures, impactions, dysphagia. *Digest Dis Sci.* 2003;48:22–29.

39. Isomoto H, Saenko VA, Kanazawa Y, et al. Enhanced expression of interleukin-8 and activation of nuclear factor kappa-B in endoscopy-negative gastroesophageal reflux disease. *Am J Gastroenterol.* 2005;99(4):596–597.

40. Yoshida N, Uchiyama K, Kuroda M, et al. Interleukin-8 expression in the esophageal mucosa of patients with gastroesophageal reflux disease. *Scand J Gastroenterol.* 2004;39(9):816–822.

41. Halasz A, Cserhati E, Kosa L, Cseh K. Relationship between the tumor necrosis factor system and the serum interleukin-4, interleukin-5, interleukin-8, eosinophil cationic protein, and immunoglobulin E levels in the bronchial hyperreactivity of adults and their children. *Allergy Asthma Proc.* 2003;24(2):111–118.

42. Betz R, Kohlhaufl M, Kassner G, Mullinger B, et al. Increased sputum IL-8 and IL-5 in asymptomatic nonspecific airway hyperresponsiveness. *Lung.* 2001;179(2):119–133.

43. Lampinen M, Rak S, Venge P. The role of interleukin-5, interleukin-8 and RANTES in the chemotactic attraction of eosinophils to the allergic lung. *Clin Exp Allergy.* 1999;29(3):314–322.

44. Benson M, Strannegard IL, Wennergren G, Strannegard O. Interleukin-5 and interleukin-8 in relation to eosinophils and neutrophils in nasal fluids from school children with seasonal allergic rhinitis. *Pediatr Allergy Immunol.* 1999;10(3):178–185.

45. Faccioli LH, Medeiros AI, Malheiro A, Pietro RC, Januario A. Vargaftig BB. Interleukin-5 modulates interleukin-8 secretion in eosinophilic inflammation. *Mediators Inflamm.* 1998;7(1):41–47.

APPENDIX A
Textbook of Laryngology Post-Test

1. A patient is unable to extend his neck because of prior cervical fusion. He requires open reduction and internal fixation of a parasymphyseal mandibular fracture. You do not believe the patient will need postoperative maxillomandibular fixation. What is your initial approach to management of the airway?
   a. Awake fiberoptic intubation
   b. Awake tracheotomy
   c. Rapid sequence induction
   d. Light wand intubation
   e. Use of a laryngeal mask airway

2. The _____ layer of the vocal fold contains mostly elastic fibers, collagen, fibronectin, and hyaluronan.
   a. epithelial
   b. superficial layer of the lamina propria
   c. intermediate layer of the lamina propria
   d. deep layer of the lamina propria
   e. muscular

3. A patient presents with signs of both UMN and LMN disease; there is some spasticity, with global weakness, atrophy, and tongue fasciculations. The patient has a weak voice and dysphagia for all consistencies. You suspect:
   a. Myasthenia gravis
   b. Multiple sclerosis
   c. Amyotrophic lateral sclerosis
   d. Essential tremor plus
   e. Oropharyngeal dystonia

4. The characteristic changes in the male voice at puberty usually correspond with the transition from Tanner stages ___ to ___.
   a. I to II
   b. II to III
   c. III to IV
   d. IV to V
   e. V to VI

5. A 44-year-old male presents with a 2-week history of hoarseness and dysphagia. He has not had any recent trauma. Your examination reveals an immobile left true vocal fold. In addition to your radiographic investigations, you order:
   a. Lyme titer
   b. Rheumatoid factor
   c. ACE level
   d. All of the above
   e. None of the above

6. Your radiographic investigation of the above patient should include:
   a. Chest radiograph only
   b. CT of the neck with contrast—from skull base to thoracic inlet
   c. MRI of the skull base with gadolinium
   d. CT of the neck and upper chest—from skull base to aortopulmonary window
   e. a and b

7. There is a direct correlation between phonatory effort and the level of systemic hydration.
   a. True
   b. False
   c. It is not known

8. Subglottic hemangiomas in children:
   a. Are usually symptomatic from birth
   b. Respond to steroids in less than 50% of cases
   c. Are exacerbated by the presence of tracheotomy
   d. Have a 2:1 female predominance
   e. Are not amenable to open resection

9. The _____ therapy technique is focused on increasing ease and quality of voice production by increasing phonatory airflow.
   a. stretch and flow
   b. yawn and sigh
   c. trill and drill
   d. breathe in/breathe out
   e. time clock

10. The image below is an example of:

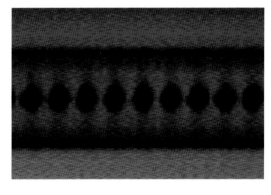

   a. Laryngeal videostroboscopy
   b. Electroglottography
   c. Spectrogram
   d. Video/airflow plot
   e. Kymography

11. During a laryngeal EMG, you note the recruitment of relatively few motor unit action potentials with a slow firing rate. You suspect:
   a. Primary myopathy
   b. CNS injury
   c. Crush injury to the RLN
   d. Complete section of the RLN
   e. Disorder of the neuromuscular junction

12. With regard to the evaluation of the neck for regional metastates from laryngeal cancer, how does ultrasound compare to computed tomography and magnetic resonance imaging?
   a. Ultrasound is better than CT
   b. Ultrasound is better than MRI *and* CT
   c. Ultrasound is better than CT but not as good as MRI
   d. Ultrasound is not as good as CT but is better than MRI
   e. Ultrasound is not as good as CT *or* MRI

13. The endoscopic examination of swallowing:
   a. Requires special equipment not found in most otolaryngology clinics
   b. Is best performed with the transoral technique to evaluate the valleculae
   c. Is less sensitive to laryngeal penetration than modified barium swallow
   d. Can be performed at the bedside
   e. Has a higher sensitivity for UES dysfunction

14. True or false? Laryngeal videostroboscopy is limited in cases of aphonia and even severe dysphonia.
   a. True
   b. False

15. Positron emission tomography (PET) is dependent on:
   a. Increased blood flow to growing tumors
   b. Decreased blood flow to necrotic tumors
   c. Increased glucose uptake in tumors
   d. Decreased glucose uptake in de-differentiated tumors
   e. Latent radioactivity from prior treatment

16. For the vast majority of patients, the ideal position for operative microlaryngoscopy is:
    a. Head flexed on the neck, neck flexed on the chest
    b. Head in neutral, neck in neutral
    c. Head extended on the neck, neck flexed on the chest
    d. Head flexed on the neck, neck extended on the chest
    e. Head extended on the neck, neck extended on the chest

17. Which tumor characteristic is a known risk factor for recurrence following laser surgery for T1 and T2 glottic lesions?
    a. Involvement of the striking zone of the vocal fold
    b. Tumor concentrated in the middle layer of the lamina propria
    c. Extension to the lateral floor of the ventricle
    d. Histologic stage of the tumor
    e. None of the above

18. Which of the following pioneers is credited with the introduction of suspension laryngoscopy?
    a. Harkins
    b. Killian
    c. Sataloff
    d. Solis-Cohen
    e. García

19. The voiceless "f" is to the "v" sound as "s" is to which sound?
    a. "sh"
    b. "ts"
    c. "z"
    d. "ch"
    e. "ss"

20. Flaccidity, atrophy, and hyporeflexia are characteristic of which type of laryngeal neurologic impairment?
    a. Extrapyramidal
    b. Upper motor neuron
    c. Lower motor neuron
    d. Neuromuscular junction
    e. End-organ (ie, muscle)

21. Phonation threshold pressure is defined as the:
    a. Maximal phonation energy that can be generated by a given person at any given frequency
    b. Minimum phonation energy that can be generated by a given person at any given frequency
    c. Minimum phonation pressure needed to drive the vocal folds into vibration
    d. The physical shear force of the apposing vocal folds
    e. The perceived auditory stimulus from a given set of phonatory constants

22. The Lee Silverman Voice Treatment is based on:
    a. Decreasing fatigue by reducing phonatory effort and minimizing adductory contact
    b. Increasing intensity through increasing phonatory effort and maximum adductory vocal tasks
    c. Combining amplification with general conditioning and hydration
    d. Very little supportive evidence
    e. Increasing articulatory precision through stretching and repetition

23. Adductor spasmodic dysphonia is _____ common than abductor spasmodic dysphonia. Generally speaking, adductor spasmodic dysphonia is _____ responsive to botulinum toxin injections.
    a. more, less
    b. less, more
    c. more, more
    d. less, less
    e. more, not

24. When applied topically to the larynx, capsaicin causes:
    a. Vocal fold abduction, hyperpnea
    b. Vocal fold adduction, hyperpnea
    c. Vocal fold abduction, central apnea
    d. Vocal fold adduction, central apnea
    e. Coprolalia

25. The right true vocal fold in these intraoperative photos is most consistent with:

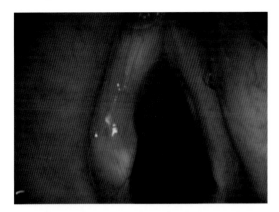

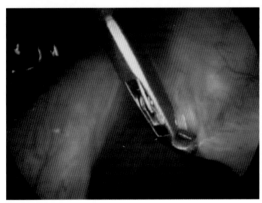

  a. Reinke's edema
  b. Pseudoparalysis
  c. Pseudosulcus
  d. Sulcus vocalis
  e. Cystica accreta laryngis

26. Tracheoesophageal speech results from:
  a. Esophageal airflow and pharyngeal resonance
  b. Pulmonary airflow and pharyngeal resonance
  c. Pharyngeal airflow and esophageal resonance
  d. Esophageal airflow and tracheal resonance
  e. Pulmonary airflow and tracheal resonance

27. Prior to puberty, there are few differences between the male and female larynx. In the male, puberty results in:
  a. Increase in vocal tract length
  b. Decrease in anteroposterior length of glottis
  c. Decrease in vocal tract length
  d. Thinning and sharpening of the glottic configuration
  e. All of the above

28. A 66-year-old woman is now 8 weeks s/p tracheal resection and primary anastomosis for a 4-cm length tracheal stenosis. She did well for the first 6 weeks but she has complained of dyspnea for the last 2 weeks. She has significant stridor on clinical examination. Laryngoscopy reveals good vocal fold motion with some edema. She doesn't tolerate further examination in clinic. In the OR, your telescopic findings are seen in this photo. You conclude that:

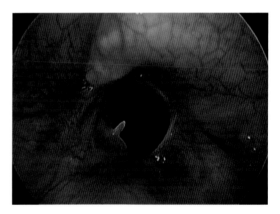

  a. Everything is healing well; her issues are related to diffuse airway edema
  b. There is an anastomotic stricture related to a technical error
  c. She has a reparative granuloma
  d. The tracheal airway is adequate; though the larynx appears normal, there must be some paradoxic motion
  e. She has a prolene allergy

29. Hirano's cover-body theory provides a critical framework to understand vocal function. In it, the cover is _____ and noncontractile whereas the body (muscle) is relatively _____ and has active contractile properties.
    a. pliable, stiff
    b. stiff, pliable
    c. pliable, elastic
    d. elastic, pliable
    e. stiff, elastic

30. Laryngotracheal separation:
    a. Is reversible
    b. Is often reversed
    c. Is contraindicated in ALS
    d. Requires the patient to be dependent on a tracheotomy tube
    e. Improves the ease and efficiency of swallowing in these patients

APPENDIX B
Answer Keys for Pre-Test, Chapter Review Tests, and Post-Test

PRETEST ANSWER KEY

1. d

2. c. Although most practitioners perform unilateral injections, low-dose bilateral injections also appear to be safe in selected patients.

3. c. The mobile arytenoid may "bump" the arytenoid on the denervated side and displace it laterally for a moment, thus impacting the mucosa of the piriform on the weak side. This will not happen if the arytenoid is mechanically fixed. This clinical observation was first described by Jackson in 1937.

4. a. This is why further technology is needed to view vocal fold motion as a synthesized moving image or (stroboscopy) or as a slowed-down replay of true motion (high-speed imaging).

5. c

6. b

7. d

8. a

9. c

10. d. The cycle-to-cycle variability in frequency is referred to as jitter. The clinical utility of these measurements is not well established.

11. d

12. c

13. d

14. e

15. b

16. d. The nucleus ambiguus is the main motor nucleus. The dorsal nucleus of X is the parasympathetic secretomotor ganglion.

17. c

18. b

19. b

20. b

21. a

22. e

23. e

24. c

25. e

26. c

27. d. With the advent of botulinum toxin therapy, the indication for postlaryngectomy cricopharyngeal myotomy has declined.

28. d

29. d. Solis-Cohen is credited with the concept of laryngofissure for open excision of laryngeal tumor in 1869.

30. d

CHAPTER REVIEW QUESTION ANSWERS

Chapter 1

1. Manuel García presented mirror laryngoscopy to the Royal Society of London in 1855. Although he was almost certainly not the first person to visualize the larynx with mirrors, his presentation created tremendous interest in laryngology. For this reason, he is generally regarded as the "Father of Laryngoscopy."

2. *Johann Czermak* and *Ludwig Turck* were among the first physicians to apply mirror laryngoscopy to systemic investigation of the larynx. Their skills as teachers, as well as their feud concerning the credit for their work, helped spur incredible growth in laryngology. Other early laryngologists who popularized indirect laryngoscopy were Morell Mackenzie in London, Louis Elsberg in New York, and Jacob Solis Cohen in Philadelphia. Elsberg and Solis Cohen helped to form the American Laryngological Association in 1878.

3. There is controversy regarding the discovery of direct laryngscopy, just as there is controversy regarding the discovery of indirect laryngoscopy. Kirstein certainly

performed direct laryngoscopy ("autoscopy") in 1895 using a spatula blade and headlight, with the patient in a sitting position. Although he did not receive much recognition at the time, Horace Green performed a similar feat in 1852; he is now considered "the Father of American Laryngology."

4. Endolaryngeal manipulation, as described by Horace Green, predates mirror laryngoscopy. Once mirror laryngoscopy was popularized, mirror-guided laryngeal instrumentation grew quickly for both biopsies and the application of caustics. Fraenkel, in 1886, was the first physician to perform a complete endolaryngeal tumor resection. Shortly thereafter advances in mucosal anesthesia and direct laryngoscopy led to the development of endolaryngeal surgery much as it is practiced today.

5. The development of the operating microscope and CO_2 laser increased operative precision greatly. Advances in stroboscopy greatly aided diagnosis of laryngeal pathology. Meanwhile, investigation into the multilayered anatomy of the vocal cord led to an increasingly sophisticated emphasis on vocal preservation. Together these advances helped to usher in the era of phonomicrosurgery.

Chapter 2

1. b. Sulcus vocalis. Sulcus vocalis, rather than being a discolored lump on the vocal folds like a polyp, has no obvious volumetric change to the vocal fold and given its fibrotic nature possess the same color (white) as the vocal ligament, making it difficult to identify.

2. c. The current method of characterizing whether the epithelium underlying the keratin (leukoplakia—Greek for "white plaque") is normal, dysplastic, or malignant is excisional surgical biopsy under microlaryngoscopy. The normally nonkeratinizing stratified squamous epithelium of the vocal

fold produces keratin when it is inflamed or genetically altered. Office endoscopy is not a reliable tool for distinguishing normal versus abnormal epithelium and office cytology is not yet widely accepted or available.

3. d. and e. Manipulation of the glottic configuration using injection or open techniques (thyroplasty and/or adytenoid adduction) are static repairs and do not address neural function. Observation may allow for spontaneous reinnervation if the original neural injury is not severe and ansa cervicalis neurorrhaphy to the recurrent laryngeal nerve can restore tone (but not mobility of the vocal folds) to the intrinsic laryngeal musculature.

2. d. proton pump inhibitors are more effective than H2 blockers in the treatment of reflux affecting the larynx and pharynx, presumably because of their ability to suppress acid production more effectively. Importantly, although the acid itself is damaging to the laryngopharynx, it is the deactivation of some of the destructive pepsin enzyme subtypes at higher pH values that likely makes acid suppression effective in preventing damage to the laryngopharynx.

3. c. As mentioned in the text, preoperative imaging and visualization of the airway are preferred and x-ray is not currently the imaging test of choice when three-dimensional reconstructions are available using CT scan.

Chapter 3

1. a

2. d

3. e

4. e

5. b

6. b

Chapter 4

1. Laryngospasm and central apnea

2. Respiration and cough

3. Laryngopharyngeal reflux and stroke

4. Expiration and the laryngeal adductor response

5. Tracheobronchial cough and laryngeal cough

Chapter 5

1. The muscles of mastication are the masseter, temporalis, and medial and lateral pterygoid. All are innervated by the trigeminal nerve, specifically the masseteric, deep temporal, and external pterygoid nerves. They function to facilitate side-to-side movement of the mandible to morselize a food bolus between the teeth. The lateral pterygoids and temporalis are key in this side-to-side motion. Other functions include translation of the mandible and jaw elevation and closure.

2. The hyoid bone is attached to the thyroid cartilage by the thyrohyoid muscle, the floor of mouth (mylohyoid), mandible (geniohyoid), sternum (sternohyoid), shoulder/scapula (omohyoid). These attachments are important to understand how multiple structures move in association with those mobilized by reflexive swallow.

3. The vagus nerve has multiple roles in coordination of swallow. It contributes to the formation of the pharyngeal plexus of nerves that innervates the constrictors and initiates reflexive passage of a food bolus. It provides sensation to portions of the laryngopharynx. It also innervates laryngeal musculature which adducts the vocal cords during swallow to prevent aspiration. Furthermore, it contributes to the esophageal plexus of nerves.

4. The trigeminal nerve innervates the muscles of mastication, allowing morselization of a food bolus. Furthermore, via the maxillary division, it provides sensation to the oral cavity, permitting clearance of food from the gingivobuccal sulcus and other areas. The trigeminal nerve also innervates the tensor veli palatini, allowing for velopharyngeal competence to prevent nasal regurgitation during deglutition.

5. The three phases of swallow are the oral (voluntary), pharyngeal (involuntary reflex), and esophageal phases. The oral preparatory phase precedes the oral phase and involves appetite and cortical influences on mastication and swallowing such as salivation.

Chapter 6

1. True
2. False
3. True
4. False
5. False
6. False
7. False
8. False
9. True

Chapter 7

1. False
2. False
3. False
4. True
5. True
6. True

Chapter 8

1. No. The complexity of vocal function is not represented by a sample of simple sustained phonation. It is imperative that a variety of tasks be elicited, including connected speech samples.

2. Yes. Therapeutic probes can provide invaluable information regarding patients' ability to modify vocal behaviors, thereby confirming their candidacy for voice therapy, as well as providing insight into the specific techniques that would be effective.

3. No. These are complementary or supplementary tools, but not the primary basis for a differential diagnosis.

4. No. Consistent with any other sophisticated discipline, the advances of knowledge in voice science and treatment of voice disorders require continual education for both otolaryngologists and SLPs.

Chapter 9

1. a
2. e
3. c
4. a, b, and c
5. a

Chapter 10

1. d
2. c
3. c
4. b
5. d

Chapter 11

1. d

2. c

3. c

4. a

5. d

Chapter 12

1. Yes. Although the two behaviors are different in their demands, they involve the same organ. Vocal abuse can damage the tissues, thereby disrupting phonatory function for either or both activities.

2. No, not directly. Swallowing beverages bypasses the larynx so the liquid does not "bathe" the tissues. However, a "soothing" effect can be realized by secondary gain through increased secretions and/or muscle relaxation facilitated by enjoying liquids.

3. This is not well studied but the answer is probably no. Generally beverages that are cool or warm are preferable to those hot or cold—particularly if extreme. The chance for tissue damage secondary to scalding or muscle contraction resulting from extreme cold should be avoided.

4. No. The physiology of whisper usually requires tight tissue contact and increased vocal fold tension, both conditions contraindicated for the inflamed tissues.

Chapter 13

1. The scope of practice for a speech-language pathologist when treating voice disorders does not include the diagnosis of organic changes that may have taken place on the vocal folds. It does include identifying the voice that presents with a current or poten-

tial problem, identifying and analyzing the problem, then providing the voice user with tools to modify vocal behaviors and use the vocal mechanism with optimal efficiency. In some cases, the larynx will be visualized and directly assessed by the SLP; in most cases, however, this is done initially by the otolaryngologist. The clinician may perceptually and acoustically identify dysphonia. It is then the clinician's responsibility to refer this patient to an otolaryngologist, ideally a laryngologist, to assess the anatomy and physiology of the larynx prior to continuing therapeutic intervention.

2. *Otolaryngologist:* The primary member of the team responsible for diagnosis and medical/surgical intervention.

   Speech-language pathologist: Conducts evaluation and treatment of the voice problem by promoting efficient use of the vocal mechanism.

   Singing voice specialist/teacher: Develops singing technique and singing voice production. This specialist may be beneficial to a nonsinger.

   Acting-voice specialist: Focuses on honing vocal skills such as projected speech and communication skills as they relate to vocally demanding professions.

   The patient: The most important member of the team. This person's role is therapeutic and educational. The patient must be motivated, knowledgeable, and involved in therapy decision-making.

   Voice researcher/scientist: Provides valuable insight and perspective with regard to the care of a voice patient because of specific knowledge and skills in acoustic measurement and voice production.

   Singing voice coach: May provide valuable knowledge and perspective following rehabilitation work and will work on the development of artistic style and repertoire for the voice user.

Psychologist or psychiatrist: Provides the patient with counseling for the management of emotional reactions to the voice disorder, as well as psychological issues that may have contributed to its occurrence.

Physiatrist: Addresses areas of tension or injury throughout the body.

Each member of the team provides valuable knowledge of voice production and treatment and care of the voice. Based on the patient's history and voice disorder, each may require different team members. It is of value to cultivate these relationships within the community to develop a network of resources not only for the patient's benefit but as a professional sounding board. The different perspectives of each discipline can provide insight in our field and aid in providing the patient with well-rounded care.

3. History taking from a professional voice user and a nonprofessional are similar in that a complete medical history and history of the onset of the voice problems should be gathered, in addition to information on possible contributing factors, vocal hygiene, and voice use. The history taking is different for a professional voice user because there are special factors to consider. These may include, learning the vocal complaints as they relate to the "performance voice," inquiring about the history of professional voice user, and probing into the extent of the professional voice user's vocal training. A professional voice user's vocal demands and expectations are higher than the nonprofessional voice user and must be delved into thoroughly.

4. Breath support during phonation ideally involves abdominal expansion during inhalation and abdominal contraction during exhalation and phonation. "Abdominal breathing" also involves appropriate and coordinated activity of muscles of the chest, back, and elsewhere. Airflow during phonation refers to the release of air to produce phonation. Airflow sets the vocal folds into motion. However, abdominal breathing does not ensure efficient phonation. An abdominal breathing pattern may be present while airflow during phonation is decreased. This may be secondary to an inefficient abdominal movement pattern or hyperfunction in the vocal tract that inhibits appropriate airflow during voice production.

5. There are multiple factors to consider when choosing a therapeutic facilitator. These include the medical diagnosis, patient's primary vocal complaints, perceptual and acoustic evaluation, and physiology of the patient's current voice production versus the targeted efficient voice production. The facilitator should be chosen with these factors in mind and then modified based on the patient's response.

Chapter 14

1. d. The "sniffing" position provides the best view of the vocal folds. Anterior cricoid pressure may be needed in some cases and may be provided by 1-inch tape stretched across the neck of the patient from the operating table.

2. c. The presence of a mass on the vocal fold does not necessarily indicate surgery is needed. All other underlying problems should be treated first. Treatment of reflux and voice therapy might provide enough improvement to satisfy the patient's needs. Other underlying factors might be considered. One might wish to consider laryngeal EMG, given the preceding URI, to see if any subtle paresis is contributing. Allergy evaluation should be considered. The decision to recommend surgical excision should be reserved until all the potentially contributing factors have been considered and medical management has been exhausted.

3. e.

4. d. The use of the laser still requires deft ability with the nondominant hand. Excellent control of the micromanipulator is required to prevent inadvertent injury to healthy tissue. CO_2 laser does introduce some uncertainty in depth of thermal injury and introduces a small risk of airway fire which is easily avoided with appropriate preparation. CO_2 laser does provide better hemostasis; however, hemostasis is achievable with cold excision too using topical epinephrine. Ultimately, individual surgeon preference and experience are the determining factors as to which technique is best to use.

5. a. Overly aggressive excision of Reinke's edema can lead to severe scarring. One should consider operating on only one vocal fold initially. If scarring occurs, the contralateral side can usually compensate and yield an improved voice. If both sides are operated on and scar excessively, the patient may be left with a pressed, breathy voice that is difficult to correct.

Chapter 15

1. All lasers have an optical resonating chamber with two mirrors, (one fully reflective and the other allowing partial transmission) and are filled with an active medium such as CO_2. Additionally, an external energy source (eg, an electrical current) is required to initiate the process by causing atoms to be raised to a higher energy state resulting in spontaneous photon emissions.

2. Endotracheal tubes must be either shielded with reflective tape or made of a reflective metal that lessens the likelihood of penetration and ignition of the anesthetic gases therein. Endotracheal tubes can be fitted with low-pressure cuffs and filled with saline tinted with methylene blue. Injury to the cuff is, therefore, detected early as methylene blue leaks into the operative field. Further

protection of the endotracheal tube cuff and distal airway structures can be accomplished by the placement of saline-soaked cottonoid pledgets between the surgical site and the endotracheal tube cuffs. Low inhaled FiO_2, (<.30), is recommended.

3. The effective extinction length in biologic tissue is usually 2 to 4 mm, making this laser ideal for indications where lateral coagulation and hemostasis are desired. On the contrary, the depth of thermal injury makes precise control and complete preservation of adjacent normal tissues practically impossible.

4. The most apparent limitation of the CO_2 laser is the inability to deliver the laser beam via a flexible fiber, necessitating the use of an articulated arm with mirrors arranged to direct the beam from the source to the target. Work on a small flexible conduit continues to be the focus of investigation. When achieved, this technology will open a far wider spectrum of applications of this user-friendly wavelength via flexible endoscopy in the sinonasal tract, trachea and bronchi as well as expanded indications within the larynx.

5. Data suggest that shorter pulse durations used with the CO_2 lasers (<0.10 second) produce less lateral thermal injury and wounds with greater tensile strength, resulting in earlier wound healing. Additionally, a pulsed CO_2 laser delivery histologically caused less thermal injury and scar formation and improved vibratory characteristics in canine vocal folds when compared to a continuous wave CO_2 laser.

Chapter 16

1. Myasthenia gravis. Characterized by fatigue with repetitive use and therefore an intermittent pattern, myasthenia gravis commonly presents in women between the second and fourth decades. Asking the patient to

repeat syllables such as "ee-ee-ee" may elicit vocal fatigue.

2. c. glottal gap. Berke et al reported that 75% of patients who had a persistent glottal gap on stroboscopic examination were satisfied with vocal fold augmentation. Parkinson's patients usually demonstrate normal vocal cord mobility. The presence of significant laryngeal tremor and poor overall neurologic status indicate more advanced disease, which is less likely to benefit from augmentation.

3. b. Voice strain is seen in lesions involving the UMN or the basal ganglia.

4. Patients with Parkinson's disease usually demonstrate normal vocal cord mobility. Patients with multiple system atrophy, however, may have stridor during sleep. This is important to elicit during history taking. If the patient or family reports stridor, the diagnosis of MSA should be seriously considered.

5. d. Patients with essential tremor of the voice report subjective reduction in vocal effort after Botox injection, according to Warrick et al.

Chapter 17

1. This is nicely summarized in Table 17–3.

2. The precise answer is not known; each patient's co-morbid conditions, such as lung cancer or a history of head and neck radiation, may play a factor. The variability in laryngeal innervation may also play a role. There is no predictable pattern based on the "site of lesion."

3. a

4. Not necessarily; synkinesis is an example of reinnervation with poor voluntary motion.

5. This is outlined in the chapter. Briefly, these include tracheotomy, posterior cordotomy, arytenoidectomy, medial arytenoidectomy, and lateralization (Lichtenberger technique).

6. c, although a may also occur depending on her degree of glottic insufficiency and likelihood of compensation

Chapter 18

1. d
2. b
3. b
4. c

Chapter 19

1. a, c, and e. When essential tremor is inherited, it is inherited in an autosomal dominant fashion. The voice appears to be affected in 25 to 30% of patients.

2. a and e. Tremor at rest, cogwheeling, and bradykinesia are signs of Parkinson's disease.

3. c. Patients with Parkinson's disease have hypophonia with articulatory difficulties. Strangled voice breaks are typical of adductor spasmodic dysphonia, and breathy breaks suggest abductor spasmodic dysphonia. "Scanning speech," which remains poorly defined, has been attributed to multiples sclerosis.

4. Flexible fiberoptic laryngoscopy.

5. d. No pharmacologic agent has a clearly documented benefit in essential voice tremor.

Chapter 20

1. a. In their review of over 900 patients with spasmodic dysphonia, Blitzer, et al[7] reported their mean dose of botulinum toxin A per visit was ~3 units. This approximates clinical practice in the majority of those that treat patients with spasmodic dysphonia.

2. This dated concept has been debunked. Voice disorders are often made worse by psychiatric illness, but psychiatric illness is not the source of dysphonia. Sometimes, a nonorganic voice disorder can be misdiagnosed as spasmodic dysphonia, and vice versa.

3. b. Abductor spasmodic dysphonia is characterized by spasms that result in an intermittent breathy voice quality. This can be highlighted by asking the patient to speak a passage loaded with voiceless consonants. Patients with spasmodic dysphonia often have minimal spasm with less complex vocal tasks such as uttering prolonged vowel sounds.

4. c. The best examiner is an experienced listener. No laboratory or imaging study is specific for the diagnosis of spasmodic dysphonia.

5. b. Speech therapy can help make spasmodic dysphonia less symptomatic in a subset of patients; however, it cannot cure the dystonia. More times then not, sending a patient with spasmodic dysphonia for speech therapy serves more to frustrate him then cure him. Speech therapy may have a small role in having patients cope with some of the negative effects of botulinum toxin treatment.

Chapter 21

1. e. The patient described has supraglottitis, Intubation and surgical airway are options, most patients can be managed without this.

2. a. Either topical or systemic antifungals may be helpful.

3. d.

4. d

5. c. There is little role for surgery in a nonsmoker with a smooth, small lesion unless other concerns arise. Botulinum toxin would be quite uncommon as an initial treatment.

Chapter 22

1. c

2. d

3. a

4. e

5. d

Chapter 23

1. b. pH probe testing is fairly reliable although it may not be "positive" in cases of minimal pH change. Surgery is not an option at this point as he has not had adequate treatment —his age and sex do not exclude him from being a candidate, however. It is generally felt that 3 to 6 months of treatment may be necessary to detect a clinical response to medical therapy.

2. b

3. d

4. d. PPIs are the mainstay of therapy along with lifestyle changes; the importance of these behavioral modifications is not well detailed, although it is reasonable to ask the patients to pursue healthy dietary choice and avoid laryngeal irritants such as tobacco, alcohol, and caffeine. H_2 blockers are widely used although their precise role in LPR patients is not clear.

Chapter 24

1. b

2. d

3. b

4. b

5. b

Chapter 25

1. d
2. d
3. c
4. d
5. e

Chapter 26

1. b. This tracheotomy-associated lesion is likely not amenable to endoscopic treatment. Primary resection has a high likelihood of success.

2. e. Mitomycin is derived from *Streptomyces caespitosus*.

3. c.

4. d. The left posterior cordotomy shown (with the usual posterior ventriculectomy) is an effective treatment in glottic airway compromise. It does, however, lead to voice impairment, which is permanent.

5. b. Diabetes is a known risk factor for failure following airway surgery. It has not been established as an independent risk factor in the development of stenosis.

Chapter 27

1. b
2. c
3. e
4. c
5. e

Chapter 28

1. d. This child's laryngomalacia is profound and requires intervention.

2. e.
3. c.
4. b.
5. e.
6. b.

Chapter 29

1. b. Successful esophageal speech rates were only about 25% in the era before TE speech became available. Although it is still an option, fewer patients are offered this form of rehabilitation today.

2. a. The other answers are relative contra-indications, since they might be associated with decreased success rates. However, severe trismus prevents the surgeon from safely passing a rigid esophagoscope to the level of the stoma.

3. c. Although esophageal speech requires more intense instruction in the early post-laryngectomy period, TE speech requires continuing visits for prosthesis replacement, resizing, and stoma troubleshooting.

4. e. A reinforcing closure can theoretically cause increase scar, spasm, and muscle tone that can make TE speech and esophageal speech more difficult.

5. d. Delaying TE formation until a secondary procedure can decrease the number of issues with which the new laryngectomy patient has to encounter. Air insufflation testing is not feasible in the setting of a primary TE fistula.

Chapter 30

1. The decrease in fundamental frequency from androgen exposure is an irreversible change. Women with hyperandrogenic

states continue with masculinized voices despite treatment, and men who undergo orchiectomy, as for gender reassignment surgery, do not experience an elevation in fundamental frequency with the decrease in testosterone levels.

2. c. The decrease in the adult male voice by one octave occurs late in puberty, during Tanner stages III and IV.

3. b. Premenstrual vocal syndrome is mostly reported in professional voice users, and is characterized by vocal fatigue, loss in vocal power, and decreased range. It is likely due to the elevation of estrogen and progesterone just prior to menses and has been shown to be further aggravated by vocal abusers.

4. a. Diabetes has been associated with serious infections of the larynx, including chronic granulomatous infections from fungal sources that can mimic carcinoma and may be improperly treated and surgically excised. Proper culture should be done before any large excisions planned in diabetic patients.

Chapter 31

1. Steroids, either oral or topical, have been used in the treatment of eosinophilic esophagitis.

2. b

3. d

4. d. Although inhaled steroids are associated with the development of laryngeal *Candida,* this may happen in immunocompetent patients as well. The beneficial effects of asthma treatment may indeed improve voice production if the local effects of the topical medication are not significant

POST-TEST ANSWER KEY

1. a

2. c

3. c

4. c

5. e

6. d. This remains somewhat controversial. CXR may miss 2- to 3-cm masses in the mediastinum, so many recommend CT for left-sided paralyses. Answer e may be appropriate for a right-sided paralysis. MRI is reasonable but the course of the nerve needs to be imaged.

7. b. There is a correlation, but it is inverse. In a double-blinded, placebo-controlled study, Verdolini and colleagues demonstrated an inverse relation between phonatory effort and hydration level.

8. d

9. a

10. e

11. b

12. e

13. d

14. a. The strobe image depends on some periodicity to the laryngeal motion so that the moving picture can be generated.

15. c. FDG (the agent administered for the study) enters cells through glucose transporters and is phosphorylated into FDG-6-phosphate. It is accumulated by metabolically active tumor cells as it cannot undergo further metabolism in this state.

16. c

17. c

18. b

19. c. This question is not presented with traditional notation.

20. c

21. c

22. b

23. c

24. d, although e may also be true

25. d

26. b

27. a

28. b

29. a

30. a

Index